illigitimi non carbondum

A Professional Study and Resource Guide for the CRNA

A PROFESSIONAL STUDY AND RESOURCE GUIDE FOR THE CRNA

Edited by

Scot D. Foster, CRNA, PhD, FAAN
Professor, Nursing
Director, Program of Nurse Anesthesia
Samuel Merritt College
Oakland, CA

Margaret Faut-Callahan, CRNA, DNSc, FAAN
Professor and Chair, Adult Health Nursing
Director, Nurse Anesthesia Program
Rush University College of Nursing
Chicago, IL

AANA

AANA Publishing, Inc.

AANA Publishing, Inc.
222 South Prospect Avenue
Park Ridge, IL 60068-4001

Printed in the United States of America

Last digit indicates print number: 10 9 8 7 6 5 4 3 2

Library of Congress Cataloging-in-Publication Data

A professional study and resource guide for the CRNA / edited by Scot D. Foster, Margaret Faut-Callahan.
p. ; cm.
Includes bibliographical references and index.
ISBN 0-9700279-2-3 (pbk.)
1. Nurse anesthetists. I. Foster, Scot Douglas. II. Faut-Callahan, Margaret.
[DNLM: 1. Nurse Anesthetists. 2. Knowledge, Attitudes, Practice. 3. Professional Practice. WY 151 P9647 2001]
RD82.P765 2001
617.9'6--dc21

2001007451

DEDICATION

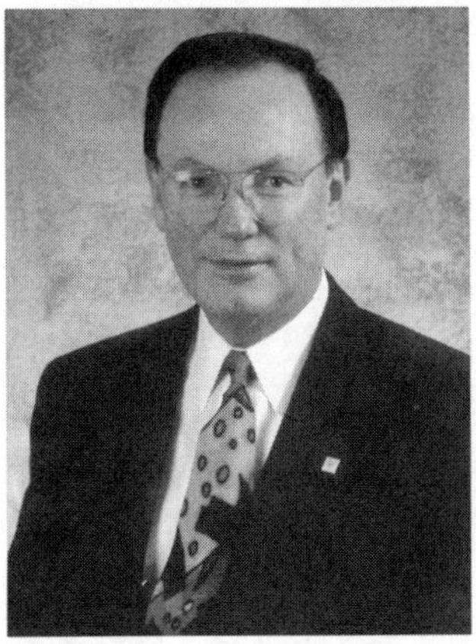

This text is dedicated to the contributions of Mr. John F. Garde, CRNA, MS, FAAN, former executive director of the American Association of Nurse Anesthetists (AANA). John retired last year, having established an unparalleled legacy of service to our profession. For many Certified Registered Nurse Anesthetists (CRNAs), he will remain the epitome of what we envision as the consummate professional and leader in healthcare. The value of this text will undoubtedly be enhanced when recalling John's contributions to CRNAs worldwide. He remains one of our finest examples of the professional spirit.

John's career spanned nearly a half century. He graduated from the Alexian Brothers Hospital School of Nursing and St. Francis Hospital School of Anesthesia, La Crosse, Wis. John received his undergraduate degree in psychology from the University of Detroit and a master's degree in physiology from Wayne State University School of Medicine. He was associate professor and chair, Department of Anesthesia, at Wayne State University, College of Pharmacy and Allied Health Profession. He became education director of the AANA in 1980 and executive director in 1983.

The CRNA community has long recognized John's leadership contributions. He was elected the first male and youngest president of the AANA in 1972. The association honored his contributions in 1981 with the Helen Lamb Outstanding Educator Award and in 2000 with AANA's most coveted honor, the Agatha Hodgins Award for professional leadership. These honors recognized John's influence in moving nurse anesthesia programs into graduate schools in colleges and universities and the establishment of the AANA's formidable federal policy role manifested in the development of the AANA Office of Federal Government Affairs based in Washington, D.C. John's tenure as an active political leader in the AANA and executive director included other accomplishments of vision including the establishment of the council system of governance, the recognition of the Council on Accreditation of Nurse Anesthesia Educational Programs by the Department of Education, formulation of several for-profit subsidiaries, and development of the AANA Foundation and the historical archives of the association.

Few CRNAs appreciate the expansive influence of the AANA as a healthcare leader within the national and international nursing community. John was at the forefront of these efforts as he guided development of the International Federation of Nurse Anesthetists and served on the boards of directors of the Nursing Organization Liaison Forum and the National Federation for Specialty Nursing Organizations. He was also a charter member of the Josiah Macy Jr. Foundation Committee for the Promotion of the Quality of Specialty Nursing Practice. For these and other contributions to nursing, John was one of the first CRNAs to be elected to the prestigious American Academy of Nursing in 1994—a group of noted nursing leaders recognized for formulating national healthcare policy based on cutting-edge nursing science.

Although John's legacy of leadership will be noted for many things, I would count as the two most important his role as mentor and his personal commitment to the value of quiet humility. During his tenure as a school director at Wayne State, his ability to mentor and nurture new CRNAs for leadership positions has long been noted. Many of John's graduates have become AANA committee and council members and chairs, noted authors and scientists, doctorally prepared CRNAs, AANA presidents, association executives, business entrepreneurs, school directors, and AANA representatives to such organizations as the Joint Commission on Accreditation of Healthcare Organizations and state boards of nursing. This profound gift for mentoring and development of others has been mirrored at the AANA where John attracted a professional staff of unparalleled talent and commitment to service.

Most appealing about John's leadership style is his humble and gracious demeanor. He has presided over some of the most expansive and positive legislative change for CRNAs of the last half century while letting others take credit. He was always there to provide subtle direction and historical perspective on issues, but never sought the spotlight. He offered alternatives which most often became solutions, yet deferred articulation to elected leadership. He always had time for every AANA member and treated each one with the same regard and attention he gave to association leaders. His attention was given totally and completely to the member.

Chapter 1 of this text talks about the indomitable spirit of CRNAs and their role as leaders in healthcare. The conclusion to that narrative provides an apt reflection of John's many gifts to us all personally and professionally:

"Professionalism is both a state of mind and commitment to action. It embodies the knowledge that our clinical work is possible only when others understand and value our service. To reach that goal requires active, life-long commitments to those ends for which we are collectively and solely responsible. Professionalism demands that CRNAs project and promote the best of what the specialty has to offer and care for things and people beyond themselves. It requires a global vision that incorporates the views of others, meeting the requirements of all stakeholders and to do so with a behavioral demeanor that is demanding of attention and respect because of the value it brings to solving problems and promoting optimal care.

"The constellation of professional skills required of every CRNA involves active participation in workplace affairs, issues forums, public relations efforts, extra-disciplinary networking and community involvement. Through these efforts, nurse anesthetists will become better informed, more effective at managing change, more satisfied with their career choice, and more adaptable to the changing healthcare environment. Most importantly, professionalism is requisite for all CRNAs today and tomorrow, as ultimately that is the only means to ensure our continued leadership in the world community of healthcare."

It is with great honor and thanks that we dedicate this book to John F. Garde.

Scot D. Foster, CRNA, PhD, FAAN
Senior Editor

PREFACE

We are delighted to introduce *A Professional Study and Resource Guide for the CRNA*. This text is, in actuality, a substantial revision of the 1994 text *Professional Aspects of Nurse Anesthesia Practice*. The title has been changed and the scope of the text broadened to reflect recent and substantial changes in healthcare, as well as the expanding influence of CRNAs in the marketplace and policy arenas.

The concept for this text came originally from recommendations of the 1992 National Commission on Nurse Anesthesia Education. Among many recommendations, there was a call to develop a text to be used in schools that spoke directly to the professional issues encountered by CRNAs in their daily lives. Although material was available from a variety of sources, there was no compendium that provided context for viewing the whole of our professional experience.

Revisions in this text hopefully reflect today's reality. There are vital content additions in the area of managed care by nationally known experts in the area. There is also a new chapter on nursing informatics and how this emerging science will change decision making and knowledge acquisition. In an effort to accommodate emerging employment and practice arrangements there are expanded chapters on reimbursement, employment contracting, and credentialing. New additions include an insightful view of managerial issues for those in leadership positions and quality improvement. Also new to this text is exciting and revealing research on the nature of the culture and value systems of CRNAs.

The text is truly meant as a resource guide for CRNAs to use on a daily basis. It addresses the pragmatics of professional regulation, legal and liability issues. It speaks to the importance of our external relationships with other agencies and organizations and importantly offers a detailed chronology of advocacy efforts of the last decade. It is an ideal companion to the *Professional Practice Manual for the Certified Registered Nurse Anesthetist,* available from the American Association of Nurse Anesthetists.

We hope not to lose sight of a common thread which unifies this text—the message that our professional growth and future standing as leaders in healthcare is challenged daily by market change, special interest pressures, competitive influences and societal demand. It will only be through vigilant attention to our professional well-being equal to the fervor of our clinical commitment to excellence, that we can secure a future for new generations of CRNAs. We trust that this text will become a useful and valued contribution to that effort.

Scot D. Foster, CRNA, PhD, FAAN
Margaret Faut-Callahan, CRNA, DNSc, FAAN

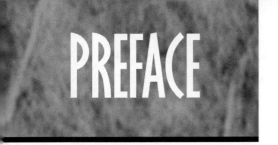

CONTRIBUTORS

Scot D. Foster, CRNA, PhD, FAAN
Senior Editor
Professor and Director
Program of Nurse Anesthesia
Samuel Merritt College
Oakland, CA

Margaret Faut-Callahan, CRNA, DNSc, FAAN
Associate Editor
Professor and Chair, Adult Health Nursing
Director, Nurse Anesthesia Program
Rush University College of Nursing
Chicago, IL

Jeffrey C. Bauer, PhD
Senior Vice President
Superior Consultant Company
Southfield, MI

Gene A. Blumenreich, JD
General Counsel
American Association of Nurse Anesthetists
Boston, MA

Marcia Bosek, DNSc, RN
Associate Professor, Adult Health Nursing
Rush University College of Nursing
Chicago, IL

Lee S. Broadston
President and CEO
BCS, Incorporated
Waconia, MN

Nancy Bruton-Maree, CRNA, MS
Program Director
Raleigh School of Nurse Anesthesia/
University of North Carolina at Greensboro
Raleigh, NC

CAPT Cynthia S. Cappello, CRNA, MAE (USN)
Acting Chair and Program Director
Department of Nurse Anesthesia
Uniformed Services University of the Health Sciences
Bethesda, MD

Ronald F. Caulk, CRNA, FAAN
Executive Director
International Federation of Nurse Anesthetists
Park Ridge, IL

Susan Smith Caulk, CRNA, MA
Director of Continuing Education, Certification and Recertification
American Association of Nurse Anesthetists
Park Ridge, IL

Kathleen Charters, PhD
Assistant Professor
University of Maryland School of Nursing
Department of Administration, Health Policy and Informatics
Columbia, MD

Russell C. Coile, Jr.
Senior Vice President
Superior Consultant Company
Southfield, MI

John F. Garde, CRNA, MS, FAAN
Executive Director, 1983-2000
American Association of Nurse Anesthetists
Park Ridge, IL

Ira P. Gunn, CRNA, MLN, FAAN
Consultant
San Antonio, TX

David E. Hebert, JD
Director of Federal Government Affairs
American Association of Nurse Anesthetists
Washington, DC

Larry G. Hornsby, CRNA, BS
Private Contractor
Birmingham, AL

Betty J. Horton, CRNA, DNSc
Director of Accreditation and Education, 1990-2002
American Association of Nurse Anesthetists
Park Ridge, IL

Michael J. Kremer, CRNA, DNSc
Assistant Professor
Rush University College of Nursing
Chicago, IL

Jeanne Learman, CRNA, MS
Director of Anesthesia
Eaton Rapids Medical Center
Eaton Rapids, MI
Director of Office Anesthesia Services
Ambulatory Surgery Consultants, Inc.
Bloomfield Hills, MI

Denise Martin-Sheridan, CRNA, PhD
Professor of Anesthesiology
Associate Graduate Director
Nurse Anesthesiology Program
Albany Medical College
Albany, NY

Cathy A. Mastropietro, CRNA, PhD
Independent Contractor
Youngstown, OH

Sandra M. Ouellette, CRNA, MEd, FAAN
Program Director, Anesthesia Program
Wake Forest University Baptist Medical/
University of North Carolina at Greensboro
Winston-Salem, NC

Diana Quinlan, CRNA, MA
Chair, AANA Peer Assistance Advisors Committee
Jacksonville, FL

Rita M. Rupp, RN, MA
Special Assistant
Office of the Executive Director
American Association of Nurse Anesthetists
Park Ridge, IL

Janet M. Simpson, JD
Holbrook, Heaven and Osborn PA
Kansas City, KS

Mitchell H. Tobin, JD
Director of State Government Affairs
American Association of Nurse Anesthetists
Park Ridge, IL

Sandra K. Tunajek, CRNA, MSN
Director of Practice
American Association of Nurse Anesthetists
Park Ridge, IL

Wynne R. Waugaman, CRNA, PhD, FAAN
Associate Professor of Nursing
Interim Chair, Department of Nursing
University of Southern California
Los Angeles, CA

Karen L. Zaglaniczny, CRNA, PhD, FAAN
Director of Education and Research
Director of Graduate Program
William Beaumont Hospital/University
Beaumont, MI

Christine S. Zambricki, CRNA, MS, FAAN
Administrative Director
William Beaumont Hospital
Royal Oak, MI

TABLE OF CONTENTS

A PROFESSIONAL STUDY AND RESOURCE GUIDE FOR THE CRNA

SECTION ONE THE ESSENCE OF PROFESSIONALISM

SECTION TWO REGULATION OF CLINICAL PRACTICE

SECTION THREE THE HEALTHCARE ENVIRONMENT

SECTION FOUR ISSUES IN PROVIDING CLINICAL SERVICES

SECTION FIVE THE POLITICS OF HEALTHCARE

SECTION SIX PRACTICE CHALLENGES

THE ESSENCE OF PROFESSIONALISM

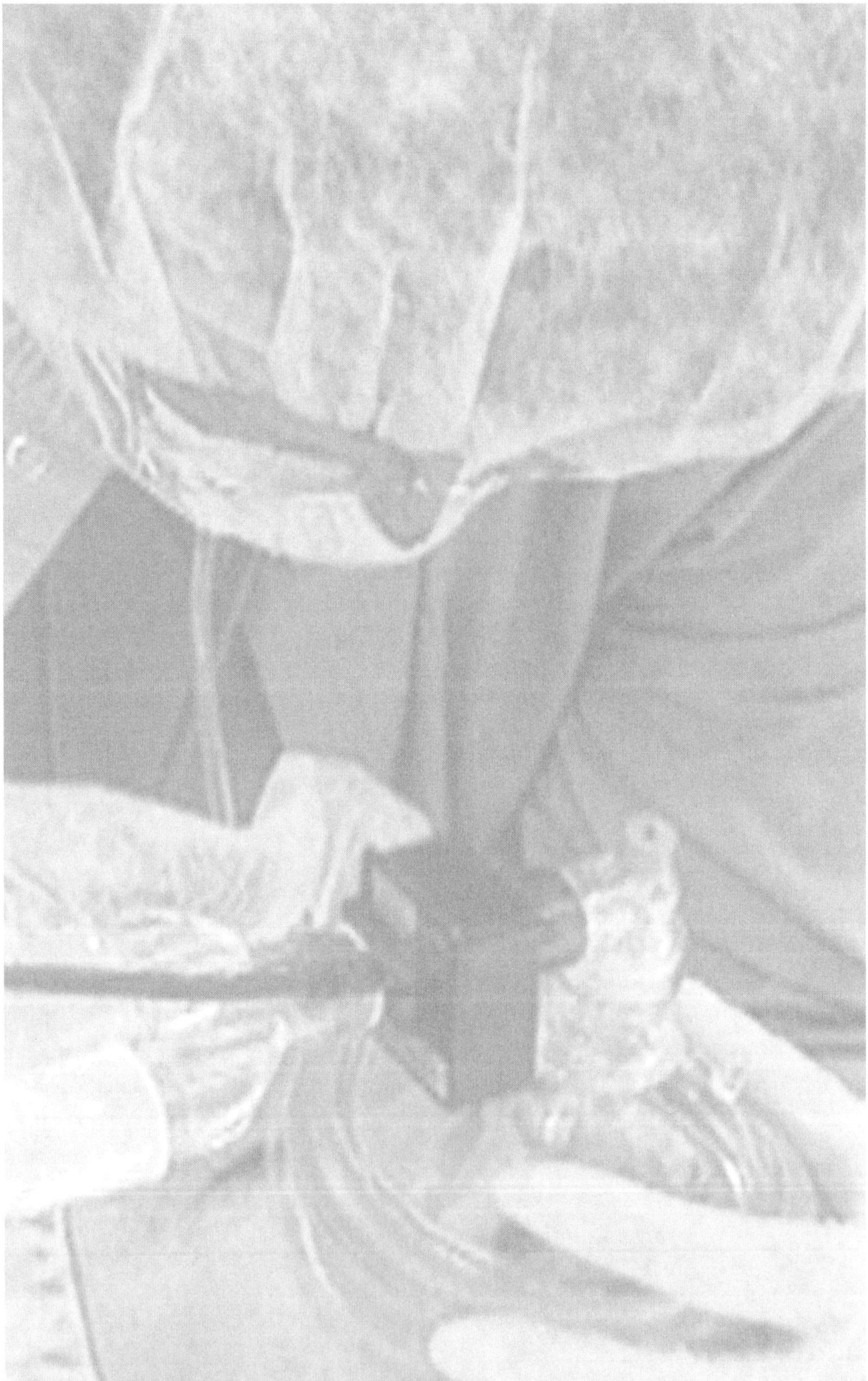

CHAPTER 1

DEFINING WORK AND THE PROFESSIONAL SPIRIT

Scot D. Foster, CRNA, PhD, FAAN

Senior Editor

Professor, Nursing
Director, Program of Nurse Anesthesia
Samuel Merritt College
Oakland, CA

KEY CONCEPTS

- Certified Registered Nurse Anesthetists (CRNAs) are advanced practice nurses certified to practice the nursing specialty of anesthesiology in all 50 states. Anesthesia practice is not a delegated act of medicine, rather a constellation of highly complex nursing skills described by a scope of practice and recognized and regulated by an appropriate state agency.
- The education of CRNAs is at the graduate level utilizing college/university-based theoretical and clinical sciences to prepare CRNAs to provide patients the full range of anesthesia services.
- Professionalism is a multidimensional set of behavioral attributes, the fundamental core value of which is integrity. Integrity is an understanding and commitment to exhibit honest, forthright, ethical, value-driven behavior that embodies skills of critical thinking, broad-based perspectives, evaluation of consequences and competent justification.
- Professionalism requires attention not only to developing clinical skills and achieving positive patient outcomes, but necessarily a commitment to serve expertly and unselfishly the interest of the public and one's self. Professionals advocate knowledgeably and act responsibly.
- Advocacy is a fundamental responsibility of the professional CRNA. Avenues of advocacy include participation in issue forums, public relations, developing and maintaining communication networks external to the profession, active involvement in legislative and regulatory activity, community service and teaching new generations of CRNAs.

The singular goal of this text is to capture in words the spirit of pride, issues in practice, and ideals of professionalism embodied in the work of the Certified Registered Nurse Anesthetist (CRNA). George Matthew Adams once wrote, "It is the spirit of a person that hangs above him like a star in the sky. People identify him at once, and join with him until there is formed a parade of men and women, thus inspired. No matter where you find this spirit working, whether in a person or an entire organization, you may know that Heaven has dropped a note of joy into the world." It is within that context that we introduce the reader to one of the most exciting and demanding of all advanced practice nursing specialties: the world of nurse anesthesia.

It is still surprising for many to learn that nurse anesthetists have provided anesthesia services in the United States for well over a century. In fact, the development of the nurse anesthesia specialty precedes that of medical anesthesiology in the United States. Today, more than 28,000 nurse anesthetists administer approximately 65 percent of the 26 million anesthetics delivered to patients in the United States each year. According to the American Association of Nurse Anesthetists (AANA), CRNAs are the sole anesthesia providers in more than two-thirds of all rural hospitals, affording these medical facilities obstetrical, surgical and trauma stabilization capabilities. CRNAs administer all types of anesthesia, from minor surgical procedures to major, complex, surgical interventions. They practice in every setting in which anesthesia is delivered, including traditional hospital surgical suites, obstetrical delivery rooms, physician offices, ambulatory surgical centers, all permutations of managed care organizations, military installations, public health service centers and Veterans Administration facilities.

Currently, the demand for CRNAs far exceeds available supply and despite the continuous and positive growth of the profession, surgical demand continues to outpace available services in most areas of the country. According to the CRNA Manpower Study from the National Center for Nursing Research, the number of CRNAs required by the year 2010 will exceed 35,000, an increase of 40 percent over the 25,000 needed in 1990 (HHS, 1990). Many observers have suggested that these numbers may be conservative estimates as we witness the continued growth and demand by managed care organizations for CRNA services. This fact, coupled with an increased surgical demand from a burgeoning geriatric population, offers bright prospects and potential for new CRNAs entering the specialty.

For those students of history, the specialty of nurse anesthesia has been richly documented in a variety of other texts and will not be repeated here. These documents provide a compelling account of the work of CRNAs since the 1870s. Virginia S. Thatcher's publication, *The History of Anesthesia with Emphasis on the Nurse Specialist* (1953), stands as the first public recognition of nurse anesthetists. The definitive history of CRNAs, *Watchful Care: A History of America's Nurse Anesthetists* by Marianne Bankert, was published in 1989. Finally, work by Evan Koch and Lee C. Fosburgh highlights pertinent historical information in "Justifiably Proud: A Brief History of Nurse Anesthetists," found in *Principles and Practice of Nurse Anesthesia* (Waugaman, Foster, and Rigor, 1999).

PROFESSIONAL DEFINITIONS

A CRNA is a licensed registered nurse who is educationally prepared at the graduate level and certified as competent to engage in the practice of anesthesiology: the art and science of rendering a patient insensible to pain by the administration of anesthetic agents and related drugs. Anesthesia and anesthesia-related care represents those services which anesthesia professionals provide upon request, assignment and referral by the patient's physician or other healthcare provider authorized by law, most often to facilitate diagnostic, therapeutic and surgical procedures. In addition to general or regional anesthesia techniques or sedation techniques required for surgery, a referral or request for consultation or assistance may be for management of pain associated with obstetrical labor and delivery, management of acute and chronic ventilatory problems, or management of acute and chronic pain through the performance of selected diagnostic and therapeutic blocks (AANA, 1996).

CRNAs are responsible and accountable for their individual professional practice and are capable of exercising independent judgment within the scope of their education (credentials), demonstrated competence (privileges) and licensure. CRNAs are recognized in all 50 states by state regulatory (licensing) bodies, primarily boards of registered nursing (BRN). The practice of CRNAs is a recognized specialty within the profession of nursing and is not a medically delegated act. In order to be a Certified Registered Nurse Anesthetist one must:

- Graduate from an approved school of nursing and hold current state licensure as a registered nurse.
- Graduate from a nurse anesthesia educational program accredited by the Council on Accreditation of Nurse Anesthesia Educational Programs (COA) or its predecessor.
- Successfully complete the certification examination administered by the Council on Certification of Nurse Anesthetists or its predecessor.
- Comply with criteria for biennial recertification, as defined by the Council on Recertification of Nurse Anesthetists. These criteria include evidence of (1) current licensure as a registered nurse, (2) active practice as a CRNA, (3) appropriate continuing education, and (4) verification of the absence of mental, physical and other problems which could interfere with the practice of anesthesia.

Scope of Practice

The scope of practice of CRNAs encompasses the professional functions, privileges and responsibilities associated with nurse anesthesia practice. These acts are nearly always performed in collaboration with other qualified and legally authorized professional healthcare providers that may or may not include surgeons, anesthesiologists or other consulting physicians, nurses, therapists or technicians who assume distinct and specialized roles required for comprehensive, perianesthetic patient care. Collaboration is a process which involves two or more parties working together, each contributing his or her respective expertise. Collaboration must necessarily exist whether a CRNA works in an anesthesiologist-lead anesthesia care team (ACT) or as an independent practitioner.

The terms "supervision" and "medical direction" most often describe a relationship between a nurse anesthetist and a physician, dentist, podiatrist or other healthcare professional with whom the nurse anesthetist collaborates to varying degrees. The specifics of these terms exist on a continuum, if they exist at all in a particular state or region. That is, a CRNA's scope of practice could potentially encompass a broad range of discretionary, independent practice rights as determined by the appropriate state regulatory agency and authorized only by the general consent of another licensed provider as established by state law. On the other end of the continuum, a CRNA's scope of practice may be limited by state or local medical staff bylaws to only approved activities (privileges). The variation in these practice roles can be substantial and requires graduating CRNAs to carefully evaluate any potential limitations imposed on their scope of practice. Finally, it should be noted that the term "collaboration" does not imply a mandated supervisory role by a physician anesthesiologist. The reader should refer to chapters 7 and 18 for details on state and federal requirements for supervision or medical direction if and where they occur.

Nurse anesthetists administer anesthesia and anesthesia-related care in four general categories: (1) preanesthetic preparation and evaluation, (2) anesthesia induction, maintenance and emergence, (3) postanesthesia care, and (4) perianesthetic and clinical support functions. A nurse anesthetist's scope of practice is detailed in Table 1.1 (1996) and additional, more specific information can be found in the "Guidelines for Granting Clinical Privileges to CRNAs" in the *Professional Practice Manual for the Certified Registered Nurse Anesthetist* (AANA, 1996).

Educational Preparation of CRNAs

From the first call in 1933 for educational standards by Gertrude Fife, president of the National Association of Nurse Anesthetists, today's nurse anesthesia programs have become increasingly sophisticated and reflective of the higher education academy. There are now nearly 90 accredited programs nationwide, all of which offer a graduate degree upon completion of a rigorous course of clinical and academic study. Approximately 52 percent of programs are housed within a department of nursing and the balance within schools of allied health, medicine or other related health disciplines. Today there are nearly 2,000 nurse anesthesia students enrolled in programs whose permanent, regular faculty is comprised of doctorally prepared faculty in nursing, education, and the physical, biological and clinical sciences. Each year approximately 975 students graduate from these programs and become eligible for certification.

Program length is a minimum of 24 months, although nearly three-quarters of all programs require a 27-month period of enrollment. Each program provides an extensive curriculum that combines academic theory and research-based clinical practice that, in many programs, approximates 1,200-1,600 hours of actual perianesthetic clinical experience. Required course work common to all programs includes upper-level anatomy, physiology and pathophysiology, chemistry and physics, pharmacology, basic and advanced practice principles, clinical conferences and professional issues. Many schools provide clinical experiences in pain management, regional anesthesia, emergency resuscitation, and intensive and emergency services such that graduates are fully competitive once in the workplace. In addition, most curricula require educational experiences in some form of research activity or other mode of scientific inquiry as well as advanced theoretical principles of nursing practice and health policy. Specific curricular requirements for program accreditation are available in the *Standards for Accreditation, Council on Accreditation of Nurse Anesthesia Educational Programs* (COA, 1994).

Although admission criteria vary among programs, minimum requirements of the COA mandate that students (1) graduate from an approved school of nursing, (2) possess a baccalaureate degree in nursing or other appropriate

TABLE 1.1: CRNA Scope of Practice

- Performing and documenting a preanesthetic assessment and evaluation of the patient, including requesting consultations and diagnostic studies; selecting, obtaining, ordering, or administering preanesthetic medications and fluids; and obtaining informed consent for anesthesia
- Developing and implementing an anesthetic plan
- Selecting and initiating the planned anesthetic technique which may include general, regional, and local anesthesia and intravenous sedation
- Selecting, applying and inserting appropriate noninvasive and invasive monitoring modalities for continuous evaluation of the patient's physical status
- Selecting, obtaining or administering the anesthetics, adjuvant drugs, and fluids necessary to manage the anesthetic
- Managing a patient's airway and pulmonary status using current practice modalities
- Facilitating emergence and recovery from anesthesia by selecting, obtaining, ordering or administering medications, fluids and ventilatory support
- Discharging the patient from a postanesthesia care area and providing postanesthesia follow-up evaluation and care
- Implementing acute and chronic pain management modalities
- Responding to emergency situations by providing airway management, administration of emergency fluids or drugs, or using basic or advanced cardiac life support techniques

Note. The functions listed above are a summary of CRNA clinical practice and are not intended to be all-inclusive. A more specific list of CRNA functions and practice parameters is detailed in the *Professional Practice Manual for the Certified Registered Nurse Anesthetist* (AANA,1996).

baccalaureate degree, (3) maintain current licensure as a registered nurse, and (4) complete one year of experience as a registered professional nurse in which they have had the opportunity to develop as independent decision makers and demonstrate psychomotor skills and the ability to use and interpret advanced monitoring techniques based on a knowledge of physiologic and pharmacologic principles.

Most often, successful applicants have acquired extensive clinical backgrounds as professional nurses in coronary, respiratory, postanesthesia and surgical intensive care units, emergency rooms or as members of a trauma or cardiac surgical team. The specifics of appropriate clinical experiences, in addition to those required by the COA, are the prerogative of the program. This and other general information about the specialty of anesthesia, a listing of all accredited programs, and educational program standards can be found on the Internet at www.aana.com or by email at info@aana.com. Many individual programs also maintain their own specific Web sites which detail educational philosophy, curricula, admission requirements and other items of interest to prospective candidates. The AANA receives over 5,000 inquiries a year from students interested in a professional career as a CRNA.

THE CHALLENGE OF PROFESSIONALISM

For CRNAs who have spent the greater part of their professional careers as educators, it becomes increasingly clear that the success of the educational endeavor hinges directly on the accomplishment of two objectives. The first, which is generally the easier of the two and requisite to clinical practice, is to equip students with the skills and abilities to conduct and manage a safe, high-quality anesthetic. The second objective, which is equally vital but often far more difficult to achieve, is to imbue in students a clear and functional appreciation for the responsibilities of professionalism—specifically, to inculcate in students personal values that promote the well-being, public image, longevity and leadership role of the specialty.

The difficulty in meeting this educational challenge stems from a variety of sources. First, the concept of "professionalism" is not an easy one to understand because over time the term has been applied so broadly and indiscriminately that a clear, unambiguous conceptual picture is often hard to formulate. The issue is further clouded because contemporary literature has yielded few new interpretations or salient applications of professional behaviors that would be useful to new students socializing into the profession. Most critically, students spend a great deal of time, necessarily perhaps, sequestered in operating rooms and have little opportunity to engage students in other programs or CRNAs in practice. Consequently, far too many graduates fail to experience the socializing influence of CRNA role models and consequently don't learn the value of their social commitment to the public or their own professional well-being.

Historical Evolution of the Professions

An informed understanding of professionalism should be based on historical perspectives. The professions derived largely from those who sought to teach or to profess. Originally, this meant to take the vows of a religious order, but by the seventeenth century had been secularized to mean the process of achieving due qualification (Stein and Kristenson, 1970). From this developed the idea that persons claiming membership in the professions profess to know better than others the nature of certain matters and to know better than their clients what aids them or their affairs (Hughes, 1963). Origins of professionalism were initially associated with the clergy, however, the professions separately organized when religion was no longer a predominate social force. Gradually, professions became formally associated with the universities of medieval Europe and most clearly resembled the more contemporary training schools for the traditional professions of law, medicine and theology.

Stein and Kristenson note that professional occupations were learned through apprenticeships or short training courses. Since both theory and practice had always been considered dual components of the learned professions, the advent of apprenticeships put renewed emphasis on the practice component. Professional candidates placed themselves under the able tutelage of a minister, lawyer or doctor and hoped by observation and imitation to be subsequently admitted to professional status. In the American colonies, early professional education came primarily from the great European universities for lack of colonist faculties or organized professional schools. Slowly the American colonists began to develop their own system of higher education from which would eventually emerge the professional school. This effort was greatly aided by the establishment of professorial chairs and special professorships in traditional academic disciplines.

Proprietary schools (staffed by teaching practitioners) were also developed during this time to help provide greater numbers of professionals. The overall quality of many of these schools was dubious at best. They did provide employment for what many considered a proliferation of doctors and lawyers so ill-trained that they could not find gainful employment elsewhere. Proprietary schools did contribute in small part to the development of professional education by emphasizing didactic instruction and relying less on apprentice-type "learning by experience." However, the actual contributions of proprietary schools to the curricular integrity of professional educational programs remains a point of historic contention.

It was not until after the Civil War that the scope and sophistication of professional schools began to fully develop. Medical practice drew increasing respectability by incorporating scientific principles and new research gleaned largely from European physicians. The medical curricula became more comprehensively based on new developments in chemistry and biology that would offer solid scientific foundations. Lawyers would come to value the need for more balanced educational approaches incorporating longer, more formalized internships under qualified mentors. Even professional faculty in schools of theology were beginning to incorporate some of the newer modes of scholarship adapted from the German models of professional education. These activities ushered the movement of professional schools into the university setting and away from the more disorganized and oftentimes ethically specious proprietary schools.

The occupations of engineering and certain of the social sciences and healthcare fields were becoming recognized and accepted as professions subsequent to the move of those disciplines into more formal education frameworks. Due to the diverse missions of emerging types of institutions of higher education, the land-grant institutions, for instance (eventually state universities), began to recognize agriculture and home economics as professional occupations. With the advent of state competence examinations, practice regulatory authorities, accreditation mechanisms, and performance standards, professional schools became more credible and reliable providers of professional services.

RESPONSIBILITIES OF PROFESSIONALISM

The student and practitioner should be reminded that abilities to practice anesthesia within the scope of what is termed a "professional capacity" is not a right afforded unconditionally. Conceptually, the traditional professions were recognized as occupational groups who, over time, gained the recognition and trust of the public for services that were highly valued by society. Consequently, professional recognition was an earned right granted solely and exclusively by the public in exchange for certain services and conduct. Society retained the right to deny recognition of any professional service provider when those services no longer met the needs, expectations or standards of the public. Too often, professional healthcare providers are under the mistaken notion that their rights to practice are afforded directly by statute or some particular licensing or regulatory body. However, these bodies are merely social conventions designed to operationalize public policy. Although this notion may appear of little importance, it should remind us that we practice anesthesia because we have earned the confidence and trust of the public. If the quality, scope and vigilance attendant to our work fails, so may the ability to claim professional status.

Chief among the responsibilities for which the public holds CRNAs responsible (in exchange for the designation, benefits and prerogatives of professional practice) is that professional activities should accrue benefit to the public, not the profession. Subsequently, the primary goal of any profession should be public service. In cases where a professional organization comes to value their financial interest over public interest, it is likely the profession will risk regulatory sanction or worse.

Most sociologists concur that the most critical features of any definition of professionalism are a mastery of skill and competence acquired by rigorous clinical training, a research-based theoretical education, and an ethical code of behavior. The AANA maintains a code of ethics espousing "right" behaviors based on a set of values or principles which the profession reveres. The code is a value-based guide for CRNAs to use as a framework for establishing and maintaining professional relationships with patients, coworkers, institutions and external agencies (AANA, 1996).

Although there is some degree of difficulty encountered in definitions of professionalism, most agree there is need for criteria that designate when any particular work group evolves to the level of professional status. Table 1.2 (Schein, 1972) provides a listing of commonly accepted characteristics of and qualifications for designation as a profession.

Pellegrino (1983) provides a humanistic perspective of what constitutes a professional. He states that the philosophical grounding of a true profession lies in the special kind of interpersonal relationship it requires between its practitioners and those who seek their assistance. Tenets of his approach include the need for healthcare providers to understand that

- Patients exist in a special and compromised state of vulnerability.
- Patient needs which the professions address are of the most sensitive kind, including mortality, freedom, human values and rights.
- The provider must always uphold the values of dignity and privacy.
- Patients trust the provider will use knowledge only in their best interest.

Pellegrino states, "To be a professional is to make a promise to hope, to keep that promise, and to do so in the best interest of patients. It is to accept the trust the patient must place in us as a moral imperative, one that the ethos of the marketplace or competition does not expect us, in our society, to honor. The special nature of the helping and healing professions is rooted in the fact that people become ill and need to trust others to help them restore health."

Although this definition deals almost exclusively with the provider-patient relationship, it is obvious that when this relationship is threatened, certain social and political activities are required to maintain it. Thus the definition of professionalism is necessarily segmentalized into a constellation of activities that address some element of the social covenant previously described. These activities can take the form of social advocacy, public education, community building, elevating standards or influencing public policy, to name only a few.

Once the commitment is made to engage in these activities, CRNAs will find themselves immediately exposed to some element of scrutiny, public exposure, controversy, and stresses from interdisciplinary conflict. Initially they may find themselves relatively uneducated about issues and needs, naive in affairs of diplomacy, and perhaps even ineffectual in debate and argument.

TABLE 1.2: Criteria for Qualification as a Profession

- The professional is engaged in a full-time occupation that comprises his principal source of income. Professionals have a strong motivation or calling to the occupation manifested by a lifetime commitment.
- The professional possesses a specialized body of knowledge and skills acquired during a prolonged period of formal education and training.
- The professional makes decisions on behalf of a client by means of a clearly defined yet broad foundation of theoretical knowledge and expertise in clinical application.
- The professional has a service orientation. This service implies diagnostic skill, competent application of general knowledge to the special needs of the client, and an absence of self interest or self promotion.
- The profession's service to the client is assumed to be based on the objective needs of the client and independent of the particular sentiments that the profession may have about the client. This promises a "detached" diagnosis and withholding of moral judgment about the client's revelations or diagnosis.
- The professional demands autonomy in actions and judgment, and subscribes to standards judged by a panel of peers. Legal protection is sought through political influence.
- Professional associations are formed which define criteria of admission, educational standards, licensing, entry examinations, and areas of jurisdiction for the profession. Ultimately, the professional association's function is to protect the autonomy of the profession; it develops reasonably strong forms of self-government by setting rules or standards for the profession.

However, in the same way that clinical skills are honed, skills of advocacy and service can also be developed. In fact, when substantive change occurs as a result of advocacy, there are accrued benefits of personal satisfaction, increased self-confidence, and a sense of personal worth and value, as well as broader visions for future change and direction.

In short, professionalism is a commitment to serve expertly and unselfishly, to advocate knowledgeably, and to act responsibly. It is a process that both exposes and promotes the philosophical underpinnings and value of work. It is through the process of exposing what we value about our work that our work will be valued by others who gain service from it. Professionalism is manifested in a variety of ways including clinical competence. However, make no mistake that clinical competence alone is an insufficient ingredient to secure the continued success of nurse anesthetists as a viable entity in the marketplace or leaders in healthcare. Success demands more: It demands professionalism.

Abuses of Professionalism

It should be evident to the most naive observer of the professional landscape that the traditional privileges and social status of the professions have been slowly eroded over the past several decades. Whether the discipline be law, medicine, religion, nursing or managed care, one can cite numerous examples which account for the downturn in public esteem the professions once enjoyed. Reasons are generally attributable to a decreasing sensitivity of providers to public need, resistance to change in the public interest, commercialization, unaffordable cost for fewer and lesser quality services, and projection of professional interests (especially financial) over those of the public.

As a result, the consuming public has been reasonably effective in initiating needed change, although many feel the hardest choices and most difficult work lie ahead. Examples of these public concerns and advocacy efforts include the need for passage of a federal patient's bill of rights, mandating access to care, rights of redress for poor quality or rationed care, and provision of affordable health insurance. Consequently, state and federal legislative agendas are contemplating legislative efforts to reverse trends the public has determined are not in their best interest. Those include caps on certain legal fees in medical liability cases, eliminating anticompetitive practices that restrict nonphysician access to patients, exclusion of prescription allowances, and lack of ability to sue HMOs for substandard, unavailable or uncompensated care.

Healthcare professionals should remain mindful of the core concepts of professionalism even when tempted by the forces of a competitive marketplace to do otherwise. Clearly, providers must recommit to traditional professional values that wisely emphasize their moral obligations and the changing needs of contemporary society.

THE CORE VALUE OF INTEGRITY

Fundamental to any definition of professionalism for either students or clinicians is the principle of integrity. In its most broadly applicable form, integrity is an understanding and commitment to honest, forthright, value-driven, behavior. The definition implies that any action taken by a clinician must be characterized by an intent to achieve excellence and to do so within an ethical context. Actions taken, or in the case of CRNAs, clinical decisions made or collegial behaviors demonstrated, should always reveal elements of critical thinking, broad-based perspectives, careful evaluation of consequences and competent justification. Actions that reveal themselves as self-centered, cursory, ill-timed, or myopic are usually characteristic of decisions made absent of any genuine commitments that value integrity.

Integrity in Student Life

For students, academic integrity is of paramount importance. That is, students should be resolved to pledge all intellectual resources to the process of learning. They should enter an educational program as an informed consumer and be clear as to their motivation and capability for pursuing a career in nurse anesthesia. Students should make a studied analysis of their educational needs, choose an appropriate learning environment and work diligently toward certification.

During a student's enrollment, faculty measure a student's commitment to academic integrity in a variety of ways: optimal classroom preparation and study, meeting deadlines, well-executed planning and organizational skills, self-motivated inquiry, self-discipline, and exceeding minimal performance standards both in the classroom and clinical area. Clearly, the experience of many educators has repeatedly confirmed the observation that a graduate is only as good as the quality effort he or she expends in pursuit of educational goals. The success students attain as clinicians is a function largely of the personal expectations and standards they set for themselves. Subsequently, the veracity, commitment and honesty to self with which students approach challenges of graduate education remain a primary key to success.

Another way in which all students should demonstrate their commitment to professional responsibility is by attending educational conferences available to them. In addition to clinical education sessions, these meetings provide opportunities to learn about advocacy issues, speak publicly, network with colleagues, perhaps manage educational programming and, importantly, learn about the values and culture that CRNAs promote. Repeatedly the observation is made that those students who actively seek opportunities to participate in state and local educational programs are those that continue to actively and productively participate in affairs of both the state and national organizations of the AANA.

Integrity in Professional Life

The most fundamental professional responsibility of CRNAs is to maintain clinical competence through a variety of mechanisms such as continuing education seminars, in-house educational conferences, and attendance at local, state and national meetings of the AANA and other qualified sponsors. It is incumbent on every CRNA to make certain that their scope of practice and expertise is constantly undergoing productive change and expansion in order to maintain skills required for the marketplace and optimally enhance patient care.

In the clinical area, a commitment to maintain competence is a form of behavioral integrity measured by the extent and manner in which CRNAs use their knowledge in the best interest of the patient, avoid breeches of patient confidentiality, and deal interpersonally with patients in an informed, supportive and unambiguous manner. Ultimately, it is about maintaining the highest possible standards of care.

Clinical skills are only as good as a provider's ability to communicate effectively both to patients and other providers. Without effective communication skills there is high probability that the provider will not be seen as an effective team member or patient advocate. Further, unskilled communications are usually the hallmark of those who lack any fundamental appreciation of the tenets of responsible, interpersonal skills. Too often the professional arrogance of healthcare providers results in written and oral communication that is misinformed, demonstrates an egregious lack of respect for others, and is often characterized by a total lack of skill for diplomacy or reasoned debate. This type of behavior is the antithesis of productive professional behavior. It should always be of concern to students and CRNAs that their professional credibility as clinicians hinges as much on their facility to communicate and project an appropriate, caring and sensitive demeanor as it does on clinical skill.

AVENUES OF PROFESSIONAL ADVOCACY

CRNAs have long revered their ability to practice with relative autonomy, to conduct patient care activities in ways they believe are most appropriate, and to participate fully in the healthcare system as respected providers. However, these privileges have neither been without cost nor will they be available in the future without continued participation by all CRNAs in activities that strengthen their public image and promote a legislative agenda designed to secure their practice rights and privileges. As will be revealed in later chapters, CRNAs have long been involved in such legislative and policy efforts via the AANA, the professional membership organization boasting a membership of approximately 95 percent of all CRNAs in the United States.

Many CRNAs have developed substantial skills in formally advocating a professional agenda that advances both the care of patients and issues affecting their own personal well-being. Countless numbers of CRNAs participate daily in a variety of nonclinical activities that enhance the standing, credibility and value of CRNAs to the healthcare community. What is key for CRNAs to appreciate about advocacy is that there is a necessary role for everyone to assume.

Providing quality patient care, while important, is not sufficient alone to maintain the leadership role of CRNAs in healthcare at the local and national levels.

The extent to which CRNAs become involved in professional advocacy efforts will change over time to accommodate activities that require more skill and dedication of time, yet there are tremendous personal and professional rewards in achieving goals that promote the welfare of all involved. Above all, it should be obvious to every CRNA that their continued ability to compete as a major health provider and enjoy the substantial professional prerogatives they currently do depends directly on personally assuming their share of work to maintain them. In the game of high-stakes competition, expansive market flux, a dwindling resource base and ever-increasing demands for better outcomes and more cost-effective work production, there will be no "big brother" to care for your needs, ensure your job security, or nurture your development. Big brother is us!

What are the important advocacy efforts in which you may find a niche?

Participation in Issue Forums

These can be local departmental meetings at your work site, hospital committees or community service organizations. They should always include attendance at state and national meetings of the AANA. It is of paramount importance that CRNAs "be at the table" when planning, negotiation and decision-making occur.

Public Relations

There are no more important activities than those directed at helping the public, policy makers and colleagues understand the nature and value of your work. Invite a legislator into the operating room to observe your interactions with patients, sponsor community health fairs, write articles for your local paper, and take every opportunity to participate on talk radio or in television clips. Always respond to inaccuracies of the press regarding your work. Establish a regular press contact and function as their primary source of information about CRNAs and anesthesia. Above all, communicate your message in an informed, accurate and responsible way.

Establish External Networks

Advocating for CRNA work necessarily includes getting the message to other persons and organizations who share your philosophies and interests. Some of the most valued relationships CRNAs have established with state and national political leaders have been through years of acquaintance as neighbors. CRNAs have established other valued communication and project networks as members of consulting teams, expert witnesses, members of city administration bureaucracies such as the school or utility board, members of state boards of nursing, representatives to other specialty nursing groups, liaisons to corporate healthcare leaders, and countless other ways. Remember, on the most basic level, personal relationships with local facility administrators is the first, best liaison to establish. Additionally, involvement with external groups demonstrates your personal willingness to be "part of the solution and not part of the problem."

Legislative and Regulatory Activity

Some CRNAs will be called upon to assume more formal relationships with policy makers to formulate or influence legislation or regulation that affects CRNA practice. Functional roles may include working directly with legislative or agency staff in state government such as the board of nursing, administrative code offices, insurance commissioners, heads of other state health regulatory agencies and boards, and congressional representatives and staff at the federal level. Most state organizations of nurse anesthetists retain professional lobbying firms whose activities depend heavily on CRNA involvement to achieve legislative or policy goals. Remember that optimum function of professional lobbyists is not possible without the direct involvement of CRNAs. Legislators want to hear directly from you about how issues affect you and your patients.

Serving the Community

Much of the provision of healthcare in the future will be decentralized and take place within the community, as opposed to large medical centers. Consequently, CRNAs need to be involved in community health projects that best expose their skills and value to society. Many CRNAs have become actively involved in teaching the public cardiopulmonary resuscitation, staffing immunization clinics, or offering missionary or volunteer work on federal or private ventures to foreign countries that provide surgical services to the underprivileged.

PROFESSIONALISM AND THE RESPONSIBILITIES OF TEACHING

It has long been appreciated that the need for education lies at the core of the human enterprise. History has demonstrated repeatedly that education is the critical component for transmitting social values, norms, and cultural traditions from generation to generation. On a more pragmatic level, education secures a competent work force and ensures a productive society and thriving economy. Education is of paramount importance to the CRNA for these reasons in addition to enhancing patient outcomes.

It is critical that CRNAs in all practice settings consider providing student nurse anesthetists some teaching-related service. These services may come in various forms, but all have immense value in the preparation of the next generation of CRNAs. The growth of programs and maintenance of national manpower requirements is singularly dependent on access of students to clinical sites where they can gain clinical experiences. For some CRNAs, participation in education and teaching may include an invitation to a student to observe or practice clinically in a hospital, outpatient surgery center, physician's office, or other environment in which the CRNA acts as a formal instructor or mentor. CRNAs may also serve as regular teaching faculty or clinical coordinators for established programs of nurse anesthesia. Virtually hundreds of CRNAs, who are not able to provide access to their clinical sites, volunteer to lecture to students or participate in continuing education programs for CRNAs and students. It is through these efforts and commitments to education that accredited programs of nurse anesthesia have increased the number of clinical sites from only a few a decade ago to nearly 800 today. As market demand continues to flourish for CRNAs, more clinical sites will be needed for supervised educational experiences, especially in community-based sites such as outpatient surgery centers and physician's offices.

SUMMARY

Professionalism is both a state of mind and commitment to action. It embodies the knowledge that our clinical work is possible only when others understand and value our service. To reach that goal requires active, life-long commitments to those ends for which we are collectively and solely responsible. Professionalism demands that CRNAs project and promote the best of what the specialty has to offer and care for things and people beyond themselves. It requires a global vision that incorporates the views of others and meets the requirements of all stakeholders, and does so with a behavioral demeanor that is demanding of attention and respect because of the value it brings to solving problems and promoting optimal care.

The constellation of professional skills required of every CRNA involves active participation in workplace affairs, issue forums, public relations efforts, extradisciplinary networking and community involvement. Through these efforts, nurse anesthetists will become better informed, more effective at managing change, more satisfied with their career choice, and more adaptable to the changing healthcare environment. Most importantly, professionalism is requisite for all CRNAs today and tomorrow, as ultimately that is the only means to ensure our continued leadership in the world community of healthcare.

REFERENCES

American Association of Nurse Anesthetists. (1997). *White Paper.* Park Ridge, IL: Author.

American Association of Nurse Anesthetists. (1996). Scope and standards for nurse anesthesia practice. In *Professional Practice Manual for the Certified Registered Nurse Anesthetist.* Park Ridge, IL: Author.

American Association of Nurse Anesthetists. (1996). Qualifications and capabilities of the Certified Registered Nurse Anesthetist. In *Professional Practice Manual for the Certified Registered Nurse Anesthetist.* Park Ridge, IL: Author.

American Association of Nurse Anesthetists. (1996). Code of ethics. In *Professional Practice Manual for the Certified Registered Nurse Anesthetist.* Park Ridge, IL: Author.

Bankert, M. (1989). *Watchful Care: A History of America's Nurse Anesthetists.* New York: Continuum Publishing.

Council on Accreditation of Nurse Anesthesia Educational Programs. (1994). *Standards for Accreditation.* Park Ridge, IL.

National Center for Nursing Research. (1990). *Study of Nurse Anesthetists Manpower Needs.* Washington, DC: U.S. Government Printing Office.

Hughes, E.C. (1963). Professions, proceedings of the American Academy of Arts and Sciences. *Daedalus*, XCII, 4, 665-68.

Koch, E., & Fosburgh, L.C. (1999). Justifiably proud: A brief history of nurse anesthetists. In W.R. Waugaman, S.D. Foster & B.M. Rigor (Eds.), *Principles and Practice of Nurse Anesthesia* (pp. 3-17). Norwalk, CT: Appleton and Lange.

Pellegrino, E.D. (1983). What is a profession? *Journal of Allied Health.* 168-176.

Schein, E.H. (1972). Professional education: Some new directions. In *Carnegie Commission Report on Higher Education.* 10, 7-14. New York, NY: McGraw-Hill.

Stein, H.D. & Kristenson, A.L. (1970). The professional schools and the university: The case of social work. *Council on Social Work Education* (p. 2). New York, NY: Author.

Thatcher, V.S. (1953). *History of Anesthesia with Emphasis on the Nurse Specialist.* Philadelphia, PA: J.B. Lippincott.

KEY REFERENCES

American Association of Nurse Anesthetists. (1996). *Professional Practice Manual for the Certified Registered Nurse Anesthetist*, Park Ridge, IL: Author.

Bankert, M. (1989). *Watchful Care: A History of America's Nurse Anesthetists.* New York: Continuum Publishing.

STUDY QUESTIONS

1. Relative to regulation of CRNAs, what are the respective functions of boards of registered nursing and the AANA or its councils?

2. Define the issues of physician supervision as they are revealed in this chapter and chapters 7 and 18. What are the implications for your own scope of practice and sense of professionalism when another work group exerts supervisory authority? What are the issues at play in this discussion?

3. Discuss the issue of autonomy, what it means, and its relevance to any healthcare discipline or specialty in today's healthcare environment.

4. Identify the basic tenets of professional work groups as they evolved historically and determine the extent to which they are applicable today.

5. List and discuss your perception of a "professional." What does it mean to you and how is it manifested in your school experience or professional life?

6. Discuss potential avenues for expressing your own skills of professional advocacy. In how many ways do you advocate for patients, yourself, colleagues, affiliations, etc. on a daily basis?

CHAPTER 2

A PHILOSOPHY OF CARING AND SERVICE

Betty J. Horton, CRNA, DNSc

Director of Accreditation and Education, 1990-2002
American Association of Nurse Anesthetists
Park Ridge, IL

KEY CONCEPTS

- Dominant cultural values in nurse anesthesia include autonomy, education, continuing education, achievement, group cohesiveness, identity as a Certified Registered Nurse Anesthetist, membership in the American Association of Nurse Anesthetists, political activism and technology.
- Foundational values of nurse anesthetists are operative to two major domains of professional activity: (1) to remain active and vigilant in defending and maintaining practice rights, and (2) dedication to patient care.
- Values inherent in providing protective care for dependent patients are individualized care, technology, touch, surveillance, vigilance and honesty.

Experiments with the inhalation of ether vapors by William Morton, a dentist, resulted in the discovery of the first effective anesthetic agent in the middle of the 19th century (Thatcher, 1953). The discovery of ether was a watershed event in history that allowed patients to undergo dental and surgical procedures without pain. Thus, the discovery of ether was a critical step leading to the practice of modern anesthesia and surgery where lengthy and complex surgical procedures are common.

After ether was discovered, a need was soon seen for a category of health-care worker to assume responsibility for the safety of patients since the administration of ether anesthesia resulted in unconsciousness as well as pain relief. Nurses were already experienced in providing care and protection to unconscious patients and anesthesia care soon became an added responsibility to the general duties of nurses in the United States (Robb, 1893). By the late 1880s some nurses began to specialize in anesthesia and became known as nurse anesthetists (Thatcher, 1953).

The first educational programs for nurse anesthetists were established in 1909 preceding the development of anesthesiology as a specialty for physicians that began following World War II (Bankert, 1989). Over the next 80 years, the education of nurse anesthetists changed dramatically from certificate training programs to degree-granting programs. By January 1, 1998, the Council on Accreditation of Nurse Anesthesia Educational Programs implemented a requirement that all accredited nurse anesthesia educational programs must offer extensive clinical and didactic experiences leading to the award of a master's or higher degree from universities.

Today, Certified Registered Nurse Anesthetists (CRNAs), nurses specializing in anesthesia, and anesthesiologists, physicians specializing in anesthesia, are the primary groups providing anesthesia care in the United States. The most common mode of practice is for CRNAs and anesthesiologists to work together, but sometimes each of the professionals work independent of the other.

More than 28,000 CRNAs work in all types of practice settings administering approximately 65 percent of all anesthetics in the United States annually. CRNAs are also the sole anesthesia providers in 65 percent of rural hospitals and nearly 50 percent of all hospitals (AANA, 2000). Thus, nurse anesthetists continue a tradition of contributing significantly to the care of patients by providing needed anesthesia and related services.

NURSE ANESTHESIA CULTURE

A comprehensive study of the worldviews of nurse anesthetists was conducted in the late 20th century to uncover implicit and explicit information about the cultural aspects of nurse anesthesia (Horton, 1998). Acquisition of knowledge about the nursing specialty revealed the meanings, values, and practices of nurse anesthetists as influenced by the cultural dimensions of social structure, technology, religion, philosophy, kinship, social factors, values, lifeways, politics, legal factors, economy, and education (Leininger, 1995). The information presented in this chapter is limited to the discovery of knowledge related to the values held by CRNAs that serve as the philosophical foundation of nurse anesthesia practice.

Values held by a group of people are part of the unique culture that binds them together. Certain values are learned, shared, and transmitted to younger generations of a group as guides for thinking, decisions, and actions (Leininger, 1995). Furthermore, the shared values and behaviors in a culture are often a result of coping with common problems. This has certainly been true for the culture of nurse anesthesia. In fact, nurse anesthetists have unconsciously developed characteristic attitudes and behaviors that have proven successful in dealing with external challenges to the profession throughout its history.

For example, strained relationships between the American Association of Nurse Anesthetists (AANA) and the American Society of Anesthesiologists (ASA) have influenced the development of the nurse anesthesia culture. Conflicts between nurse anesthetists and anesthesiologists began in earnest in the middle of the 20th century when the physicians began concerted attempts to claim anesthesia practice from nurses and to establish anesthesiology as the practice of medicine in the United States. As events unfolded over the years it became apparent that the organized group of anesthesiologists wanted to gain control over the education and practice of nurse anesthetists. However, anesthesiologists were faced with problems in gaining control. One problem was that nurse anesthetists and anesthesiologists had similar scopes of anesthesia practice. This meant that the anesthesiologists needed to establish their identity and practice as different from that of the nurses.

Another problem facing the physicians was that nurse anesthetists did not wish to relinquish any part of their practice or any control over nurse anesthesia. Instead, the nurses refused to cooperate with the plan and actively resisted efforts at domination by developing the problem-solving skills necessary to defend their scope of practice. Thus, the scene was set for ongoing tensions, struggles, and cultural clashes between the two groups.

The acceptance of certain rules of behavior as norms by a group of people and transmitting that knowledge to the next generation is characteristic of a culture. Cultural norms serve as unwritten guidelines to show individuals how to act appropriately in a variety of situations. Importantly, nurse anesthetists have adopted certain attitudes and behaviors to facilitate the provision of effective patient care (Table 2.1) in addition to adopting norms utilized to defend the scope of practice.

Among the norms is a high degree of self-confidence, being in control, and using assertiveness to facilitate the role of nurse anesthetist as a patient advocate. Other accepted norms are to demonstrate skill, efficiency, and clinical competence in carrying out multiple responsibilities. A tendency toward compulsive behavior is said to be beneficial in complying with a rule for organization and meticulous attention to detail. All of these unwritten rules of behavior are derived from values held by nurse anesthetists that help to continue the culture.

VALUES HELD BY CRNAS

Nurse anesthetists share the vast majority of American values. These values include achievement, goal attainment, assertiveness, materialism, technology, equal rights, action orientation, and reliance on scientific facts (Leininger, 1995). However, nurse anesthesia differs from the American culture in valuing group cohesiveness over individualism and equality for race, religion, and sexual preference in addition to the American value for gender equality.

Importantly, there are dominant shared cultural values held among nurse anesthetists that set the group apart from other nurses (Table 2.2). These values are autonomy, education, continuing education, achievement, group cohesiveness, identity as a CRNA, membership in AANA, political activism, and technology.

Table 2.1: Dominant Rules of Behavior of Nurse Anesthesia in the United States

- Able to control and manage stressful clinical situations
- Able to make independent judgments quickly
- Accepts a high degree of responsibility
- Belongs to a professional organization (AANA)
- Committed to life-long learning of scientific facts
- Demonstrates self-confidence
- Effective in using assertiveness to facilitate role as patient advocate
- Engages in political activities
- Enjoys short-term patient care
- Functions effectively and calmly in life and death situations
- Ability to be organized with meticulous attention to detail
- Possesses intelligence and current knowledge
- Technically skilled, efficient, and clinically competent
- Upholds patient care values
- Willing to work hard and dedicate long hours to the job

Note. From Nurse anesthesia as a subculture of nursing in the United States, by Horton, B.J., 1998, (Doctoral dissertation, Rush University). *Dissertation Abstratica International, 9912475.* Copyright 1998 by B. J. Horton. Adapted with permission.

Autonomy

CRNAs value autonomy or the ability to be self-governing in decision making whether or not they are supervised by anesthesiologists. Autonomy is reflected in the split-second decisions and quick actions inherent in the administration of anesthesia.

A CRNA described how autonomy was important in all work settings:

> "Whether you are working for anesthesiologists [or] working for a hospital, you are still independent. You are at the head of the table. You are thinking and you are still making decisions."

Another CRNA agreed, saying:

> "Even though we work in collaboration with physicians, for the moment to moment basis, we are making independent decisions."

Education and Continuing Education

The importance of acquiring scientific knowledge on which to base decisions for patient care is a dominant value in nurse anesthesia. The schooling to become a nurse anesthetist is rigorous, with research emerging as a value within educational programs.

Education does not stop with graduation but continues as a mandatory continuing education requirement. CRNAs talk frequently about the need to continue learning to fulfill continuing education requirements for recertification. A CRNA commented:

> "I think as a group that we have a higher regard for education than others do. Maybe it's because we have mandatory continuing education."

Another CRNA noted that nurse

Table 2.2: Dominant Cultural Values of Nurse Anesthesia in the United States

- Achievement—education and personal life
- Autonomy—right to be self-governing
- Continuing education—commitment to life-long learning
- Education—control and standard setting
- Group cohesiveness—institutional and professional organization
- Identity as a CRNA—a way of life
- Membership in AANA—strength in numbers
- Political activism—state and national
- Technology—efficiency and safety

Note. From Nurse anesthesia as a subculture of nursing in the United States, by Horton, B.J., 1998, (Doctoral dissertation, Rush University). *Dissertation Abstratica International, 9912475.* Copyright 1998 by B. J. Horton. Adapted with permission.

anesthetists were not simply motivated to continue learning in order to earn continuing education credits:

> "I see nurse anesthetists all the time in my department talking about cases, learning from each other. How would you have handled this? And they are not being tested and no one is giving CE credit for it. Life-long learning, I think, is really critical."

Thus, both education and continuing education are embraced as dominant values in nurse anesthesia.

Achievement

The selection process for entry into nurse anesthesia programs favors the selection of high achievers. Good grades and high admission test scores are expectations. Student nurse anesthetists are often competitive with other students for grades. CRNAs also value achievement such as the acquisition of academic credentials.

Nurse anesthetists show pride in achievement in both their personal and professional lives. Behavior typically identified with nurse anesthesia is often valued in family relationships as noted by a CRNA:

> "One of the things that I see as positive is that it allows me to be a good role model for my children and they have even said that to me. They admire what I have accomplished and want to be like me. They see me as a role model."

Group Identity

There is a dominant value for group cohesiveness in nurse anesthesia. The strong value for assuring the welfare of nurse anesthetists as a group likely emanates from the need for "strength in numbers" to fend off challenges to practice rights. The large number of AANA members also confirms the value for group cohesiveness to foster solidarity and group action. Membership is said to be an expectation as a professional duty within the culture. A seasoned CRNA commented:

> "They join the association. It's kind of like a family and they want to share the values. There are [almost] 28,000 CRNAs that make up this fairly close-knit family."

Nurse anesthetists also take great pride in being identified as CRNAs.

Identity as a CRNA takes precedence over being an instructor, practitioner, or any other subgroup of anesthetists. In fact, the need to remain unified, as a group of CRNAs within the professional organization, is very great.

Political Activism

Nurse anesthesia has learned to value and embrace politics as an important factor in thinking, decision making, and actions. Politics influence the behavior of nurse anesthetists at federal, state, and local levels and within work environments. Behavior focuses on the defense of a full scope of practice for nurse anesthetists when challenged by others. This behavior can be detected in the response of CRNAs to requests for assistance with lobbying as described in an account from a CRNA:

> "I know that we generated thousands of letters from CRNAs to our governor last spring about our practice act. Nationally, if you measure outcomes [from lobbying efforts] and look at our funding history, the amount of money the government has put into our education efforts, student traineeships, program development, and faculty development has been pretty impressive."

Technology

A cultural value of nurse anesthesia in the United States is the use of technology for its efficiency and enhancement of patient safety. The rapid development of complex machines occurred during the last quarter of the 20th century resulting in sophisticated equipment for the delivery of anesthesia and for monitoring patients. A CRNA commented on the issue:

> "When I first started, we did not need to troubleshoot a monitor or zero a monitor. It [the use of equipment] was pretty simple. Most of that time you didn't have an EKG. You had a precordial stethoscope and a regular blood pressure cuff, and now you have one machine after another machine after another machine routinely everyday."

Technology has a great influence on nurse anesthesia practice because so much equipment is necessary to administer anesthesia and monitor patients. However, good clinical judgment is said to far outweigh the technological aspect of care. A CRNA explained:

> "They have the perception of anesthesia being things that we do and equipment we use. I tell them that if you put together everything that we do, putting in lines, intubating people, etc., those mechanical skills are really only about 5 percent of the practice. The other 95 percent is really an intellectual exercise in planning and staying out of trouble. To plan alternatives for any consequence is mental work that nobody ever sees us do and that is one reason that anesthetists don't get credit for the real amount of work that they do to keep patients out of trouble. Instead people focus on us as being technicians and that certainly is not the essence of the practice."

CRNAs also consider technology a mixed blessing since sophisticated equipment facilitates the provision of protective care yet places a barrier between CRNAs and patients. As one CRNA expressed:

> "I worry that technology takes away the closeness we have had with our patients. I always have my hands on the patient during an anesthetic, others haven't really touched the patient because of what the monitoring is telling you. The human part, the human involvement ... must be maintained."

MORAL CODE

Unwritten moral codes set the boundaries for accepted behavior in any culture. This is also true for nurse anesthetists who function with a moral code and action patterns that support that code (Table 2.3). Patient care values, honesty, loyalty, and equality are part of the expected behavior in nurse anesthesia.

Honesty

Honesty is highly valued as a philosophical concept. Nurse anesthetists consistently base patient care decisions and actions on honesty, which is believed to foster safe patient care. Honesty guides thinking, decision making, and behavior in both education and practice. Admitting mistakes, acknowledging a lack of knowledge, acceptance of responsibility for personal action, and telling the truth at all times are part of the unwritten moral code.

The importance of honesty is stressed over and over again by nurse anesthetists. A nurse anesthetist recounted:

> "My patients are entitled to integrity and honesty on my part. Being fair, honest and ethical I think all have to do with integrity. You need to be able to understand when you've made an error and admit it."

Instructors say they teach the value of honesty to student nurse anesthetists. Honesty is considered so important that acts of dishonesty can result in the dismissal of a student from school, according to some experienced educators.

A clinician talked of the high value placed on honesty in practice:

> "I look for someone with honesty and integrity when I pick out someone to give my anesthetic or my kid's anesthetic. I want to know if I take over a case from somebody that I can feel sure that what is documented on that record is truly what has happened. And that if they've made an error in judgment, they're not going to cover it up or they're not going to tell me. Maybe it's something I need to know because maybe there will be repercussions down the line from something that she or he did. I just want to know that I can trust what they're telling me."

Honesty also includes accepting responsibility for personal actions as conveyed by a CRNA:

> "When people don't take responsibility for themselves, I really question whether or not they can do the same with patients. I think honesty is an important aspect because of the inordinate level of trust which patients bestow on you. There has to be total trust."

Loyalty

Another part of the moral code of nurse anesthesia is loyalty to colleagues. The overall loyalty of nurse anesthetists to colleagues helps to maintain the cohesiveness of the organized group. Unlike the larger group of nurses who have created multiple special interest groups, nurse anesthetists have prevented reduction of power by resisting division of the group due to internal differences. Nurse anesthetists believe it is right to offer support to colleagues in a crisis. Additionally, there is little evidence of jealousy among nurse anesthetists in contrast to reports in the literature that identify jealousies and a power hierarchy in the larger group of nurses (Dougherty, 1985; Leininger, 1995).

Equality

Interestingly, stories told by CRNAs reveal a belief in equality that is not often verbalized yet sets the culture apart as unique. This seems to originate from the fact that being a nurse anesthetist overshadows any

Table 2.3: Moral Code of Nurse Anesthesia in the United States

- Patient care values must be honored
- Nurse anesthetists must be honest
  - Admit mistakes
  - Be able to say, "I don't know"
  - Accept personal responsibility for actions
  - Tell the truth at all times
- Nurse anesthetists are loyal
  - Allegiance to the larger group of nurse anesthetists
  - Supportive of individual colleagues in a crisis
  - Supportive of accomplishments of colleagues
- Nurse anesthetists believe in equal opportunities for individuals
  - Equality for gender and sexual preference
  - Equality for race and religion
- Nurse anesthetists do not anesthetize family members except in an emergency

Note. From Nurse anesthesia as a subculture of nursing in the United States, by Horton, B.J., 1998, (Doctoral dissertation, Rush University). *Dissertation Abstratica International*, 9912475. Copyright 1998 by B. J. Horton. Adapted with permission.

other characteristic of an individual. Thus, gender, race, religion and sexual preference become insignificant in relationships among nurse anesthetists.

This quote from a CRNA represents the belief in equality:

> "I think as a whole we do not see each other as males and females. We see each other as anesthetists without gender or racial differences. We are a tight professional group and willing to accept each other's differences."

Another CRNA reported:

> "When you look at nurse anesthesia you will realize that you don't see women and men, black and white—you see anesthetists."

PATIENT CARE VALUES

Dedication to patients is a recurrent finding when talking with nurse anesthetists and observing them in practice. CRNAs are particularly serious about the important responsibility of caring for dependent patients. The ability to focus on the needs of one patient at a time is valued. Accepted norms for patient care are a distinct part of the unwritten moral code. The importance of protective care is demonstrated through adherence to upholding values for individualized care, technology, touch, surveillance, and vigilance (Table 2.4).

Anesthetists actually accept responsibility for being surrogates for patients during anesthesia when patients are unable to protect themselves or maintain normal physical homeostasis. As a patient surrogate, the nurse anesthetist fills a temporary role as the consciousness for unconscious patients and for maintenance of respirations and other vital functions.

The value of acting as a patient surrogate was emphasized by a CRNA:

> "You have to feel the pulse, whether the skin is wet or dry, change the patient's position to prevent muscle soreness. Has that arm been there too long?

Table 2.4: Patient Care Values of Nurse Anesthesia in the United States

- Individualized care
- Serving as a patient surrogate
- Protective care
- Surveillance and vigilance
- Using touch to communicate caring

Note. From Nurse anesthesia as a subculture of nursing in the United States, by Horton, B.J., 1998, (Doctoral dissertation, Rush University). *Dissertation Abstratica International, 9912475.* Copyright 1998 by B. J. Horton. Adapted with permission.

> Should I move it or massage it? You are thinking of the things the patients would think of if they had been awake."

CRNAs teach students the importance of constant surveillance and vigilance when administering anesthesia. As one instructor said to a student:

> "The minute we take their cognition away, it is unique in nursing. Patients are totally dependent, 100 percent. You are not only their monitor; you are responsible for maintaining their vital signs. Nobody else has information [about the condition of the patient] like you have."

The importance of protective care was also related by a clinical CRNA:

> "It all comes back to the patient being the focus. The basic theme is always present in any decision, like a basic philosophical belief. The safety of the patient should drive whatever you do.... All of a sudden you have an unconscious patient totally dependent on you.... I say to them when I put them to sleep, I will protect you. That is my job."

Observations in anesthetizing areas show that a great deal of attention is given to the safety of patients, thereby confirming the value of protective care. Nurse anesthetists can be seen assuring the well-being of patients through continuous visual surveys. Frequent assessments of physical status are also performed through technological and tactile means.

Talking to unconscious patients is often used as an important act of caring. However, the use of touch to convey caring to conscious and unconscious patients was identified repeatedly by CRNAs as a dominant value in nurse anesthesia. Touch is viewed as an important way to communicate care to patients in a highly technical environment.

The rationale for using touch to demonstrate care is identified in the classical writings of Montagu (1971) and Leininger (1980). Montagu documented the importance of an increased need for body contact during stressful situations. Montagu also noted that the skin remained most sensitive during normal sleep and touch was the first sense to recover during reawakening. Leininger listed touch as one of a multitude of terms used to describe caring behavior.

A CRNA remembered her first anesthetic as a child with a broken leg:

> "I remember him [the anesthetist] talking with me in a very quiet low voice and rubbing my arm and telling me it was going to be OK. That sensation of touch was so soothing to me at the time. That's how I put all my patients

> to sleep. I always touch them, hold them, or rub their arm. You have to let the patient know that you are there with them."

SUMMARY

A study of the cultural aspects of nurse anesthesia found that historical events strongly influenced the development of values, attitudes, and behaviors that are accepted as appropriate for nurse anesthetists (Horton, 1998). Some of the values held by nurse anesthetists originate from the middle- and upper-class American culture, while other values are held by the larger group of nurses. Certain values, however, are part of the unique culture of nurse anesthesia that binds individual nurse anesthetists together as a group.

The dominant cultural values in nurse anesthesia are for autonomy, education, continuing education, achievement, group cohesiveness, identity as a CRNA, membership in AANA, political activism, and technology. Some of these values help nurse anesthetists remain active and vigilant to defend and maintain their practice rights while many other values reflect a dedication to patient care. Upholding patient care values is an expectation in nurse anesthesia, with a particular emphasis on providing protective care for dependent patients. Individualized care, technology, touch, surveillance, and vigilance are important values underlying the provision of protective care. Honesty is also believed to foster safe patient care and is part of the unwritten moral code.

The values shared by nurse anesthetists are the philosophical foundation underlying the provision of effective patient care and anesthesia services. Therefore, it is vitally important for each generation of nurse anesthetists to pass the values on to the next generation in order to perpetuate the culture.

REFERENCES

American Association of Nurse Anesthetists. (1999). *Nurse Anesthetists at a Glance.* (Available from the American Association of Nurse Anesthetists, 222 S. Prospect Ave., Park Ridge, IL 60068).

Bankert, M. (1989). *Watchful Care: A History of America's Nurse Anesthetists.* New York: Continuum Publishing.

Dougherty, M.C. (1985). The interface of nursing and anthropology. *Annual Review of Anthropology.* 14, 219-241.

Horton, B.J. (1998). Nurse anesthesia as a subculture of nursing in the United States (Doctoral dissertation, Rush University). *Dissertation Abstratica International,* 9912475.

Leininger, M.M. (1980). Caring: A central focus of nursing and health care services. *Nursing and Health Care.* 1(3), 135-143, 176.

Montagu, A. (1971). *Touching: The Human Significance of Skin.* New York: Columbia University Press.

Robb, I. (1893). *Nursing: Its Principles and Practices for Hospital and Private Use.* Toronto: J. A. Carveth & Co.

Thatcher, V.S. (1953). *History of Anesthesia with Emphasis on the Nurse Specialist.* Philadelphia, PA: J.B. Lippincott.

STUDY QUESTIONS

1. How have historical events influenced the development of nurse anesthesia as a culture?

2. How are values developed in a culture and why are they important?

3. What are the dominant cultural and patient care values shared by nurse anesthetists?

4. Describe the importance of the accepted rules of behavior or norms that are characteristic of nurse anesthesia.

5. Discuss the value of the unwritten moral codes that are part of the nurse anesthesia culture.

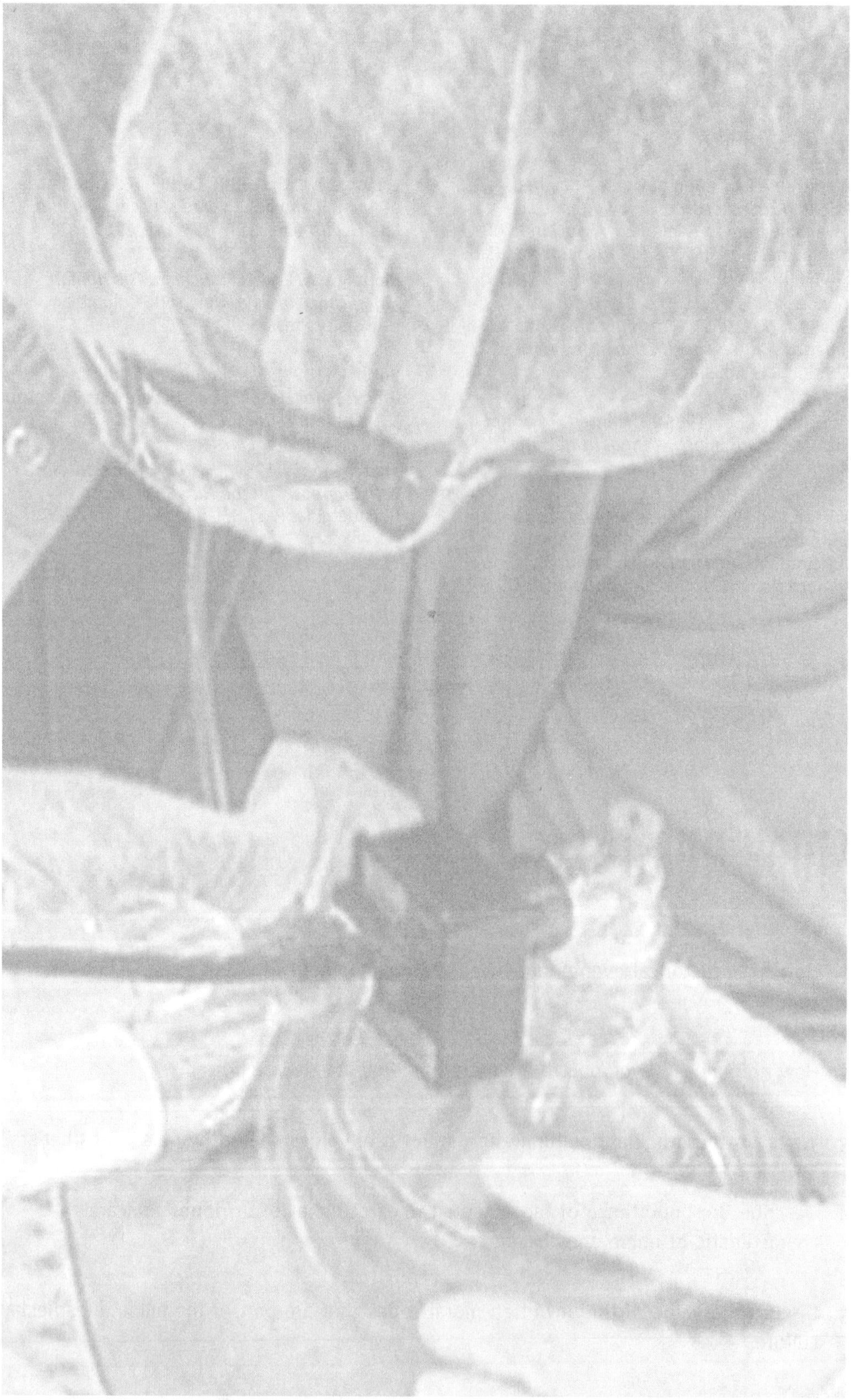

CHAPTER 3

THE SOCIALIZATION AND PROFESSIONAL ROLES OF CRNAS

Wynne R. Waugaman, CRNA, PhD, FAAN

Associate Professor of Nursing
Interim Chair, Department of Nursing
University of Southern California
Los Angeles, CA

KEY CONCEPTS

- Professional socialization is the essence of how nurses become nurse anesthetists by developing skills, knowledge, professional behavior, and career commitment, all of which occur concurrently with the educational process.
- Personal motivation is a key factor in promoting professional membership and the lifetime continuance of the professional career.
- Professional socialization and career commitment among nurse anesthetists are facilitated by early exposure to professional role models during clinical education.
- Age, gender, culture, and race/ethnicity all influence professional socialization.
- The utilization of research in evidence-based practice will significantly influence Certified Registered Nurse Anesthetist (CRNA) practice in the 21st century.
- To enhance their value to the healthcare team, CRNAs must develop new skills to become multiskilled professionals and must strengthen their clinical management and leadership roles.
- Professional success requires CRNAs to demonstrate expertise in financial/business management, critical thinking and decision making, computer literacy, and multilingual communications.
- Emerging roles for CRNAs include opportunities as acute care and pain management specialists, business entrepreneurs, administrators, alternative therapy experts, blended or combined advanced practice nurses, educators, researchers, writers, and legislators.

Opportunities for new work roles and professional positions will evolve for Certified Registered Nurse Anesthetists (CRNAs) in the new millennium, by virtue of their rich education and practice experience. This expansion will evolve within the context of a new focus in healthcare—that of basing care on a model of wellness, rather than disease. This raises logical questions about our future, considering the fact that much of our work is based on care models designed to ameliorate or palliate disease. How will CRNAs in the future accommodate these changes? How will we move nurse anesthesia care into a community-based model of service? To explore a new vision of practice and service, we must carefully analyze trends in healthcare with critical attention given to new and pervasive market influences and the rapidly changing U.S. demographic. In short, CRNAs of the new millennium will be socializing into the profession of nurse anesthesia in a markedly changed environment from that which existed only several decades ago.

PROFESSIONAL SOCIALIZATION

The concept of professional socialization describes how nurses are "molded" into their new role as nurse anesthetists by developing knowledge, skills, behavior, and career commitment appropriate to the profession. This process occurs during the educational period and is influenced by both intentional and unplanned circumstances of the academic environment. Professional socialization is the process of "becoming" a nurse anesthetist through exposure to experiences regarded by members as a prerequisite for inclusion into the profession. Socialization involves active membership in the professional group and acquisition of the cultural attributes of the profession (Simpson, 1979). Personal motivation is a key factor in promoting professional membership and a lifetime commitment to a professional career.

The process of professional socialization enables graduate students to identify with and acquire behaviors and attitudes of the CRNA group to which they are seeking membership. This includes assuming the group's organizational goals, social mission and knowledge advancement (Scholtfeldt, 1987; Waugaman, 1988). Critical components of professional socialization include learning the technology and language of the profession, internalizing values and norms, and integrating the professional role into one's professional identity and other life roles (Cohen, 1981).

Numerous models and conceptual frameworks have been used to study the socialization process in nurses. Waugaman (1981, 1983) adapted the multi-dimensional model of Simpson (1979) to study the socialization process of nurse anesthetists. This model describes professional socialization as consisting of three analytically distinct dimensions or categories of variables: education or the imparting of occupational knowledge and skills; development of occupational orientations; and forming personal relatedness to the occupation. The first two dimensions are mainly cognitive while the third dimension is motivational. Each dimension is comprised of one or more scales which describe the components of each dimension (Table 3.1).

A change in any one of the dimensions does not necessarily influence another. For example, a temporary decline in professional commitment to the job itself may occur because of changing family roles, while those identifying features important to the work role remain stable (Waugaman, 1999). In other words, life experiences can influence some of the variables that influence socialization, but these are temporary effects.

Professional socialization and career commitment among nurse anesthetists are facilitated by early exposure to professional role models during clinical education (Waugaman, 1983). The emphasis in nurse anesthesia education on practical experience during the curriculum enables students to visualize their professional roles with a high degree of realism very early in the program. Role modeling by nurse and physician anesthetists throughout the program is a valuable tool of professional socialization (Waugaman, 1988). The mentoring role is especially important in the helping professions because of the interdependent working conditions among these professionals. Educational program content, design, and faculty/practitioner/mentor role models all play a vital role in the professional socialization of nurse anesthetists. These factors directly influence the degree to which students are socialized into the profession, and the continuation of the socialization process influences the degree of professional career commitment as people mature from nurses to nurse anesthetists (Waugaman, 1988).

In general, it is important to note that the process of professional socialization of nurse anesthetists has been especially important in the development of the specialty profession of nurse anesthesia. Clearly, it is because of this process that CRNAs have built a formidable national professional organization representing 95 percent of all practicing CRNAs. It is also because of the socialization process that the American Association of Nurse Anesthetists (AANA) has emerged as a potent lobbying group influencing a myriad of state and national issues that have had profound and beneficial effects for individual practitioners and patients alike.

THE CHANGING DEMOGRAPHICS OF NURSE ANESTHESIA STUDENTS

Nurse anesthesia students, unlike some other professional students, identify with their professional role very early in their professional education. Sixty-seven percent of the U.S. nurse anesthesia students enrolled during the 1998-99 academic year reported thinking of themselves as nurse anesthetists within the first six months of their graduate program. By 24-30 months of enrollment, 95 percent identified completely with the nurse anesthetist professional role

Table 3.1: The Dimensions and Scales of Professional Socialization of Nurse Anesthetists

DIMENSION	SCALES
Education	Orientation to nurse anesthesia
Cognitive occupational orientations	Holistic vs. bureaucratic view of patient care
	Administration and supervision
	Collegialism
Relatedness to the professional role	Attraction to nurse anesthesia
	Socioeconomic rewards
	Commitment to nurse anesthesia
	Self-identification as a nurse anesthetist

(Waugaman and Lohren, 1999). A number of factors influence the professional socialization process including age, gender, culture and race/ethnicity.

Waugaman and Lu (1999) found in their study of professional socialization of more than 1,000 U.S. student nurse anesthetists that culture and race/ethnicity both correlated significantly ($p < 0.05$) for all nondominant nurse anesthesia student groups (Asian-Pacific Islanders, Hispanics, African Americans, and Native American/Alaskan Natives) compared to the dominant European/American groups. Overall, Asian-Pacific Islanders responded more positively to the process of professional socialization, which is consistent with cultural beliefs of Eastern cultures. Hispanics responded negatively to the point of statistical significance (compared to all other cultural groups) to the educational dimension which describes the skills and knowledge of nurse anesthesia practice. This may imply more difficulty for Hispanics in learning the professional tasks in the same manner as the dominant culture. Asian-Pacific Islanders valued collegialism and were more likely to pursue administrative and supervisory roles than were African Americans, which may confirm the historical isolation of African Americans from non-African American peers. Hispanics responded negatively (to the point of statistical significance) to the dimension of personal-relatedness, which identifies the relationship of the individual to the occupation through status identification, professional commitment, attraction to the job, and socioeconomic rewards. The profound negative response by Hispanics also indicates that there may be difficulty with professional recruitment and retention of this ethnic group into nursing, specifically advanced practice nursing specialties.

Emerging majority cultures are changing the U.S. demographic and that, in turn, profoundly influences both the education and practice of all advanced practice nursing specialties. As a result of longer life expectancy, as well as a growing number of refugees, students, and immigrants residing in the United States, one in every three Americans belongs to one of these emerging majority cultures (Ferrell, 1988). By the year 2050, it is projected that 56 percent of the population will be White, while the remaining 44 percent will be comprised of 22 percent Hispanic, 14 percent African American, 7 percent Asian-Pacific Islander, and 1 percent American Indian/Alaskan Native (U.S. Bureau of the Census, 1996). In California, it is predicted that by 2020 the Hispanic population will surpass the White population and that by 2040 Hispanics will become the majority group within the state (McLeon, 1998). Interestingly, the U.S. population of registered nurses (RNs) does not mirror changing national demographics. Nearly 90 percent of U.S. RNs are White while the remaining 10 percent are comprised of 4.2 percent African Americans, 3.4 percent Asian-Pacific Islanders, 1.6 percent Hispanics, and 0.5 percent American Indian/Alaskan Native (U.S. Department of Health and Human Services, 1996).

As the population continues to change, the nursing and nurse anesthesia population will also change. To meet the educational needs of future nurse anesthesia students, faculty must evaluate how curricular and instructional design influences the degree of professional socialization attained, particularly in emerging majority cultures. Even more fundamental is the fact that nurse anesthesia faculty must appreciate the values and cultural mores of diverse groups, especially as they relate to learning style. Without this, faculty may inadvertently impede professional socialization and student learning by imposing teaching methods deemed successful for the dominant culture, but unproved for diverse populations. Demonstration of cultural competence in teaching is key to enhancing recruitment and retention among diverse populations in graduate specialty nursing, particularly nurse anesthesia.

The general population of nurses and nurse anesthetists is aging. Entering students are often older and enter nursing as a mid-life career change. The ratio of men to women (40:60) in nurse anesthesia is vastly different from the generic nursing population. Factors of age and gender also influence professional socialization. In the U.S. population of student nurse anesthetists, older students (>40 years of age) responded less positively to the scales comprising the dimensions of socialization (Waugaman and Lohren, 2000). The older student is less related to the occupation through status identification, commitment, and attraction to nurse anesthesia as a career. Students over 40 years of age are less concerned with the socioeconomic rewards of the profession as a component of socialization when compared to students under 30 years of age. Older students also believe that age is a factor in how they respond to their educational process, in how instructors evaluate them, and in their own ability to provide patient-centered anesthesia care (Waugaman and Lohren, 2000). Male nurse anesthesia students strongly associate with characteristics typified in bureaucratic organizations, such as following rules and regulations, the importance of technology, distancing oneself from patients, and the importance of proper physical care irrespective of the patient's feelings (Waugaman and Lohren, 2000). Men also are more positively oriented toward assuming administrative and supervisory roles, while women are more focused on holistic care and providing culturally congruent anesthesia care.

THE EFFECTS OF GRADUATE EDUCATION ON SOCIALIZATION

Educational programs have a profound influence on the socialization of CRNAs. It is during the educational program that students are first exposed to a very different culture than what they have been used to as practicing, highly experienced intensive care nurses. Often, students entering nurse anesthesia programs undergo tremendous adjustments to graduate study. For many students, sitting in a classroom each day for one or more academic terms, when accustomed to active clinical practice, is at best difficult. Some students may have been away from the academic setting for a decade or more and must develop new study habits to ensure success in graduate school.

For a variety of reasons, a nurse anesthesia educational program is unlike most other forms of higher education in that it mixes a highly rigorous academic curriculum with demands for accomplished performance in a high stress clinical environment. Further, many students of nursing come to the educational experience unprepared for the demands of critical thinking. It is common for many nurses to have assumed a role, in the course of their daily work, as master technicians and largely observers and recorders of patient problems. They are not, by and large, prepared to be problem solvers and to think through multidimensional problems in systematic ways to yield usable solutions. The concept that they will be ultimately responsible for all decisions regarding a patient's care is often foreign as they have depended on physicians to assume that role. In addition, there is a substantial amount of new, didactic information that they are required to sort through, prioritize and recall in appropriate circumstances. These are significant stressors for students embarking on the process of socializing to a new role as an anesthetist.

Graduate education in nurse anesthesia demands that students be self-motivated, independent thinkers. Pedagogic teaching styles, where teachers impart knowledge to passive students, is essentially nonexistent. Specialist education requires that students take primary responsibility for learning under expert guidance, developing skills of critical thinking and integration of theory into practice. Nurse anesthetists must learn to apply useful theoretic principles to clinical practice in order to make rational, justifiable decisions relative to patient care problems. Instruction requires that students be actively engaged in learning through independent study, small group discussions, case analysis presentations, research presentations, and a vast amount of reading from books and periodic literature. Education imparts the values of socialization through self-discipline, resourcefulness, responsibility, and setting standards of academic and clinical performance.

THE INFLUENCE OF HEALTHCARE CHANGES ON CRNA ROLES

A number of factors are predicted to significantly influence healthcare and nursing practice in the 21st century. Chinn (1991) predicts that these changes will be largely related to the technology explosion, an evolution of drastic disease trajectories, increasing scarcity of healthcare resources, and an increasing demand for new and still unmet services. Other sources of change impacting nursing will come from the increased use and management of information, movement of care to outpatient and home environments, demand for evidenced-based care, emerging quality measurement mandates, and heightened compliance requirements for clinical credentialing and privileging.

What will these changes imply for the evolving clinical role of nurse anesthetists in the future? How will CRNAs need to change in order to remain competitive and viable in the marketplace?

- Education: CRNAs in the future will need to have substantially more formal preparation in the social demographics of their patients in order to provide culturally competent care. There will need to be more curricular attention given to biomedical engineering and information management to master new clinical technology and data-base driven mechanisms for clinical decision making. There will be increasing use of human simulation as an instructional technique and more attention given to engendering skills of critical thinking and incorporation of intellectual standards.
- Practice: CRNAs will be required to not only maintain their scope of practice, but to expand it to areas of acute and chronic pain management, critical care, and home delivery of care to chronically ill patients requiring pain blocks and specialized ventilatory care. Some CRNAs will be examining potential roles in administration of alternative therapies such as herbal and aromatherapy, acupuncture, hypnosis, and massage techniques. All CRNAs will increasingly be required to document anesthesia care in ways that demonstrate competence, productivity and quality. They will have to learn to manage and interpret a new generation of monitoring modalities that dimensionally display vital organ function. They will increasingly be administering anesthesia services as a sole provider, utilizing physicians in consultant roles.

- Credentialing: CRNAs will eventually be required to recertify by simulated testing or other means to demonstrate clinical competence beyond initial certification. Graduate education for all practitioners will likely be a requirement in all states for the next generation of providers.
- Surgery: All CRNAs should be aware of how changes in surgical technique influence demand for their services. What are the implications for CRNAs relative to the increasing use of endoscopic techniques in surgery, use of specialized catheter access procedures, laser technology, and advanced imaging procedures? Coupled with frequent changes in the numbers and types of cases that qualify for reimbursement in general, how will the nature of CRNA services necessarily change?
- Work setting: CRNAs will be increasingly employed under contractual arrangements that do not include the traditional package of employee benefits. CRNAs will be hired on the basis of proven expertise. They must be mobile and functionally crossed-trained to assume a variety of care roles. Care settings will increasingly utilize community-based clinics, physician offices, schools, skilled nursing facilities and the home environment.
- Communication: CRNAs will be required to demonstrate increasingly sophisticated communication skills that facilitate critical thinking, effective problem solving, negotiation, and fulfillment of organizational goals, primarily within some form of integrated managed-care organization.
- Professional advocacy: In order to remain competitive, all CRNAs must be able to demonstrate some effectiveness in advocacy efforts that promote their own well-being and that of their patients. These are skills that are learned through systematic study of the profession, within the social context.

EMERGING PROFESSIONAL ROLES

In addition to clinical roles, CRNAs often assume employment roles in pharmaceutical or manufacturing companies or a host of other public and private agencies that deal with healthcare products and services. The unique educational background and clinical expertise of CRNAs make them particularly well suited to positions in education, marketing, or sales with companies that manufacture and sell anesthesia equipment, devices, and pharmaceutical agents and adjuncts used in anesthesia practice. Some nurse anesthetists have assumed positions as advisors to public and private agencies such as the Food and Drug Administration. These professional contributions by CRNAs enhance public awareness of CRNA services as well as promote the importance of our role in healthcare planning and delivery.

CRNAs are increasingly involved in creating and managing entrepreneurial enterprises. CRNA-owned practices, group or individual, have proven track records of success. Some CRNAs have become successful as educational conference or seminar providers, while others have developed and marketed computer software. Consulting for organizational and management entities, the legal profession, or educational institutions is frequently a full- or part-time professional option for qualified CRNAs. Advanced degrees in education, business, finance, and economics often provide the skills and experiences on which to base entrepreneurial efforts.

The field of administration has been embraced by countless nurse anesthetists who serve as department managers, chief nurse anesthetists, or directors of clinical services. These professionals are responsible for general administrative management, budgeting, resource procurement and distribution, human resource activities, and frequently institutional committee work including quality management. CRNAs have also assumed positions in educational administration. These professional opportunities include deanships or other academic administrative roles, department or division chairs, and program directorships. Nurse anesthesia administrators in higher education must be well-versed in accreditation and certification requirements in nurse anesthesia, graduate and university policies, and public and case law, all of which have an impact on higher education. Educational administrators are responsible for developing and deploying the curriculum, recruiting and retaining students, and in most cases demonstrating accomplishment in service, teaching and research.

Increasingly, CRNAs in the academy as well as in clinical practice are becoming involved in the promulgation of research, either as a full-time or part-time professional role. CRNAs with doctoral degrees in the basic sciences are more likely to conduct research in a basic science laboratory, often using an animal model. Some CRNAs prefer applied research that involves testing and evaluation of clinical theories and modes of practice and therapy. Clinical studies may include testing anesthesia products or equipment, or managing clinical trials of new pharmaceutical agents or other relevant clinical applications. Opportunities are available for nurse anesthetists to complete degree or certificate programs in clinical research, enabling them to participate in and lead the conduct of clinical drug trials.

CRNAs who have doctoral degrees in behavioral sciences or education may prefer to conduct research that evaluates educational models and theories applied to nurse anesthesia practice or professional behavioral adjustments such as socialization. Since nurse anesthesia education has moved into the graduate framework, most curricula include some course preparation in theory and research. Some programs offer research opportunities for master's level students while other programs reserve this experience for doctoral students. However, the conduct of research need not be reserved for doctoral students and doctorally prepared CRNAs. Practicing CRNAs are frequently and actively involved in the research programs of the department in which they are employed.

Professions are often measured by their scholarly works and peer-reviewed publications and not exclusively by the quality of their clinical practice (Waugaman, 1991). More CRNAs are required to conduct original research and author publications that enhance the professional standing of the nurse anesthesia community as a valued contributor to the body of anesthesia knowledge and, in turn, raise the level of consumer awareness and value placed on nurse anesthesia services. Although nurse anesthesia is the oldest nursing specialty, it regrettably has the smallest number of publications, both textbooks and journals, when compared with other nursing specialties. CRNAs have a professional obligation to share new knowledge with professional colleagues and consumers so that all can benefit from their findings or message. This dissemination of knowledge is a link to the next generation, our legacy.

SUMMARY

Nurse anesthetists have been leaders in

healthcare for more than a century and our roles have continually evolved to meet societal needs. As CRNAs, we must be visionary in identifying our future professional directions and make deliberate choices that move us toward those realities. It is not sufficient to react to challenge and opportunity or expect that change will not occur. We must be proactive in designing the future. For nurse anesthetists, there is no status quo. We must be evolving in a continuous, planned and creative way.

REFERENCES

Chinn, P.L. (1991). Looking into the crystal ball: Positioning ourselves for the year 2000. *Nursing Outlook.* 7, 251-256.

Cohen, H.A. (1980). Authoritarianism and dependency: Problems in nursing socialization. In F. Flynn & M. Miller (Eds.), *Current Perspective in Nursing Social Issues and Trends.* St. Louis, MO: C.V. Mosby.

Ferrell, J. (1988). Education: The changing world of candidates for nursing. *Journal of Professional Nursing.* 4(3), 145-153.

Schlotfeldt, R.M. (1987). Structuring nursing knowledge: A priority for creating nursing's future. *Nursing Science Quarterly.* 35-38.

Simpson, I.H. (1979). *From Student to Nurse.* Cambridge, UK: Cambridge University Press. 3-326.

U.S. Bureau of the Census. (1996). *Population projections of the United States by age, sex, race, and Hispanic origin: 1995-2050.* (Current Population Reports, P25-1,130, pp. 4,017). Washington, DC: Government Printing Office.

U.S. Department of Health and Human Services, Bureau of Health Professions. (1996). *The Registered Nurse Population.* Washington, DC: Government Printing Office.

Waugaman, W.R. (1983). From nurse to nurse anesthetist: Effects of professional socialization on career commitment (Doctoral dissertation, University of Pittsburgh, 1981). *Dissertation Abstracts International.* 43(9).

Waugaman, W.R. (1988). From nurse to nurse anesthetist. In W.R. Waugaman, B.M. Rigor, L.E. Katz, H.M. Bradshaw, & J.F. Garde (Eds.), *Principles and Practice of Nurse Anesthesia* (pp. 3-5). Norwalk, CT: Appleton & Lange.

Waugaman, W.R. & Lu, J. (1999). From nurse to nurse anesthetist: The relationship of culture, race, and ethnicity to professional socialization and career commitment of advanced practice nurses. *Journal of Transcultural Nursing.* 10(3), 237-247.

Waugaman, W.R. & Lohren, D.J. (1999). Factors influencing status identification as a nurse anesthetist among graduate students. *AANA Journal.* (6), 527, A43.

Waugaman, W.R. & Lohren, D.J. (2000). From nurse to nurse anesthetist: The influence of age and gender on professional socialization and career commitment of advanced practice nurses. *Journal of Professional Nursing.* 16 (1), 47-56.

KEY REFERENCES

Taskforce on Health Care Workforce Regulation. (1995). *Reforming Health Care Workforce Regulation: Policy Considerations for the 21st Century.* San Francisco, CA: Pew Health Professions Commission.

Waugaman, W.R. (1988). From nurse to nurse anesthetist. In W.R. Waugaman, B.M. Rigor, L.E. Katz, H.M. Bradshaw, & J.F. Garde (Eds.), *Principles and Practice of Nurse Anesthesia* (pp. 3-5). Norwalk, CT: Appleton & Lange.

Waugaman, W.R. & Lu, J. (1999). From nurse to nurse anesthetist: The relationship of culture, race, and ethnicity to professional socialization and career commitment of advanced practice nurses. *Journal of Transcultural Nursing.* 10(3), 237-247.

Waugaman, W.R. & Lohren, D.J. (2000). From nurse to nurse anesthetist: The influence of age and gender on professional socialization and career commitment of advanced practice nurses. *Journal of Professional Nursing.* 16 (1).

STUDY QUESTIONS

1. What is professional socialization and how does it influence how CRNAs view their profession?

2. How do age, gender, culture, race, and ethnicity factors influence the professional socialization of nurse anesthetists?

3. How will changes in healthcare affect CRNA roles in the future?

4. What are examples of extended or emerging CRNA roles beyond that of clinician?

5. What are the advantages of pursuing the extended nontraditional roles available in nurse anesthesia?

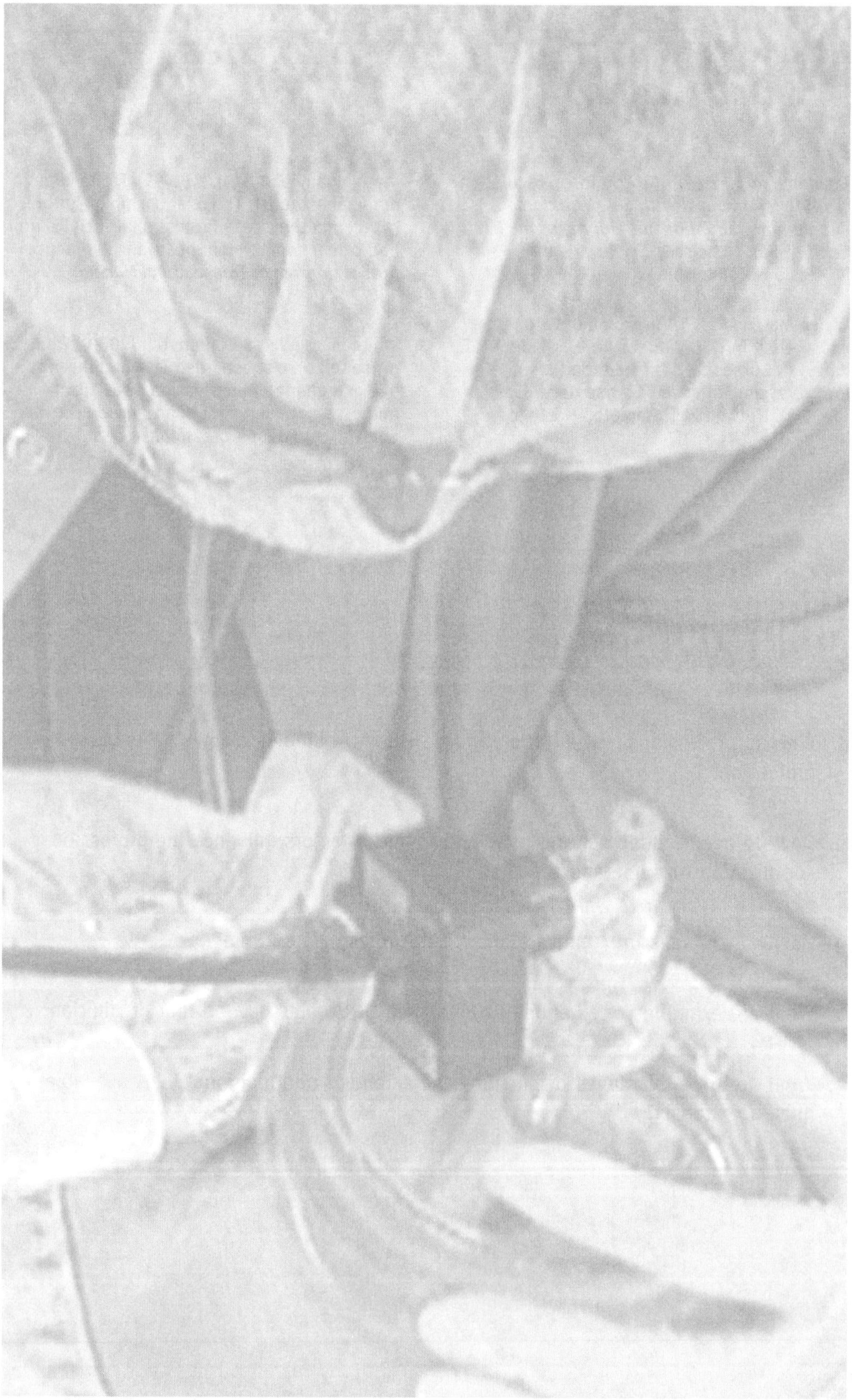

CHAPTER 4

THE AMERICAN ASSOCIATION OF NURSE ANESTHETISTS: THE ROLE OF THE PROFESSIONAL ORGANIZATION

John F. Garde, CRNA, MS, FAAN

Executive Director, 1983-2000
American Association of Nurse Anesthetists
Park Ridge, IL

KEY CONCEPTS

- The American Association of Nurse Anesthetists (AANA) is the single professional organization in the United States that represents the interests of Certified Registered Nurse Anesthetists (CRNAs). Its mission is to promote the full scope of practice for CRNAs and promote healthcare policy that supports nurse anesthesia practice.

- The AANA is based in Park Ridge, Illinois. The national headquarters supports approximately 75 full-time staff members. In addition, the Federal Government Affairs office in Washington, D.C. has five staff members.

- The national association staff works under the direction of the executive director, who in turn works at the pleasure of the Board of Directors. All Board members, including officers, are elected by member CRNAs.

- The AANA represents approximately 95 percent of all CRNAs.

- State organizations of the AANA are independent organizations supported by national dues that access a variety of support services from the national association on issues related to state and federal government affairs, practice, managed care and reimbursement, public relations, education, continuing education, research, and membership.

It has been claimed by many that, since the inception of nurse anesthesia more than 100 years ago, our collective strength and influence in the healthcare arena today has been largely the result of two factors: first and foremost, the quality of anesthesia services provided by Certified Registered Nurse Anesthetists (CRNAs), and second, the strength of the professional association of CRNAs, the American Association of Nurse Anesthetists (AANA). Given birth and guided by such towering and legendary figures as Agatha Hodgins, Helen Lamb, Hilda Salomon, Adeline Curtis, and Gertrude Fife, the AANA has evolved into a professional organization of substantial influence. This chapter charts that growth since 1931 and acquaints the anesthesia student with the organizational structure of the AANA, the role members play in its continued development, and the services accrued from active participation in association business.

A PHILOSOPHIC PERSPECTIVE

Professional organizations, regardless of the discipline with which they are associated, play a unique and demanding role in society. Often the roles they assume are complex, multifaceted, and seemingly contradictory; yet they have become the necessary vehicle by which professional healthcare providers are able to promote their interests, interface with the public, maintain relationships with external healthcare agencies, and effectively influence health policy in both state and federal legislatures.

There are several basic tenets that every student of nurse anesthesia should come to appreciate about professional organizations. First, organizations are established by members for the pursuit of collective goals that serve the self-interest of the provider. Organizations such as the AANA would not exist if not for the support and mandate of its members; therefore, organizational goals should be based largely on the basic tenets, philosophies, and values of its membership. Second, professional organizations cannot exist apart from the underlying fabric of social norms and values. As stated in the initial chapter of this book, professions exist only at the behest of society; that is, they are given the rights and privileges of practice because they remain accountable to the public. Consequently, professional organizations are required to "walk a fine line" between member and consumer interest. It is largely this ambiguity that can result in the perception by the public of overriding self-interest on the part of the profession. If not managed with great care, this situation can lead to public skepticism and mistrust. This results in increased public advocacy via legislative action intended to shift the balance back toward the public good. When a profession fails its public responsibility, society will usually demand, and obtain, change.

Some have claimed that professional organizations are inherently in conflict with the greater good of society and as such should be abolished. However, for all the justification that could support this argument, few alternatives have been suggested to adequately substitute for the work of professional organizations. The fact remains that a strong, visionary professional association is one of the best means of securing the rights and privileges of practice for its members. All CRNAs should appreciate, however, the need to maintain the delicate balance between self-interest and the public good.

The AANA remains unique in several respects when compared to other professional organizations. The AANA was among the first nursing specialty organizations to be recognized within nursing. Few other professional specialty organizations in nursing can claim its tenure, experience, or stature. The AANA also claims an active membership of 95 percent of all CRNAs in the country. This statistic is unparalleled in any other professional organization of healthcare providers. Given the fact that CRNAs are not required to join the professional organization to practice, it would appear obvious that the vast majority of CRNAs value highly the role and productivity of the AANA.

Finally, the success of the AANA may be predicated on the unique relationship between its members, the executive office, and its elected leadership. Decision-making relative to AANA business is encouraged at every level. Individual members have direct access to communicate with their elected state or national leaders and exercise direct voting privileges; that is, membership sentiment is not funneled through a delegate system in which individual opinions may be diluted or distilled into a group or consensus opinion. CRNAs remain singularly individual in their ability to participate and be heard on issues affecting their practice.

HISTORICAL DEVELOPMENT

In 1926, the first meeting of the Lakeside alumnae group of nurse anesthetists was held in Cleveland, Ohio. There, Agatha Hodgins announced her vision of establishing a national association of nurse anesthetists. Prior to this time, a few states had had varying success with establishing small groups of CRNAs in which to discuss difficult cases, yet none were organized to the extent that they could claim a national following.

Hodgins maintained the philosophy that nurse anesthesia should not be considered a part of nursing service, rather a part of general hospital service. On several occasions she approached the American Nurses Association (ANA) in regard to nurse anesthetists being recognized within that group. However, the ANA failed to approve the proposition and required more study of the AANA proposal. Headstrong and tiring of inattention by the ANA, Hodgins called CRNAs around the country to convene at Lakeside Hospital in Cleveland "for the purpose of considering the organization of the nurse anesthetists group." Forty-four CRNAs from 12 states agreed to form the National Association of Nurse Anesthetists (NANA) and to continue their efforts to affiliate with the ANA.

Over the next several years, Hodgins again attempted affiliation with the ANA but to no avail. Its board of directors finally rejected the proposal of the NANA, stating that affiliate membership could be accomplished through regular, established channels at the state level. Few of the AANA's early leaders were surprised at this outcome, none less than Hodgins, who by now was in ill health and left a small, fledgling organization still without the national recognition she fervently sought.

By 1933, the NANA had still not convened its first national meeting and suffered from general disarray organizationally. However, Gertrude Fife, the recently elected president of the organization, was encouraged by John Mannix, a department of anesthesia administrator at Lakeside Hospital, to seek recognition from the American Hospital Association (AHA). Given the fact that this group readily recognized the value of nurse anesthetists to their hospitals, the AHA invited NANA to present its first national meeting in conjunction with them. Fife stated, "We were going to put on the first convention. Who was going to make out the program? We had very little time. And Mannix said that we had to meet ...

we had to put that convention on. And, consequently, Helen Lamb and Walter Powell came to Cleveland and we made out the program over my kitchen...my dining room table. The three of us (Bankert, 1989)." And so was born a renewed, vibrant, and committed organization of nurse anesthetists in Milwaukee, Wisconsin, September 13-15, 1933. By the close of the first annual meeting of the NANA, Gertrude Fife, the newly elected second president of the association, declared, "I feel that we are making history and that we are laying the foundation for a fine organization that will be a great benefit to the future of the work (Bankert, 1989)."

After this meeting, Fife was faced with the first and most important issue facing nurse anesthetists—education. She called for a committee to investigate all schools of nurse anesthesia with the object of creating a list of "accredited" schools. Additionally, she called for the establishment of national board examinations for nurse anesthetists. With this agenda set for the NANA in 1933, the members continued to move forward. In 1939, the organization's name was changed to the American Association of Nurse Anesthetists. In 1955, the commissioner of education recognized the AANA as the national accrediting authority for nurse anesthesia education. This was a major milestone for the AANA as recognition afforded students of accredited programs eligibility for federal funds such as grant or loan programs.

MISSION, VALUES, PHILOSOPHY AND OBJECTIVES

The mission of the American Association of Nurse Anesthetists has guided the development of its strategic plan and operational priorities. According to the strategic plan, the mission of the association is "To advance excellence in anesthesia services through meeting its members' professional needs and increasing public awareness that CRNAs provide patients with high-quality anesthesia services in all practice settings (AANA, 2000)."

The bylaws and standing rules of the AANA state, "The members of this professional association are dedicated to the precept that its members are committed to the advancement of educational standards and practices, which will advance the art and science of anesthesiology and thereby support and enhance quality patient care (AANA, 2000)."

Since the founding of the association, its objectives have changed very little from those presented at the first annual meeting in Milwaukee. As required by law in Illinois, the objectives appear in the original certificate of incorporation of the AANA notarized October 11, 1939, and filed with Edward J. Hughes, then secretary of state of Illinois, on October 17, 1939. The certificate is renewed annually. The objectives were amended at the AANA 1978 Annual Meeting to read as follows:

- To promote continual high-quality patient care.
- To advance the science and art of anesthesiology.
- To develop and promote educational standards in the field of nurse anesthesia.
- To develop and promote standards of practice in the field of nurse anesthesia.
- To facilitate effective cooperation between nurse anesthetists, anesthesiologists, and other members of the medical professions, the nursing profession, hospitals, and agencies representing a community of interest in nurse anesthesia.
- To publish scientific journals, bulletins, and other publications per-

tinent to the objectives of the association.

- To maintain informational and statistical data for reference and assistance in matters pertaining to the profession or its practice.
- To provide opportunities for continuing education in anesthesia.
- To provide members with direction pertaining to governmental policy, legislation, or judicial decisions of importance to anesthesia.

THE RESPONSIBILITIES AND QUALIFICATIONS OF MEMBERSHIP

The ability of CRNAs to become involved in their professional association is not without cost and responsibility. First and foremost is the responsibility each CRNA has to carefully assess his or her professional commitment by making the decision whether to become an active, dues-paying member. This decision should be based largely on careful study of what the professional association can provide to the member by way of services and the extent to which the individual CRNA shares the values, philosophy and objectives promoted by the membership. Active membership requires that all CRNAs who become involved in association activities be conversant with current issues in order to effectively engage in discussions and decision-making activities. As students will soon realize, most CRNAs have little problem voicing their opinions; however, as with any professional organization, the quality of those decisions is predicated largely on an informed position, one that not only serves the individual member but also recognizes the needs and priorities of colleagues and stakeholders in our services who are external to the organization.

There are five categories of active membership:

1. Active Certified — Individuals who have been granted initial certification by the Council on Certification of Nurse Anesthetists. Once certified, membership is automatic for the remainder of said fiscal year and then only until the individual is eligible for membership as an active recertified member.
2. Active Recertified — Individuals who are currently recertified by the Council on Recertification of Nurse Anesthetists.
3. Active Nonrecertified — Individuals who are required to be recertified but are not currently recertified and desire to enjoy the rights and privileges of active membership. Individuals who are actively practicing anesthesia may not remain in this category of membership for a period to exceed two years or one recertification period following the date of expiration of their recertification. Individuals who are not actively practicing anesthesia may remain in this category. Upon recertification, active nonrecertified members shall become active recertified members provided they have met all criteria for recertification.
4. Life — This is a closed category of membership comprised of individuals who have held this category of membership since August 31, 1976, and will do so for the remainder of their lifetime. Life members shall be granted the category of active membership for which they qualify. Life members shall be exempt from payment of dues.
5. Emeritus — Individuals who have held active membership for a minimum of 25 years and who desire to enjoy the privileges of active membership but have retired from the practice of anesthesia.

Qualifications for active membership are graduation from an accredited program in nurse anesthesia, successful completion of the certification examination, and compliance with association guidelines, standards, or other qualifications set forth in the bylaws of the association. Students who are enrolled in accredited programs of nurse anesthesia are eligible for student associate membership at a fraction of the cost of full membership. One third of the current dues for membership in the AANA is allocated to the state association in which the CRNA resides. Membership in the AANA constitutes automatic recognition of membership of the CRNA in his or her respective state organization. The privileges and rights of members will be addressed in a later section of this chapter.

ORGANIZATIONAL STRUCTURE AND FUNCTION

The AANA was incorporated on October 17, 1939, in Illinois and designated as a tax exempt organization by Subsection 501(C)(6) of the Internal Revenue Service. AANA's Education and Research Foundation was incorporated on July 15, 1981, and designated as a tax-exempt organization by Subsection 501(C)(3) of the Internal Revenue Code.

The AANA bylaws are essentially the AANA's working constitution and dictate how the association operates functionally. The bylaws consist of 23 articles that in turn have a number of important subheadings, called "sections," that further detail important facts about the association and its policies. Articles address areas such as the different classes of membership available, decision-making procedures, the responsibilities of AANA's elected officials, and configurations of committees and function of their members.

Proposed amendments to the bylaws of the AANA must be submitted in writing by five active members to the association's executive director not less than 90 days prior to the next annual meeting. Proposed amendments must be referred to the Bylaws Committee for review and recommendations and then are forwarded to the membership at least 30 days prior to the annual meeting. Amendments to the bylaws may be adopted by an affirmative vote of two-thirds of those members present and voting at a business meeting.

The AANA Foundation

The AANA Foundation was formed in 1981. Its mission is to be "the champion of research and development for the profession of nurse anesthesia." The foundation consists of seven CRNA and four lay members whose job it is to direct the various activities of the foundation, specifically to work in cooperation with the AANA to meet its mission of promoting research in areas of professional development and outcomes. Foundation activities include a grants program for research in anesthesia, student scholarships, fellowships to assist CRNAs to attain graduate degrees, and cutting-edge workshops that advance the practice of anesthesia in clinical settings. To date, the foundation has supported the research and educational efforts of virtually hundreds of students and CRNAs throughout the country. The foundation provides a planned-giving program and many CRNAs have recognized the valuable work of the foundation by making substantial financial gifts through the Friends for Life program.

National Headquarters

The AANA executive office moved from Cleveland to Chicago in 1937. After being situated in downtown Chicago for many years, the office moved to 216 Higgins Road in Park Ridge, Illinois, a northwest suburb of Chicago, in 1980. In 1992, due to limited space, expanding staff, and increased member services, the AANA purchased a 43,000 square-foot building at 222 South Prospect Avenue, in the downtown area of Park Ridge (below). This new building nearly tripled the size of the AANA's national headquarters, allowing the housing of all member services and subsidiaries at one site, including a new learning center from which continuing education seminars became available to members on a variety of clinical and professional topics. The AANA Archives and the International Federation of Nurse Anesthetists are also housed at the Prospect address.

Due to the increased attention given to federal-level issues affecting nurse anesthetists, the AANA recognized a need to have continuous representation in Washington, D.C. In 1991, the AANA established a Federal Government Affairs office to increase nurse anesthetists' visibility nationally and to deal with relevant practice issues. Currently, the Washington, D.C. office has a professional staff of five, headed by the director of Federal Government Affairs, working on behalf of members regarding a wide variety of federal issues that impact CRNA practice. These office personnel report to the association's executive director. It should be noted that in 1999, the AANA was recognized by *Fortune* magazine as having one of the most effective lobbying organizations in Washington, D.C. among major healthcare associations.

Departmental Organization

The AANA executive office consists of approximately 75 professional and clerical staff. The organization of the association is composed of the following departments, each with its own director, who reports to the executive director and ultimately to the association's elected Board of Directors: the Executive Unit; Managed Care and Reimbursement; Accreditation and Education; Continuing Education; Certification and Recertification; Membership, State Associations, and Information Systems; Research and

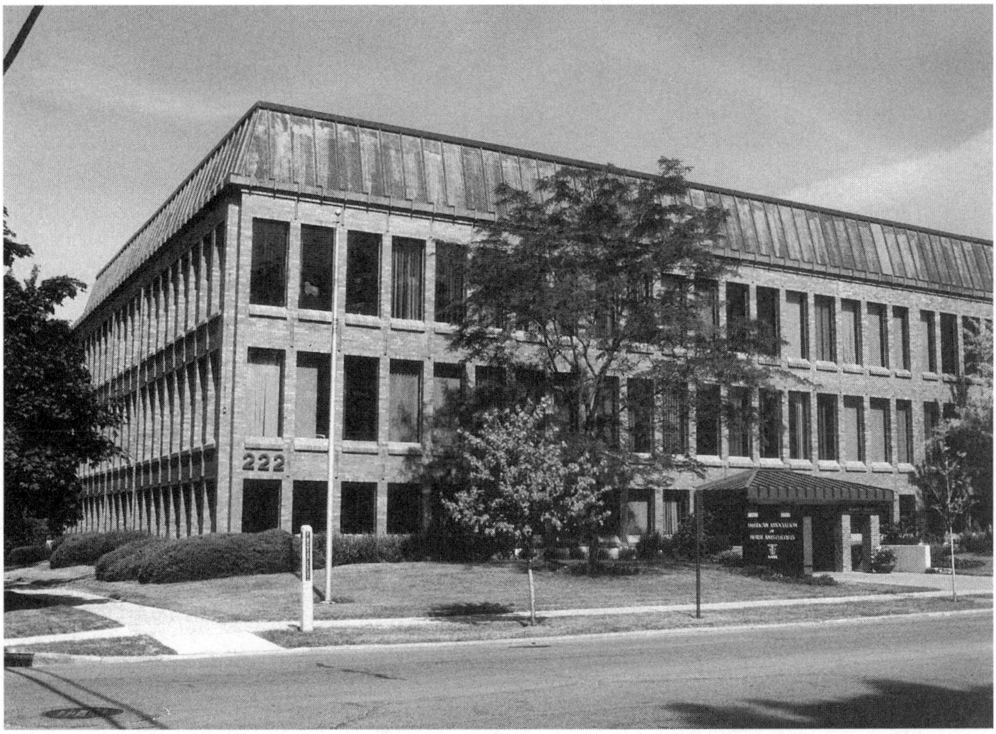

Figure 4.1: American Association of Nurse Anesthetists Executive Office Staff Structure, January 2002

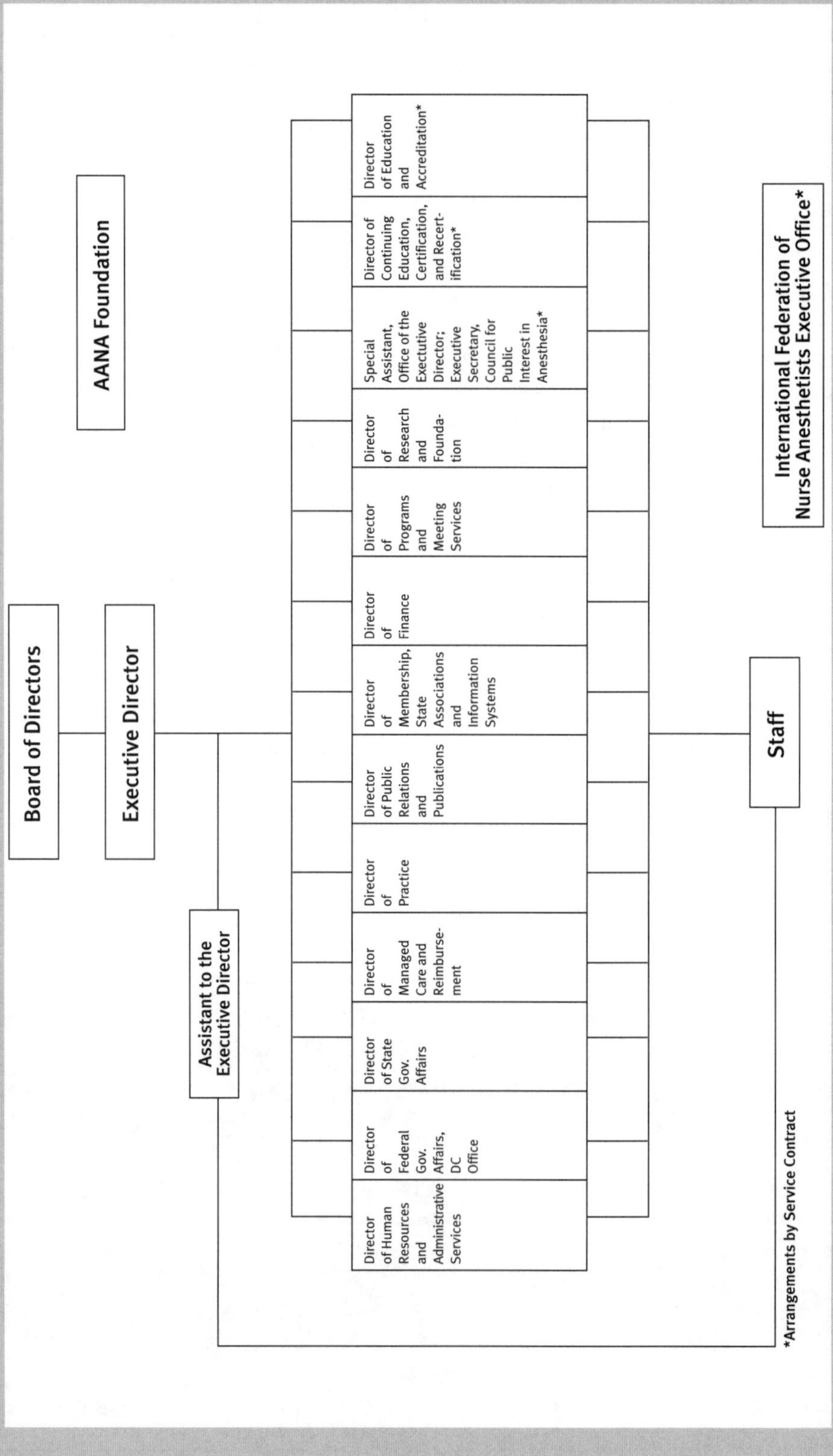

Foundation; Finance; Practice; State Government Affairs; Federal Government Affairs; Public Relations/Publications; Human Resources/Administrative Services; and Programs and Meeting Services (Figure 4.1). Within each of these major departments are member service sections. The executive staff serves in many capacities, including staff functions connected with each of the standing and ad hoc committees of the association.

The executive director remains responsible for the administrative functions of the national office and reports directly to the Board of Directors. The executive director, a position created by President Lucy Richards in 1948, is responsible for keeping minutes of all AANA meetings, attending meetings of the Board of Directors and the Executive Committee, and any other activities designated by the president. The executive director has no voting privileges on the Board of Directors. He or she provides advice and guidance on policy formulation, maintains professional AANA staff, negotiates and renews necessary service contracts for the AANA, oversees all financial decisions for the national office at the direction of the board, and provides leadership to educational, legal, and legislative entities of the AANA, as well as serving as a representative of the AANA to external organizations.

Council Configurations and Relationships

Within the AANA bylaws, there are provisions allowing for the establishment of four separate, independent councils: the Council on Certification of Nurse Anesthetists, the Council on Recertification of Nurse Anesthetists, the Council on Accreditation of Nurse Anesthesia Educational Programs, and the Council for Public Interest in Anesthesia. These councils are solely responsible for their own internal affairs, including the election of officers and the direction of financial activities. The councils do not report to the association president or executive director, with the exception of evaluation oversight. Membership on the councils includes CRNAs, students, physicians, and lay representatives, appointed or elected according to their own internal set of bylaws. The councils were established in the mid-1970s to ensure the public that certification, recertification, accreditation, and public interest functions of the discipline of nurse anesthesia were separate from and not unduly influenced by the national professional association. Most professional healthcare organizations of similar type to the AANA have made provisions within their operational bylaws to establish these requisite bodies which, although supported financially in part or whole by the professional organization, do not interfere with their basic functions. Communication between the AANA and the councils takes place through a formal liaison committee of council chairs and association officers to facilitate discussion of issues of mutual concern.

The Council on Accreditation of Nurse Anesthesia Educational Programs (COA) consists of 11 individuals representing the community of interest involved in the accreditation process of educational programs. The purpose of the COA is to (1) advise, formulate and/or adopt standards, guidelines, procedures, and criteria for the accreditation of nurse anesthesia educational programs, subject to review and comment by all constituencies that are significantly affected by them, and (2) accredit entry into nurse anesthesia practice educational programs. In essence, the COA is the body responsible for ensuring to the public that educational programs of nurse anesthesia are of quality as evidenced by compliance with a set of minimum education performance standards. The COA is recognized by the Commission on Recognition of Postsecondary Accreditation and the U.S. Department of Education as the sole agency empowered with the right to confer accreditation status to member programs.

The Council on Certification of Nurse Anesthetists consists of 11 individuals representing the community of interest involved in the process of certification of nurse anesthetists. The purpose of this council is to formulate and adopt requirements, guidelines, and prerequisites for certification and for eligibility to take the certification examination. The council is also responsible for administering each certification examination and evaluating the candidate's performance. The council grants initial certification to those candidates who successfully complete the certifying examination and who meet the other criteria for eligibility.

The Council on Recertification of Nurse Anesthetists consists of nine individuals representing the community of interest involved in the process of recertification of nurse anesthetists. Its purpose is to formulate and adopt criteria for eligibility for recertification of CRNAs based on participation in approved continuing education activities and other recognized activities conducive to professional proficiency. The council is also responsible for formulating and adopting criteria for recertification requirements recommended by the AANA Continuing Education Committee.

In response to increasing interactions between the communities of interest in anesthesia, the general public, and external healthcare organizations, the AANA Board of Directors in 1974 appointed an Ad Hoc Council on Nurse Anesthesia Practice. In 1975, the council was officially established and named the Council on Nurse Anesthesia Practice. In 1988, it was renamed the Council for Public Interest in Anesthesia and charged with the responsibility of monitoring issues that affect the public interest in matters regarding nurse anesthesia practice. Few other professional healthcare organizations have addressed the issue of public accountability in the manner of referring such issues to an autonomous body. This action again serves to ensure that public interest issues are not subordinated to the self-interest of the professional organization.

Subsidiaries

The AANA owns three subsidiaries that provide a source of nondues revenue for the association as well as services to the general membership. These subsidiaries are AANA Publishing Inc. (API), AANA Insurance Services Inc. and AANA Management Corporation. API is the publishing company for the *AANA Journal* and various other publications of the association. The *AANA Journal* disseminates original research, information on current issues, and serves as a source of information for persons interested in the art and science of anesthesia and the role and functions of the nurse anesthetist. AANA Insurance Services Inc., incorporated in 1988 as the AANA-owned insurance brokerage for professional liability programs for CRNAs, currently provides approximately 5,000 CRNAs with various product lines of professional liability insurance. It also provides liability insurance for many nurse midwives in the United States. AANA Insurance Services' agents are appropriately licensed and undergo continuing education to maintain their positions. The newest subsidiary is AANA Management Corporation. Formed in 1995, the company provides administrative and management related services. It currently provides such services to the International Federation of Nurse Anesthetists.

ELECTED LEADERSHIP

Board of Directors

The affairs of the AANA are conducted and lead by an elected Board of Directors. The Board consists of the president, president-elect, vice-president, treasurer, and seven regional directors. Officers serve for one year and directors serve a two-year term. To be eligible to serve as a director, an individual must have served at least one term as an officer or director of a state association and must have been active in state or AANA affairs. The Nominating Committee presents a slate of candidates for the Board of Directors at the Mid-Year Assembly. All CRNA members are allowed to vote for all officers and directors regardless of the region in which they hold membership. The newly elected Board of Directors is introduced to the membership at the Annual Business Meeting in August.

The Board of Directors is the administrative authority of the AANA. It receives and considers the reports of committees and directs the president to prepare an annual report reviewing the work of the preceding year that is submitted to the AANA membership. The Board of Directors assumes many other responsibilities on behalf of the association, including the responsibility of contracts and all budgetary and related financial matters, promoting position statements, promulgating clinical standards, managing the association standing committees, and maintaining a liaison with a myriad of external governmental and professional agencies. The Executive Committee of the Board of Directors is composed of the president, president-elect, vice-president, and treasurer, and manages the affairs of the AANA between meetings of the Board.

Committee Configurations

The appointed committees of the AANA include Administrative Management, Program, Bylaws, Continuing Education, Education, Finance, Government Relations, Strategic Planning, Minutes, Practice, Public Relations and Occupational Safety and Hazard. Committee members are appointed by the president with approval of the Board of Directors. All committees consist of at least three active members appointed for a one-year term by the president, who designates their committee chair subject to the approval of the Board of Directors. The committees conduct their business as directed by the AANA Strategic Plan, with input and guidance from the Board. Committees usually meet two to three times per year, often in conjunction with other major association-related meetings.

The elected committees of the association are the Nominating Committee and the Resolutions Committee. Election of these two committees is by mailed ballot, in conjunction with the election of officers and regional directors. The Nominating Committee is responsible for slating and determining eligibility of candidates for the AANA Board of Directors and the elected committees. Members of the Resolutions Committee submit resolutions (a resolution is a written "main motion" that contains subject matter potentially having significant impact on the policies of the AANA) signed by at least five active members to the executive director no less than 90 days prior to the AANA Annual Meeting. At the Annual Meeting, the Resolutions Committee holds an open hearing at which time all submitted resolutions may be discussed. The Board of Directors is responsible for implementing any resolutions approved by the general membership.

CONDUCTING THE BUSINESS OF THE ASSOCIATION

In addition to the daily activities of the national office, the business of the association is conducted largely via primary meetings of different membership segments of the association. These include the Assembly of School Faculty, Fall Assembly of States, Mid-Year Assembly, and Annual Meeting. All members are invited to attend and fully participate in these activities.

Assembly of School Faculty

The Assembly of School Faculty takes place twice per year, once in February and again in conjunction with the Annual Meeting. Participants generally include program directors, associate directors, physician and CRNA faculty, PhD faculty, educational advisors, students, and other interested individuals. Participants of the assembly discuss affairs pertinent to the conduct of educational programs including current issues, standards, legal implications, legislative trends, clinical practice, teaching/instruction, and research. The meeting is conducted by the Education Committee of the AANA.

Assembly of States

The Assembly of States is held each year in the fall. Attendees of this meeting include the Board of Directors, members of the standing AANA committees, officers and board members of affiliated state associations, and other interested members.

Assemblies usually take place over an extended weekend and are held to disseminate information on current issues affecting practice and other programming to assist state organizations in the conduct of their business. Both the Assembly of School Faculty and Fall Assembly of States provide ample open forums during which any member may speak to issues of his or her concern.

Mid-Year Assembly

Each year the AANA hosts a Mid-Year Assembly in the Washington, D.C. area to provide opportunity for CRNAs to meet their elected national congressional delegation and lobby directly the AANA federal legislative agenda. These sessions also present nationally and internationally recognized political and bureaucratic leaders as speakers in addition to providing instructional workshops for CRNAs to improve their lobbying skills. This meeting provides an opportunity for participants to experience a rare behind-the-scenes look at the legislative process and learn first-hand about federal legislative activities and how important CRNAs are to the process of shaping national healthcare legislation.

Topics discussed at this meeting include healthcare reform, Medicare reimbursement for anesthesia services, and federal policies and law affecting healthcare cost, access, and quality as well as current issues affecting practice patterns of CRNAs. Most CRNAs attending the meeting meet personally with their members of Congress on the final day of the conference to discuss their positions on proposed legislation. Much of the assembly is given to preparing CRNAs on the issues and how to best deal with congressional members and staff during face to face meetings.

Annual Meeting

One of the most popular meetings the AANA holds is its Annual Meeting, which typically lasts for five days in early to mid-August in a major metropolitan city. Attendance at this meeting typically reaches nearly 3,000, of which approximately 700 are students. Members cite many benefits of attending the Annual Meeting, such as earning continuing education credits from more than 100 scientific sessions, networking with fellow

CRNAs, observing the latest in technology and equipment, hearing nationally and internationally known speakers, and sharing ideas and positions with colleagues and elected leaders of the profession. The meeting includes an entire day of activities for students, including the Anesthesia College Bowl and student luncheon. The student program is managed by the Education Committee and its elected student representative. In addition, the meeting includes the AANA Opening Ceremonies, general business session, bylaws hearings, scientific sessions and workshops, focus sessions concentrating on special issues, exhibits, receptions, and the glittering Annual Banquet which plays only to sold-out crowds.

STATE ORGANIZATIONS

State Organizational Configurations

State associations are formed by members who live and work in a particular state and are recognized by the Board of Directors as a duly incorporated entity. State associations are responsible for organizing their own committees, electing state officers, and handling their own financial affairs. States are supported financially by state membership dues which are collected by the AANA and paid back to the state association. Officer and board configurations of state associations are similar to the national organization. State organizations deal with many local issues, such as CRNA access to hospitals and other healthcare institutions, clinical privileges, and ability to receive adequate reimbursement from a variety of payers. Activity of the state association is dependent largely on the volunteer effort of CRNAs and is of primary importance to the profession, as most of the legislative activity affecting CRNA practice is conducted at the state level. Further, an active state association is vital for optimal function of the AANA Federal Government Affairs office. Without the state level contacts and networks that state organizations have with their elected state executive and legislative leaders, the national legislative agenda of the AANA would be significantly less effective. Participation by CRNAs in their state association is usually considered the point of entry into activities and offices at the national level.

State Relationship to the AANA

Members from each state association maintain contact with the national office by providing them annually with a list of its officers, committee members, and current bylaws. Officers and members of individual state associations often contact executive office staff, seeking advice and counsel on issues related to practice, government affairs, education, public relations, and membership. In addition, a complete library located in the AANA executive office and staffed by a full-time librarian/archivist serves as a central repository of information for state associations when devising position statements, conducting research, or proposing legislative language.

Membership Services

There are many reasons to become a member of the AANA or to renew one's membership annually. Table 4.1 provides a list of the benefits CRNAs enjoy through active participation in the AANA. It is also important to recognize that AANA membership provides another substantial benefit to interested members. Because AANA is a voluntary organization, it values and requires the active participation of members on its standing committees and in its ad hoc work groups, continuing education programs, consultant activities, and the AANA Foundation, to mention only a few. These

TABLE 4.1
Benefits and Services Provided to AANA Members

PRACTICE ISSUES

1) Valuable employment and salary information on a nationwide basis
2) Consultation services in employment practice matters
3) Assistance with regulatory and accreditation issues
4) National representation with external health agencies that impact nurse anesthesia practice
5) Development of guidelines and standards for practice
6) Preparation of numerous practice monographs
7) Legal commentary on practice and quality of care issues
8) Information and assistance on numerous practice settings
9) Assistance in obtaining equitable reimbursement from third-party insurers
10) *Professional Practice Manual* development and updates; manual includes the following documents
    a) Guidelines for Nurse Anesthesia Practice
    b) Qualifications and Capabilities of CRNAs
    c) Professional and Legal Issues
    d) Guidelines for Infection Control
    e) Informed Consent
    f) Implementing Quality Assurance Programs in Anesthesia
    g) Risk Management Guide
    h) AANA Position Statements
    i) Code of Ethics
    j) Documenting Standard of Care, Anesthesia Record
    k) Anesthesia Outcome by Provider Studies
11) Expert witness referral program
12) Anesthesia department consultation referrals
13) AANA hotline for chemically impaired professionals (800-654-5167)

GOVERNMENTAL REPRESENTATION

1) National representation on governmental issues through the AANA Washington, D.C. office
2) Broad legal interpretation of events that impact the profession
3) AANA government relations hotline (800-423-0625)
4) Assistance for Medicare carriers in obtaining equitable reimbursement
5) State legislative/regulatory tracking service
6) Analysis of state legislation/regulations for state associations
7) Legislative updates in each *AANA NewsBulletin* and *AANA Journal*
8) Political Action Committee furthering nurse anesthesia causes

(continued)

TABLE 4.1 (continued)
Benefits and Services Provided to AANA Members

PUBLICATIONS

1) Bimonthly *AANA Journal* containing the latest in scientific and educational advancements
2) Monthly *AANA NewsBulletin* containing timely information on healthcare policy and issues facing nurse anesthetists
3) Bimonthly *Quality Review in Anesthesia* discussing quality assurance/risk management policies
4) *NewsBulletin* classified advertisements listing open positions and professionals seeking new positions
5) Calendar of continuing education program events
6) Annual *AANA Journal* course for six continuing education credits

PUBLIC AWARENESS

1) Professional recognition and identity
2) Public relations campaigns focused on educating the general public on the role of nurse anesthetists
3) National campaign to purchasers of anesthesia services, expanding employment possibilities for nurse anesthetists
4) Development of patient information brochures for use by CRNAs in practice

MEETINGS

1) Reduced registration fees for AANA events
2) AANA Annual Meeting, which represents the single largest gathering of CRNAs, colleagues, and past classmates each year
3) Annual Fall Assembly of States, which focuses on state association management and national issues
4) Two Assemblies of School Faculty, which are specifically targeted at educators
5) Annual Mid-Year Assembly, which is held in Washington, D.C., and focuses on the lobbying efforts of CRNAs on healthcare issues

EDUCATION

1) Recruitment of nurses into the profession through exhibits, speaking engagements, and printed material
2) Standards and guidelines for educating CRNAs
3) Securement of funding from governmental sources for nurse anesthesia programs and students
4) Numerous national professional and educational workshops, seminars, and meetings
5) Maintenance of continuing education records for easy submission to the Council on Recertification
6) Identification of funding sources and procurement of funding for research
7) Faculty development programs
8) Fellowship programs for CRNAs obtaining further education
9) Consultative services for potential new nurse anesthesia program sites

(continued)

TABLE 4.1 (continued)
Benefits and Services Provided to AANA Members

10) Review and approval of continuing education programs
11) School transcripts
12) Consultation for research activities

MEMBER SERVICES

1) Group insurance programs including health, life, and income protection
2) Affinity credit card program
3) Partial payment of biennial recertification fee
4) AANA-owned professional liability insurance agency dedicated to malpractice insurance for nurse anesthetists nationwide
5) Maintenance of database of CRNAs appropriately credentialed to obtain Medicare reimbursement from the Centers for Medicare & Medicaid Services
6) Emergency student loan program for nurse anesthesia students and CRNAs furthering their education
7) Financial support for Council on Accreditation of Nurse Anesthesia Educational Programs
8) Educational programs and Council on Public Interest in Anesthesia

opportunities provide invaluable experiences for CRNAs to expand their own professional development and skill base as administrators, managers, team members, educators, researchers and leaders by working together to achieve organizational goals. CRNAs then bring back benefits of these experiences to the workplace, which undoubtedly enhance their potential for promoting the interests of nurse anesthesia more effectively, expanding their own personal and professional roles, or even achieving promotion. There is no doubt that these voluntary experiences play a vital role in socializing CRNAs into a more satisfying professional role.

SUMMARY

As the healthcare field continues to grow and change, so does the AANA, thanks to its loyal members, who continue to serve with the dedication, enthusiasm, and perseverance characteristic of its founding members. The AANA is a unique organization that owes its success to the support of 95 percent of the nation's CRNAs. Each CRNA has something of importance to contribute to the AANA, and the diversity among its members is a vital key to its continued growth and success. To meet the challenges of the future, we must remain an informed and unified organization that serves all its members and extends its promise of quality and caring service to the public.

REFERENCES

American Association of Nurse Anesthetists. (1996). *Professional Practice Manual for the Certified Registered Nurse Anesthetist.* Park Ridge, IL: Author.

Bankert, M. (1993). *Watchful Care: A History of America's Nurse Anesthetists.* New York: Continuum Publishing.

Malone, B.L. (1996). Clinical and Professional Leadership. In Hamric, A.B., Spross, J.A, & Hanson, C.M. (Eds.), *Advanced Nursing Practice: An Integrative Approach.* Philadelphia, PA: Saunders.

STUDY QUESTIONS

1. Discuss the philosophical questions and potential conflicts that could arise relative to the dual mission of a professional organization serving the interests of both patients and providers. Give examples.

2. Discuss issues or problems you have observed as a student that CRNAs have in the workplace and conjecture ways in which the AANA or state organizations could help solve the issues.

3. Design a plan of action and rationale that you would use to convince a fellow CRNA of the value of membership and need to belong to the AANA.

4. Describe the organizational relationship of the four councils to the AANA and the rationale for why they are constituted in such a manner.

REGULATION OF CLINICAL PRACTICE

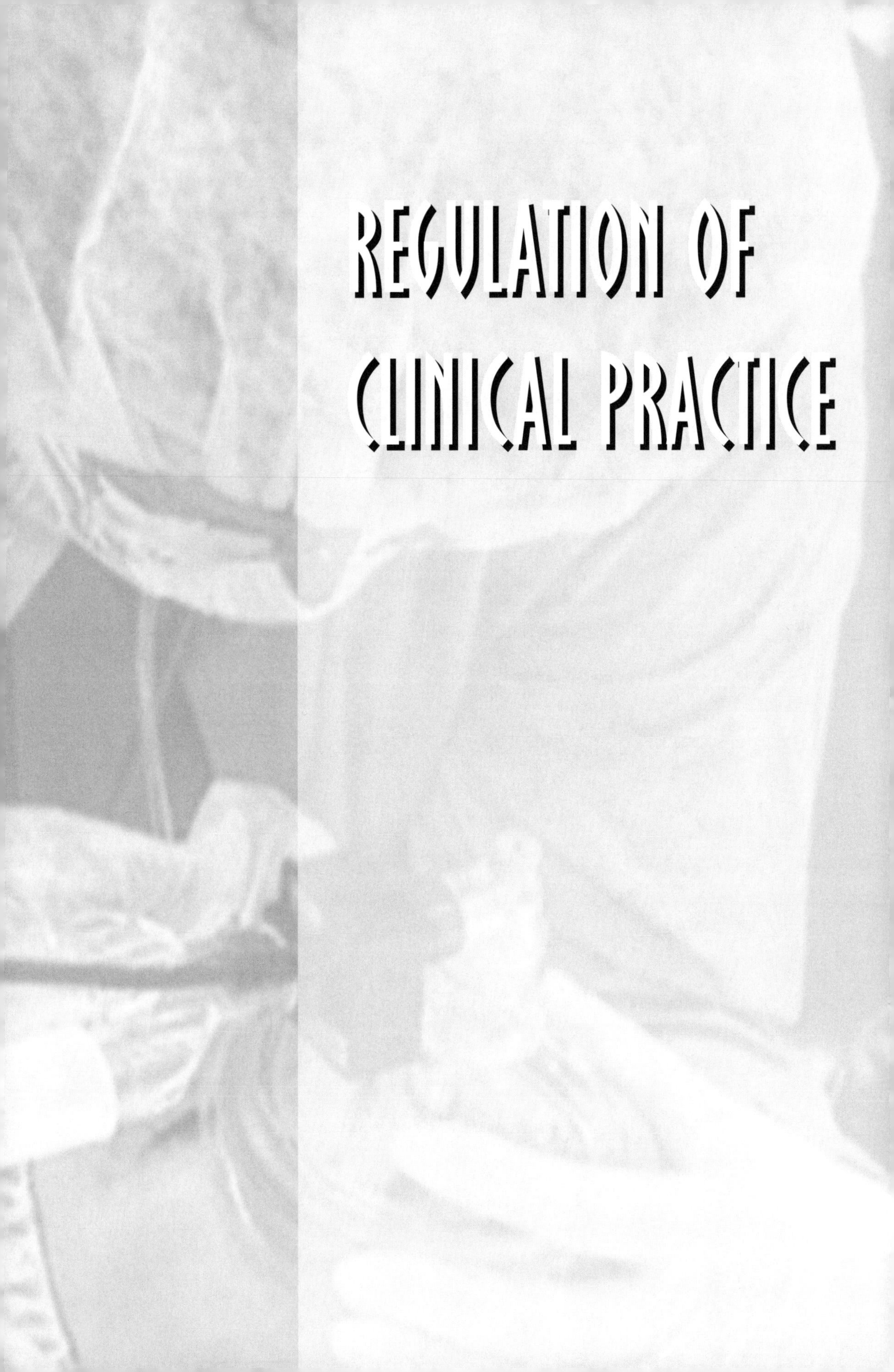

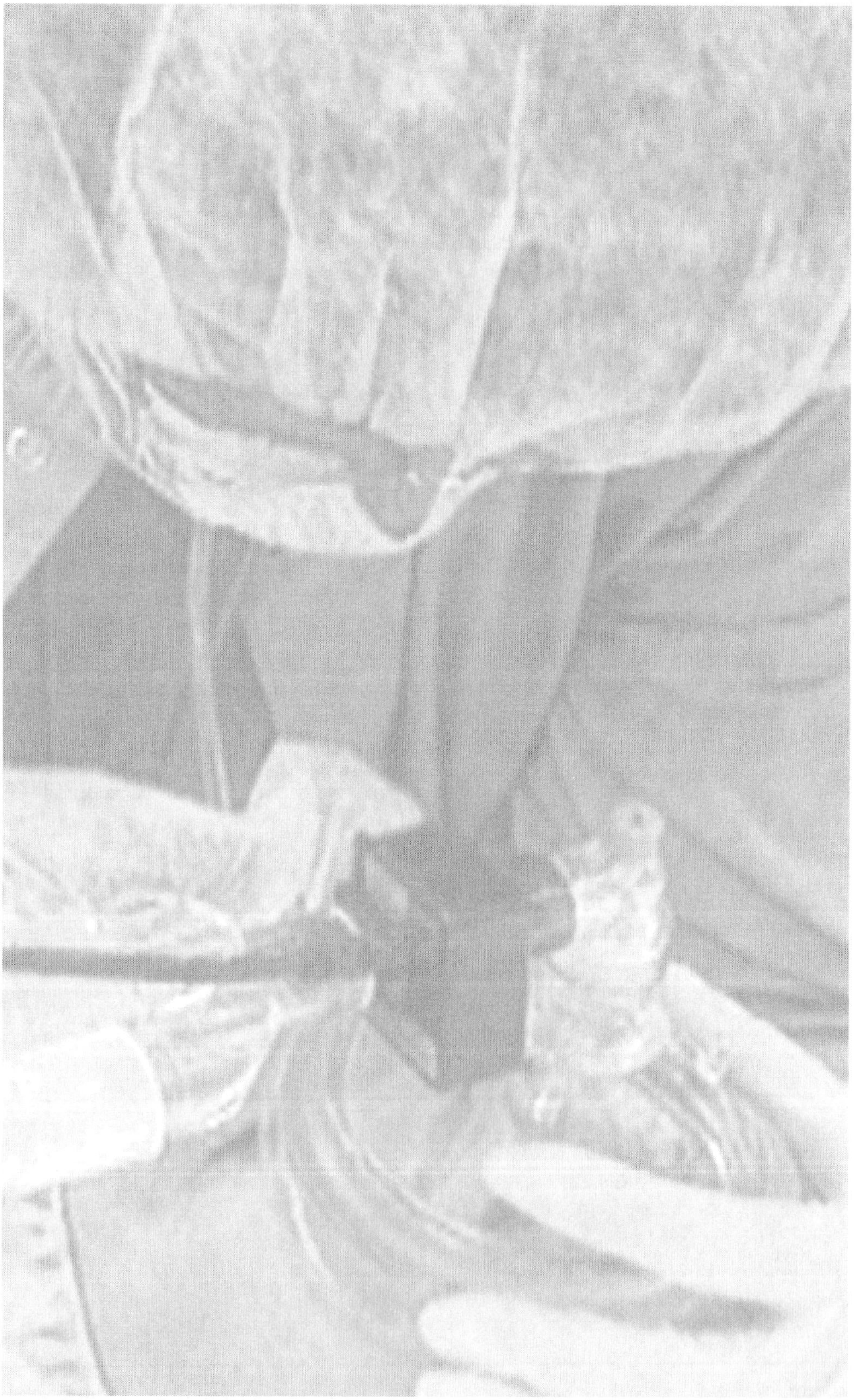

CHAPTER 5

THE U.S. LEGAL SYSTEM AND ISSUES AFFECTING CLINICAL PRACTICE

Gene A. Blumenreich, JD

General Counsel
American Association of Nurse Anesthetists
Boston, MA

KEY CONCEPTS

- State and federal courts differ from one another in jurisdiction, traditions, rules and body of law. The federal system deals with issues that broadly affect interstate commerce, actions involving federal property, and actions between states. Matters affecting the health, safety and welfare of citizens generally come with the "police" powers of states and are reserved for state government and their courts.

- Courts do not make law the way a legislature does. Court decisions are applicable to actions that occur both before and after their decisions. Legislation affects matters which arise only after it is enacted. In choosing between conflicting parties, the judicial system applies its goals of fairness, consistency, predictability and the effectuation of public policy.

- It is the members of the professions themselves who are responsible for promulgating standards of care by which quality of care is measured. Both the courts and the legislature can change these standards should the profession render care at a lower standard than is acceptable.

- There is a single standard of care against which both anesthesiologists and Certified Registered Nurse Anesthetists (CRNAs) are measured.

- A professional must render care not only as a reasonable person would act, but with the same degree of skill and care as would be practiced by a reasonable member of the profession in similar circumstances. In specialty areas, such as anesthesia, there is a nationwide standard of care that does not vary from community to community.

- The theoretic basis of negligence or malpractice is that the defendant should pay for damages caused to the plaintiff because, as between the two parties, the one who was at fault should bear the damage. Anesthesia accidents involving CRNAs have become prime examples for the application of the doctrine of *res ipsa loquitur.*

Nurse anesthesia is legally recognized as a specialty in the profession of nursing. Consequently, it is important for Certified Registered Nurse Anesthetists (CRNAs) to have an informed understanding of the legal system because it profoundly affects the way the profession is practiced. Because many challenges to nurse anesthesia practice are commonly based on misinformation concerning the legal status of CRNAs, an understanding of the legal system and tenets guiding its function is vitally important.

As the reader will become aware in subsequent chapters, nurse anesthesia is regulated by licensing boards and by the courts which illuminate the standard of care. It is important to note at this point that the hallmark of a profession is its ability to set its own standard of care. Courts learn of the standard of care through expert testimony. Since experts may disagree, the courts may have to choose between conflicting testimony. Moreover, the legislature may require new standards of care through legislation. Consequently, even though standards are set by the profession, the standard of care is affected by many aspects of the legal system, including regulatory bodies of the state, the legislature through statute and, of course, the court.

DEFERENCE TO THE HEALTHCARE PROFESSION

Regulation of healthcare differs significantly from regulation of other industries. In most areas, regulation clearly and specifically sets forth powers, duties, and procedures. However, in medical and nursing regulation there is a large degree of deference afforded the healthcare community by both legislatures and courts. This deference is expressed in the California Nursing Act (Cal. Business and Professions Code, 1974):

> "...the legislature recognizes that nursing is a dynamic field, the practice of which is continually evolving to include more sophisticated patient care activities. It is the intent of the legislature in amending this section at the 1973-74 session to provide clear legal authority for functions and procedures which have common acceptance and usage."

Law school students learn very early that during a trial, "law" is determined by the judge, whereas "facts" are determined by the jury if there is one or by the judge in the absence of a jury. Evidence is offered by the parties to establish the facts. However, in some cases involving the healthcare field, judges appear to rely on expert testimony for interpretation of statutes as well as facts (*Chalmers-Francis v. Nelson*, 1936), [nurse anesthesia practice is not diagnosing nor prescribing ... within the meaning of the California Medical Practice Act] and (*Bentley v. Langley*, 1978), [an anesthesiologist was permitted to testify (incorrectly) that a doctor who supervised a nurse anesthetist was responsible for the anesthesia services administered].

This special position the courts give to healthcare can sometimes be taken advantage of. In the case of *Sermchief v. Gonzales* (1983), the Missouri legislature amended the Missouri statute on nursing so as to permit advanced practice nurses to give routine examinations and dispense medications within a medical protocol, without being under the direct supervision of a physician. The Missouri Medical Board, known as the Board of Registration for the Healing Arts, threatened criminal prosecution of nurses who carried out these activities, claiming that the nurses were engaged in the illegal practice of medicine. A group of nurses sought protection against the Board of Registration for the Healing Arts. Both the nurses and physicians presented the case in such a manner as to ask the court to draw what the court referred to as "that thin and elusive line that separates the practice of medicine and the practice of professional nursing in modern day delivery of health services." Instead, the court pointed out that what the nurses were doing was, in fact, exactly what the legislature intended them to do. Because licensing is the prerogative of the legislature, the fact that the legislature had authorized nurses to do something that physicians thought might have been the practice of medicine was irrelevant. If the legislature said that nurses could do it, it was the practice of nursing and the medical board had no right to interfere with their practice of it.

SOURCES OF LAW

Legislature

The powers of the legislature are limited only by constitutional restrictions and the political control of the voting public. Legislation is forward looking; it affects actions taking place after its effective date. When legislation is passed, courts interpret it by trying to determine what the legislature intended. Court decisions, on the other hand, state what the law is and, theoretically, what the law always has been. When a court determines that a judicial doctrine, such as "captain of the ship," is no longer the law, every undecided case is governed by the decision, regardless of when it arose. If a state was still following the captain of the ship doctrine, and the legislature wanted to, it could pass a law that, after a certain date, surgeons would no longer be assumed to control all actions in an operating room. Cases arising before the effective date would be decided assuming surgeons were in control and cases after the date would be decided assuming surgeons were not in control. Only the legislature has the authority to change the law and only the legislature can say that after a specific date the law will be something else. The legislature can reverse decisions made by the judiciary. The legislature is limited by constitutional restrictions (e.g., a legislature could not adopt a law making something that has already happened a crime, or taking property, or imposing punishment without following due process and having a fair hearing). The judiciary interprets existing law, the Constitution, statutes and prior court decisions. Judicial interpretations of the Constitution cannot be overruled by the legislature, they can only be changed by changing the Constitution.

Executive Branch

The executive branch enforces laws made by the legislature and interpreted by the courts. Before the American Revolution, the executive branch was headed by the monarch or his or her representative. Now the executive branch is headed by the president or a state governor.

A part of the executive branch of government is the attorney general, who serves as the lawyer for the government. The attorney general serves two functions: first, as the government's lawyer, the attorney general brings lawsuits and represents the country or the state in court; second, the attorney general gives advice to administrative agencies or departments by interpreting the law. Interpretations of the law by the attorney general are not binding on the courts. They are important, however, because they tell how the attorney general's client, the executive branch of the government, will act.

An example of an attorney general

interpretation important to nurse anesthetists is the opinion of the California attorney general on whether nurse anesthetists could administer regional anesthetics. The attorney general is often asked to give opinions when there is very little authority or precedent. In 1972, the attorney general of California was asked if it was legal for nurse anesthetists to give regional anesthetics. The attorney general searched the case law and found only an isolated statement by the California Supreme Court in the case of *Magit v. State of California* (1961). In *Magit*, three foreign anesthesiologists were administering anesthesia without medical licenses. The chief anesthesiologist who employed them was prosecuted for aiding and abetting the unauthorized practice of medicine. His defense was based on the case of *Chalmers-Francis v. Nelson* (1936), one of the fundamental cases upholding nurse anesthetist practice. The chief anesthesiologist claimed that since California courts permitted Dagmar Nelson, who was a nurse, not a licensed physician, to administer anesthesia, California law should permit nonlicensed anesthesiologists to provide anesthesia as well. The California Supreme Court noted the special position that nurses have in the healthcare system, and pointed out that the Dagmar Nelson case had been decided at a time when California did not have a nurse practice act (a nurse practice act has since been enacted). Therefore, as precedent, the Dagmar Nelson case was limited to its facts. The court found a nurse anesthetist administering a general anesthetic was not illegally practicing medicine.

From this simple statement in *Magit*, the California attorney general developed a theory that under California law, nurse anesthetists could only administer general anesthesia and could not administer regional anesthetics. While the ruling was patently absurd, nurse anesthetists in California were uneasy that the decision would be enforced by the board of nursing. Very few nurse anesthetists continued to administer regional anesthesia, although most believed that the attorney general's decision was incorrect. In 1976, the California Association of Nurse Anesthetists went back to the attorney general and asked for a reversal of his prior decision. The attorney general agreed that the *Magit* case was not authority for his ruling. Unfortunately, the attorney general found a new problem. The legislature had passed a bill specifically giving nurse anesthetists the ability to administer regional anesthetics, but the bill had been vetoed by the governor. The attorney general decided that the California legislature must have believed that nurse anesthetists required additional statutory authority to give regional anesthetics or the legislature would not have passed the bill. Since the bill had been vetoed, nurse anesthetists did not receive the additional authority and must still lack the power to administer regional anesthetics (the California governor vetoed the bill because he thought it was unnecessary).

The attorney general's ruling stood for eight more years until, in 1984, the office finally issued an opinion that there was no prohibition against nurse anesthetists giving regional anesthesia. As can be seen, the attorney general rendered two incorrect decisions that were not subject to review or correction. The decisions were troublesome because they were binding on administrative agencies. Although they were not binding on the courts, nurse anesthesia practice was harmed in California in the years the ruling stood.

Administrative Agencies

Another part of the executive branch is the administrative agency. An administrative agency combines elements of all three branches of government. An administrative agency such as the Food and Drug Administration (FDA) has a legislative function in that it adopts regulations that have the force of law, an executive function in that healthcare institutions that violate the regulations are prosecuted by the FDA, and a judicial function in that the agency conducts hearings on charges and determines guilt or innocence. Regulations issued by an administrative agency must be consistent with enabling acts and other legislation. While an agency may clarify unclear or ambiguous terms, it cannot adopt interpretations which are inconsistent with the clear language of legislation. Licensing agencies such as boards of nursing, boards of medicine, and boards of pharmacy are administrative agencies and combine functions of each of the branches of government.

Courts

Courts do not make law the way a legislature does. Court decisions are applicable to actions that occur both before and after their decisions. A court interpretation of a statute affects all actions subject to the statute, whether the action occurred before or after the decision. Even though courts interpret what the law always was, the fact is that society changes, and its institutions change. Consequently, statutes and the Constitution are constantly reexamined and reinterpreted by the courts in light of current events and situations. For example, when the antitrust laws were passed in 1890, they were intended to prevent the excesses of the robber barons of the late 19th century who manipulated prices of oil, steel, and other products. Probably very few people in 1890 could have imagined that antitrust laws would ever be applicable to services, especially professional services. It was not until 1942, 52 years after passage of the original legislation, that the Supreme Court held that the antitrust laws applied (and had always applied) to restraint of trade by physicians. Today, the antitrust laws are often applied to matters involving the healthcare professions.

COMMON LAW

In some countries, the judicial system is based entirely on interpretation of statutes. English speaking countries, including the United States, inherited a tradition of judge-made law. In feudal times in England, the courts decided disputes between persons when there were no statutes or legislation. The courts decided these matters using the goals of consistency, fairness, predictability, and effectuation of policy. These decisions eventually resulted in a large body of common law legal principles and precedents the courts used to make individual decisions in areas not governed by statute. The English system, including the tradition of common law dating back to feudal times, forms the basis of law in every state of the United States except Louisiana. At the time of its acquisition by the United States, Louisiana had a thriving commercial port with important commercial transactions. Fairness and consistency required that Louisiana continue its system based on the continental system of statutory interpretation, rather than common law.

In feudal times, the king rode from location to location resolving disputes between his subjects. These disputes often involved the ownership and use of land. It was important to the feudal economy that there be quick and consistent resolution of these disputes because land represented wealth and capital. If land was properly used, the kingdom would prosper, but if land was unused, the kingdom would suffer. Determination of disputes between individual citizens was an important function for the king. Over time, the process of dispute resolution became institutionalized and certain of the king's assistants became specialists in dispute resolution, or judges. The tradition (largely oral) of these judges became the basis of common law. Eventually, persons seeking justice in the king's legal system were allowed to confer with other persons with experience in the system. Thus, the profession of law developed.

The Goals of Judicial Decisions

In choosing between conflicting parties, the judicial system applies its goals of fairness, consistency, predictability, and the effectuation of public policy. In a democracy, the courts draw their authority from the consent of the governed. While the judicial system must make unpopular decisions from time to time, it must always appear to be fair in its process or it will lose support. It must be predictable as well. Those who are governed by the system must be able to understand what the system expects and how the system will operate. The system must also be consistent. It would be unfair to hold one person negligent in one case and to exonerate a person in another when both were engaged in identical conduct. A system that lacks consistency is neither predictable nor fair. The legal system also attempts to encourage actions that benefit society as a whole and to discourage actions that harm society. Consequently, the common law that was inherited from England had at its heart that all members of society must act as reasonable people would act. When a member does not, he or she is responsible for any damage caused.

While individual court decisions may be difficult to justify, these decisions must be judged by whether they carry out the goals of fairness, consistency, predictability, and effectuation of policy. Sometimes, to carry out its ultimate goals, the legal system may produce decisions that seem incorrect. Courts may find decisions difficult when fundamental principles are in conflict. For many years, courts held surgeons liable for any activity in an operating room because the surgeon was like the "captain of a ship" and theoretically could control any action in the room. Even when it was clear that the surgeon was not in control but dependent on a number of specialists, some courts continued to apply the captain of the ship doctrine, weighing consistency and predictability more heavily than fairness. Sometimes the system simply yields incorrect decisions, as does any human system.

STATE VERSUS FEDERAL COURTS

The U.S. legal system is divided into two separate and largely independent systems. The first is the legal system of the federal government, and the second is legal systems belonging to each of the 50 states and the District of Columbia. While there is some overlap in jurisdiction, the federal and state governments have their own laws, traditions, judges, courtrooms, rules, and body of law. Certain areas have been reserved exclusively for the federal system, including matters affecting interstate commerce. Over the years, the level of impact these activities have had on interstate commerce, to justify federal regulation, has been more and more liberally interpreted so today the federal government has numerous programs affecting the health, safety, and welfare of citizens. Courts have held that they are proper because of their impact on interstate commerce.

Federal Courts

Litigants have only limited rights to choose between federal and state courts. The jurisdiction of the federal courts is limited to actions brought under federal statutes, actions involving federal property, and actions between citizens of different states (diversity). The perception (which may or may not be accurate) is that plaintiffs get larger awards in federal courts.

State Courts

Matters affecting the health, safety, and welfare of citizens generally come within the "police" powers of states and are reserved for state government. This includes not only states but also cities, towns, and other local governments. As part of their police powers, states have primary jurisdiction in licensing the healthcare industry. Disputes between people arising out of agreements or contracts are decided by state laws as are claims by one person that he or she may have been damaged by the negligence or actions of another.

Lawsuits Arising Under Federal Legislation

Lawsuits based on federal statutes may be brought in federal courts, and if there are related state issues to be decided, the federal courts may decide the related state issue. Federal laws take precedence over state and local laws. If both the federal and state governments enact legislation in a particular area, the federal act prevails. Under the doctrine of "preemption," once the federal government has enacted legislation in an area, state laws may no longer be enforced unless the federal government specifically permits states to enact legislation in the area. The doctrine of preemption ensures that the purpose of federal legislation will be carried out and not be affected by inconsistent state laws. Sometimes Congress determines that state acts would promote and not interfere with federal policy. In such cases, Congress may permit states to adopt their own regulations. For example, in the field of antitrust law, the federal government has indicated that states may also adopt legislation prohibiting restraints of trade. Numerous states have adopted "baby antitrust statutes."

Federal Property

The second area of jurisdiction of the federal courts is that of disputes relating to federal property or to which the federal government is a party. In feudal England, the king was always right so a person could not have a dispute with the king. The king was immune from suit. Today, this doctrine of "sovereign immunity" protects the government from being sued without its consent. However, most citizens would be very unhappy if they were to suffer damage because of the negligence of a government worker and could not be compensated because of sovereign immunity. The federal government permits lawsuits to be brought against it under most circumstances, but these lawsuits must be brought in federal courts.

Diversity

Finally, the federal government is committed to promoting interstate commerce. Because of the founding fathers' concern that state courts would give unfair advantage to citizens of their own states, the third area of federal court jurisdiction consists of situations in which a citizen of one state sues a citizen of another. Even though a matter may involve only a state issue, if the plaintiff is a resident of one state and the defendant is a resident of another, the lawsuit may be brought in the federal court if the matter involved in the controversy exceeds $50,000.

Until 1938, the federal courts had developed their own common law and disputes in diversity cases could have different outcomes depending on whether suit was brought in state or federal court. Since 1938, federal courts have applied state law to diversity cases as best they can. In diversity cases, federal courts are obligated to try to reach the same result as would the state court.

Trial and Appellate Courts

Courts are either trial courts or appellate courts. Trial courts are where cases are brought and facts presented. The trial court makes determinations of the facts of the case as well as the applicable law. In certain circumstances, the trier of facts is not a judge, but a jury. The Seventh Amendment to the Constitution preserves the right of a citizen to trial by jury. Over the years, the Seventh Amendment has been interpreted to mean that in those matters in which a trial by jury was provided when the Bill of Rights was adopted, citizens still have rights to trial by jury. In other cases, litigants can choose trial by jury, but it is not guaranteed.

Trial courts are required to make decisions quickly, and in the heat of litigation mistakes sometimes occur. In both federal and state systems, decisions of trial courts can be appealed to appellate courts. The appeals process provides time for consideration and research and is intended to lead to more uniformity in court decisions. In some states there may only be one appellate court, which would be the highest court in the state. In other states, the volume of litigation may be very large and there may be levels of appellate courts. In the federal system, decisions of the trial or district courts are appealed to a court of appeals for the region in which the state is located. Decisions of the courts of appeals may be appealed to the Supreme Court of the United States, although in some circumstances cases may be appealed directly from the trial court to the Supreme Court. The Supreme Court has the right to set its own agenda and, as such, has the right to decide which cases it will hear of the many presented to it.

In general, decisions by the trial court as to facts made either by the judge or jury are accepted because the judge or jury has had the opportunity to see the witness and determine credibility. Testimony that is reproduced in written form does not give a reader the chance to make observations. Did the witness look people in the eye, squirm, seem uncertain, appear uneasy, or otherwise indicate that the testimony was unreliable? Consequently, the appellate courts often defer to the fact finding of lower courts unless it is clear from the record that the finder of fact was erroneous or prejudiced. In matters of law, appellate courts are free to review any decision made by a trial court and to come to their own conclusion. Decisions of an appellate court are binding on all courts within its jurisdiction. Consequently, many of the decisions of the appellate courts are collected and published so that people will have a chance to see the law as adopted by the court.

Each state is free not only to adopt legislation that differs from that of other states but also to have its courts make their own interpretation of nonstatutory common law. While states may be interested in what other state legislatures and courts may have done in addressing common problems, they are not obligated to follow their decisions. Obviously, because of common backgrounds and restraints, there is more uniformity than diversity among states, but diversity does exist.

Civil/Criminal Matters

The judicial system distinguishes between civil and criminal matters. A civil matter is a dispute between two parties. Criminal matters are proceedings in which criminal statutes are at issue. Legislatures enact criminal penalties providing for jail or monetary punishments for violation of the basic fundamentals of societal living (murder, robbery, etc.). Another application of criminal punishment is to facilitate the enforcement of regulatory matters. In order to give administrative agencies authority, the legislature provides that violation of regulatory acts or rules are criminal and can be punished by monetary penalties or incarceration. For example, in *Chalmers-Francis v. Nelson* (1936), one of the fundamental cases upholding nurse anesthetist practice, Dagmar Nelson was prosecuted under a criminal statute for illegally practicing medicine.

In a civil case, the courts are more concerned with compensating people for damages they have suffered because of improper actions than with punishment. It is difficult to provide absolute distinctions between criminal and civil matters, however, because legislatures have recognized that private litigation may also play an important role in public policy. To encourage private litigation, some statutes provide that litigants are entitled to a multiple of their damages. If the behavior of the defendant is reprehensible or careless, the courts sometimes impose punitive damages to discourage the defendant. In the antitrust area, Congress recognized that the attorney general did not have the budget to bring every possible antitrust suit. To encourage private parties to bring antitrust actions, Congress provided that private litigants could recover not only their damages but three times their damages and receive reimbursement of attorneys' fees as well.

Civil Litigation

The two basic forms of civil litigation are disputes over contracts and claims for negligent or intentional infliction of injury, known as torts. The law of contracts allows private parties to create their own legal framework to govern their behavior. When parties enter into a contract, both parties are expected to perform their obligations. If one of the parties fails to perform the agreed obligation, the court will award damages based on the value of the performance the injured party did not receive. Tort liability, on the other hand, recognizes that each of us has a duty to act in a reasonable manner and that where our failure to act in a reasonable manner hurts or damages someone, and the damage was reasonably foreseeable, the court will award a monetary payment intended to equal damages caused.

An illustration of the difference between contracts and torts can be seen in the case of *Hawkins v. McGee* (1929), where a physician told a patient that the physician would transplant skin to replace damaged skin on the palm of the hand. The physician promised that he would make the hand perfect. In fact, the physician transplanted skin from a hairy part of the body to the palm with the result that the plaintiff had a hairy palm. The patient sued. In this classic case, which many law schools use to illustrate the difference between torts and contracts, the question was not whether the physician was negligent for using skin from a hairy part of the body but only whether the physician had promised (contracted) to give the patient a perfect hand, and if so, had he carried out the contract. The court held that the physician had not made good on his promise and awarded damages. Damages were not based on the damage the physician had caused (the tort standard) but on the difference between a hand with hair on the palm and one that was perfect (the damage resulting from the physician's breach of contract).

TORT LIABILITY

Standard of Care

The law of contracts governs many things concerning nurse anesthetists, including their employment, relationships with hospitals and physicians, purchases of drugs and equipment, and numerous other matters. However, when most nurse anesthetists think about the legal system, they think of the law of torts. Tort liability affects nurse anesthetists as it affects any member of society. When engaged in activities during which a failure to act reasonably can reasonably be foreseen to result in harm, each of us owes a duty of care to others to act in the way in which a reasonable person would act. For example, careless operation of an automobile can kill or severely maim other people. We are expected to drive automobiles as reasonably prudent persons would drive their vehicles.

Because the courts do not understand what nurse anesthetists do, they designate nurse anesthesia as a profession. For a professional, the standard of care becomes more complicated. A professional must render care not only as a reasonable person would act, but with the same degree of skill and care as would be practiced by a reasonable member of the profession in similar circumstances. A nurse anesthetist has expertise and education that ordinary members of society do not have. A nurse anesthetist has an obligation to render care to patients that is not merely what a reasonably prudent member of society would render, but care at a level which other nurse anesthetists would render. This gives members of the profession the ability to largely determine the quality of care to be rendered by the profession. When a plaintiff questions whether the nurse anesthetist has rendered appropriate care, the court hears expert testimony as to what that standard is. In some areas of healthcare, the quality of care may vary from geographic community to community. In those cases, practitioners are only held to the standard of care within their community. In specialty areas, such as anesthesia, there is a nationwide standard of care that does not vary from community to community.

Normally, only members of the profession are competent to testify as to the standard of care for their profession. Nurses testify to the standard of care in nursing; physicians testify to the standard of care in medicine. Some people erroneously assume or question whether there is a dual standard of care in the anesthesia field, one for anesthesiologists and one for nurse anesthetists. In fact, because of the nature of anesthesia and the fact that attention and proper monitoring of patients is the overwhelming factor in the safety of anesthesia, there is a single standard of care. The single standard of care is reflected not only in the reality of practice but also in the decided cases that discuss the standard of care. Standard of care is closely related to the quality of care. A profession that renders care at a lower standard than another will necessarily have a different quality of care. In the anesthesia field there is a rather uniform quality of care between nurse anesthetists and anesthesiologists, and that is further evidence that the standard of care is the same. In the area of anesthesia, even though care is given by members of both groups, there is only one standard of care to be followed by both nurse anesthetists and anesthesiologists. Consequently, there are cases when courts have permitted anesthesiologists to testify as to the standard of care to be followed by nurse anesthetists and cases where nurse anesthetists have been allowed to testify as to the standard of care for anesthesiologists (*Carolan v. Hill*, 1977).

The standard of care for nurses is "to apply that degree of skill and learning in treating and nursing a patient which is customarily applied in treating or caring for the sick or wounded who are suffering in the same community." The Michigan case of *Whitney v. Day* (1980) is interesting because it was claimed that nurses were not entitled to a shortened statute of limitations available for professionals sued for malpractice. The charge was made that nurses had to be examined on the same negligence standard as the general population. In *Whitney v. Day*, the court specifically discussed the profession of nurse anesthetists. The court said:

> "... nurse anesthetists are licensed as nurses and then they are certified after an 18 month period of study [this has, of course, been increased since the case was decided in 1980] in their specialty. Thus, they are professionals who have expertise in an area that is akin to the practice of medicine. Because a nurse anesthetist possesses responsibilities greater than those possessed by an ordinary nurse, and because those responsibilities lie in an area of expertise in which some physicians receive full residency training, we conclude that it was not an error for the trial court to set forth a standard which ... [incorporates the malpractice standard] (p. 711)."

The court pointed out that the Michigan statute had been amended so that malpractice limitations were specifically made effective to nurses.

Since nurse anesthetists have been recognized as a separate professional group that establishes its own standard of care, it is understandable that the uninformed would assume that this standard of care would be different than that of an anesthesiologist. For example, in another Michigan case, *Theophelis v. Lansing General Hospital* (1985), there had been a suit against a hospital where both the nurse anesthetists and the anesthesiologist had been released from liability prior to trial. In what really amounted to legal maneuvering in the absence of any factual information, the hospital argued that a release of the nurse anesthetists and the anesthesiologist implied that the hospital was innocent as well. The court, attempting to justify the trial court's determination to let trial proceed against the hospital, wrote:

> ". . . we note for example that it would have been possible for the jury to determine that Nurse Palmer, given her limited training, was not negligent in failing to use a precordial stethoscope but that the hospital was negligent in not requiring the use of one (p. 252)."

This is sheer speculation on the part of the court and does not in any way determine that there is a different standard of care for nurse anesthetists. It does, however, illustrate what can happen when laypersons (who unfortunately include judges) are allowed to speculate, in the absence of information, about the nature of nurse anesthetists and nurse anesthesia.

More typical is the case of *Webb v. Jorns* (1971). In this case involving a cardiac arrest during the course of administering the anesthetic, the court turned its attention to whether the nurse anesthetist had been negligent, specifically whether the patient had received an overdose of halothane. The expert testimony introduced was that of a physician. The testimony did not concern what a nurse anesthetist would or would not have done under the circumstances but rather whether in the physician's judgment there had been an overdose of halothane. The physician had testified that a mixture in excess of 1.5 percent halothane would have been an overdose, but the facts supported the position of the nurse anesthetist that the mixture had never exceeded 1.5 percent. Thus, the standard by which negligence was judged was a general standard based on what happens in the anesthesia area and not one that focused on whether nurse anesthetists follow different standards than anesthesiologists. It is not conceivable that nurse anesthetists would consider a maximum dosage to be 1.5 percent while anesthesiologists would have another maximum dose limitation.

Other cases which support the view of a single standard of care in anesthesia are: *Parks v. Perry* (1984), [numbness and weakness in a patient's hand submitted to the jury under the doctrine of *res ipsa loquitur* based on expert testimony that the damage would not have occurred in the absence of negligent administration of an anesthetic. No reference to the standard of care by nurse anesthetists or that of anesthesiologists] and *Yoos v. Jewish Hospital of St. Louis* (1982), [the court did not look at separate standards of care, but at what should and should not occur in the field of anesthesia].

Why is there only one standard of care in the anesthesia field? Because there is only one quality of care. Studies have shown that anesthesia incidents tend to occur because of human error or failure, not because of lack of education. Care and attentiveness are not attributes that depend on whether the practitioner is a nurse or a physician. Therefore, the standard of care in anesthesia is to be as careful and attentive as the human mind will permit.

The issue of the standard of care is a factual matter because it depends on the testimony of expert witnesses. What the expert testifies to and what the jury believes can vary from case to case. Disquieting though it may be, as a practical matter it must be recognized that the standard of professional care is determined on an individual basis for each case. Thus, to discuss whether something is or is not required by the standard of care is really to make a prediction as to what experts will testify to and what will be believed by both jury and judge during the malpractice trial.

This point is illustrated by the case of *Washington v. Washington Hospital Center, et al.* (1990). Expert testimony as to what constitutes the standard of care cannot be based on mere speculation or conjecture but should have a factual basis. "While absolute certainty is not required, opinion evidence that is conjectural or speculative is not permitted (*Washington v. Washington Hospital Center* quoting from *Sponaugle v. Pre-term, Inc.*, 1980)." The testimony must show what the standard is as practiced by the profession. What a single practitioner would do does not establish the standard of care. Similarly, the testimony should not be what the expert would have done under similar circumstances, but what members of the profession would do.

In the *Washington* case, the plaintiff was a healthy 36-year-old woman who underwent elective surgery at the Washington Hospital Center on November 7, 1987. An endotracheal tube was inserted into the esophagus rather than the trachea. It was not noticed until it was too late and the plaintiff suffered catastrophic brain injury. The nurse anesthetist and anesthesiologist settled and the case proceeded only against the hospital. It was claimed that the hospital was negligent in failing to provide an end-tidal CO_2 monitor which would have allowed early detection of insufficient oxygen, arguably in time to prevent the brain injury. After a jury verdict in favor of the plaintiff, the hospital asked the trial court to rule that the expert testimony offered was insufficient and that judgment should have been entered in the hospital's favor, notwithstanding the jury verdict. The trial court refused and the hospital appealed the decision to the District of Columbia Court of Appeals.

The plaintiff's expert had testified that the hospital deviated from the standard of care by failing to supply a CO_2 monitoring device. Among other things, the hospital claimed that the plaintiff's expert lacked an adequate factual basis for his testimony. The court noted that the standard of care was as follows:

> "...the course of action that a reasonably prudent [professional] with the defendant's specialty would have taken under the same or similar circumstances.... Thus the question for decision is whether the evidence as a whole and reasonable inferences therefrom, would allow a reasonable juror to find that a reasonably prudent tertiary care hospital ... at the time of [plaintiff's] injury in November 1987 and according to national standards, would have supplied a carbon dioxide monitor to a patient undergoing general anesthesia for elective surgery."

The plaintiff's expert had testified that the standard of care in November 1987 required a hospital to provide an end-tidal CO_2 monitor. The hospital charged that the plaintiff's expert based his opinion on inadequate facts. Even though the expert gave no testimony on the number of hospitals having end-tidal CO_2 monitors in place in 1987 and never referred to any written standards or authority as the basis of his opinion, the court concluded that his opinion, combined with other evidence concerning the standard of care, was sufficient to create an issue for the jury.

The hospital argued that end-tidal CO_2 monitors were not the standard of care. It pointed to an American Society of Anesthesiologists (ASA) policy that recommended but did not require them and standards adopted by Harvard Medical School teaching hospitals which referred to CO_2 monitors only as an "emerging" standard. The court indicated nonetheless that the jury's conclusion should be allowed to stand based on other testimony introduced at trial. The question was what a reasonably prudent hospital would do and "Hence, care and foresight exceeding the minimum required by law or mandatory professional regulation may be necessary to meet that standard." Thus, the fact that neither the ASA nor Harvard Medical School recognized CO_2 monitors as a standard of care was irrelevant if a reasonably prudent hospital would have provided them.

To someone not familiar with anesthesia as it was practiced in 1987, the principles underlying the *Washington* case seem straightforward. To those familiar with anesthesia in this period, the proof that was offered in the *Washington* case that CO_2 monitors were the standard of care seems pretty thin. Most practitioners would have agreed that end-tidal CO_2 monitors were not widely used in 1987 and were not part of the standard of care. Thus, a valuable lesson about the legal standard of care must be learned. Even though the standard of care is determined by practitioners, it must be found and applied by courts and juries who are subject to their own emotional demands. Those entities have substantial discretion to believe or not believe evidence and sources practitioners might weigh differently. Standards set by professional organizations may be evidence of the standard of care, but they are not necessarily accepted as the standard of care. In addition, the courts reserve the right to determine that the level of care practiced by an entire profession may be inadequate, although this has been rare in the healthcare field.

Failure to Comply with Law or Regulation

The court's right to determine that a level of care is inadequate is similar to the ability of the legislature to set a standard of care without regard to the practices previously followed by a majority of the profession. Once the legislature enacts legislation creating the standard, it is the standard. Failure to follow a standard of care set forth in a statute is negligence in and of itself. This is known as "negligence per se." The principle of negligence per se is helpful to a plaintiff because the plaintiff does not have to offer expert testimony on the standard of care followed by the profession. *Central Anesthesia Associates, P.C., et al. v. Worthy, et al.* (1985) demonstrates the application of this legal principle.

In the *Worthy* case, anesthesia was administered by a registered nurse enrolled as a student nurse anesthetist in a school operating at a hospital. The student nurse anesthetist was under the supervision of a physician assistant. During a tubal ligation procedure, the patient, Ms. Worthy, suffered a cardiac arrest resulting in brain damage. During the cardiac arrest, only the obstetrician/gynecologist, the physician assistant, and the student nurse anesthetist were in the operating room where the surgery was being performed. At the time, Georgia had a statute that required that a CRNA administer anesthesia "under the direction and responsibility of a duly licensed physician with training or experience in anesthesia." The requirement that the supervising physician have "training or experience in anesthesia" is unusual: In states where statutes require supervision, they usually only require that the supervisor be a physician. Large numbers of nurse anesthetists work with surgeons who have no training or experience in anesthesia (in fact, Georgia has since changed its law). Moreover, there is no indication as to whether this standard is higher or lower than normal practice standards. However, whatever Georgia's statute means, it does not mean that a physician assistant can supervise a student nurse anesthetist.

The *Worthy* court held that the Georgia statute created a standard of conduct for those who are authorized to administer anesthesia. For negligence per se to apply, the person injured must be someone the statute was trying to protect. The court also held that the standard of conduct was created by the legislature to protect patients, such as the plaintiff, from unreasonable risks associated with the administration of anesthesia. The court held that under the statute, the role of supervising a nurse administering anesthesia could not be delegated to a physician assistant. As a result, the court concluded that the defendants had violated the statute and were, therefore, negligent per se.

Other Evidence of the Standard of Care

The standard of care is set by the profession except when courts may require a higher standard, if the profession sets it at an inadequate level. The legislature may also establish a standard of care in its discretion. Nonetheless, nongovernmental bodies, such as professional and accrediting agencies, hospitals and institutions may establish rules or policies that can be considered by the judge or jury as evidence of the standard of care. In certain cases, hospital or institutional rules can become binding by contract. In

Williams v. St. Claire Medical Center (1983), the issue presented to the court was whether a hospital owed a duty to its patients to enforce its policies and bylaws and, if so, whether a violation of these policies and bylaws constituted negligence per se. The patient suffered permanent brain damage while being administered an anesthetic by a nurse anesthetist who was not a CRNA.

The hospital's policy required that anesthetics be administered by a CRNA or a qualified physician. In addition, CRNAs were required to be supervised by the chairperson of anesthesia services and be in communication with an anesthesiologist and surgeon or obstetrician, except in emergency procedures, when an anesthesiologist was not available. At the time of the incident, the hospital, contrary to its own policies, did not have an anesthesiologist on staff and the nurse anesthetist, who had graduated from school only one month prior to the incident, had not yet taken the examination for certification and was not a CRNA.

The court held that when a patient consents to and authorizes an operation, he or she thereby accepts all the rules and regulations of the particular hospital at which the operation is performed. The court further held that while a patient must accept the hospital's particular rules and regulations, the patient should be able to rely on the hospital to follow its rules and regulations, ostensibly established for the patient's care. The plaintiff in this case argued that the hospital's violation of its own policies constituted negligence per se. The court refused to extend negligence per se to a hospital's policies but allowed the policies to be admitted as evidence of negligence. Similarly, in *Castillo v. United States* (1975), violation of institutional policy was not negligence per se but could be considered as a relevant factor in determining the extent of the duty owed to the patient.

Proving that an anesthetist failed to meet the standard of care can be difficult and expensive. Plaintiff's lawyers must obtain testimony as to the standard of care, must obtain and present evidence that the standard of care was breached, and must be able to present this to a jury in a way that will be understandable. This makes the trial of malpractice cases difficult and demanding for plaintiffs' lawyers. The economics of litigation push plaintiffs' lawyers to look for "magic bullets" which allow plaintiffs to recover, without expending the effort and costs of proving negligence. After the decision in the Worthy case was published, a number of cases followed claiming that various routine aspects of nurse anesthesia practice violated state statutes and gave rise to negligence per se. For example, in *Mitchell v. Amarillo Hospital District* (1993), the Texas Court of Appeals dismissed a negligence per se case that had argued that nurse anesthesia constituted a denial of constitutionally guaranteed civil rights, and in *Drennan v. Community Health Investment Corporation* (1995, 1996), the Texas appellate courts dismissed yet another negligence per se claim that it was negligence per se for a pharmacy to dispense drugs to a CRNA.

SPECIFIC TOPICS

Vicarious Liability

As hospitals evolved in the later part of the 19th century, the courts were confronted with a new entity. How they dealt with this entity demonstrates the application of fairness, consistency, predictability and the effectuation of public policy. Part of the public policy in assessing damage for tort liability is to discourage dangerous conduct. Persons held liable should be able to adjust their conduct to avoid situations that cause damage. Moreover, persons liable should either be able to afford the damage or should be in a position to pass the cost of reimbursing injured parties on to other users of the products or services.

How did the courts award damage caused by nurses employed by hospitals but who were assisting independent contracting physicians? While nurses were liable for their own negligence, this was often little help to patients since the nurses were often paid too little to be capable of paying for the damage their negligence might have caused. At the same time, the nurses were employed by hospitals that frequently were charitable institutions. Hospitals seldom made sufficient profit to absorb the cost of negligence of their employees. Much of a hospital's operating budget was dependent on charitable contributions. Holding hospitals liable for the negligence of the nurses they employed really meant asking contributors to the hospitals to pay patients for damages incurred. Consequently, the courts borrowed "sovereign immunity," an ancient English legal doctrine that the king could not be liable because the king could do no wrong. This developed into the doctrine of "charitable immunity": hospitals would not be liable for the negligence of their employees.

The doctrine of charitable immunity can be traced back to 1876 and the Massachusetts case of *McDonald v. Massachusetts General Hospital* (1876). In *McDonald*, a patient claimed that he had been damaged by the actions of a doctor on the staff of Massachusetts General Hospital. The patient was receiving free care at the hospital and the physicians and surgeons were also providing free services. Moreover, funds for Massachusetts General Hospital were derived primarily from grants and donations. Patients paid only according to their ability and not according to services they received. The Massachusetts court reasoned that the hospital was acting as if it were a government agency. Just as a government has sovereign immunity (meaning neither the king nor his government can be sued), the court held that a charity engaged in similar activities had charitable immunity. If the grants and donations the charity solicited from the public were used to pay malpractice claims, the court worried that the public would not support the hospital, and a worthwhile activity would be denied the public. The result of this policy was that patients themselves would bear the risk of negligence encountered. However, the courts were not willing to agree that patients who were injured at charitable hospitals could have no recourse.

One of the principles of tort law was the doctrine of "respondeat superior": let the master answer. When damage is caused by a servant (later referred to as an employee), the master (later referred to as an employer) should be held responsible for it. It was the employer who controlled the way things were done and was in the best position to see that the action giving rise to negligence was avoided. It was the employer who sold the product, set the price, and earned the profit. When respondeat superior was applied to hospitals, the idea of holding the hospital responsible was not appealing. Who served in the role of "master" with regard to a nurse's negligence that occurred in a hospital? Ultimately, the courts agreed that the answer was the surgeon. It was the surgeon who attracted patients to a hospital, the surgeon who profited from the services of the hospital and its nursing employees, and the surgeon who had the apparent authority to be responsible to see that negligent actions were controlled and did not cause damage. Although the surgeon was not the employer in a strict sense, negligence of the nurse and other hospital employees was attributed to the surgeon.

In a number of cases, including *Schloendorf v. Society of New York Hospital* (1914), the courts held that physicians who were on the hospital's staff were not employees of the hospital and the physician's negligence could not be blamed on the hospital. Similarly, nurses engaged in treating patients, even though paid by the hospital, were acting to benefit the surgeon and should be treated as servants of the surgeon. This developed into doctrines known as "captain of the ship" (which holds that once the surgeon assumes control of the operating room, the surgeon is responsible for everything, including negligence that occurs) and "borrowed servant" (which holds that a doctor may be held liable for the negligence of a hospital employee who is subject to the doctor's control).

But what of the hospital's administrative employees who are not engaged in patient care? They could not be said to be borrowed by surgeons no matter what simile or metaphor was suggested. Moreover, nurses did not spend all of their time on patient care; time was spent on administrative matters, as well. Despite the doctrines of captain of the ship and borrowed servant, there were some activities of hospital employees for which only the hospital could be liable. In some states, persons damaged by administrative acts of hospital employees were unable to recover. In other states, the courts attempted to deal with this problem by developing exceptions to charitable immunity and captain of the ship. When a nurse negligently injured a patient while engaged in administrative activities the hospital was liable, but when a nurse injured a patient while engaged in medical duties, the surgeon was liable. Because even in the earliest days of the 20th century, the healthcare field was quite complicated and because lawyers and courts do not understand healthcare, these fine distinctions led to a number of seemingly inconsistent holdings about the liability of nurses and hospital employees. Because there were activities of their employees for which the hospitals were liable and a sense that charitable immunity would not last forever, hospitals began to purchase liability insurance. In 1957, New York began to roll back its support of the doctrines of charitable immunity and captain of the ship (*Bing v. Thunig*, 1957). The court in *Bing v. Thunig* emphasized the inconsistent results of charitable immunity.

As charitable immunity died, one would have expected its companions, captain of the ship and borrowed servant, to die with it. However, they continued as the courts made difficult decisions between consistency and predictability on the one hand and fairness on the other. As the captain of the ship doctrine unfolded and was further developed by the courts, the courts realized that what was important about the relationship of the surgeon to the hospital staff was not the legal status of employer/employee (which everyone knew was a fiction) but the nature of control established by the surgeon. Where the surgeon actually controlled the negligent act, the nurse or other assistant was acting as the surgeon's agent and the negligence of the nurse or other assistant should properly be charged to the surgeon. Because anesthesia is a specialized area requiring additional education, surgeons do not normally control the actions of nurse anesthetists. Captain of the ship and its fellow travelers, such as borrowed servant, have fallen out of favor in recent years as courts have more clearly seen that an operating room is a complex byplay of professionals with areas of specialty, and that the surgeon's role is one of coordination rather than control. Increasingly, surgeons are held liable only when they actually control the action that gives rise to the negligence and not when they are deemed to have assumed the helm of the operating room or to satisfy other nautical or military analogies.

Misrepresentations Concerning Vicarious Liability of Nurse Anesthetists

In the early part of the 1980s, the number of anesthesiologists in the United States increased dramatically. Certain anesthesiologists had believed that when there was a sufficient number of anesthesiologists, the healthcare community would turn to physician anesthesia and the practice of nurse anesthesia would die out. When that did not happen, some anesthesiologists began to compete with nurse anesthetists by warning surgeons of the so-called significant risks that surgeons took when operating with a nurse anesthetist rather than an anesthesiologist. This risk was based in large part on the captain of the ship theory of legal liability even though fewer and fewer states recognized it.

In holding physicians liable for the negligence of anesthetists, the courts, except in states still following captain of the ship, do not look at whether the anesthesia administrator is a nurse or a physician but at the degree of control the physician exercises over the anesthesia administrator. Thus, a court may render different conclusions for cases that involve a physician working with a CRNA or, for that matter, a physician working with an anesthesiologist, if the physician controlled the anesthetist in one case but not in the other. A physician or authorized provider is neither automatically liable when working with a CRNA, nor is the physician immune from liability when working with an anesthesiologist. In *Schneider v. Einstein Medical Center* (1978)) and *Kitto v. Gilbert* (1977), the court found surgeons liable for the negligence of anesthesiologists because the surgeons controlled the anesthesiologists' actions. The question, as in cases of a physician working with CRNAs, is whether the physician was in control of the acts of the anesthesiologists. This is a factual inquiry and not a conclusion of law. There are many cases in which courts have found that the surgeon was not in control of the CRNA and, therefore, not liable for the negligence of the CRNA: *Cavero v. Franklin Benevolence Society* (1950); *Kemalyan v. Henderson* (1954); *Sesselman v. Mulenberg Hospital* (1954); *Hughes v. St. Paul Fire and Marine Insurance Company* (1981); *Fortson v. McNamara* (1987); *Pierre v. Lavallie Kamp Charity Hospital* (1987); and *Thomas v. Raleigh General Hospital* (1987).

Even in cases in which the surgeon was held liable there is often evidence of individual wrongdoing on the part of the surgeon. Moreover, numerous cases hold that mere supervision or direction of a CRNA is insufficient evidence to hold a physician liable for the CRNA's negligence. See, for example, *Whitfield v. Whittaker Memorial Hospital* (1969); *Foster v. Englewood Hospital* (1974); *Elizondo v. Tavarez* (1980); *Baird v. Sickler* (1982); *McCullough v. Bethany Medical Center* (1984); and *Parker v. Vanderbilt* (1988). It is clear from the case law that in order for a physician to be liable for the acts of the anesthesia administrator, the physician must be in control of the administrator's actions and not merely be supervising or directing the administrator.

Consequently, court decisions concerning liability of surgeons for the negligence of nurse anesthetists have varied depending on the facts of the particular case. Where surgeons have been held to be in control they have been held liable, and where they have not, they have not been held liable. The same principles govern liability of surgeons for negligence of anesthesiologists.

It does not make sense for either nurse anesthetists or anesthesiologists to attempt to capitalize on the errors of the other. Not only can anesthesiologists make mistakes, but surgeons can be sued when they work with anesthesiologists just as easily as they can when they work with nurse anesthetists: *Seneris v. Haas* (1955); *Medvecz v. Choi* (1977); *Thompson v. Presbyterian Hospital* (1982); *Kerber v. Sarles* (1989); *Menzie v. Windom Community Memorial Hospital* (1991); *Brown v. Bozorgi* (1992); *Ruby Jones v. Neuroscience Associates, Inc.* (1992); *Adams v. Childrens Mercy Hospital* (1993); *Szabo v. Bryn Mawr Hospital* (1994); *Costell v. Toledo Hospital* (1994); *Robertson v. Hospital Corporation of America* (1995); *Dunn v. Maras* (1995); *Tiburzio-Kelly v. Montgomery* (1996); and *Bert v. Meyer* (1997).

The Lawyer

Although anesthesia is very safe, nurse anesthetists face occasional litigation or may require assistance to deal with regulatory boards. Courts and administrative agencies have their own rules to make their tasks flow more efficiently. Thus, nurse anesthetists may meet another element of the legal system, the lawyer. One of the biggest benefits of professional liability insurance is that it will cover the cost of a lawyer to represent the nurse anesthetist who faces suit. The lawyer provided by professional liability insurance will face a number of important, if conflicting, concerns as he or she addresses a case. Litigation can be and often is extremely expensive. Litigation is also uncertain. We all like to think that we govern our activities solely on the basis of logic, however, human beings, including those who serve on juries, are complicated. Sometimes they are affected by things which are not logical, including emotions such as sympathy for a severely damaged patient.

Finally, the parties in any given litigation matter are engaged in a complex drama in which interests and relationships often are not what they appear to be. For example, the nurse anesthetist involved in a malpractice lawsuit is provided a lawyer by the insurance carrier. The nurse anesthetist's attorney has a duty of loyalty to the nurse anesthetist. However, the lawyer is hired by the insurance company and the attorney's bills will be paid by the insurance company. Usually, this will not be the only matter referred to the attorney by the insurance company. On the other hand, nurse anesthetists are rarely involved in more than one malpractice claim. A nurse anesthetist whose practice creates enough malpractice claims to have a regular relationship with a malpractice attorney will probably lose the ability to practice either because of the inability to obtain malpractice insurance or as a result of a licensing decision. Human nature makes it likely that the attorney will have more loyalty to the insurance company than to the insured.

Sometimes there can be a conflict between the insurance company and the insured. To an insurance company, litigation is often a simple financial decision. If it is going to cost a lot in legal fees to defend a case and if a jury is likely to award a large recovery regardless of fault, then business concerns suggest that the case be settled and the risk of greater loss avoided. To a healthcare practitioner, who views himself or herself as innocent, deciding whether to settle may not be that easy. Agreeing to a settlement carries with it a number of unpleasant ramifications. The practitioner's name will be referred to the National Practitioner Data Bank. People may assume that if a practitioner settled, he or she must have done something wrong. A settlement can cause problems later on and may have to be explained to future employers. How willing will the insurance company be to continue to provide insurance coverage for a practitioner who has cost them a lot of money? From the insurance company's standpoint, it is easy for insureds to want the insurance company to defend their honor, no matter the cost. Insureds do not have to pay for it.

Because of these conflicts inherent in the insurance relationship, the question sometimes arises: Who does the lawyer represent? The case of *Trementozzi vs. Safety Insurance Co.* (1991) stated that the duty of a lawyer provided by an insurance company is to represent the insured and not the insurance company even though the insurance company may pay the bills. Both the lawyer and the insurance company are obligated to act in the best interests of the insured.

Lawyers are not supposed to represent clients with different interests at the same time. The Model Code of Professional Responsibility (1980) of the American Bar Association has been adopted by many states. It provides that:

> "The professional judgment of a lawyer should be exercised within the bounds of the law, solely for the benefit of his client and free of compromising influences and loyalties. Neither his personal interests, the interests of other clients, nor the desires of third persons should be permitted to dilute his loyalty to his client.... Maintaining the independence of professional judgment required of a lawyer precludes his acceptance or continuation of employment that will adversely affect his judgment on behalf of or dilute his loyalty to a client. This problem arises whenever a lawyer is asked to represent two or more clients who may have differing interests, whether such interests be conflicting, inconsistent, diverse or otherwise discordant."

Nurse anesthetists must be aware of and involved in their legal defense. Even knowledgeable healthcare defense attorneys may not be familiar with the capabilities of nurse anesthetists. The insurance company may also be providing coverage for multiple defendants. Nurse anesthetists must be vigilant that their interests are being protected and that they are entitled to a defense that protects their best interests, not the interests of the insurance company paying the bills.

The attorney/client privilege protects one of the oldest confidential relationships in society. Communication between attorney and client is protected because of the need of attorneys and their clients to have open, full and frank discussions. What happens to this privilege when the attorney is representing conflicting clients? The attorney/client privilege only protects documents and disclosures that are not disclosed to third parties. If someone discloses information to persons with whom there is no privilege, then the information is not confidential and it is no longer privileged even if his or her attorney were part of the group to whom the information was disclosed.

Damages

The amount of damages awarded to a successful plaintiff depends on the type of case. In a suit based on a breach of contract, damages are based on the difference between what was promised or agreed to and what was delivered. In a tort case, damages are measured by the value of the damage inflicted by the defendant. In the healthcare field, trying to value the damage caused is a significant area of dispute. As with many other areas for which there cannot be precise answers, damages are an area for the jury to answer as best it can. In the case of bodily injury, monetary damages are awarded to compensate people for damage that has no monetary value. What is the value of a chipped tooth? How do you compensate for the loss of eyesight or death with a monetary award? Some lawyers have been quite successful in refining techniques to increase jury awards for damage to the body. Awarding damages when harm results from a failure to meet the standard of care compensates the individual who was damaged and encourages practitioners to be careful. Damages based on the value of the injury caused, even if it is difficult to value, are called compensatory damages.

If the wrongdoing has been intentional or gives a sense of outrage, courts may award punitive or exemplary damages. Something more than mere negligence is required for punitive damages. There must be circumstances of aggravation, spite, or malice; a fraudulent or evil motive; or a conscious disregard of the interests of others (Prosser, 1995). Punitive damages are private fines imposed to punish reprehensible conduct and to deter its future occurrence.

An important aspect of punitive damages is the lack of insurance coverage. Many professional liability insurance policies do not insure against intentional acts. Punitive damages are imposed for intentional actions and therefore are not covered by insurance. Critics of the legal system contend that, in the healthcare field, when juries award punitive damages, they merely multiply their award. Since awarding compensatory damage for bodily damage has little basis in reality anyway, compensatory damage already punishes the defendant. Awarding punitive damages is just another opportunity to invite a jury to grant large awards.

Cases imposing punitive damages against nurse anesthetists are rare. The Georgia Court of Appeals, in a close 5:4 split, reversed the award of punitive damages in a case where, apparently, the anesthesia machine ran out of agent and had to be refilled during the operation. Running out of an anesthetic agent in the middle of surgery is, obviously, a violation of the standard of care.

Four of the nine judges would have upheld the award of punitive damages. They reasoned that the jury had determined that the anesthesia machine would not have run out of agent if it had been checked. The failure to check the level of anesthetic was similar to failing to check the level of gas before flying an airplane. It shows such a conscious indifference to the patient's well-being that the jury was entitled to award punitive damages. On the other hand, the majority of the Court of Appeals held that there was no evidence of an intentional disregard of the rights of the patient nor was there any evidence that the anesthesia providers knowingly or willfully disregarded the rights of the patient so as to authorize a finding of conscious indifference to consequences (1991).

Another case involving punitive damages arose in Arkansas, where a jury assessed $3 million in punitive damages against the manufacturer of a ventilator. There was evidence that the manufacturer was aware that anesthetists using a selector valve could easily place hoses on the wrong unmarked valve with disastrous results. In the Arkansas case, someone had incorrectly put a hose where a bag should have been connected. When the nurse anesthetist decided to change bags, she attached a hose to the wrong port. The effect of the improper connection was to permit the anesthesia machine to continue to pump air into the patient's lungs, with no way for the air to escape. The ensuing buildup of pressure and lack of oxygen resulted in damage to the patient's lungs and brain. The rule for imposing punitive damages in Arkansas is that the defendant must have known, or ought to have known, in light of the surrounding circumstances, that its conduct would naturally or probably result in injury and that the defendant continued such conduct in reckless disregard. The manufacturer claimed it was not at fault because separate acts of negligence had to occur for the accident to result. Many witnesses testified that the accident was foreseeable. The unmarked valve had been criticized in premarket tests, and other similar incidents involving the machine had been reported. The appeals court upheld the jury award of punitive damages because the manufacturer knew that the patient's life always depended on the artificial breathing supplied by the ventilator (*Airco, Inc., Appellant, v. Simmons First National Bank, Guardian*, 1982).

Because of the great risks involved in anesthesia, even the smallest moment of carelessness can have disastrous consequences. Nurse anesthetists can avoid the imposition of punitive damages by being able to prove that they followed procedures, such as the use of checklists designed to minimize the possibility of lapses, and by being able to document that they acted in the best interest of their patient, even after an incident occurred.

Res Ipsa Loquitur

A key element of the law of negligence is fault: Awards are made against a defendant because the defendant caused the damage. The theoretic basis of negligence or malpractice is that the defendant should pay for damages caused to the plaintiff because, between the two parties, the one who was at fault should bear the damage. In terms of prevention, the knowledge that one can be held liable for malpractice or negligence is supposed to make people more careful and avoid negligent actions in the future. In cases involving anesthesia, how does the patient show that the anesthetist was at fault? The field is too complicated for the average patient to understand. Sometimes the patient does not even know what happened because they were unconscious. As a result, many cases involving malpractice of anesthetists are decided under the legal doctrine of *res ipsa loquitur*.

Res ipsa loquitur, literally translated as "the thing speaks for itself," had its basis in a case decided in 1863 in which a barrel of flour rolled out of a warehouse window and fell on a passing pedestrian (*Byrne v. Boadle*,1863). Although the injured pedestrian had not personally observed whatever went wrong on the upper floor of the warehouse, it was clear that this type of accident would not have happened without someone's negligence. Whoever caused it must have been under the control of the warehouse owner (Prosser, 1995).

The doctrine of *res ipsa loquitur* depends on three things: (1) the injury must occur under circumstances such that in the ordinary course of events the injury would not have occurred if someone had not been negligent, (2) the injury must be caused by something within the exclusive control of the defendant, and (3) the injury must not have been due to any voluntary action or contribution on the part of the plaintiff. Classic examples are exploding boilers, defective food in sealed containers, and various types of falling objects including not only barrels of flour, but elevators and, in one case, a 600-pound cow.

Anesthesia accidents have become prime examples for the application of the doctrine of *res ipsa loquitur*. In an anesthesia accident, the third requisite, that the plaintiff did not contribute to the accident, is almost always true, especially where the patient is unconscious. Similarly, if an anesthesia injury has occurred, the instrumentality that caused the damage will often have been within the exclusive control of the anesthetist. It is the application of the first requisite, that the event must be of a kind that ordinarily does not occur in the absence of someone's negligence, that has caused whatever theoretic disputes there may be over the application of the doctrine to anesthesia.

The basis of the law of negligence is fault. Many accidents can occur without anyone being at fault. Someone slipping and falling, a blowout of a tire, skidding cars, and fires of unknown origin have all been held to be situations where the doctrine of *res ipsa loquitur* would not apply because it could not be said that the injury could not have occurred without negligence (Prosser, 1995).

Theoretically, laypeople are supposed to understand that anesthesia is an area where accidents can happen without anyone being at fault. Realistically, however, it is a tribute to anesthetists that anesthesia accidents occur so infrequently that there is a common tendency, albeit incorrect, to believe that the accident would not have occurred without someone being negligent. There is also a financial incentive for the patient to base the case on *res ipsa loquitur*. Lawsuits can be very expensive and part of the expense is hiring expert witnesses to testify as to the standard of care. The major benefit to a patient of the doctrine of *res ipsa loquitur* is that it moves the burden of proof to the defendant.

How can a defendant-anesthetist defend a case of *res ipsa loquitur*? The defendant must introduce proof that (1) whatever instrumentalities were in the defendant's exclusive control during the operation were not those that caused the injuries, and/or (2) there were ways in which the incident could have occurred other than as a result of the anesthetist's negligence. Thus, in anesthesia cases, the role of the jury becomes one of choosing to believe the defendant's expert witnesses or the plaintiff's expert witnesses as to whether the injury would have occurred without negligence.

SUMMARY

The legal system is imperfect, as are all human systems, in its attempts to resolve disputes in a fair, consistent, and predictable manner. Nurse anesthetists should be aware of their status as professionals and the principle that the system expects them to act as other nurse anesthetists would act.

The author would like to thank Betsy L. Wolf for her assistance with the material on negligence per se, which appeared in the AANA Journal.

REFERENCES

Adams v. Childrens Mercy Hospital (848 S.W. 2d 535, Missouri Court of Appeals, 1993).

Airco Inc., Appellant, v. Simmons First National Bank, Guardian (2765 Ark. 486, 638 S.W. 2d 660, 1982).

American Bar Association, Model Code of Professional Responsibility, EC5-14, 1980.

Baird v. Sickler (69 Ohio St. 2d 652 1982).

Bentley v. Langley (249 S.E. 2d 481, N.C. 1978).

Bert v. Meyer (663 N.Y.S. 2d 99, N.Y., 1997).

Bing v. Thunig (2 N.Y. 2d 656, 143 N.E. 2d 3, 1957).

Brown v. Bozorgi (234 Il. App. 3d 972, 602 N.E. 2d 48, 1992).

Byrne v. Boadle (1863 159 Eng. Rep. 299).

California Nursing Act (Calif. Business and Professions Code, Chapter 6, Code 2725, 1974).

Carolan v. Hill (553 N.W. 2d 882, Iowa, 1996).

Castillo v. U.S. (406 F. Supp. 585 N.M., 1975).

Central Anesthesia Associates, P.C., et al. v. Worth, et al. (254 Ga. 728, 333 S.E. 2d 829, 1985).

Chalmers-Francis v. Nelson (6 Calif. 2d 402, 1936).

Cornfeldt v. Tongen (262 N.W. 2d 684, Minn., 1977).

Costell v. Toledo Hospital (98 Ohio App. 3d 586, 649 N.E. 2d 35, 1994).

Davero v. Franklin Benevolence Society (223 p.2d 471, Calif., 1950).

Drennan v. Community Health Investment Corporation (905 S.W. 2d 811, Texas, 1995).

Dunn v. Maras (182 Ariz. 412, 897 p.2d 714 1995).

Elizondo v. Tavarez (596 S.W. 2d 667, Texas, 1980).

Fortson v. McNamara (508 S. 2d 35, Fla., 1987).

Foster v. Englewood Hospital (19 Il. App. 3d 1055 1974).

Hawkins v. McGee (84 N.H. 114, 146 A. 641, N.H., 1929).

Hughes v. St. Paul Fire and Marine Insurance Company (401 S. 2d 35, Fla., 1987).

Kemalyan v. Henderson (277 p.2d 372, Wash., 1954).

Kerber v. Sarles (542 N.Y.S. 2d 94, 151 Ad.2d 1031, (N.Y., 1989).

Kitto v. Gilbert (570 p.2d 544, Colo., 1977).

Magit v. State of California (57 Calif. 2d 74, 1961).

McCullough v. Bethany Medical Center (235 Kan. 732 1984).

McDonald v. Massachusetts General Hospital (120 Mass. 432, 1879).

Medvecz v. Choi (569 F. 2d 1221, U.S. Ct. of App., 3d Cir., 1977).

Menzie v. Windom Community Memorial Hospital (774 F. Supp. 91 U.S.D.C.,Conn., 1991).

Mitchell v. Amarillo Hospital District (885 S.W. 2d 857, Texas, 1993).

Parker v. Vanderbilt (767 S.W. 2d 412, Tenn., 1988).

Parks v. Perry (68 N.C. App. 202, N.C., 1984).

Pierre v. Lavallie Kamp Charity Hospital (515 S. 2d 614, La., 1987).

Prosser, W.L. (Ed.), Keeton, W.P., & Dobbs, W.B. (1995). *Law of Torts, West Group* (5th ed., p. 9,217). West Publishers.

Robertson v. Hospital Corporation of America (653 S. 2d 1265, Court of Appeals of La., 1995.

Ruby Jones v. Neuroscience Associates, Inc. (250 Kan. 477, 827 p.2d 51, 1992).

Schloendorf v. Society of New York Hospital (211 N.Y. 125, 105 N.E. 92, 1914).

Schneider v. Einstein Medical Center (390 A. 2d 1271, Pa., 1978).

Seneris v. Haas (45 Calif. 2d 811, 291 p.2d 915, Calif., 1955).

Sermchief v. Gonzales, (660 S.W. 2d 683, Mo., 1983).

Sesselman v. Mulenberg Hospital (306 A. 2d 474, N.J., 1954).

Sponaugle v. Pre-term, Inc., (411 A. 2d 366, District of Columbia, 1980).

Szabo v. Bryn Mawr Hospital (432 Pa. super. 409, 638 A. 2d 1004, 1994).

Theophelis v. Lansing General Hospital (355 N.W. 2d 249, 1985).

Thomas v. Raleigh General Hospital (358 W.E. 2d 222, W.Va., 1987).

Thompson v. Presbyterian Hospital (652 p.2d 260, Okla., 1982).

Tiburzio-Kelly v. Montgomery (452 Pa. Super. 158, 681 A. 2d 757, 1996).

Trementozzi v. Safety Insurance Co. (Mass. Suffolk Superior Court Civil Action No. 90-1017B, June 26, 1991).

Washington v. Washington Hospital Center, et al (579 A. 2d 177, District of Columbia Court of Appeals, 1990).

Webb v. Jorns (473 S.W. 2d Texas, 1971).

Whitfield v. Whittaker Memorial Hospital (210 Va. 176, 1969).

Whitney v. Day (100 Mich. App. 707, 1980).

Williams v. St. Claire Medical Center (657 S.W. 2d 590 Ky. Ct. App. 1983).

Yoos v. Jewish Hospital of St. Louis (645 S.W. 2d 177, Mo., 1982).

KEY REFERENCES

A broad variety of legal issues involving CRNA practice, employment and other professional issues can be found in the "Legal Briefs" section of the *AANA Journal*. Articles by Gene Blumenreich and other noted legal experts can be reviewed through the annual index of the *Journal*. All publications are available in the library or archives of the AANA in Park Ridge, Illinois.

STUDY QUESTIONS

1. Why is it that courts generally grant substantial deference to the healthcare community? What relationship does this behavior have to traditional definitions of professionalism?

2. Identify which court cases involving CRNAs have had major implications for the profession since the turn of the century. What is their enduring legacy to contemporary practice?

3. Using the AANA standards of care as a reference, discuss how standards developed, what external agencies have influenced them, and how technology and scientific advances have influenced their refinement.

4. Propose reasons why there is a single standard of care in anesthesia for all providers. What benefits does this fact accrue to CRNAs?

5. List the state bureaucratic agencies/bodies and other professional organizations or institutions that have a direct and compelling influence on the standard of care of CRNAs.

6. What argument would you provide a surgeon who is refusing to work with you because of the issue of vicarious liability? What is your rationale and what are the facts?

7. Define and discuss the relevance in practice of the legal doctrines of respondeat superior, captain of the ship, borrowed servant, charitable immunity and *res ipsa loquitur.*

CHAPTER 6

UNDERSTANDING MALPRACTICE LITIGATION

Janet M. Simpson, JD

Holbrook, Heaven and Osborn PA
Kansas City, KS

Gene A. Blumenreich, JD

General Counsel
American Association of Nurse Anesthetists
Boston, MA

KEY CONCEPTS

- Standard of care can be defined as that level of care generally practiced by members of the profession in the same or similar circumstances (community), a deviation from which represents a risk of injury to the patient/plaintiff. Medical negligence may be considered operative when a Certified Registered Nurse Anesthetist (CRNA) does not exercise the required degree of skill and reasonable care espoused by this standard and the action is inclusive of "duty, breach and causation."

- The most commonly considered evidence of whether an appropriate standard of care was upheld comes from the expert witness, who must testify in terms of medical probabilities, events or deviations.

- CRNAs bear the responsibility in tort action to report notice of receipt of a claim or lawsuit to their carrier, be available to meet with an assigned attorney, and actively assist the legal team in preparing the facts, evidence and plan for defense.

- There are several types of depositions in which CRNAs may be involved, all of which require detailed preparation. Depositions are guided by strict protocol and can best be prepared for with careful study and planning.

- Occurrence insurance is by far the preferable type of liability product covering all acts occurring within the policy period, regardless of when the lawsuit is filed.

In the course of an active clinical career, most Certified Registered Nurse Anesthetists (CRNAs) are likely to come into contact with the civil justice system; hopefully not, however, as a defendant. If such an occasion does arise, the CRNA must understand in detail the course of malpractice litigation and how best to defend oneself in that event. In this chapter, the reader is introduced to the most common sources of claims and lawsuits filed against anesthetists. Details are presented regarding the frequency of suits, assertions of negligence, causes of injuries, types of injuries, and amounts of money paid in damages to the plaintiff. By studying this data, one can draw general conclusions regarding the prevention and defense of medical negligence actions. The chapter also acquaints the reader with the process of a medical negligence lawsuit and what to expect during the proceedings, including guidance from the insurance carrier and attorney, depositions and trial testimony, acting as an expert witness, confidential and privileged communications, and settlement and trial considerations. Issues involving professional liability insurance and coverage benefits also are discussed.

Most importantly, the reader will come to appreciate the importance of communication with families as a primary defense against malpractice litigation. Even as the trend nationally has demonstrated a decrease in the number of anesthesia mishaps and complications, the severity of injury from complications may be devastating. Since the risk potential for CRNAs remains the highest of any nursing specialty, it is paramount that CRNAs appreciate the fact that effective, attentive communication with families and patients attenuates litigation risk, but only when accompanied by comprehensive and legible documentation of perioperative events.

CONSIDERATIONS IN NEGLIGENCE

The ever-present threat of a medical negligence lawsuit substantially influences the day-to-day delivery of healthcare. Reasons are numerous, but related generally to consumer dissatisfaction and frustration with the healthcare system at large. The system appears insensitive and often fails to consider the effects of its actions or nonactions on the patient and the patient's family. In addition, adequate healthcare is priced beyond the means of many in society. In the United States today, there are nearly 45 million people who cannot afford health insurance or are underinsured. We spend nearly one trillion dollars a year on healthcare yet provide no universal coverage. With these statistics, it is no wonder that many citizens hold great contempt for the system in general, as well as for the providers who seemingly represent this flawed and unresponsive system. It should also be noted that patients and their families frequently have unrealistic expectations of both the healthcare system and providers. Complicated medical and surgical procedures that do not produce desired outcomes reinforce the public's perception that failure to obtain ideal medical results constitutes negligence. In addition, litigants have unrealistic expectations both of the monetary awards that can be secured in negligence cases and the total cost of litigation itself.

These notions often overshadow the fact that, beginning in the 1980s, anesthesia mishaps have been in steady decline for both nurse and physician providers of anesthesia resulting in an overall mortality rate that has dropped from approximately two deaths for every 10,000 anesthetics given 20 years ago to approximately one death for every 240,000 anesthetics given today. As is consistently shown, there is no statistically significant difference between CRNA and anesthesiologist rates of injury and death attributable to anesthesia-related causes (AANA, 1996).

Components of Medical Negligence

Often one hears the term "medical malpractice" used more frequently in popular jargon than the term "medical negligence." The former is technically incorrect as there is no legal theory of malpractice, be it medical, legal, architectural, or related to any other discipline. There is, however, a legal theory of negligence about which the CRNA must become familiar.

Legal theories are comprised of specific elements and the plaintiff has the burden of proof for all elements of negligence. The first element in negligence is duty. The plaintiff must prove that a duty to exercise reasonable care existed between the plaintiff and the defendant, in this case the anesthetist. Anytime an anesthetist undertakes patient care, he or she must exercise reasonable care. If debate arises on this element it generally involves whether the anesthetist entered into a professional relationship with the patient.

As an example, if two anesthetists with the same last name are working in the same hospital and a plaintiff sues the one who did not provide anesthetic care, the claim fails because there is no duty to exercise reasonable care flowing from the anesthetist sued by the plaintiff. That is, no patient-anesthetist relationship was ever established. Taking a less obvious example, if an anesthetic is planned for 1300 hours, and the patient was visited preoperatively by the anesthetist at 0900 hours, can the patient prevail in a suit if her appendix ruptures between 0900 and 1300 hours? Does a duty exist between the patient and CRNA? The simple answer is probably. However, circumstances involving other required elements will likely arise to make this case defensible as well.

The second element involves breach of the anesthetist's duty to exercise reasonable care with the patient. This is the negligent act, error, or omission part of the formula. The anesthetist must act within the appropriate standard of care in providing anesthesia services to the patient. The patient's petition or complaint filed to initiate the lawsuit generally sets out the allegations of negligence. A plaintiff asserts that several actions were carried out improperly or were omitted, thus making a claim that these actions, errors, and/or omissions constituted negligence on the part of the anesthetist.

For example, the plaintiff may claim the defendant should have employed a regional anesthetic rather than a general technique. This allegation involves negligent professional judgment. A plaintiff may allege the anesthetist improperly placed an endotracheal tube in the esophagus and failed to recognize its misplacement. This involves an allegation of technical error and a judgment or diagnostic error.

In all instances, the breach must have caused physical injury to the plaintiff, or the plaintiff's decedent, as the case may be. This represents the third element of negligence, causation. The anesthetist may have negligently administered the anesthetic, but the patient had no injury. For example, if the CRNA anesthetized the patient with a general anesthetic agent, turned on the ventilator, and left the room, this would constitute improper care. Yet, if the patient awoke at the end of the case without sequelae, a lawsuit based on these circumstances would fail for lack of a causation element as there was no physical injury.

Assume the same conduct by the anesthetist, but this time the patient is injured. The surgeon nicked a ureter. Still, the case of medical negligence fails as to the anesthetist because the nicked ureter and the anesthetist leaving the operating room are not linked. Again, there is no causation element. The plaintiff must prove he or she was injured as a result of the negligent conduct. An unfortunate result, in and of itself, does not raise the question of negligence. In fact, law is to the contrary. In most jurisdictions, the healthcare provider is entitled to exercise his or her best judgment as the public and courts understand that medicine is not an exact science. In some jurisdictions, if the healthcare provider exercises the required degree of skill, he or she is not liable for any honest error in judgment (*Brown v. U.S.*, 1969). This assumes that the action carried out was an action that a reasonable healthcare provider might elect as a treatment option.

ASSESSING STANDARDS OF CARE

For a plaintiff to proceed to a point where a jury can consider the case, he or she must establish what the appropriate standard of care is in relation to the alleged negligent acts or omissions. The standard of care can be defined as that level of care generally practiced by members of the profession in the same or similar circumstances, a deviation from which represents a risk of injury to the patient/plaintiff. The "same or similar community" is also referenced by many when describing the appropriate standard of care. Be aware that the definition of community has expanded dramatically because of continuing education requirements and because national professional groups have promulgated standards and goals for safe practice. Professional groups publishing and endorsing standards hope that by reducing patient injury, the number of medical negligence claims and lawsuits will decrease through improved practice techniques. This will focus the issues and merits for attorney consideration before suits are filed, and shorten the time and expense associated with litigation (Garnick, Hendricks, and Brennan, 1991).

There are a variety of means available to establish, for a jury's consideration, the appropriate standard of care. These include but are not limited to textbooks, authoritative treatises, professional journal articles, facility policy and procedures, standards or policy statements of professional organizations, expert witnesses, state or federal statutes, and prior case law. Textbooks, treatises, and journal articles, however, may not be sufficient by themselves to override the professionals' general practice patterns. This evidence often must be supported with expert testimony (*Mohr v. Jenkins*, 1980). An individual facility's policies and procedures are actually self-imposed standards. They make a statement of the standard of care that is expected of its healthcare providers.

The rationale for these standards is generally patient safety. Therefore, if an anesthetist fails to follow anesthesia departmental policies and procedures, and an adverse result occurs, there is little justification for the deviation. Such cases are difficult to defend successfully. State or federal statutes and prior case law come into play somewhat less frequently. However, consider the statute enacted in Massachusetts, which requires that end-tidal CO_2 monitors and pulse oximeters be used in all general anesthetics. An anesthesia mishap that can be tied to a failure to use one of these legally required monitors would be devastating from a defense standpoint. Legal cases that have been appealed through the appellate courts sometimes make blanket statements of what the court considers the appropriate standard of care to be. This statement can be translated into law in future cases.

DAMAGES

To collect money for negligent conduct, the plaintiff must establish damages. Damages may be of several forms: economic (sometimes called compensatory), noneconomic, or punitive. The petition or complaint also sets out in general terms the damages claimed in the lawsuit. Economic or compensable damages include all things lost to the plaintiff as a result of the alleged negligence and resultant injury that can be measured through economic calculations. Economic damages may include medical expenses attributable to the injury, both past and future; lost wages due to time off work to recover from the injury; and future lost wages. If the patient has died, heirs may be entitled to recover the patient's projected lifetime wages through a claim filed by the deceased's estate.

Loss of household services are routinely compensated as economic damages. Some courts allow economists to testify for the plaintiff as to the economic value of more esoteric functions such as the loss of guidance a parent provides to a child. If the parent has died as a result of medical negligence, that person's minor child may be able to recover the economic loss associated with the parent's guidance and counseling. The precise calculation of economic damages varies considerably among jurisdictions. Calculations change dramatically depending on the circumstances of the parties as well. Look to your attorney for specific information on the calculation of economic damages if you are a defendant and compare this calculation with the amount of professional negligence insurance coverage you have available.

Noneconomic damages are the intangible elements of life. They include pain, suffering, loss of enjoyment of life, and disfigurement. As between a husband and wife, noneconomic damages also include loss of consortium, or loss of sexual or other marital relations, between the two. Some jurisdictions rule that loss of affection, guidance, and counseling to an injured party's minor child fall within noneconomic damages. It is the noneconomic damage portion of awards that the plaintiff has historically tried to inflate. By injecting a medical negligence case with extreme sympathy for the injured party, the plaintiff's attorney seeks to inflate the verdict far in excess of the actual economic damages. Some courts have recently placed caps or maximum recovery limits on the amount of noneconomic damages a plaintiff may recover. The jury is generally allowed to render any verdict it selects. The court then applies the cap, if appropriate, to reduce the noneconomic portion of the verdict.

Occasionally a defendant's conduct will be such that the plaintiff will seek punitive damages. The key words generally found in a petition or complaint that indicate punitive damages requested include gross, willful, and/or wanton. A specific request or prayer for punitive damages may or may not be articulated in the petition or complaint. Seldom does a claim of medical negligence rise to a punitive level. Generally a court must decide whether the evidence is sufficient to allow a jury to consider awarding punitive damages. A court might allow punitive damages when a patient who is under a general anesthetic and on a mechanical ventilator is abandoned by the anesthetist during the course of anesthesia. Habitual negligent conduct may also rise to punitive levels. As the word indicates, punitive damages are meant to punish the offending defendant. These damages are not covered by professional liability insurance and cannot be discharged through bankruptcy proceedings. The defendant is obligated to pay them personally.

ISSUES OF TORT JUSTICE

The original purpose for the tort justice system was to provide compensation and deterrence. In recent years the system has come under more frequent attack for several reasons. Critics claim the system affords variable and unpredictable compensation for injuries. Because a jury determines the dollar award, if any is to be awarded, plaintiffs with similar injuries may receive vastly different awards. Another criticism proposes that too much of the professional liability insurance premium does not reach the injured party. Rather, the premiums are used for defense costs, operating the insurance company, or as profit for the company's shareholders. Finally, critics of the current system assert that too much of the jury award goes to the plaintiff's attorney in fees, generally 33 percent to 50 percent. Deterrence can more readily be handled, it is claimed, through effective risk management and quality improvement efforts.

There are justifications for leaving the basic tort system in place, however. If inequities exist, adjustments in the law can compensate. Allowing a jury to consider evidence on an individual's injuries provides compensation, if deserved, in an amount appropriate for the plaintiff's circumstances. A no-fault compensation system would likely decrease the costs of defending medical negligence claims, but the number of claims would likely rise dramatically, perhaps not saving any money because of the increased overall payout. There are certainly inequities and abuses in the current tort system, but without it, the healthcare provider would have no opportunity to defend his or her reputation, and providers in high-risk healthcare areas might decide to leave practice. Also, checks in the current system make portions of the award paid to a plaintiff's attorney subject to court approval in some jurisdictions. This at least prevents the plaintiff's attorney from blatant overcharging.

THE EXPERT WITNESS

The most commonly considered evidence of whether an appropriate standard of care was upheld comes from the expert witness. The court makes the determination of whether a proposed expert witness qualifies as such and may testify. Some states have statutory limitations on who may testify. For instance, Kansas requires that the expert testifying on liability issues must practice in the same profession at least 50 percent of the time within two years of the incident in question. This is meant to prevent physicians from retiring and spending their golden years in the courtroom supporting or criticizing the actions of others. This does not prevent a retired professional from giving an opinion on causation. All testimony must be offered on the standard of care in place at the time of the incident. This is difficult at times, as several years may pass between the incident and the filing of the lawsuit. Additional years may pass before the case comes to trial. This is especially true in cases where minors are involved and the statute of limitations, in some states, allows filing lawsuits up to 19 years after the alleged negligent conduct.

An expert witness must testify in terms of medical probabilities or events that are more likely than not. An expert may not speculate to establish the alleged deviation. An expert must also indicate a familiarity with the standard of care. To simply advise a jury, "I administer anesthesia this way," is not sufficient. One individual's practice does not comport with the definition of an appropriate standard of care. Expert witness testimony is generally required to show both liability and causation. Causation testimony deals with what medical injuries have been incurred to date as a result of the negligent act and what will likely be suffered in the future.

An expert witness serves the purpose of informing jurors on specialized areas not within the knowledge of laypersons. Occasionally medical negligence cases are filed that can be analyzed without the assistance of medical expert testimony. As an example, if a patient falls from the operating room table and is injured, a jury could well assess whether this could occur absent negligence on the part of the professionals attending the patient in the operating room. Another common example involves the retained sponge or instrument. A jury can assess without expert testimony whether items should be left in a body cavity following surgery. Jurors are encouraged to rely on their own common sense and life experiences when making such judgments.

As medical negligence actions often involve more than one defendant, and patient care generally involves more than one provider, comparative fault becomes a critical issue. Strict comparative fault means the plaintiff collects the percentage of the award assessed against each defendant. Variations apply. For example, some states do not allow the plaintiff to collect at all if that plaintiff is judged to be 50 percent or 51 percent negligent. Instances where the plaintiff's fault may be compared include failure to return for follow-up treatment, smoking with knowledge that the same causes lung cancer, or failure to follow rehabilitation instructions. The rules also vary on whether nondefendant healthcare providers' fault can be compared. Some states allow this and some do not. However, if a party settles with the plaintiff before trial, his or her negligence can be compared unless the remaining defendants have agreed to the contrary.

WHAT TO DO IF NAMED IN A SUIT

Process Service

The first involvement with a new lawsuit is service of process, meaning the delivery of the lawsuit petition or complaint to the provider. This is the document filed by the plaintiff with the court setting out the complaint of negligence or other alleged wrongdoing. This document may be served personally. A court representative actually locates you, generally at home or work, and personally delivers the petition or complaint along with information indicating when you must respond to the allegations to avoid a default judgment. A default judgment results when the defendant fails to respond in a timely fashion to the petition or complaint. The plaintiff's allegations are therefore deemed admitted and judgment in the amount requested by the plaintiff is entered. As one can see, the appropriate response or answer to the service of process is very important.

There are other means of receiving notice of the lawsuit, including delivery via certified mail. This too is an appropriate way to effect service on a defendant in most jurisdictions. Occasionally service of process is improper. The precise rules dictating proper and improper service and remedies for improper service vary among jurisdictions. Generally, if the plaintiff is trying to carry out personal service and someone leaves the documents with an office or hospital employee who is not designated with authority to receive such documents, the service is invalid. However, if the court representative leaves the documents with someone of suitable age at your home, service is valid.

There are two important points to keep in mind when one is served with process. First, make a note of the date, time, and manner in which the documents were delivered and the date and time you received the documents if it is different from the former. An attorney will need this information. Second, notify your professional liability insurance carrier immediately that you have been named in a lawsuit and served with process. Notify your carrier initially by telephone and follow this notice with a letter advising the company of the lawsuit and enclose a copy of the suit papers received. Next, open a personal records file to keep copies of documents, letters, and other papers that will be generated during the course of litigation.

One should not ignore the service of process, as a default judgment can be entered following the time allowed for your answer to be filed with the court. In addition to the risk of default judgment, ignoring service of process places your professional liability insurance coverage at risk. Most policies contain a clause requiring you to notify the company of a claim or lawsuit so that a defense can be undertaken. Failure to comply with this requirement may void your coverage. Above all, the CRNA should speak to no one about the allegations or the case. The plaintiff's attorney may ask in deposition or trial who you have spoken with about this case. By talking about the lawsuit with others, you may be involving them unnecessarily in the litigation process.

Some professionals want to undertake an immediate and independent investigation of the facts. Avoid this urge until you have consulted with the attorney that your insurance company appoints to the case. Certain privileged status attaches to an investigation undertaken at the direction of your counsel. Embarking on an independent investigation before conferring with counsel regarding your intended efforts may result in your work ending up in the hands of the plaintiff and plaintiff's counsel. In summary, when served with process advise your insurance carrier of this fact. Do not speak with others regarding the lawsuit and do not undertake an investigation of the matter without first speaking with and clearing your proposed action with your appointed attorney.

Selection of Counsel

Once advised of the lawsuit, a claims adjustor with your professional liability carrier will appoint an attorney to defend you. Selection of counsel is obviously an important aspect of defense. Some professionals in seeking a level of comfort with the whole process will request that a friend, neighbor, or relative be appointed to handle the case. Most adjustors resist this suggestion with good reason. Attorneys, similar to healthcare providers, specialize in their practice area. It takes years to acquire the knowledge of medicine necessary to defend medical negligence actions. Likewise, it takes years to develop networks with potential experts around the country. It is not in your best interest for the insurance company to accede to your request and appoint an attorney friend or acquaintance.

One should feel comfortable with inquiring into the proposed attorney's background and qualifications. Professional liability carriers generally have a limited list of attorneys who they have previously investigated relative to qualifications and past work performance. These attorneys generally limit their practice to medical negligence defense. You may want to inquire in some general areas such as an attorney's prior experience with medical negligence cases and anesthesia cases in particular.

Often more than one defendant is named in a medical negligence action and one attorney represents more than one defendant. If you find yourself being represented by an attorney who also represents a co-defendant in your lawsuit, you can question this arrangement with your adjustor and the attorney if the arrangement seems inappropriate to you. The analysis made in this situation is twofold. First, do you and the co-defendant have the same interests; that is, are you both employed by the same hospital or professional group and did you both provide care to the allegedly injured party? Second, do you have conflicting interests that could result in compromising the defense of one to bolster the defense of the other? For example, did the two of you disagree regarding the method of anesthesia used with the allegedly injured party?

CRNA Responsibilities in Tort Action

Professional liability insurance finances your defense and provides coverage in case of monetary settlement or verdict. However, in addition to paying premiums, you have other duties under the terms of the insurance contract. As mentioned earlier in this section, you have a duty to report receipt of a claim or lawsuit so that an investigation and defense can be set in motion. You also have a duty to assist and cooperate in preparing your defense. This includes being available to meet with your attorney to discuss the facts of the case, plan a defense, and prepare for your deposition and trial. Failure to make yourself reasonably available may result in a warning that your company will no longer finance your defense and will not be responsible for a settlement or judgment. Continued failure to cooperate and make yourself reasonably available will result in the warning being carried out.

Generally, nurse anesthetists are interested in being involved in the process of discovery and in assisting with the defense. Early in the relationship, you should enter into an understanding with your attorney regarding your level of involvement. Always feel free to contact your attorney with questions or comments. You may wish to limit your involvement to periodic reports from the attorney of discovery schedules, important court dates, and settlement discussions. You may wish to assist in selecting expert witnesses, by attending key depositions, or by suggesting demonstrative ways to explain the technical aspects of the case to the jury. Your attorney will welcome your interest and participation. Keep in mind that anesthesia liability cases are not common and that many important issues are based on what occurs in actual anesthesia practice. Your attorney may not be familiar with anesthesia practice. Consequently, you should actively monitor your case and be aware of positions being taken.

Certain privileges attach once your attorney becomes involved in the litigation. As with the privilege of confidentiality between a healthcare provider and patient, often called the physician-patient privilege, there is a privilege of confidentiality between an attorney and client. In order to qualify under the attorney-client privilege, there must be true confidentiality of communications. Therefore, when you meet with your counsel, do not take your spouse or best friend along for moral support. As your attorney does not represent this person, the confidential nature of the attorney-client communications would be destroyed. A plaintiff's attorney would be entitled to ask what was said during the meeting. Also do not describe the content of the communications between yourself and your attorney to third persons later. This too destroys the confidential nature of the communication and opens the possibility of disclosure to the opposing side.

A second privilege that attaches after your attorney is appointed to represent you deals with attorney work product. This means that all efforts undertaken by the attorney or someone under his or her direction and acting on the attorney's behalf are privileged and cannot be discovered by the opposing side. Therefore, any investigation that you assist with should be specifically requested by your attorney in order to remain protected and thus confidential. Investigation you may assist with includes literature searches on relevant standards of care or causation issues, review of the patient's lifetime medical records, or review of literature authored by plaintiff and defense experts.

Peer review, quality assurance, and risk management activities may or may not be protected from discovery, depending on the state and jurisdiction. However, if these activities are to be protected under the laws of any jurisdiction, they must be handled in a confidential manner. If you participated in a peer review activity or know that one was conducted on your case, advise your attorney of this fact to allow him or her an opportunity to deal with the issue before it becomes a problem.

The Process of Planning for Litigation

Within the time allowed, your attorney will prepare an answer denying the plaintiff's allegations of negligence and file this with the court. This document is general in nature and requires little, if any, input from the defendant to complete. As soon as practical, your attorney will want to meet with you to discuss the case. Be prepared to review the anesthetic record with your attorney in detail. Even experienced medical negligence attorneys have difficulty deciphering the symbols and abbreviations used on an anesthetic record. Also be prepared to discuss other parts of the patient record that contain your notations or to which you refer when preparing for or administering an anesthetic. If you have the opportunity, review the entire patient record before the initial meeting. You may be able to isolate events or conditions that explain the patient's condition that may or may not have to do with anesthetic management.

In addition to the thorough record review, your attorney will want your best recollection of the events at issue. Do not prepare a written chronology unless asked to do so by your attorney. Include as much detail as possible in your oral description. Your attorney may also want a description of formal and informal relationships among all operating room personnel. Laws vary from state to state regarding lines of responsibility and comparative fault principles. The better defense is one with all defendants agreeing there is no liability among themselves. If the defendants point fingers at one another and claim the other is at fault, the plaintiff wins automatically. The plaintiff does not care where the money comes from, only that money is recovered. Therefore, the best defense is a joint defense, whenever possible. Confide in your attorney any suspicions that other healthcare providers may have been at fault. Discuss this matter thoroughly with your attorney before offering testimony at deposition or trial to this effect.

During the initial interview with your attorney, a preliminary list of the plaintiff's specific allegations of negligence will be discussed. Your input into weaknesses in the case is important. Also, your attorney will ask your opinion of standard of care matters at issue. Sources of standards which support your care can be identified, namely standards of the American Association of Nurse Anesthetists (AANA), American Society of Anesthesiologists, facility policies and procedures, textbooks, and noted journal articles. Be certain to point out portions of the patient record that support your defense and refute the plaintiff's theories. This is the time for a frank, open discussion of the case. It is best to make a sound preliminary judgment as soon as practical regarding the likelihood of prevailing, should the case proceed to trial.

Your initial interview will also include a discussion of potential expert witnesses. Because of your expertise, you can suggest local anesthetists who are familiar with the standard of care, are articulate, and are not intimidated by direct questioning. Nationally recognized experts may also be considered, depending on the issues to be addressed. Because the standard of care for administering anesthesia is the same for both physician and nurse anesthetists, either CRNAs or physicians may be used as expert witnesses. Friends are generally not preferred as potential expert witnesses, because the jury may discount their testimony as biased. Areas of expertise beyond anesthesia may be required to fully support your patient care in a case. The causation element may be addressed by others such as a forensic pathologist, neurologist, and so on. Finally, in an initial interview, you will probably discuss the course of the litigation. This is a time for you to learn what to expect and over what time frame. Expect delays and cancellations through the discovery process. It is not clear whether these are due to the nature of litigation or the nature of attorneys. Whatever the reason, flexibility is a must. During the pendency of the litigation there will be many occasions to rediscuss and refine the items mentioned thus far. A specific discussion of the discovery process and deposition testimony is found later in this chapter.

Sometime during the course of the action, the plaintiff will make a demand for settlement, meaning payment of a specific dollar payment that will resolve the matter without trial. Settlement discussions can take on many formats, both formal and informal. Formal settlement discussions may be held outside the courtroom through mediation or arbitration. Mediation often takes on a form of shuttle diplomacy. Each side presents the strengths of his or her case and points out the weaknesses in the other side's case. This is generally done through statements of counsel. Clients are generally in attendance, along with representatives of the professional liability carriers. After listening to both sides make a presentation, the plaintiff and defense sides often separate. The mediator then meets with each side to discuss privately and candidly their chances of prevailing at trial. Demands and offers to settle are made and conveyed by the mediator.

Arbitration is different from mediation in that the independent arbitrator may be an individual or a group. The sides present their arguments and the arbitrator arrives at an opinion regarding the value of the case and proportionate shares of contribution, if any. Arbitration may be binding or nonbinding, depending on the agreement made before the process is undertaken. If the arbitration is binding, the parties are agreeing in advance to accept the arbitrator's judgment and forgo a trial. If negligence is found by the arbitrator, money in the amount and proportions suggested by the arbitrator is paid. Nonbinding arbitration is advisory only. It allows the parties to consider how a jury might react to the facts of the case. Both mediation and arbitration are generally undertaken when both parties are genuinely interested in settlement.

Court-managed settlement conferences are mandated in some states. A judge serves in a role similar to the mediator. The judge's status often influences the parties to accommodate and makes the parties feel they have aired their relative positions in open court. Both are obvious advantages when dealing with the emotions that often charge a party's judgment.

Informal settlement negotiations are generally conducted between the attorneys. You have the right to inquire about and be kept advised of this process. You may not have the right to prevent settlement under the terms of your insurance contract. When considering whether to support settlement efforts or proceed to trial and a jury verdict, there are considerations beyond the merits of the case. Is there a large sympathy factor for the plaintiff? Will trial pose a significant personal expense in terms of time away from employment? Is there a significant chance there could be a verdict in excess of policy limits?

This last item, excess verdict, brings the subject of personal counsel into discussion. Even though your attorney, paid by the insurance company, represents your interests, there may be times when it is prudent to undertake the personal expense of consulting with additional counsel. If punitive damages are claimed or if there is a significant chance that a jury could reach a verdict against you in excess of your policy limits, your personal assets are exposed to judgment. Punitive damages are generally not covered by insurance and the company may be reluctant to offer the money necessary to settle the case. A personal attorney can make an independent evaluation of these factors and advise you accordingly. You may request that the personal attorney press the insurance company to settle the case so that you avoid exposure of personal assets.

Assuming the lawsuit is moving on to trial, anticipate extensive preparation beforehand. You will need to review the medical records and know their contents thoroughly. Allow time to read depositions of all witnesses before the trial begins. Feel free to take notes regarding aspects of testimony that can be improved or attacked. Note the style of questions posed by plaintiff's counsel. Conduct any final research and review your attorney's research as it applies to standard of care and causation issues.

Assist in gathering anesthesia equipment, anatomical models, or other items that will help educate the jury about your role as an anesthetist. Juries appreciate a witness who takes time and effort to teach them about the subject matter. Your testimony has a much greater impact on the jury when you use demonstrative aids. The jury remembers what you show them longer than what you tell them. This way you demonstrate to the jury that you are knowledgeable about the equipment and procedures. Be absolutely positive all demonstrative aids brought to the courtroom function properly.

Make yourself available for extensive conferences with your attorney before trial, as your attorney will want to prepare you for testimony before the jury. Generally this includes actual practice situations where you are asked to respond to questioning. All of the exhibits and means to use each will be reviewed. Preparation is a key element to success at trial. Spend the time necessary to prepare adequately. Know the medical record and listen to your attorney.

Personal attendance is required every day of the trial and it is important for you to assist your attorney with the defense. Attendance also shows the jury that you care about the outcome of the litigation. Depending on the complexity of the issues and the number of parties, an average medical negligence case may last one to four weeks. If you do not live in the city where the trial will be conducted, discuss your personal expenses associated with room, meals, and so on ahead of time. Your insurance policy probably does not cover these items. They will likely be your personal responsibility.

Dress professionally for the trial. This means a jacket and tie for the men and suits or dresses for the women. Avoid flashy clothing, jewelry and driving an expensive car to the courthouse. Jurors can become offended by an obviously expensive lifestyle. Always conduct yourself professionally in the courtroom. Appear interested in the proceedings and remember that the jurors are constantly evaluating you, whether you are testifying or not. After a verdict is rendered, the losing side may take an appeal to a higher court. The specific circumstances and implications of an appeal are so individual that we cannot speak to them here. Should an appeal be taken in your case, look to your attorney to explain all possible results and ramifications.

DEPOSITION AND TRIAL TESTIMONY

Types and Purposes of Depositions

Depositions are used by attorneys in the discovery process of any major piece of litigation. Specific rules governing the procedure are set out in every state and vary somewhat among the jurisdictions. Generally, depositions are conducted outside the courthouse, by agreement of the parties. The witness swears to tell the truth and a certified court reporter takes down every word spoken during the deposition. Attorneys ask questions and the witness, or deponent, answers. The stress of these proceedings is most often relieved by adequate study and preparation prior to the event.

The deponent may provide valuable information to a medical negligence case for several reasons. First, the deponent may have been present when the events in question occurred. The deponent may have treated the individual at another time, making him or her knowledgeable about the plaintiff's condition. In these types of situations, the deponent is a fact witness. There is no anticipation on anyone's part that the anesthetist will become a defendant in the lawsuit. A fact deposition is limited to questions involving who, what, when, and where. A second form of deposition involves the defendant who has knowledge about the facts, but also a rationale for decisions, treatment, and judgments carried out with the patient. As a defendant, your answers to questions are the crux of the case. You will spend a significant amount of time preparing for the deposition before it occurs. Tips for depositions, included in this section, are particularly applicable to the defendant deponent.

In a third type of deposition, the deponent may be an expert witness, someone with no personal knowledge of the facts. The expert witness generally has been selected by a party to testify because of his or her background and education. This makes the person uniquely qualified to offer opinions about the facts of the lawsuit. The expert witness reviews medical records, other deposition testimony, procedural documents, and any other relevant information. He or she then offers opinions on the appropriate standard of care, causation, damages, or other related topics which are beyond the knowledge of laypersons.

Depositions are not always exclusively categorized within one of the three areas mentioned above. For instance, a fact witness may later become a defendant. The fact witness may also have opinions about the appropriate standard of care or causation based on his or her knowledge of the events or experience. A defendant certainly testifies about facts, but may also have opinions about the appropriate standard of care or causation. The expert witness must interpret facts in order to supply the opinion testimony. The boundaries of your testimony should be considered before the deposition begins.

There are multiple reasons for taking depositions and multiple uses for them once they have been completed. Understanding an attorney's intent helps prepare you to offer testimony in the most favorable light. Beginning with the fact witness deposition, the testimony establishes a sequence of events that can later be evaluated. Did the healthcare providers make appropriate judgments in treating the patient? Did any single act or series of actions lead to the injury? The deposition makes the testimony immortal. If a witness is unavailable for live trial testimony, the deposition can be read to the jury. A witness may be unavailable because of distance from the trial location, death, or injury. If the deponent does appear at trial and changes his or her testimony from the sworn statements given in the deposition, an attorney can point out the changes to the jury. The attorney may suggest a variety of reasons for changing the testimony, such as the deponent has a poor memory, is trying to protect someone, or is simply lying at one time or the other. An attorney may suggest to the jury that the witness is not credible.

Before agreeing to give deposition testimony, a nondefendant anesthetist should fully investigate the possible ramifications of the deposition. Could you become a defendant after the testimony? If the answer is yes, you should advise your professional liability insurance carrier that your deposition has been requested. Tell the insurance representative that you are concerned you may become a party to the lawsuit. Request that an attorney be appointed to prepare you for the deposition and represent you at that proceeding. If there is no chance or likelihood that you will be added to the lawsuit, you will probably work with a defense attorney who represents another healthcare provider to prepare for the deposition. Note, however, that rules allowing contact between a healthcare provider and attorney vary from state to state and must be considered before discussions of a patient's treatment are undertaken.

Documents reviewed in direct preparation for your deposition and relied on for testimony can be reviewed by opposing counsel. Therefore, only review documents before your deposition which your attorney agrees are appropriate. As an example, if your attorney has asked you to provide a narrative of the events at issue and you review this document to refresh your recollection for the deposition, that document may be discoverable by opposing counsel. The same is true for research materials you may locate and review to support your actions and opinions.

If you have an opportunity to attend one or more depositions before yours, it will help you to be comfortable with the process. You will be able to appreciate the attorney's manner of questioning and direction for theories of liability. In general, a deposition is not a time to explain everything that you believe is relevant. Save that detail for trial. Rather, in a deposition, answer only the question that is asked. Answer truthfully, but answer yes or no when possible. Avoid nods of the head and gestures as the reporter can only take down actual words. Explain your answer with detail only when necessary. Any explanation you give will prompt further questions. You are not giving a deposition to help the opposing side. Do not suggest areas of questioning or help the attorney ask the question. If you do not understand a question, say so.

Do not answer a question that you do not understand. Ask the attorney to rephrase it. You are not required to answer all questions. There may be occasions when you do not know or remember the answer. Respond accordingly. Do not guess or speculate about an answer. If at the conclusion of the process you believe the plaintiff's attorney has failed to ask you questions on an important aspect of the case, do not worry. That does not preclude you from commenting on the subject at trial. This is the plaintiff's attorney's opportunity to learn all information that he or she believes is relevant and important to the plaintiff's case. Deposition is generally not the time for you to win the case. Save your arguments for the jury.

There are three means to testify regarding involvement with a patient. First, you can testify to things you remember. If an event was catastrophic, you may well remember details clearly. If the patient's care was not appreciably different from that of any other patient and a significant amount of time has passed, you may not remember the case at all. Second, you may testify to what is found in the patient care record. While you may not specifically remember that the patient's blood pressure was 120/80 on arrival in the postanesthesia recovery area, the chart indicates that is the fact. Therefore you can say without hesitation what the blood pressure reading was at that time. Similarly, with other aspects of your documentation, you can refer to the record when answering questions. Third, you can testify from habitual conduct. Many things that you do everyday are not documented. One cannot document every single aspect of care. However, if you routinely perform a function, you can say you are sure to have performed that act in this case simply because it is your habit. Do not hesitate to testify to facts that fall within your habit, routine, or custom of practice. On the other hand, if you claim something is your habit when it is not, you open the door to otherwise irrelevant but potentially harmful testimony of what you may or may not have done on certain other occasions.

Because brain injury or death and other respiratory complications are often the issues when an anesthetist is a defendant in a medical negligence action, a plaintiff's attorney will try to establish events on a minute by minute basis. Discuss with your attorney before the deposition how to approach this subject. Hypoxia and injury occur and become permanent within a very few minutes. Therefore, the plaintiff's attorney will attempt to show inappropriate judgments, inattention, or negligent conduct during the critical minutes. Anesthetic records generally provide an accounting of vital signs every 5 minutes. Establishing exactly what occurred between the recorded vital signs is often difficult. Healthcare personnel use terms that may seem harsh to laypersons. Consider your phraseology and discuss key terms with your counsel before a deposition. As an example, brain-damaged infants are often called "bad babies" in loose conversation. A plaintiff's attorney can make you seem cruel and insensitive for associating a negative term with a helpless infant who has been irreparably damaged due to negligence.

Only parties to the lawsuit—the plaintiff and defendant, their attorneys, the court reporter, and the witness—may attend depositions, absent agreement among the parties to the contrary. It is common to take a short break every hour or so. As a witness, you do not want to become overly tired when answering questions. Breaks help refresh you and help keep your mind focused. You can confer with your counsel out of earshot of all others anytime you desire. You have the opportunity to review your deposition after the reporter has transcribed it. Take that opportunity to make careful and detailed reviews and correct any errors that have been made.

Your second opportunity to testify is at trial. Needless to say you will spend considerable time with your attorney in preparation. The same cautions apply at trial as in your deposition. In addition to your words, the jury will evaluate your demeanor. You may be called to testify by the plaintiff to establish the events at issue. Seldom can the plaintiff describe to the jury what transpired in the operating room. Healthcare providers must set the stage for the plaintiff to attempt to prove his or her theories of negligence and show the injury and damage that resulted. Trial testimony is extremely individualized depending on the facts, attorney preference, strengths of the witness, and trial strategy, among other things. This is the main event. Do not spare time in preparation, and be sure to listen to your attorney's advice.

Tips For Avoiding Litigation

Goals set by every CRNA include helping patients to the best of one's ability, avoiding injury, and avoiding involvement as a defendant in a medical negligence action. Avoiding litigation begins with anesthesia education. Attitudes of respect for the patient and caution in treatment decisions set the stage for your career and impact directly your involvement in situations where medical negligence might occur. One cannot prevent a patient from suing. One can, however, be in the best possible position to defend oneself should a suit be filed. This attitude and manner of conducting oneself may deter some attorney from actually filing the lawsuit.

Communication with Patients and Families

Patients and families should all be treated with respect. Surgery and an anesthetic are significant events in a person's lifetime; consequently, the patient and family deserve time and attention to properly prepare and decrease their anxiety. It cannot be stressed enough that should significant patient complications arise perioperatively, especially those associated with a negative patient outcome, families should be informed immediately. Events can be described in general terms and the CRNA should provide a clear description of what treatments, therapies, interventions, and follow-up care has been planned for the patient. The CRNA should be available periodically throughout follow-up care and should be actively involved in discussions with the family regarding the patient's progress. Often patients and families sue based not on patient outcome alone, but rather on a perceived lack of sensitivity or understanding of the gravity of the situation by the provider.

OBTAINING INFORMED CONSENT

A patient's memory for details and discussions of informed consent is poor (Cassileth, 1980). However, the discussion should go forward with family members in attendance if the patient desires. The entire process should be documented. List the family members present, for example, husband, aunt, adult daughter, and so on. List the risks of the anesthetic that are discussed. Death, although a rare event, should also be mentioned. List the options of anesthetics discussed. If one option is discarded in favor of another based on patient preference, document this fact. If the option of anesthetic technique selected by the patient is not as advisable as the discarded option, detail this discussion in the patient record.

Anesthetic options assume that more than one technique can satisfactorily be accomplished taking into account the patient's condition and requirements of the surgeon.

Many institutions are employing a consent form for the anesthetic similar to the one the patient signs authorizing the surgical procedure. The consent form validates that the anesthetist explained the risks and options associated with the procedure and that the patient knew and accepted this information before agreeing to proceed. These forms are helpful in defending patient claims of no knowledge of possible death or injury associated with the anesthetic. If an institution provides separate surgical and anesthesia consent forms, both should be signed by the patient. In those cases, the surgical consent alone may not provide sufficiently broad consent for anesthesia.

DOCUMENTING REVIEW OF PATIENT RECORDS

The patient's medical history should be taken carefully and comprehensively and compared with the documented physician history (by surgeon or referral physician). If an anesthesiologist or other CRNA has completed the patient's history and physical, be sure to document on the chart or operating room record that you have been apprised of that information before you administer the anesthetic. By assuming duty for the case, you assume responsibility for all perioperative activities including a competent anesthesia workup.

The respiratory, cardiovascular, and airway examinations are most relevant for anesthetists as failed intubations account for a significant number of anesthetic mishaps. Anticipating potential airway difficulties via a competent and documented airway examination will generally result in avoiding patient injury and exposing oneself to litigation. A special anesthesia checklist with blanks for elaborating on information received is an excellent method for documenting the procedure. As always, equipment and machine checks should be documented on the anesthetic record, as this information attests to proper function and acquisition of baseline physiologic data.

Do not limit your ability to prove that you provided standard of care services to a patient by failing to document actions in the operating room or any other anesthetic setting. Fill out the record completely regardless of whether the case involves sedation and monitoring or a complicated general anesthetic. Sophisticated monitoring of cardio-respiratory status is now commonplace. The information from these monitors must be recorded on the patient record frequently to show you were aware of the readings and that they fell within normal parameters. If the readings are outside normal parameters, an adjustment in the anesthetic should be reflected on the record as well.

In an emergency situation the patient becomes the priority, providing less time for detailed record keeping. During these periods, make short and cryptic notes of vital signs, monitor readings and medications. Once the emergency has passed, complete the anesthetic record as soon as possible. If the patient can safely be left in the care of others, find a quiet place to sit and complete your anesthetic record without distraction. If the timing of events is only approximate, indicate that fact. Review the record carefully to see if all information available has been included. Avoid leaving large gaps in vital signs or monitoring readings. If the original record is illegible, rewrite the entire anesthetic record in clear handwriting immediately after the crisis has passed and place it with the patient record. The legible record should contain the same information, but with more detail, than the illegible original. Discard the illegible copy. Do not confuse completing a record with altering an already completed record.

Do not feel restricted to document only on the anesthetic record after a crisis has occurred. In order to fully document the situation, a dictated or longhand progress note may be indicated. This note should also reflect any conferences with family members after the emergency. Again, list the individuals present for the conference and the general nature of the information you relayed. Note the family response if it seems threatening or out of the ordinary for the circumstances.

Routine Postoperative Patient Follow-up

Crisis or no crisis, you will want to follow up with your patient after he or she has recovered from the anesthetic. If the patient has a complaint, you may be able to explain why the discomfort was necessary. Your obvious concern for the patient goes far toward avoiding a formal lawsuit. As before, document the substance of the postoperative visit, including all patient complaints and your response. Occasionally a patient complains and files suit much later, alleging memories of pain during the procedure. However, if the patient voiced no such complaint to anesthesia or hospital personnel, the claim is not likely to prevail. Always make a note of this factor after an anesthetic. Also be sure you have documented that you have transferred care to appropriately licensed individuals in the postanesthesia care unit or intensive care unit before beginning another case. Remember to maintain continuity in care.

Maintaining and Documenting Standards of Care

At all times, maintain familiarity with standards of care promulgated by anesthesia specialty organizations. These are the academic and clinical constructs against which your performance will be measured. Always pattern your practice in accordance with these standards and fashion your anesthesia record to reflect their implementation. If a patient wishes to file a medical negligence action, an attorney will review the case before proceeding to determine its merits. In addition, before the filing of a lawsuit an expert review is obtained by most reputable plaintiff's attorneys, again to assess merit. If the attorney and expert consultant can find no deviation from the appropriate standard of care on your part, based on the patient's record, there is an excellent chance the lawsuit will never be filed.

As a final point in discussing documentation, the question arises as to whether the anesthetist should prepare a set of personal notes describing some crisis event. The better response is no. The patient record should reflect the patient's condition, treatment provided, and patient's response. A set of personal notes should not elaborate on these items. Generally, an anesthetist considers writing personal notes when disagreement or conflict has occurred. Again the better suggestion is not to undertake the effort of detailing a conflict. Personal notes prepared without advice and direction of counsel are generally subject to discovery if a lawsuit results. Calmer heads will prevail later. Memorialized conflicts will little serve anyone's purpose at that time.

Professional and community participation play a role in one's likelihood of involvement in a medical negligence lawsuit. This is especially true if one lives and works in a smaller community. If one lives a lifestyle of helping and caring for others, and maintains high personal and professional standards, prospective plaintiffs are less likely to sue, prospective plaintiff's attorneys are less likely to pursue the case, and prospective expert witnesses for the plaintiff are less likely to agree to testify. Hesitation at any one of the three links in the chain may result in no medical negligence action, or a failed or abandoned action.

PROFESSIONAL LIABILITY INSURANCE

In general, there are two types of policies written by professional liability insurance companies: occurrence and claims made. Occurrence is by far the preferable type. This type of policy was available generally through the mid-to-late 1970s when medical negligence insurance became difficult to obtain.

An occurrence policy covers the insured for all acts occurring within the policy period, regardless of when the lawsuit is filed. If you purchased an occurrence policy for the calendar year 1995 and a minor child filed a negligence claim in 2000, you would be covered under your 1995 policy assuming that is when the alleged negligence occurred. This is obviously favorable to the CRNA. It does, however, make long-range risk and liability planning difficult for the entity that provided coverage. In this circumstance you may have had insurance coverage with this company only one year (1995) and only paid one premium, yet the company is responsible for defending the lawsuit filed against you in 2000.

A claims-made policy is much less favorable for the insured CRNA. Under a claims-made policy, you must have coverage at the time of the incident and continuously through the date the claim is made or the lawsuit is filed. To have coverage in the preceding example, you would have to purchase the insurance in 1995 and maintain coverage continuously with that company through 2000, the time the lawsuit is filed. Obviously the insurance company has several advantages. The early years with an insurance company are relatively low risk. It is not often that an act leading to a lawsuit and the lawsuit occur in the same policy year. Therefore, the company can collect several years of premiums before having to defend a lawsuit. Also, the company's risk begins, as above, in 1995. If you had any anesthetic mishap before 1995, it is not the responsibility of this company as you have no negative history to begin the policy period. This type of policy also encourages the CRNA to remain with one company over a long period of time, stabilizing the market from the company's point of view. Terminating coverage with the company terminates the company's risk with respect to future claims or lawsuits.

There are ways for a CRNA to change professional liability insurance carriers and maintain continuous coverage. This brings into play two additional insurance terms: retroactive date, often called retro date, and tail coverage. The retroactive date is the date on which coverage for incidents begins. One can purchase liability coverage for a time period preceding the actual date coverage is purchased. For example, if you purchase claims-made insurance on January 1, 1992, but have practiced anesthesia since 1990, you may want to purchase coverage for events that may materialize into claims or lawsuits from 1990. In your policy, the retro date would read January 1, 1990. Any number of years of retroactive coverage is available for a quoted price. The length of time you purchase will depend on a number of individual factors, including your state's statutes of limitation and the length of time you have practiced.

At the other end of the picture is tail coverage. When one is canceling insurance for any reason, it is possible to purchase tail coverage. Tail coverage provides insurance benefits in the future for events that may have occurred during the time the insurance you are now canceling was in effect. Using the same years as before, if you maintained claims-made insurance with the same company from 1995 through 2000 and canceled, you may be able to purchase tail coverage from that company at the time of cancellation. The tail coverage would provide benefits for a specified number of years into the future, for claims and suits arising from care rendered during the policy years 1995 through 2000. The number of years for which you should have tail coverage varies as with retro dates. Many people purchase tail coverage upon retirement or when moving to a different state where their prior company does not sell insurance. Obviously, one would want to price shop to see if tail coverage or retroactive coverage is the most economical, assuming one is continuing to practice.

Limits of professional liability coverage have two components. The limits are indicated with a slash mark between two numbers, for example, $1,000,000/ $3,000,000. This means $1 million in liability coverage is available for any one event in a policy year. Remember, one event may have more than one plaintiff; for example, a husband is injured and sues for physical injuries, and his wife sues for loss of consortium. Three million dollars in coverage is available for any number of events in the policy year. These limits concern the payment of verdicts and settlements only. They are not depleted by the expenses incurred in litigation, for example, attorney's fees, deposition and expert charges, and so on. Injuries sustained as a result of anesthesia negligence can have catastrophic results. Therefore, large limits in liability coverage are recommended. An active practicing CRNA should generally not carry insurance limits below $1 million/ $3 million. Some individuals recommend that the limits of liability be tailored to your geographic area and work setting. If lower limits are selected, the CRNA should understand that there may be some exposure of personal assets to attachment and liquidation in order to pay a large judgment.

Your policy details what is and is not covered in your defense. In general, however, all judgments and settlements within the limits are covered. Expenses of litigation are covered and these include fees paid to your attorney, fees paid to expert witnesses, costs of depositions, costs of creating demonstrative exhibits, costs associated with collecting medical records, and numerous other expenses which amount to a significant expenditure when added together. Your insurance covers events occurring within the course and scope of your duties as an anesthetist. Specific exclusions may exist in your policy and you should be aware of these to avoid practicing in a setting where you have no coverage. A policy may cover you while you practice in one state only. This would limit crossing state lines or moving about the nation in a locum tenens arrangement. A policy may cover you while working for your employer only. This would limit freelance arrangements in your spare time. Policies are limited to acts falling within the scope and practice of anesthesia services. While not seen frequently in the anesthesia profession, a claim of improper touching or fondling of a patient may not be covered under your policy.

Professional liability insurance coverage is available from several types of companies and sources. An obvious first choice for the CRNA to consider for medical liability insurance is AANA Insurance Services, a wholly owned subsidiary of the AANA. This service agency was established specifically for CRNAs to obtain high-quality insurance products and as a source of expert guidance on insurance matters. Many groups of physicians or hospitals have collaborated to form privately owned and operated mutual insurance companies. Some groups with substantial financial backing have self-insured their prospective liability expenses and exposure. These are often health maintenance organizations, hospital chains, or state university facilities. If coverage is not available to a CRNA through one of these means, there may be a patient compensation fund in your state. Some states operate such funds to assure the public that healthcare providers in the state will have liability coverage should a judgment be entered against them. Finally, a joint underwriting association (JUA) may be available. This may also be referred to as a high-risk pool. The purpose of a JUA is to provide professional liability insurance for providers who in good faith are entitled to coverage but who are unable to procure even basic insurance from traditional markets.

SUMMARY

It should be obvious to every CRNA and student anesthetist that an in-depth knowledge of the legal system of this country, especially as it relates to medical negligence litigation, is mandatory. Both time and care should be taken by the CRNA to meticulously document his/her standard of care, become familiar with the processes of deposition and trial testimony, and know how to effectively support the attorney's effort to procure a positive outcome for the provider.

References

American Association of Nurse Anesthetists. (1996). *Professional Practice Manual for the Certified Registered Nurse Anesthetist*. Park Ridge, IL: Author.

Brown v. United States (419 F.2d 337, 341, Mo. cite—66085 [2] Mo., E.D., 1969).

Cassileth, B.R. (1980). Informed consent—why are its goals imperfectly realized? *N Engl J Med*, 302(16): 910.

Garnick, D.W., Hendricks, A.M., & Brennan, T.A. (1991). Can practice guidelines reduce the number and costs of malpractice claims? *JAMA*, 226:2856.

Mohr v. Jenkins (393 S.2d 245, Court of Appeals of La., First Circuit, 1980). K.S.A. 60-3412.

Key References

Blumenreich, G. (1999). Legal foundations of nurse anesthesia practice. In Waugaman, W.R., Foster, S.D., & Rigor, B.M. (Eds.), *Principles and Practice of Nurse Anesthesia*. Norwalk, CT: Appleton and Lange.

Study Questions

1. Define the common elements that constitute claims of negligence and give practical examples of how each are operative in the anesthesia setting.

2. Discuss the different forms of damages and in what cases punitive judgments against an anesthesia provider may be upheld.

3. List and discuss some of the major roles and responsibilities that a CRNA may have in helping prepare for trial with his or her attorney.

4. What advice would you give a colleague as tips for avoiding litigation?

5. What are the differences between occurrence and claims-made liability insurance? Which is most advantageous and why?

CHAPTER 7

STATE GOVERNMENTAL REGULATION OF NURSE ANESTHESIA PRACTICE

Mitchell H. Tobin, JD

Director of State Government Affairs
American Association of Nurse Anesthetists
Park Ridge, IL

The author wishes to acknowledge the assistance of Jana L. Conover, BA, in compiling the numerical summaries in the section of the chapter regarding state statutory and regulatory requirements concerning nurse anesthetists. In addition, Ms. Conover's input and editorial suggestions were invaluable in updating the chapter. Ms. Conover is the American Association of Nurse Anesthetists' State Legislative Affairs Analyst.

KEY CONCEPTS

- State laws and regulations concerning nursing developed in the 20th century. While state regulation of nursing initially dealt with registered nurses, from the 1970s to the present most states adopted explicit statutory and regulatory provisions concerning nursing specialties such as nurse anesthesia.

- Advanced practice nurses such as nurse anesthetists have sometimes encountered difficult battles in defining scope of practice in state laws and regulations; this is in part a result of organized medicine having successfully defined the practice of medicine broadly in state laws and regulations prior to formal recognition of nursing practice.

- While state laws and regulations often set forth requirements nurse anesthetists must meet in order to be recognized or to practice, local institutional policies and procedures often affect practice significantly as well. Facilities (such as hospitals) have wide latitude to impose policies more restrictive than state law.

- The primary sources of state statutory and regulatory recognition for nurse anesthetists are state nursing statutes and board of nursing regulations. Other state statutes and regulations, such as state hospital or ambulatory surgical center regulations, can also have important practice implications.

- The manner or type of statutory and regulatory recognition of nurse anesthetists varies considerably from state to state. In addition, the qualifications a nurse anesthetist must possess to practice, as well as how scope of practice is addressed, are not uniform in every state.

HISTORICAL BACKGROUND

Formal state regulation of nursing practice in the United States is so entrenched that it is easy to assume it always existed. State laws and regulations concerning nursing, however, are a 20th century phenomenon. To understand why and how nurse anesthetists are formally recognized in states today, it is necessary to first explore the development of state regulation of medicine, then nursing.

Spurred by the efforts of the American Medical Association (AMA), Texas passed the first modern medical practice act in 1873 (Clayton, 1999). The enactment of this state law was significant, because it heralded the beginning of an era in which physicians would have to obtain a license to practice medicine. The legitimacy of compulsory licensure for physicians did not go unchallenged, however. There were those who did not believe government had the right to require healthcare professionals to be licensed to practice. The U.S. Supreme Court put the issue to rest in the 1889 case of *Dent v. West Virginia* (1889).

In *Dent,* the court upheld the constitutionality of the West Virginia Medical Practice Act. In doing so, the court relied on the Tenth Amendment to the U.S. Constitution, which states that: "The powers not delegated to the United States by the Constitution, nor prohibited by it to the States, are reserved to the States respectively, or to the people." The Tenth Amendment is the source of the states' "police power," or right to regulate the public health, welfare, and safety. As *Dent* confirmed, states have the authority as part of their police power to regulate and license healthcare professionals. Following the *Dent* decision in 1889, states moved quickly to adopt compulsory licensure laws for physicians. By 1905, 39 states had enacted medical practice laws that required physicians to obtain a license before practicing medicine (Bullough, 1984).

Medical licensure led the way for formal state regulation of nursing. As Bullough noted, because organized medicine had already fought the battle concerning the legitimacy of state licensing laws, nursing's path was easier. Further, medicine's efforts in state legislatures constituted a guide for the political actions necessary for adoption of state nursing laws. Basic state regulatory terms are explained in Table 7.1.

The fact that medical licensure preceded nursing's regulatory attempts also had negative implications. Physician medical practice laws defined the practice of medicine broadly. As Bullough stated, "authors of the early registration laws and those who worked on subsequent revisions in the early twentieth century assumed that medicine was the only health profession, and the language they used in the registration statutes often reflected that assumption. This meant that nursing and the other health professions had to consciously avoid that area previously carved out by medicine or, if they intruded therein, had to be prepared to face a battle. The nursing profession, as a result, avoided challenging the position of medicine. Only recently have things begun to change."

THE DEVELOPMENT OF NURSING LICENSURE

With medical licensure well established, the stage was set for formal state regulation of nursing. Bullough (1984) identified three primary phases in the development of nursing regulation in the United States:

1903 - 1938 Enactment of nurse registration acts in numerous states.

In 16 yrs

Table 7.1: Basic State Regulatory Terms

Throughout this chapter, terms such as statutes, laws, regulations, and the like are used. It is important to understand these terms, because they represent the building blocks states use to recognize nursing professionals. The following section defines some of the more common terms you will encounter in this area.

Jurisdiction

A jurisdiction is a geographic area having the power to adopt, implement, and enforce laws. All states are jurisdictions, as are entities such as the District of Columbia, Puerto Rico, and the Virgin Islands.

Statutes

Statutes are also known as laws. Statutes are enacted, that is, passed, by state legislatures. The level of specificity of statutes varies. They are often general, leaving the specifics to administrative regulations. Every state has a primary law governing nursing practice. The law is usually called the "nurse practice act," "nursing practice act," or a similar designation.

Regulations

Regulations are also frequently referred to as "rules." Regulations are specific written policies adopted by an administrative agency. States typically have a law (often known as the "administrative procedure act") that sets forth the procedures state administrative agencies must follow to adopt regulations. Commonly, an administrative agency must publish a regulation, accept written comments, and hold hearings before the regulation can be finalized. Specific administrative rulemaking procedures, however, vary from state to state. In some states, for example, there are legislative oversight committees comprised of state legislators who review proposed rules. The particular powers of such committees vary. An oversight committee may or may not have the power to reject a rule that an administrative agency has adopted; in other states, the committee may have the power to only recommend whether a rule should be adopted or not. In still other states, there are administrative oversight commissions or similar bodies whose task is to review proposed regulations and recommend whether the regulations should be adopted or modified. State nurse anesthetist associations should become conversant with the particular administrative procedures in their respective states. It is difficult to effectively play the rulemaking "game" without understanding the rules.

State administrative agencies derive their rulemaking authority from an *enabling law.* An enabling law is one in which the state legislature delegates to an administrative agency the authority to adopt regulations to implement the law's purposes. The nurse practice act in every state is an enabling statute in that it commonly authorizes the state board of nursing or similarly named entity to adopt regulations to implement the nurse practice act's provisions. In a few jurisdictions, board of nursing rules sometimes must be either jointly promulgated or adopted with the state board of medicine.

Once finalized, regulations generally have the force of law. To be valid, however, regulations must be consistent with the enabling statute under whose authority they were adopted. To the extent a regulation is inconsistent with an enabling law, the law will control. Regulations often contain a severance or savings clause that states that to the extent any particular provision of the regulations proves invalid, the remainder of the regulations will still be in effect.

1938 - 1971	State legislatures began defining the scope of nursing practice.
1971 - present	Increasing state recognition of the expanded roles and advanced practice specialties (such as nurse anesthesia) of registered nurses (RNs).

copy of IL nurse practice

First Phase

In 1903, North Carolina enacted the first nurse registration act in the United States (Bullough, 1984). The act provided that, beginning in 1904, only persons that the North Carolina Board of Examiners certified could be listed as registered nurses (Bullough, 1984). By 1923, similar laws had been passed in all states and the District of Columbia (Greenlaw, 1985). Greenlaw identified four weaknesses that characterized these laws: "(1) These laws were title protection or 'certification' laws in nature. The laws regulated the titles 'registered nurse' and 'RN' rather than the practice of nursing itself. Nurses who had not registered with the state as 'registered nurses' could still practice as long as they did not refer to themselves as registered nurses or use the title RN. (2) The nursing boards created to implement registration laws often had physician members as well as nurses. As late as 1938, 17 state nursing boards still included at least one physician. (3) The registration laws required minimal educational requirements. As of 1938, 19 states did not require graduation from high school as a prerequisite of nursing registration. (4) Nursing practice was not defined in the registration laws. Registered nurses were defined exclusively by their qualifications rather than the functions they performed."

Second Phase

In 1938, New York passed the first mandatory nursing licensure law (Bullough, 1984). As Hadley (1989) notes, the law contained two attributes that became the hallmark of all modern nursing statutes—a definition of what constitutes nursing practice and a prohibition against unauthorized practice. Bullough (1984) states, "It was necessary to specify the scope of practice of the occupation that was being protected against encroachment. The older nursing laws made it illegal for an unauthorized person to use the title 'registered nurse,' but not illegal for such a person to practice nursing. Once the new mandatory laws made it illegal for an unauthorized person to practice nursing, a definition of the scope of practice had to be written into those laws."

The New York definition of the practice of nursing became a model for many other states. The New York statute (Bullough, 1984) defined the practice of nursing as, "A person practices nursing within the meaning of this article who for compensation or personal profit (a) performs any professional service requiring the application of principles of nursing based on biological, physical and social sciences, such as responsible supervision of a patient requiring skill in observation of symptoms and reactions and the accurate recording of the facts, and carrying out of treatments and medications as prescribed by a licensed physician, and the application of such nursing procedures as involve understanding of cause and effect in order to safeguard life and health of a patient and others; or (b) performs such duties as are required in the physical care of a patient and in carrying out of medical orders as prescribed by a licensed physician, requiring an understanding of nursing but not requiring the professional service as outlined in (a)." The New York definition did not refer to specialty nursing practice per se or identify specific specialties such as nurse anesthesia. Formal recognition of advanced practice would not emerge in the states for some time to come.

By 1946, 10 states had adopted a definition of nursing (Bullough, 1984). In 1955, while the trend to define nursing practice and adopt mandatory licensure laws gained momentum, the American Nurses' Association (ANA) adopted a model definition of nursing (Bullough, 1984). Like the seminal New York law of 1938, the ANA model definition did not refer to specialty nursing or identify specific specialties such as nurse anesthesia. The ANA's model definition of nursing practice stated that "practice of professional nursing means the performance for compensation of any acts in the observation, care, and counsel of the ill, injured, or infirm, or in the maintenance of health or prevention of illness of others, or in the supervision and teaching of other personnel, or the administration of medications and treatments as prescribed by a licensed physician or dentist; requiring substantial specialized judgment and skill and based on knowledge and application of the principles of biological, physical, and social science. The foregoing shall not be deemed to include acts of diagnosis or prescription of therapeutic or corrective measures."

The ANA's definition of nursing practice became the new model for state nurse practice acts. Fifteen states adopted the definition verbatim, and six states adopted the language with slight modifications (Bullough, 1984). Bullough criticized the definition's specific exclusion from nursing practice of "acts of diagnosis or prescription of therapeutic or corrective measures." It is notable that this disclaimer was made by the ANA, not the AMA. Although a reasonable assumption might be that the nurses believed the disclaimer necessary to avoid medical opposition to the new practice acts, there is little evidence of overt pressure by physicians. In effect, organized nursing surrendered without any battle over boundaries (Bullough, 1984).

Greenlaw (1985) writes that the disclaimer was troublesome for nurses who were already practicing independently. She also notes that the disclaimer failed to take into account that many nurses were currently performing acts constituting diagnosis and treatment. To reconcile discrepancies between the definition of nursing and existing practice, joint statements were often adopted by nursing, hospital, and medical organizations and associations. The joint statements typically specified activities qualified nurses could perform in certain settings. Interestingly, the joint statements were usually considered authoritative even though they were not legislatively authorized (Greenlaw, 1985).

Third Phase

The third and current phase of state regulation of nursing involves an increasing recognition of the role of RNs such as Certified Registered Nurse Anesthetists (CRNAs) practicing in an advanced or expanded role. Bullough noted that factors influencing this growing formal recognition for nursing specialties were discussed and encouraged by a special committee appointed by the secretary of the U.S. Department of Health, Education and Welfare in 1971. The special committee's report supported an extended scope of function for registered nurses. Bullough stated that in "response to that request and to those forces that stimulated it, the state nurse practice acts began to change (Bullough, 1984)."

Some of the factors Bullough noted that influenced the growth of specialty nursing included upgrading of educational standards, increased complexity of practice because of developments in science and technology, and an aging population that required competent and affordable care. She also noted that the women's movement was a factor, because it helped reduce the sexual stereotyping that classified medicine as men's work and nursing as women's work. More men entered nursing specialties such as nurse anesthesia, and nurses in general assumed functions previously performed exclusively by physicians.

Another significant impetus for the third phase of nursing practice legislation was the ANA's amending of its model nursing definition in 1970. The ANA definition now stated that a professional nurse may also perform such additional acts, under emergency or other special conditions, which may include special training, as are recognized by the medical and nursing professions as proper to be performed by a professional nurse under such conditions, even though such acts might otherwise be considered diagnosis and prescription (Greenlaw, 1985).

The reference to "additional acts" performed "under emergency or other special conditions" marked a recognition, albeit somewhat oblique, that RNs with advanced education (such as CRNAs) existed and were practicing. The ANA's choice of language was unfortunate, however. The definition required that the additional acts be ones recognized by both the "medical and nursing professions." This implied that nursing could not legitimately be the sole arbiter of appropriate advanced nursing practice and needed medicine's consent to do so.

In 1990, the ANA's model nursing practice act no longer contained the reference to "additional acts" or the requirement that such acts be ones recognized by both the medical and nursing professions. The ANA's 1990 model act defined "professional nursing practice" as encompassing "the full scope of nursing practice and includes all its specialties and consists of application of nursing theory to the development, implementation, and evaluation of plans of nursing care for individuals, families, and communities. Professional nursing practice requires substantial knowledge of nursing theory and related scientific, behavioral, and humanistic disciplines. Professional nursing practice includes, but is not limited to... (p. 8, section 201[d])."

As of 1990, the ANA's model definition of nursing practice contained explicit reference to nursing's "specialties." As of that time, it had been the ANA's longstanding philosophy that nurse practice acts should not refer to specific areas of specialized nursing practice, such as nurse anesthesia. In the comments section to its 1990 model nursing practice act, the ANA stated explicitly that acts "should not provide for recognition of particular clinical specialists in nursing or require certification or other recognition or credentialing beyond the minimum qualifications established for licensure. Standards for specialized areas of practice and the certification of individuals as competent to practice in specialized areas is the domain of the professional association (p. 9)."

The ANA's current model practice act, last revised in 1996, includes both a broad definition of nursing, as well as specific recognition of advanced practice registered nurses, including CRNAs. This represents a shift from the ANA's previous philosophy of not mentioning specific nursing specialties in the ANA's model practice act. In the discussion section to its model practice act, the ANA states that, while previous ANA model acts regulated only registered nurse practice, the current model act's intent is to regulate licensed practical/vocational nurses, registered nurses and advanced practice registered nurses under one statute. Consistent with the ANA's policy that all of these nurses should be regulated under a common scope of nursing practice, the model practice act is intended to include advanced practice registered nurses in the definition of "nursing," allowing boards of nursing to "make professional distinctions in tasks by levels of practice."

The ANA's model act now defines "nursing" in part as "the performance of any acts to care for the health of the patient that require substantial, specialized or general knowledge, judgment and skill based upon principles of the biological, physical, behavioral and social sciences as defined through rules promulgated by the Board of Nursing.... The Board of Nursing shall determine the skill level and scope of practice for each type of nurse licensed under this Act (section 2[I])."

In addition, the model practice act now includes a definition of "advanced practice registered nurse" as "a registered professional nurse who has specialized knowledge, education and skills to provide health care as determined appropriate by the Board of Nursing through administrative rule making and by fulfillment of all qualifications outlined in this Act. They are registered professional nurses with national certification as deemed appropriate by the Board of Nursing, and include nurse practitioners, nurse anesthetists, nurse-midwives and clinical nurse specialists (section 2[B])."

The ANA believes that a broad, general definition of nursing scope remains necessary to provide "expansiveness and flexibility [that] allows the profession—not the [board of nursing]—to define the practice (p. 12)." This also allows nursing educators to "re-tool and restructure programs to reflect health care delivery needs and not the requirements of licensure and, if necessary, to redesign the requirements for each level of practice (p. 12)." The trend in recent years has been for states to increasingly grant specific recognition to identifiable nursing specialists such as CRNAs, nurse practitioners, nurse-midwives, and clinical nurse specialists. Later in this chapter we explore this phenomenon in detail as it relates to CRNAs. As is reflected in the changes to the ANA model practice acts, many aspects of the ANA's philosophy on state regulation of nursing have changed over time, along with state trends. Most nursing specialties have applauded the trend toward specific recognition in state nurse practice acts or board of nursing regulations, as opposed to exclusive reliance on broad definitions of nursing. As Greenlaw (1985) states, "Nurses relying upon broad statutory language do not always feel confident that their practice will go unchallenged by physicians and, indeed, challenges have occurred."

States continue to defer in great measure to professional organizations regarding certification of specialties, as well as accreditation of educational programs. Greenlaw (1985) notes that: "In the mid-1970s, when the states began to recognize advanced nursing practice through statutory and regulatory provisions, the states also began to require that nurses in advanced practice obtain certification by the appropriate national nursing specialty organizations.... [This] can be viewed as a reasonable compromise between the authority of the state and the function of the professional association. The state is not usurping the functions of the professional associations; rather, the state, exercising its power to safeguard the public, is giving statutory recognition, or deferring, to the role of the professional associations."

The Debate Over Mandatory Licensure

Mandatory licensure of RNs and physicians is so well established that its necessity might seem a given. This is not the case, however, as many commentators have debated whether mandatory licensure per se should be eliminated. Licensure is the most restrictive type of state-granted credential. Mandatory licensure laws require individuals to obtain a license before practicing a specified profession. The scope of practice of the profession is commonly defined. Persons who do not possess the requisite license may neither use the title of the profession (e.g., RN) nor practice the profession as it is defined. In this sense, mandatory licensure laws protect both titles and practice. Unauthorized practice is commonly punishable by sanctions handed down by the state administrative board that oversees the profession (e.g., the board of nursing).

Depending on the specifics of state law, sanctions may include letters of reprimand, license suspension or revocation, fines, or other appropriate penalties. Criminal sanctions may also apply.

The primary rationale for mandatory licensure laws is the protection of the public's health and welfare and not individual professions. It has been argued that patients are sometimes unable to obtain sufficient information to adequately judge healthcare practitioner competence and therefore benefit by licensure. Further, patients arguably do not possess the knowledge to accurately gauge the risks to their health from inadequate or incompetent care. Clayton (1999) argues that "[b]y setting minimum standards for the qualifications and training required of health care personnel, licensure laws attempt to control the quality of health care. Competent health care is, in turn, more likely to preserve the health and well being of patients and to save society the costs of unnecessary injuries and deaths that may result from bad medical care."

Despite its purported benefits, mandatory licensure has been criticized, as Clayton notes. Commentators have questioned whether it actually improves patient care and have expressed concerns about its economic impact. Further, by granting a monopoly over the practice of a profession to those individuals who meet state-defined standards, the state in effect outlaws competition by other individuals who might also deliver good medical care even though they cannot satisfy the criteria required for licensure. State licensing boards have also been accused of being slow to accept changes in technology, are prone to establishing professional practice standards that bear little relationship to an applicant's actual ability to take care of patients, and are overly protective of licensed professionals' vested interest in maintaining their own privileged status. State disciplinary and licensure bodies are also criticized for having little success in controlling professionals who either do not practice competently or practice in an unethical fashion. Licensure, it has been argued, contributes to high healthcare costs and reduces innovation and consumer choice. Alternatives to licensure, such as a voluntary accreditation system or a complete abolition of licensure, have been suggested (Clayton, 1999).

Gunn (1986) has also discussed the criticisms of mandatory licensure. She points out that some have argued for allowing institutions such as hospitals to assume the responsibility for screening healthcare professionals and eliminating government involvement. Gunn states, however, that opponents of institutional licensure have cited the possibility that institutions may sacrifice quality to assure fiscal soundness and profits, thereby engaging in marginal or unsafe care. Other major concerns about institutional licensure include the fear that there would be no consistency of healthcare standards or qualifications of providers, such as educational requirements; decreased geographic mobility for providers; and no way for consumers to make truly informed choices about their care. At least in part because of criticism of the proliferation of mandatory licensure, some states now require groups seeking passage of mandatory licensure legislation to demonstrate why licensure, rather than registration, certification, or no regulation, is necessary (Clayton, 1999). Despite criticisms of mandatory licensure, no state has eliminated licensure for either RNs or physicians. Mandatory licensure appears here to stay, absent a profound shift in how states view this area.

STATE RECOGNITION AND REGULATION OF CRNA PRACTICE

As with RNs in general, formal state recognition of nurse anesthetists followed well-established practice. It is important to bear in mind that CRNA practice was widely regarded as legal and legitimate long before states formally regulated the profession. For the most part, formal state recognition and regulation of CRNAs have ratified existing practice rather than reshaping the parameters of the profession. On a day-to-day basis, institutional policies and procedures sometimes have a greater impact on practice than state statutes and regulations. An example of this practical reality is regional anesthesia practice. Although no state laws or regulations prohibit CRNAs from administering regional anesthesia, some hospitals have institutional policies prohibiting CRNAs from administering regional anesthesia.

This example demonstrates another facet of state laws and regulations. Merely because a particular activity may be legal under state law does not compel institutions to permit practitioners to engage in the activity. In other words, employers such as hospitals and private anesthesiologist groups have wide latitude to impose policies more restrictive than state law. Employer policies may not violate antitrust, civil rights, and other types of laws potentially applicable to the workplace, but such laws often provide less protection than the unwary employee suspects. Although institutional and employer policies often have a more immediate impact on practice than state law, this does not mean state statutes and regulations are irrelevant. First, state nurse practice acts and board of nursing regulations often specify qualifications CRNAs must possess in order to practice. Second, while state statutes and regulations usually do not restrict actual practice in significant ways, the potential for such restriction always exists. CRNAs must always be vigilant concerning proposed legislation or regulations that affect practice.

In addition, CRNAs must be alert to statutory or regulatory proposals to mandate anesthesiologist supervision. Currently some states require that CRNAs be "supervised" by a "licensed physician." No state, however, specifically requires in either its nurse practice act or board of nursing regulations that the supervising physician be an anesthesiologist. The supervision issue is a subject of continuing debate between state nurse anesthetist associations and their anesthesiologist counterparts. Anesthesiologist societies continually insist that CRNAs are technicians who must be supervised by anesthesiologists to ensure quality care. The American Association of Nurse Anesthetists (AANA) disagrees, and opposes any statutory or regulatory proposal requiring that CRNAs be supervised by anesthesiologists. It is important to preserve the right of CRNAs to choose the practice situation in which they are most comfortable. Once anesthesiologist supervision is mandated in a statute or regulation, that choice is lost or seriously compromised, particularly for those who would like to be self-employed.

Significance of Nonnursing Statutes and Regulations

To the extent CRNAs are specifically regulated in a state's statutes and regulations, the most significant provisions concerning the type and manner of nurse anesthetist recognition usually appear in a state's nurse practice act or board of nursing regulations. Other state statutes and regulations can affect nurse anesthesia practice, albeit in less obvious ways. For example, every state has hospital licensing regulations commonly promulgated and adopted by the state department of health. Hospitals must comply with these regulations to receive a license to provide patient care. Hospital licensing regulations frequently contain provisions concerning anesthesia. For example, some hospital licensing regulations require that CRNAs perform anesthesia under the supervision of a physician. Suppose such a provision appeared in the hospital licensing regulations of a state that did not specifically require physician supervision in its nurse practice act or board of nursing regulations. A hospital would nevertheless have to require physician supervision of CRNAs in order to comply with the state's hospital licensing requirements. To do otherwise would jeopardize the hospital's state license. Individual CRNAs and state nurse anesthetist associations cannot afford to restrict their attention to proposals amending state nursing statutes and regulations. An anesthesiologist supervision requirement in a state's hospital licensing regulations would leave as much potential for damage as would one found in a state's nurse practice act or board or nursing regulations.

There is considerable reason to believe that CRNAs are potentially more vulnerable to restrictions in state facility licensing regulations than in board of nursing regulations. Boards of nursing are typically much less inclined to entertain proposals to restrict CRNA practice than are state departments of health that regulate hospitals and ambulatory surgery centers. Departments of health are less likely than nursing boards to understand the nature of nurse anesthesia practice.

The preceding discussion illustrates that there are state statutes and regulations other than nursing statutes and regulations that can affect CRNAs. Individual states sometimes use different names for the various statutes, regulations, and regulatory agencies that can affect CRNAs. In addition to a nurse practice act, most states have at least the generic equivalent of the following:

Board of Nursing Regulations

In some states, these are jointly developed or approved with the state board of medicine.

Medical Practice Acts/Board of Medicine Regulations

Medical practice acts or their generic equivalents are the state laws setting forth the scope of practice for physicians.

Hospital Licensing Statutes and Regulations

Although many states do not have a hospital licensing statute, virtually every state has hospital licensing regulations. These regulations are commonly promulgated by a state's department of health.

Ambulatory Surgery Center (ASC) Licensing Statutes and Regulations

Although relatively few states have ASC licensing laws, many states have ASC regulations. As with hospital licensing regulations, ASC regulations are usually promulgated and adopted by a state's department of health.

Trauma Center Statutes or Regulations

Some states have specific statutes or regulations concerning trauma centers; those that do tend to emulate the guidelines of the American College of Surgeons (ACS). These guidelines are problematic in some respects. In Level I and II trauma centers, the ACS guidelines require that anesthesia services must be available in house 24 hours a day. Although this requirement may be fulfilled by a CRNA or an anesthesiology resident, when CRNAs or residents are used, a staff anesthesiologist must be promptly available and present for all operations. In Level III trauma centers, the anesthesia services requirement may be fulfilled by either anesthesiologists or CRNAs, but CRNAs are required to be under physician supervision. To the extent that state regulation of trauma centers increases, CRNAs must prevent widespread adoption of the objectionable features of the ACS guidelines.

The 1999 ACS guidelines for Level I trauma centers added an explicit reference to CRNAs, affirming the validity of CRNA practice in those centers.

Dental Practice Acts/Board of Dentistry Regulations

These statutes and regulations are often relevant because they frequently contain specific provisions concerning anesthesia. It is very common for states to require dentists who use anesthesia in the office to have advanced anesthesia education and training and obtain a special permit, even if the dentist uses a CRNA to administer the anesthesia. The AANA believes that dentists who use CRNAs or anesthesiologists to administer anesthesia should be exempted from advanced anesthesia education and training requirements. While a handful of states have such exemptions, most do not. CRNAs who work with dentists, therefore, particularly in dental offices, should make certain that such dentists meet any applicable state requirements. In addition to requirements concerning who may administer anesthesia in the dental office, there are often equipment requirements as well.

A final caveat concerning CRNAs and dentists is relevant. As noted previously, state-imposed supervision requirements concerning CRNAs vary. States having supervision requirements sometimes specifically state that CRNAs can work under dental supervision. Other states, however, merely state that CRNAs must practice under the supervision of a licensed physician. Taken literally, this would preclude CRNAs from working with dentists absent physician supervision. In some states, however, it may be possible to argue that the term "licensed physician" in the context of CRNA supervision was intended to include dentists as well as medical doctors. This is a legally intricate argument that can be made only after careful research.

Podiatry Statutes or Regulations

In some states, podiatrist practice is addressed in a statute or regulation specific to podiatrists. In other states, podiatry provisions are found as sections of the medical practice act or board of medicine regulations. Like dentists, whether podiatrists may supervise nurse anesthetists in the absence of a licensed medical doctor depends on state law. Questions sometimes occur concerning the range of services a podiatrist can order a CRNA to perform. For example, podiatry statutes often restrict podiatrists from administering any type of anesthesia other than local. While a podiatrist clearly could not personally administer regional anesthesia, would a nurse anesthetist working with a podiatrist be precluded from administering regional anesthesia as well? This is a difficult legal question, the answer to which will depend on interpretation of a particular state's laws and regulations.

Pharmacy/Drug Statutes or Regulations

States usually have statutes and regulations that address various aspects of drug use including distinguishing between controlled and noncontrolled substances. In addition, states commonly have statutes governing pharmacies and regulations adopted by the board of pharmacy. State statutes and regulations governing drug use can affect nurse anesthetists, particularly if questions are raised concerning whether a nurse anesthetist is properly handling drugs or has the authority to engage in certain practices.

Attorney General Opinions

Attorney general (AG) opinions are not statutes or regulations, but are mentioned here because of their relation to them. As the state's chief legal officer, an AG often provides interpretations of state laws or regulations. For example, a state administrative entity such as a board of nursing might ask an AG to render an opinion concerning whether the agency has exceeded the scope of its statutory authority. In addition, a board of nursing could ask an AG whether a specific activity of a nurse was permitted or prohibited by state law. An AG opinion is not binding in the manner of a court's decision but often carries significant weight. For this reason, CRNAs must carefully consider the advisability and ramifications of seeking an AG opinion.

State Recognition of Nurse Anesthesia Practice

Few states formally recognized nurse anesthetists in statutes and regulations until the 1970s. That decade marked the beginning of an era of increased formal and specific state recognition of nursing specialties. Currently, all 50 states mention nurse anesthetists in at least one state statute or regulation. Puerto Rico does not appear to specifically refer to nurse anesthetists, but does mention nurses practicing in a "specialized area," which implicitly recognizes nurse anesthesia practice. The Virgin Islands mentions nurse anesthetists in board of nursing regulations. Finally, the District of Columbia recognizes nurse anesthetists in both its statute governing health occupations and in Department of Consumer and Regulatory Affairs regulations.

Although it is clear that the legitimacy of nurse anesthesia as a profession is widely accepted, the manner, type, and frequency of statutory and regulatory recognition of CRNA practice varies considerably. State statutes and regulations sometimes refer to nurse anesthetists as a type of "advanced registered nurse practitioner," or "advanced practitioner of nursing," or as nurses practicing in an "expanded role" or "specialty area." States use these categories to describe nurses such as CRNAs who have qualifications beyond those required of RNs. In some states, CRNAs are named both specifically as a discrete nursing specialty and more generally as one of several specialties that fall within a broader generic category such as "advanced registered nurse practitioner." In addition, some states have general statutory or regulatory provisions that apply to all specialty nurses, and additional provisions that apply specifically to individual specialists such as nurse anesthetists.

As Table 7.2 indicates, nurse anesthetists are specifically mentioned in all 50 states. Figures are estimates based on the AANA's review of pertinent state laws and regulations. In many states, nurse anesthetists are mentioned in statutes and regulations other than nurse practice acts or board of nursing rules or regulations. The table does not attempt to categorize every statutory and regulatory reference to nurse anesthetists. The table demonstrates, though, that nurse anesthetists are recognized in every state, even if there is not a specific reference in the nurse practice act or board of nursing rules or regulations. The following is an explanation of each of the table's categories.

Nurse Practice Act Only

Approximately three states explicitly mention nurse anesthetists in the nurse practice act (NPA) but not in state board of nursing rules or regulations (SBON R&R).

State Board of Nursing Rules or Regulations Only

Approximately eight states (and the Virgin Islands) explicitly mention nurse anesthetists in SBON R&R but not in the nurse practice act.

Nurse Practice Act and State Board of Nursing Rules or Regulations

Approximately 37 states explicitly mention nurse anesthetists in both the NPA and SBON R&R. This is a dramatic increase since 1993, when only 21 states mentioned nurse anesthetists in both the NPA and SBON R&R. Taking the preceding three categories together, 48 states explicitly mention nurse anesthetists in either the NPA or SBON R&R. This is a significant increase since 1993, when 40 states explicitly mentioned nurse anesthetists in either the NPA or the SBON R&R. Clearly, formal state recognition of nurse anesthesia as a specialty is now the rule, as opposed to being the rare exception in the early 1970s.

Medical Practice Act

Indiana recognizes nurse anesthesia in the medical practice act (MPA) as an exception to the unauthorized practice of medicine. This is an antiquated approach at best. Indiana also mentions nurse anesthetists briefly in its NPA and is included in the "NPA only" category of Table 7.2, in addition to the MPA category. This accounts for the 51-state total for all categories combined in Table 7.2. Ohio also recognizes nurse anesthesia in the MPA as an exception to the unauthorized practice of medicine, but now has extensive provisions concerning nurse anesthetists in both its NPA and SBON R&R. The MPA is no longer the primary source of statutory or regulatory recognition for Ohio CRNAs.

Although no state currently uses the medical practice act as the sole source of recognition for nurse anesthetists, a few state medical practice acts do include provisions concerning nurse anesthetists, or advanced practice nurses generally. For example, the Medical Practice Act of Texas includes provisions regarding the ordering of drugs and devices by a CRNA in a licensed hospital or ambulatory surgery center. Nurse anesthetists need to be aware that, even if their primary source of recognition is the nurse practice act or board of nursing rules, provisions in other statutes, such as the medical practice act, may affect nurse anesthesia practice as well.

Department of Health

Two states (New York and Tennessee) that do not recognize nurse anesthetists

TABLE 7.2: Primary State Statutory/Regulatory Sources of Recognition

PRIMARY SOURCES OF RECOGNITION	NUMBER OF STATES
NPA Only	3
SBON R&R Only	8
NPA and SBON R&R	37
MPA	1
Department of Health	2

NPA = Nurse Practice Act; SBON R&R = State Board of Nursing Rules or Regulations; MPA = Medical Practice Act.

in NPAs, SBON R&R, or MPAs, nevertheless explicitly mention nurse anesthetists in state department of health facility licensing regulations.

Methods of State Regulation of Nurse Anesthesia Practice

Every state requires that RNs apply for and receive a state-issued license before practicing. Although licensure is the uniform method of state recognition of RNs, there is no such consistency concerning the way states recognize specialty nurses such as nurse anesthetists. It does not appear that any state deems the mere possession of a license as an RN sufficient authority to administer anesthesia. In every state, there appears to be statutory or regulatory language of some sort that enables only certain RNs to practice nurse anesthesia. States vary widely in the specific method of regulation they use to authorize nurse anesthesia practice. Some states require RNs to obtain a specialty license, in addition to the RN license, before they can practice nurse anesthesia. Other states require nurse anesthetists to register, obtain a certificate, or to apply for "recognition," "authorization," or "approval" to practice. Finally, some states do not identify a specific method by which they authorize nurses to administer anesthesia. These states, however, generally state qualifications needed to practice as a nurse anesthetist.

Commentators frequently refer to licensure as the only method of state regulation that protects both a profession's practice and title, because licensure is the only method that ensures that unauthorized persons do not practice a profession. Other methods of state regulation of professions such as recognition, certification, and registration are often thought of as forms of title protection only. In other words, these methods are sometimes thought to merely prohibit individuals who do not possess certain qualifications from using a protected title, such as "CRNA." Individuals who do not use the protected title may still supposedly practice the profession. A close examination of the state statutes and regulations in which nurse anesthetists are recognized reveals the potential danger of relying on classic definitions of licensure, registration, or other methods of state regulation. There is no substitute for examining these terms as they are actually used in a particular state and evaluating their substantive effect.

In contrast to the definitions used by commentators, methods of regulation thought of as conferring only "title protection" often appear to be something more than that as they are actually used in state laws and regulations. For example, in many states in which "recognition" is the method of regulating nurse anesthesia practice, it is clear that nurses may not administer anesthetics unless they possess certain state delineated qualifications. This is the case regardless of whether a nurse is called a nurse anesthetist or a CRNA. In these states, recognition is actually being implemented in a way that resembles licensure in the sense that both the practice and title of a profession are being protected. The practical reality is that regardless of what a state calls its particular method of regulating nurse anesthesia practice, the goal of the method is usually the same: to allow and authorize only those nurses with certain qualifications to administer anesthesia. Table 7.3 summarizes the methods states use to authorize nurse anesthesia practice based on AANA's review of pertinent state laws and regulations. Five states use multiple terms for the regulation process (e.g., "licensure and recognition" as a CRNA). This accounts for the 55-state total for all categories combined in

TABLE 7.3: State Methods or Types of Recognition for Nurse Anesthetists

METHOD/TYPE OF RECOGNITION	NUMBER OF STATES
Licensure	16
Certification	9
Authorization or Approval	9
Registration or Recognition	11
Method Not Specified	10

Table 7.3. Combining all categories but the last (method not specified), approximately 40 states explicitly mention a specific process in which nurse anesthetists participate before practicing as CRNAs. These state mechanisms are described in state NPAs or more commonly, SBON R&R. The mechanisms summarized in Table 7.3 are in addition to whatever state procedures nurse anesthetists must comply with to obtain their RN licenses.

While the ostensible purpose of formal state processes for CRNA recognition is to ensure that only qualified RNs administer anesthesia, the practical importance of these state requirements is diminished by a key factor. Most hospitals require that, apart from students and new graduates, nurse anesthetists be graduates of an accredited nurse anesthesia educational program and be certified by the Council on Certification of Nurse Anesthetists. Apart from quality of care considerations, hospitals are motivated by liability concerns. Regardless of whether states required CRNAs to possess certain qualifications, most nurse anesthetists would ultimately be forced to pass the Council on Certification of Nurse Anesthetists' certification examination if they wished to continue to practice. The following is an explanation of each of the categories in Table 7.3.

Licensure

Approximately 16 states require that nurse anesthetists obtain a state license in addition to licensure as an RN. This is an increase from 1993, when only seven states required an additional license. The nature of the additional license varies. In some states, the additional license is as a CRNA. In others, the license is more general, such as an advanced registered nurse practitioner (ARNP) license. States that require additional licensure do not necessarily delineate stricter qualifications for practice than states that do not require additional licensure. In no way are CRNAs who receive additional licensure better qualified than those who do not.

An example of this method of recognition is Arkansas. There, RNs are granted a license as an advanced practice nurse in the category of Certified Registered Nurse Anesthetist after providing proof of completion of a nurse anesthesia educational program that meets the standards of the Council on Accreditation of Nurse Anesthesia Educational Programs (COA) or other nationally recognized accrediting body. The applicant must also provide documentation demonstrating current certification from the Council on Certification of Nurse Anesthetists or recertification from the Council on Recertification of Nurse Anesthetists or other nationally recognized certifying body.

Certification

Approximately nine states, the District of

Columbia, Puerto Rico, and the Virgin Islands require that nurse anesthetists apply for and receive certification as a CRNA or in a particular kind of general specialty nurse category such as advanced registered nurse practitioner. The certification is not a license. Further, the certification is issued by the state and should not be confused with the certification conferred by the Council on Certification of Nurse Anesthetists on passage of the council's examination. The state certification is granted after the CRNA provides evidence that he or she possesses certain qualifications.

In South Dakota, for example, an applicant for certification as a CRNA must provide written evidence to the board of nursing that the applicant has completed an approved program of nurse anesthesia accredited by the COA. The applicant must also provide written evidence that he or she has passed a board-approved examination that has been validated and scored in accordance with generally accepted testing procedures. To renew certification, the applicant must show evidence of meeting the recertification requirements of the Council on Recertification of Nurse Anesthetists.

Authorization or Approval

Approximately nine states require that nurse anesthetists formally apply for and receive "approval" or "authorization" to practice. In Alabama, for example, CRNAs apply to the board of nursing for approval to practice. The CRNA must submit documentation that he or she has graduated from a school of anesthesia accredited by the COA and has been certified by the Council on Certification of Nurse Anesthetists or recertified by the Council on Recertification of Nurse Anesthetists. The board of nursing then notifies the CRNA that he or she has been approved to practice and endorses the CRNA's registered nurse license card with the letters "CRNA."

Registration or Recognition

Approximately 11 states, after receipt of appropriate documentation concerning qualifications, formally recognize or register nurse anesthetists. The documentation required is typically similar to documentation required in states that approve, authorize, or certify nurse anesthetists to practice. After receiving such documentation, Montana, for example, recognizes that an advanced practice registered nurse such as a CRNA may practice in his or her area of specialty. The board of nursing lists the area of specialty on the nurse's RN license.

Method Not Specified

The remaining 10 states do not delineate a specific method or process by which they authorize nurses to administer anesthesia. Many of these states nevertheless state qualifications needed to practice as a nurse anesthetist. In Arizona, for example, the NPA merely states that a licensed RN may administer anesthetics if the nurse has completed a nationally accredited program in the science of anesthesia. Arizona, therefore, does not delineate a specific process, such as authorization or approval, that nurse anesthetists must observe to practice. To legally practice in Arizona, however, nurse anesthetists must possess the requisite qualification of graduation from a nationally accredited nurse anesthesia educational program.

QUALIFICATIONS REQUIRED FOR PRACTICE

Regardless of whether a state has a specific process by which nurse anesthetists are recognized (e.g., licensure, authorization, or approval), most states specify qualifications nurse anesthetists must possess to practice. These requirements are generally delineated in nurse practice acts or board of nursing rules or regulations; the requirements specified vary. Before practicing in a state, it is prudent for a nurse anesthetist to obtain copies of the state's nurse practice act and board of nursing rules or regulations. These documents are commonly available from the board of nursing either at no charge or for a minimal fee. In addition, when contacting a board of nursing for these documents, it is advisable to ask whether there are any particular forms or applications that must be completed to practice as a nurse anesthetist. Regardless of any requirements a nurse anesthetist must meet to practice in a particular state, he or she must also comply with requirements for practice as an RN.

The most common qualifications that states specify a nurse anesthetist possess to practice concern education, certification, and recertification. Many states also address new graduate practice. In addition, most states delineate nurse anesthetist scope of practice.

Education

Approximately 46 states require that nurse anesthetists graduate from a nurse anesthesia educational program in order to practice. The balance of states do not specifically require graduation from a nurse anesthesia educational program. Of the 46 states that require graduation, approximately 34 states (and the District of Columbia, Puerto Rico, and the Virgin Islands) require nurse anesthetists to have graduated from an accredited program. Approximately 12 of the 46 states require graduation from a nurse anesthesia educational program but either do not specifically refer to accreditation or have ambiguous language concerning whether the program must be accredited. In practice, the omission of a specific requirement that the nurse anesthesia educational program be "accredited" is not meaningful, because all existing programs are presently accredited.

The specific language states use to require graduation from a nurse anesthesia educational program varies. Many states require that a nurse anesthetist graduate from a program accredited by the COA. Some states do not specifically refer to the council but instead require graduation from a program that is nationally recognized or nationally accredited. These states sometimes add the caveat that the national accrediting body must be approved by the board of nursing. Language of this sort is in effect a requirement that one graduate from a program accredited by the COA, since there is no other national entity that accredits nurse anesthesia educational programs. In addition, in states that require the national accrediting body be approved by the board of nursing, no state has failed to approve the Council on Accreditation of Nurse Anesthesia Educational Programs as the appropriate accrediting body.

Master's degree requirements

In recent years, a trend toward requiring master's degrees for nurse anesthetists and other advanced practice nurses has emerged in state laws and regulations. As of December 2001, 20 states had enacted laws or adopted regulations that require master's degrees either currently or at a future date. State requirements vary widely regarding when degree requirements will be implemented, required degree concentration, and the potential effect on CRNAs who wish to practice in states having such requirements. The COA required that, as of 1998, all programs be at the graduate level, i.e., awarding at least a master's degree. Consequently, all nurse anesthetists entering nurse anesthesia educational programs in or after 1998 will graduate with a minimum of a master's degree. As a result, graduates after that date should meet current state master's degree requirements.

Most states that have adopted a master's degree requirement have included a grandfather clause concerning nurse anesthetists without master's degrees. Generally, in the context of recognition or licensure of healthcare providers, a grandfather clause is a provision in a law or regulation that exempts a provider from having to comply with a new requirement that would otherwise affect prior rights or privileges. In other words, a grandfather clause allows practitioners to continue to practice, even if additional restrictions imposed by a law or regulation would otherwise prohibit their practice. In the case of a master's degree requirement, a grandfather clause would allow nurse anesthetists without master's degrees who are currently recognized by a state to continue to practice with their existing educational credentials. For additional information regarding state master's degree requirements for nurse anesthetists, see the article titled, "State Master's Degree Requirements for Nurse Anesthetists" in the *AANA Journal* (1998; 66:351-357). The article discusses implications of state master's degree requirements for nurse anesthetists, including those who have master's degrees and those who do not.

Certification

Approximately 45 states (and the District of Columbia and the Virgin Islands) require nurse anesthetists to be certified to practice. This is an increase from the approximately 40 states that required certification as of 1993. Some of these states exempt new graduates from the certification requirement for varying periods of time. Approximately five states (and Puerto Rico) do not specifically require nurse anesthetists to be certified to practice, but nurse anesthetists must bear in mind that many individual institutions will require certification even if a particular state does not.

As with state educational requirements, the language of certification requirements varies; the manner in which certification requirements vary tends to parallel language variations in educational requirements. For example, just as many states require graduation from a program accredited by the COA, many states require that a nurse anesthetist be certified by the Council on Certification of Nurse Anesthetists. Some states do not specifically refer to the certification council but instead require certification from a nationally recognized or national certifying body. These states sometimes also require that the national certifying body must be approved by or be acceptable to the board of nursing. This is in effect a requirement that one be certified by the Council on Certification of Nurse Anesthetists, since there is no other national entity that certifies nurse anesthetists. In states that require that the national certifying body must be approved by the board of nursing, no state with such a requirement has failed to approve the Council on Certification of Nurse Anesthetists as the appropriate certifying body.

Recertification

Approximately 44 states (and the District of Columbia) require nurse anesthetists to maintain certification, that is, to be recertified at appropriate intervals. This is an increase from the approximately 37 states that had such a requirement as of 1993. The Virgin Islands Board of Nurse Licensure rules are somewhat ambiguous concerning whether recertification is required, merely stating that CRNAs shall be "afforded every opportunity" to maintain their certification status.

The comments in the preceding section of this chapter regarding variation in language used to require certification apply to recertification as well. In other words, some states specifically require that nurse anesthetists be recertified by the Council on Recertification of Nurse Anesthetists, but other states merely refer to a "nationally recognized" or "national" recertifying body. The recertifying body sometimes must be approved or accepted by the board of nursing. In these states, the Council on Recertification of Nurse Anesthetists has uniformly been the entity approved or accepted. Again, bear in mind that regardless of state requirements, most institutions will require that nurse anesthetists maintain certification.

New Graduates

New graduates of nurse anesthesia educational programs are not certified at the time of graduation; that is, they have not yet taken and passed the national examination of the Council on Certification of Nurse Anesthetists. Consequently, in states that require nurse anesthetists to be certified, the question arises as to whether new graduates are allowed to practice for a period of time following graduation prior to certification.

In approximately 38 states (and the District of Columbia and Puerto Rico), there are explicit provisions in the NPA or SBON R&R regarding new graduate practice. This is an increase from 29 states in 1993. Of the 38 states, approximately 26 states and the District of Columbia permit new graduates to practice while they are awaiting results of the first certification examination. In these states, however, a new graduate who fails the examination must stop practicing until he or she passes the examination. Four of these 26 states permit new graduates who fail the first examination to petition the board of nursing for an extension until a second examination is taken. This extension is granted at the discretion of the board of nursing. Approximately eight states permit new graduates to practice for up to one year. Commonly, this allows graduates multiple opportunities to pass the certification examination. Finally, approximately three states permit new graduates to practice for more than one year while awaiting results of the certification examination. Of these three states, one permits new graduates to practice for up to 18 months and two allow new graduates to practice for up to two years.

The remaining 12 states (and the Virgin Islands) do not have explicit new graduate provisions in the NPA or SBON R&R. This does not mean, however, that new graduates in such states may not practice. At least four of the 12 states clearly do not require certification as a prerequisite to practice. In the approximately eight remaining states in which certification appears to be required, a state board of nursing may or may not feel that the requirement can be interpreted to permit new graduate practice for a period of time. Questions regarding specifics of new graduate practice in any particular state should be directed to the applicable board of nursing.

Scope of Practice

Although there is a lack of uniformity concerning how states regulate nurse anesthetist scope of practice, nearly every state does address or define scope of practice in some manner. The majority of states define it broadly and others define it via a "laundry list" of permitted activities. Still other states say that nurse anesthetists must practice in accordance with the AANA's guidelines or standards for practice.

Every state, although not always

explicitly, permits nurse anesthetists to administer local, regional, and general anesthesia. As a practical matter, nurse anesthetists are not prohibited by state law from engaging in the common anesthesia practices they were educated to perform. State law, of course, can change. Nurse anesthetists must always be alert to the possibility of proposals to change state statutes or regulations to restrict their scope of practice. While state laws and regulations are generally not an impediment to nurse anesthetists providing the full range of anesthesia services for which they are qualified, the same cannot be said for institutional policies. Institutions sometimes do not permit all functions permitted by state law. Even in states with a broadly state-defined scope of practice, CRNAs must still be prepared to address scope of practice issues at the institutional level, because institutions are generally free to define scope of practice more restrictively than does the state.

SUMMARY

Formal state regulation of the nursing profession in the United States evolved in the 20th century from the rare occurence to the commonplace. While state regulation of nursing initially focused on registered nurses, from the 1970s to the present most states adopted additional statutory and regulatory provisions specific to nursing specialties, such as nurse anesthesia. Institutional and employer policies may have a more immediate effect on practice than do state laws or regulations. Nevertheless, because formal state regulation of nurse anesthesia practice is widespread, the possibility always exists for adoption of state laws or regulations that could restrict or undermine nurse anesthesia practice. For this reason, it is imperative that state nurse anesthetist associations, as well as individual CRNAs, closely monitor and be involved with pertinent state statutory and regulatory developments.

REFERENCES

American Nurses Association. (1990). *Nursing Practice Act: Suggested State Legislation.* Kansas City, MO: Author.

American Nurses' Association. (1996). *Model Practice Act.* Washington, DC: Author.

Bullough, B. (1984). The current phase in the development of nurse practice acts. *St. Louis University Law Journal.* 28:365.

Clayton, J.E. (1999). Licensure of health care professionals. In Becker, S. (Ed.). *Health Care Law: A Practice Guide* (2nd ed.). New York, NY: Matthew Bender.

Conover, J. & Tobin, M.H. (1998). State master's degree requirements for nurse anesthetists. *AANA Journal.* 66:351-357.

Dent v. West Virginia, 129 US 114 (1889).

Greenlaw, J. (1985). Definition and regulation of nursing practice: An historical survey. *Law, Medicine, & Health Care.* 13:117.

Gunn, I.P. (1986). Professional credentialing: Tying hands while protecting the public. *CRNA Forum.* 2:11.

Hadley, E.H. (1989). Nurses and prescriptive authority: A legal and economic analysis. *Am Journ of Law and Medicine.* 15:245.

STUDY QUESTIONS

1. How does the definition of the practice of medicine in a state potentially affect the scope of practice of a nurse anesthetist?

2. What are common qualifications that states require nurse anesthetists to possess before they may practice?

3. How do institutional (such as hospital) policies and procedures affect nurse anesthetist practice, and are such policies and procedures similar to or different from state statutory and regulatory requirements?

4. What are the types or methods of recognition that states use for nurse anesthetists and how are those types or methods similar or different?

5. What might be some of the implications for a nurse anesthetist who is unaware of state statutory and regulatory provisions that mention nurse anesthetists?

6. What is a statute or law, and what is a rule or regulation? If a statute and rule deal with the identical subject, which will take precedence if there are inconsistencies between them, and why?

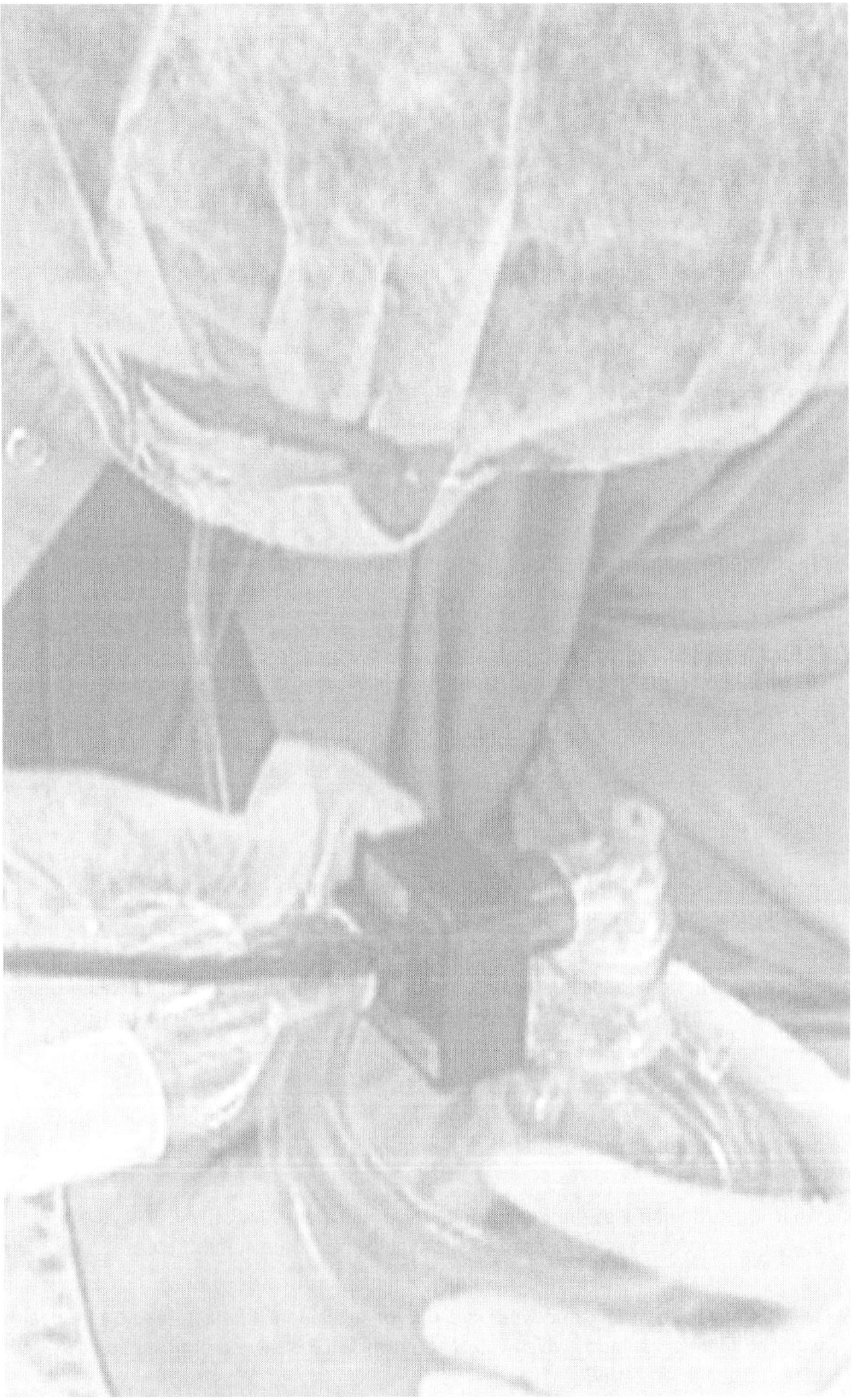

CHAPTER 8

PROFESSIONAL REGULATION OF NURSE ANESTHESIA PRACTICE

Karen L. Zaglaniczny, CRNA, PhD, FAAN

Director of Education and Research
Director of Graduate Program
William Beaumont Hospital/University
Beaumont, MI

Susan Smith Caulk, CRNA, MA

Director of Continuing Education, Certification and Recertification
American Association of Nurse Anesthetists
Park Ridge, IL

KEY CONCEPTS

- Certification and recertification processes developed and managed by the respective councils of the American Association of Nurse Anesthetists (AANA) conduct two important functions attributed to any recognized professional group. If the professional group, such as the AANA, does not develop and manage these systems, external organizations will move to impose standards.
- Continuing education is a common mechanism adopted by many professional organizations through which their members can demonstrate continued competence in their specialty.
- Although organizationally under the corporate umbrella of the AANA, the Councils on Certification and Recertification of Nurse Anesthetists maintain autonomous function relative to their governance, decision-making capability and finance.
- External agencies involved in facility certification or accreditation may, and often do, exert some control on the regulation of Certified Registered Nurse Anesthetists (CRNAs), in addition to the controls required by the councils. Often, however, these agencies "recognize" the authority and function of the councils in statute or regulation as the sole authority for regulation issues. This is often the case with regulatory issues involving CRNAs by state boards of nursing.

This chapter describes the professional regulation of clinical practice for Certified Registered Nurse Anesthetists (CRNAs). For this discussion, professional regulation of clinical practice will pertain to national credentialing procedures for CRNAs, including certification and recertification through mandatory continuing education (CE). These regulatory requirements for CRNA practice are congruent with standards of the Joint Commission on Accreditation of Healthcare Organizations, the Accreditation Association for Ambulatory Health Care Inc., the American Association for Accreditation of Ambulatory Surgery Facilities, and total quality management standards. This discussion focuses on describing these credentialing procedures and the facilitatory role of the American Association of Nurse Anesthetists (AANA).

HISTORICAL PERSPECTIVES

The AANA has fostered the professional growth and continued competency of CRNAs since its inception. As stated in the organizational philosophy, "The members of this professional association are dedicated to the precept that its members are committed to the advancement of educational standards and practices, which will advance the art and science of anesthesiology and thereby support and enhance quality patient care (AANA Bylaws, 1999)." Advancement of CRNA practice has been promulgated by the AANA through the certification and recertification processes, implementation of mandatory CE, and the publication of standards and guidelines related to clinical anesthesia.

One of the educational objectives of the AANA is to provide CE opportunities for CRNAs. This objective has been met primarily through the use of CE lectures related to nurse anesthesia practice at state and national nurse anesthesia meetings. The historical precedence for CE was established at the first AANA Annual Meeting held in 1933. Clinical lectures were presented by anesthesia practitioners and included such topics as "The Induction of an Anesthetic, Intratracheal Anesthesia, Ethylene Anesthesia and Carbon Dioxide Filtration of Anesthesia (Bankert, 1989)." At this meeting, AANA President Agatha Hodgins identified the need for continued growth of the nurse anesthesia profession, stating that "This present meeting is the first fruit of what might be called an adventure. This spirit of adventure is then the dynamic force that keeps us constantly contrasting what we are and what we may be and supplies the necessary courage to change from static to growing conditions (Bankert, 1989)." Nurse anesthesia practice has continued its dynamic growth due to the historic leadership of the AANA and opportunities provided by the constant evolution of technologic and scientific advances. The promotion by AANA of performance standards relating to both education and practice have since served as a paradigm for other professions to pattern their own developement.

In 1967 and early 1968, the AANA Board of Directors realized the increasing importance of documenting continued professional excellence and that continuing education was essential to maintain that measure of competence. Further, the growth of consumer knowledge and demand for quality care required all professional associations, such as the AANA, to be accountable for the competence of practitioners. As a result, the AANA Board directed the Education Committee to study how new requirements for CE for nurse anesthetists should evolve (CE Programs, 1998).

The committee recommended awarding certificates to CRNAs who voluntarily attended CE meetings related to anesthesia practice. At the AANA Annual Meeting in 1969, a bylaw amendment was adopted providing certificates of professional excellence at five-year intervals to members with documented completion of additional clinical and didactic experiences. Participation in this optional program indicated that nurse anesthetists were highly motivated to maintain current knowledge and skills for practice (CE Programs, 1998). However, throughout the 1970s, the public began to require more of the health professions in terms of provider competency than what volunteer efforts would provide.

In 1975, the AANA established the Councils on Accreditation, Certification, and Practice. This restructuring occurred partially from awareness of the 1975 U.S. Department of Health, Education, and Welfare proposal related to credentialing for healthcare. In the final report published in July 1977, two recommendations relating to competency measurement and continued competence were pertinent to nurse anesthesia. The recommendation on competency measurement stated, "Certification organizations, licensure boards, and professional associations should take steps to recognize and promote the wide spread adoption of effective competency measures to determine the qualifications of health personnel. Special attention should be given to the further development of proficiency and equivalency measures for appropriate categories of health manpower (*Credentialing Health Manpower,* 1977)."

The recommendation on continued competence stated, "Certification organizations, licensure boards, and professional associations should adopt requirements and procedures that will assure the continued competence of health personnel. Additional studies of the best mechanisms to assure continued competence should be supported on a high-priority basis by professional associations, the proposed national certification commission, state agencies and the federal government (*Credentialing Health Manpower,* 1977)."

The reorganization of the AANA to include the formation of the councils was a result of the visionary insights of the Board of Directors and membership to further advance the profession of nurse anesthesia. The goals of restructuring were to:

- Overcome questions of conjugation of membership and recertification by external agencies.
- Allow the AANA to respond more freely to members' requests for increased activities in political and economic arenas.
- Provide a mechanism that would separate the evaluation of professional competence from association activities. (*AANA NewsBulletin,* 1978)

At the 1976 AANA Annual Meeting, members amended the bylaws to provide for mandatory CE for recertification of active practicing nurse anesthetists. The CE program was developed by the CE Committee and adopted by the membership at the AANA Annual Meeting on August 22, 1977, to be implemented August 1, 1978. As healthcare professionals, CRNAs were motivated to support and participate in this credentialing process. Their support was echoed in the introductory statements of the AANA CE program, "The rapidly changing character and increasing complexity of nurse anesthesia practice demands continuous updating of the practitioner's knowledge, understanding and skills. Any improvement in standards and expectations could not be accomplished without the ongoing involvement of knowledgeable and skillful professionals who were engaged in a lifelong growth process. Nurse anesthesia practitioners accepted responsibility for their individual actions and for participation in quality CE activities. Nurse anesthetists have always been ethically and legally responsible for the quality of their individual practice. And as a profession, nurse anesthetists have accepted collective responsibility for the quality of service they offer to the public (CE Programs, 1978)."

To facilitate implementation of the program, an ad hoc committee on recertification was appointed by the AANA Board of Directors. This committee drafted the initial standards, criteria, and procedures for recertification. At the 1978 AANA Annual Meeting, the members approved the formation of the Council on Recertification of Nurse Anesthetists.

CERTIFICATION

Certification has been a requirement for nurse anesthesia practice since 1945. One of the early leaders of the profession, Gertrude Fife, identified the need to establish a national board examination for nurse anesthetists. The national board examination was chosen "to safeguard the surgeon's interest, the interest of the hospitals and the interest of the public. (Bankert, 1989)." The Credentials Committee of the AANA was organized in 1941. This committee drafted the qualifying examination and administered it to all eligible nurse anesthesia graduates of approved schools. The qualifying examination was renamed the certification examination in 1982.

Certification is defined as a process by which a professional agency or association certifies that an individual licensed to practice a profession has met certain standards specified by that profession for specialty practice (ANA, 1979). The purpose of certification is to assure the public that an individual has mastered a body of knowledge and acquired skills in a particular specialty. Licensure refers to a process by which a state government grants permission to individuals to practice their occupation as a way of ensuring that the public health, safety, and welfare will be reasonably protected. Licensure and certification are both mandated mechanisms of regulating nurse anesthesia practice, however, certification goes beyond licensure by recognizing the acquisition of additional specialized knowledge and establishing certain professional standards (Scofield, 1988).

Council on Certification

The responsibilities for the development and administration of the National Certification Examination (NCE) were transferred to the Council on Certification of Nurse Anesthetists (CCNA) in 1975. The council is an autonomous, certifying agency under the corporate structure of the AANA. The certification program has been accredited by the National Commission for Certifying Agencies (NCCA) since 1980. The NCCA approval provides recognition that the council's certification program has met the highest national voluntary standards for private certification. It indicates that the program has been reviewed by an impartial commission and deemed to have met the nationally accepted criteria and guidelines of the NCCA (CCNA, 2000).

The American Board of Nursing Specialties (ABNS), established in 1991, is a national peer review program for specialty nursing certification bodies. ABNS serves as the national umbrella organization for nursing specialty boards authorized and recognized to certify nurse specialists in the United States. It promotes the highest quality of specialty nursing practice through the establishment of standards of professional specialty nursing certification. The Council on

Certification of Nurse Anesthetists was one of the first national certification bodies to be recognized by the ABNS (CCNA, 2000).

The council is charged with protecting and serving the public by assuring that individuals who are credentialed have met predetermined qualifications or standards for providing nurse anesthesia services. The purposes of the council are to:

- Formulate and adopt requirements for eligibility for admission to the certification examination and for the certification of registered nurse anesthetists.
- Formulate, adopt and administer the certification examination to those registered nurse anesthetists who have met all requirements for examination and have been found eligible by the council.
- Evaluate candidates' performance on the certification examination.
- Grant initial certification to those candidates who pass the certification examination and fulfill all other requirements for certification. (CCNA, 2000)

The membership of the council includes three CRNA educators, three CRNA practitioners, two anesthesiologists, a nurse anesthesia student, one public member, and one hospital administrator. Members are elected to the council for a term of three years with eligibility to be re-elected for one additional term.

The eligibility criteria for admission to take the NCE are listed in Table 8.1. To be certified by the council, the applicant must meet all of the eligibility requirements and successfully pass the NCE. If an applicant does not pass the NCE, he or she may retake the examination. Currently, the NCE is administered year round at national testing centers.

Table 8.1: Eligibility Requirements for the National Certification Examination

- Maintain current and unrestricted licensure as a registered professional nurse
- Complete a nurse anesthesia educational program accredited by the Council on Accreditation of Nurse Anesthesia Educational Programs
- Submit application form with an official notarized transcript which documents the candidate's academic and clinical experiences
- Payment of application fee
- Sign and agree to the eligibility certifications:

  That his or her license has never been revoked, restricted, suspended or limited by any state, has never been surrendered, and is not the subject of a pending action or investigation

  That he or she does not currently suffer from a mental or physical condition which might interfere with the practice of anesthesia

  That he or she does not currently suffer from drug or alcohol addiction or abuse

  That he or she has not been convicted of and is not currently under indictment for any felony

  That he or she has not been the subject of any documented allegations of misconduct, incompetent practice or unethical behavior

Note. From *Council on Certification of Nurse Anesthetists 2000 Candidate Handbook, 107th Certification Examination*, pp. 4-5. AANA. Park Ridge, IL. Copyright 2000 by the Council on Certification of Nurse Anesthetists. Reprinted with permission.

Content Validation Procedures for the NCE

The Council on Certification has collaborated with national testing agencies to aid in the administration of the NCE. Previous testing agencies used by the council included the Psychological Corporation (1975-1984), Assessment Systems, Inc. (1984-1991), and the American College Testing (1991-1996). In 1995, Computer Adaptive Technologies Inc. was selected to serve as the testing agency to facilitate the transition of the NCE from paper and pencil to computerized testing.

Representatives from the testing agencies and the council have collaborated on the procedures to build a valid, job-related examination to comply with the Uniform Guidelines on Employee Selection Procedures. These guidelines established a uniform federal position prohibiting discrimination in employment practices, particularly in the use of tests (Civil Service Commission, 1978). The guidelines address the importance of test validation procedures and documentation of a job analysis. Although the guidelines were unclear with respect to voluntary certifying organizations, it is well established in the courts that a validated test is a solid defense against allegations of discrimination (Bryant, 1981). The council recognized that the guidelines could apply to those employers who use the certification credential for employment purposes.

In the Standards for Educational and Psychological Testing, validity is described as the appropriateness, meaningfulness, and usefulness of specific inferences made from test scores. Test validation is the process of accumulating evidence to support such inferences (American Psychological Association, 1985). Credentialing examinations are validated through content, criteria, or construct validation strategies. Content validation is the most frequently used strategy for professional certification examinations. Since certification reflects the acquisition of the knowledge, skills, and abilities (KSA) required for specialty practice, the content validation procedure can link the KSAs to the certification examination.

The content validation procedures for the NCE were documented through a job analysis in 1987 and a professional practice analysis (PPA) in 1992 and in 1996 (Zaglaniczny, 1993, 1998). The goal of a PPA is to define performances critical to the definition of credentialed behavior and to delineate the knowledge, skills and abilities underlying these performances (Schoon, 1996). Content validity refers to the degree to which the content of the examination is representative of the area of work about which the inference is to be made. Content validation studies are used to assess whether the questions on the examination adequately represent a performance domain (Henderson, 1996). According to national testing standards, credentialing agencies should repeat their validation studies every three to five years.

The PPA survey instrument used in 1992 and 1996 included information related to demographics, practice setting, education, and fundamental knowledge of nurse anesthesia practitioners. Areas of the survey were organized to identify the frequency and level of expertise related to patient conditions, procedures, anesthesia agents, techniques, equipment, instrumentation and technology encountered in practice. All of the survey items were considered important to practice. Assessment of the relative importance of the responses is used in determining appropriate test specifications. The surveys were mailed to practitioners with one to two years of anesthesia experience, the AANA Board of Directors, coun-

Table 8.2: Content Outline National Certification Examination

CONTENT	PERCENT
I. Basic Sciences	30
II. Equipment, Instrumentation, Technology	5
III. Basic Principles of Anesthesia	31
IV. Advanced Principles of Anesthesia	30
V. Professional Issues	4

Note. From *Council on Certification of Nurse Anesthetists 2000 Candidate Handbook, 107th Certification Examination*, pp. 14-20. AANA. Park Ridge, IL. Copyright 2000 by the Council on Certification of Nurse Anesthetists. Reprinted with permission.

cil representatives, and committee members (Zaglaniczny, 1993, 1998).

Data obtained from the 1996 surveys were tabulated and analyzed by representatives from Computer Adaptive Technologies, Inc. using Rasch rating calibrations. The Rasch rating scale calibrations are a log-linear transformation of the ordinal data onto a linear, equal-interval scale. The Rasch rating scale model is a measurement model that places all of the observations on a common linear scale so that a comparison between items can be obtained (Wright, 1982). This measurement model facilitates the understanding, interpretation and meaningful inferences that can be made from the PPA. The Rasch calibrations also provide the basis for making a meaningful transformation of all the responses to the items on the NCE. A positive Rasch calibration indicates an item of relatively high importance, while a negative calibration indicates an item of relatively low importance (Wright, 1982). The results revealed that there was agreement between respondents in most areas surveyed as indicated by high correlations obtained in each section. The results of the 1996 survey were consistent with the frequency and level of expertise rating results from the 1992 PPA and support the current blueprint of the NCE.

Content validation is provided by linkages between the PPA, knowledge and skill statements, and the test items. The current content outline and percentage of the examination tested in each area are listed in Table 8.2. A conceptual overview of the relationship of each candidate's computerized adaptive testing (CAT) to CRNA practice is presented in Figure 8.1.

Development of the NCE

The NCE for nurse anesthetists was administered in paper and pencil format from 1945-1996 based on the standard criterion-referenced testing process. In April 1996, the Council on Certification implemented computer adaptive testing procedures for their examinations (Zaglaniczny, 1996). The council administers two adaptive tests: the NCE and the Self-Evaluation Examination (SEE). The purpose of the NCE is to assess the entry-level knowledge and skills required for nurse anesthesia practice. The purposes of the SEE are to allow students to assess their knowledge of the fundamental aspects of nurse anesthesia and provide them with the opportunity to prepare for the computer adaptive certification examination.

CAT is a method of administering tests that uses current technology and is based on the psychometric framework of item response theory (IRT). IRT uses a

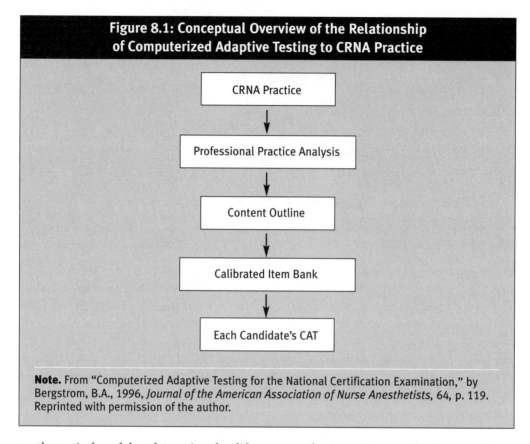

Figure 8.1: Conceptual Overview of the Relationship of Computerized Adaptive Testing to CRNA Practice

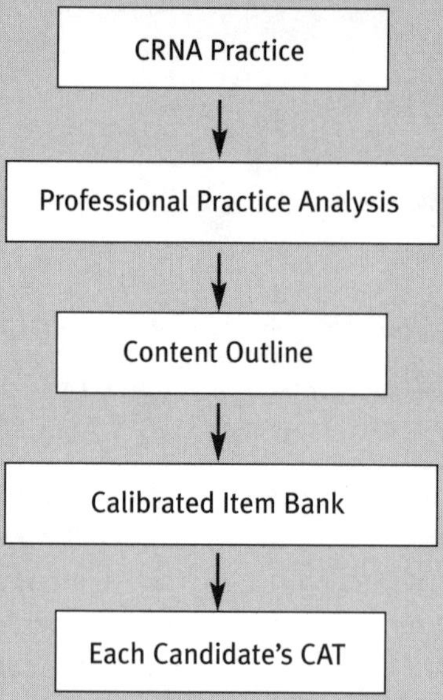

Note. From "Computerized Adaptive Testing for the National Certification Examination," by Bergstrom, B.A., 1996, *Journal of the American Association of Nurse Anesthetists, 64,* p. 119. Reprinted with permission of the author.

mathematical model to determine the difficulty of test questions and estimate the ability of candidates (Wright, 1979). With CAT, each candidate's test is individualized; it is assembled interactively as the candidate is tested (Bergstrom, 1992). Test questions are stored in a large item bank and classified by content category and level of difficulty. After the candidate answers a question, the computer calculates an estimate of competence and chooses a next question of appropriate content and difficulty. This process is repeated for each question, thus creating an examination that is tailored to each individual's knowledge and skills and also fulfills the council's test plan requirements (CCNA, 2000).

Each test conforms to the NCE outline which assures inclusion of test questions in the content areas of basic sciences, basic and advanced principles of anesthesia, equipment, instrumentation and technology, and professional aspects. All of the questions are chosen from the same item bank. The item bank contains all of the questions necessary to meet the test specifications. The passing score remains identical for all candidates, assuring the difficulty level to pass the NCE is consistent for all candidates. All candidates have the opportunity to demonstrate their ability or competence level, as the certification examination will not end until a pass or fail decision is determined (CCNA, 2000).

The NCE is a variable length, computerized, adaptive, multiple-choice test. The examination is for entry into nurse anesthesia practice. Each candidate takes a minimum of 90 questions, 70 questions representing the certification content outline and 20 pretest questions. The maximum number of questions is 160, which includes 20 pretest questions. A maximum of three hours is allowed for the test period (CCNA, 2000). Questions are submitted by members of the Examination Committee which consists of CRNA and physician representatives. This committee meets annually to write and review test questions for the approved item bank and update the item bank each year. Performance statistics for questions are continuously monitored by the council and testing agency.

Determination of the Passing Score

CAT examinations are scored based on the candidate's performance relative to the difficulty of items administered. A candidate must obtain a scaled score of 450 to pass the examination. A pass/fail decision is made when one of the following conditions has been met:

1. The candidate has clearly demonstrated competence. This decision may be reached at any point between 90 and 160 items.
2. The candidate has clearly demonstrated incompetence. This decision may be reached at any point between 90 and 160 items.
3. The maximum number of questions (160) has been administered, and the pass/fail decision is based on whether the candidate's level of competence is above or below the pass/fail point.
4. The maximum amount of time (three hours) is reached. A fail decision is made if the candidate has not completed more than 90 questions. If the candidate has completed more than 90 questions, the pass/fail decision is based on whether the candidate's level of competence is above or below the pass/fail point. (CCNA, 2000)

Future Directions

The Council on Certification is committed to continually investigating avenues to keep current with new developments related to testing procedures. These include updating the content validation process, investigating computerized testing techniques and promoting research activities related to testing. Representatives from the council participate in meetings with other agencies associated with professional certification issues. These agencies include the National Organization for Competency Assurance, National Council of State Boards of Nursing, National Specialty Nursing Certifying Organizations, the NCCA, and the ABNS.

RECERTIFICATION

Following initial certification, a CRNA is eligible to apply for recertification on July 31 and accumulate CE credits for two years beginning the August 1 following the date of initial certification. Recertification is a voluntary process. CRNAs apply for recertification biennially. Through the recertification process, the Council on Recertification of Nurse Anesthetists (COR) seeks to advance the quality of anesthesia care provided to patients. Specifically, it endeavors to make certain that nurse anesthetists maintain their skills and keep current with scientific and technological developments. It also strives to assure that appropriate limitations are placed on those who are known to have developed conditions that might adversely affect their ability to practice anesthesia (COR, 1998).

A nurse anesthetist who has satisfied the council's objective criteria receives recertification for a period of two years. Recertification, of course, is not and cannot be a guarantee of competence to perform all anesthesia procedures. Full recertification is, however, an indication that the CRNA has maintained a current license to practice, has exercised his or her skills, has participated in approved CE activities, and is not known to have developed any impairment that could interfere with the administration of anesthesia (COR, 1998). The council has set forth established guidelines and criteria for recertification with input from the AANA membership.

Council on Recertification

The purposes of this council are to:

- Recertify qualified CRNAs on a biennial basis.
- Formulate and adopt criteria for eligibility for recertification of CRNAs based on the current licensure, maintenance of practice skills, participation in approved CE activities, and other recognized activities conducive to professional proficiency and freedom from known mental or physical impairments that may interfere or prevent the professional practice of nurse anesthesia. The practice of nurse anesthesia may include clinical practice and anesthesia-related administrative, educational, and research activities.
- Formulate and adopt criteria for approval of CE programs and offerings.
- Develop and maintain mechanisms to provide for a hearing and appellate review for individuals seeking recertification.
- Develop and maintain a mechanism for the investigation and final resolution of charges or other allegations against individuals currently holding recertification by the council.
- Make recommendations to the Board of Directors, councils, and committees in conformity with stated purposes.
(COR, 2000)

The membership of the council includes four CRNA practitioners, one CRNA educator, the chairman of the CE Committee, one anesthesiologist, one surgeon, and one public representative. Members are elected to the council for a term of three years with eligibility to be re-elected for one additional term.

Categories of Recertification

Two categories of recertification have been established by the council: full recertification and interim recertification. The criteria for full recertification are listed in Table 8.3. The process of recertification includes meeting all of the criteria and completing the application procedures.

A CRNA applying for recertification needs to submit the following information to the council: completed application and fee, documentation of current nursing licensure, completion of 40 hours of approved CE, and documentation of practice by the July 31 deadline. The recertification period is effective for a two-year period from August 1 through July 31. The recertification status is renewed every two years and expires automatically at the end of the recertification period unless renewed.

The category of interim recertification includes provisional recertification and conditional recertification. Provisional recertification may be granted for any of five reasons: pending review of an application, pending fulfillment of the practice requirements, pending completion of a treatment or rehabilitation program, pending completion of probation, and pending the outcome of an investigation or disciplinary or legal action. The council will grant a CRNA provisional status while reviewing an application if questions arise as to the fulfillment of the established criteria. After completion of the investigation, the council may grant

Table 8.3: Criteria for Full Recertification

- Initial certification by the Council on Recertification
- Current and unrestricted licensure as a registered professional nurse
- Documentation of completion of 40 hours of approved CE within the two-year period prior to the applicant's recertification date
- Certification of substantial engagement in the practice of nurse anesthesia during the two-year period prior to the applicant's recertification date
- Certification by the applicant:

  That his or her license has never been revoked, restricted, suspended or limited by any state, has never been surrendered, and is not the subject of a pending action or investigation

  That he or she does not currently suffer from a mental or physical condition which might interfere with the practice of nurse anesthesia

  That he or she does not currently suffer from drug or alcohol addiction or abuse

  That he or she has not been convicted of and is not currently under indictment for any felony

  That he or she has not been the subject of any documented allegations of misconduct, incompetent practice or unethical behavior

Note. From *Council on Recertification of Nurse Anesthetists Criteria for Recertification 1978-1998*, pp. 5-6. AANA. Park Ridge, IL. Copyright 1998 by the Council on Recertification of Nurse Anesthetists. Reprinted with permission.

or deny recertification (COR, 1998).

For a CRNA who is currently able to practice nurse anesthesia, but has not been substantially engaged in practice during the two-year period prior to recertification, provisional recertification may be granted. A CRNA who is participating in a drug, alcohol, or other type of treatment or rehabilitation program may be assigned provisional recertification if all of the other recertification criteria are met. After completion of the rehabilitation or treatment program, the CRNA may receive full recertification (COR, 1998).

Conditional recertification is granted to those CRNAs who meet the recertification criteria but have restrictions placed on their professional nursing license. The conditional recertification will reflect any conditions imposed by the appropriate state licensure authority. Examples of a restricted license include a license to practice only under supervision, and a license to practice provided the individual remains in a drug, alcohol, or other type of treatment program for a stated period. The status may be changed to full recertification when the restrictions are removed from the license (COR, 1998).

The council has the authority and the ability to revoke or modify the recertification status of an anesthesia practitioner. Reasons for automatic revocation of recertification include the failure to maintain licensure as a registered nurse, adjudication by a court that the individual is mentally incompetent, and conviction of or pleading no contest to a felony that is, in the view of the council, related to the practice of nursing or nurse anesthesia. Discretionary revocation of recertification is used for the following reasons:

- Failure of the individual to maintain licensure as a registered nurse, with authority to practice nurse anesthesia if such authority is granted in all states in which the individual practices.

- Conviction of or pleading no contest to a felony.
(COR, 1998)

The recertification status of a CRNA may be modified at anytime to reflect applicable information which comes to the attention of the council. The COR has established procedures for reconsideration of any modification in the recertification status of a CRNA. These include prompt notification and guidelines for appeal through the Council for Public Interest in Anesthesia. The council strives to maintain the integrity of the nurse anesthesia profession and to protect the welfare of the public in its decisions about the recertification status of CRNAs (COR, 1998).

Future Directions

The Council on Recertification is dedicated to consistently evaluating and updating the criteria and procedures related to recertification. Through the established recertification process, the council seeks to ensure that nurse anesthesia practitioners maintain the high level of knowledge and skill required for practice. It also aims to ensure that appropriate limitations are placed on those CRNAs who are known to have developed conditions that might adversely affect their ability to practice. The council will continue to explore strategies to meet its goals and the needs of the profession.

CONTINUING EDUCATION

CE for CRNAs has been a requirement for recertification since 1978. The AANA CE Committee defines CE as those learning activities intended to build on the educational and experiential bases of the professional nurse anesthetist for the enhancement of clinical, education, administration, research, or theory development to improve public health. The CE program for CRNAs enhances the professional competence of healthcare providers in the specialty of nurse anesthesia practice. CE is an organized and evaluative process that extends beyond basic preparation, and promotes the enrichment of knowledge toward the goal of maintaining anesthesia expertise. The AANA assists each member in accepting personal responsibility for safe anesthesia practice (CE Programs, 1998).

Continuing Education Committee

The CE Committee is a standing committee of the AANA. Members are appointed by the president-elect with approval from the Board of Directors. According to AANA bylaws, the committee shall formulate criteria for eligibility for recertification. Such criteria shall be submitted to the Council on Recertification for evaluation and adoption. The committee shall also supervise CE projects conducted by the association, evaluate applications for program approval, and approve refresher courses based on established criteria that are required prior to transference to active recertified membership (CE Programs, 1998).

The philosophy of the committee describes the vital importance of CE to nurse anesthesia practice. The AANA believes that nursing is accountable to the public for promulgating standards of nursing practice that will improve the delivery of nursing services and promote quality patient care. As the national professional association for nurses specializing in anesthesia, the AANA holds itself responsible for providing CE activities that will help maintain excellence in practice. It further meets this commitment to society and the profession by establishing standards that foster quality

CE activities offered by other providers of nurse anesthesia programs (CE Programs, 1998).

The CE Committee is primarily responsible for providing opportunities for continued learning by individual and groups of nurse anesthetists. It believes that lifelong learning is essential for the continued acquisition of knowledge and skills required to maintain competence. The committee maintains that nurses, by entering the field of anesthesia, hold themselves accountable and responsible for seeking out learning experiences that will improve and advance the practice of anesthesia and the quality of care they provide (CE Programs, 1998). The committee believes that CE activities are most effective when the learning needs of participants are taken into consideration and when principles of adult learning are applied. It supports these beliefs by providing, developing and upholding standards of CE that include those basic concepts. Furthermore, the committee monitors and appraises the CE activities of other providers to ensure their adherence to the established standards that promote quality CE for nurse anesthetists (CE Programs, 1998).

Continuing Education Program

The purpose of the CE program of the AANA is to support and promote quality CE for nurse anesthetists. The program includes standards and criteria for the review, approval, and recognition of CE activities. The CE Committee, under the guidance of the director of Continuing Education, oversees the program and continually monitors the system to ensure that the standards and criteria are maintained.

The goals of the CE program facilitate the promotion of quality CE for nurse anesthetists. They include:

- Promoting high-quality CE by implementing a review and recognition process that includes standards and criteria for CE providers.
- Providing a clearly defined application process as well as procedures for review and approval.
- Assisting state associations and other providers of CE to develop quality CE offerings in nurse anesthesia.
- Implementing an ongoing process for evaluating the policies, procedures, and criteria of the CE program to better assess the effectiveness of services provided.
- Engaging in strategic long-range planning activities to ensure the continued growth and viability of the AANA's CE program.
(CE Programs, 1998)

Each CRNA is required to obtain 40 CE credits every two years as part of the recertification criteria. One CE credit is equal to 50 minutes or one contact hour. Individual CRNAs must first perform a self-assessment to identify the areas and types of CE activity that correspond to their need in professional practice. CRNAs elect to participate in the CE activity that provides the most benefit to them in terms of content, location, and cost. The provider of the CE activity is responsible for securing approval for the educational opportunity. The CE program has two types of approval for CE activities: prior approval and nonprior approval. Table 8.4 lists the types of educational activities available for CE credit.

The AANA has established standards and criteria for CE programs that are used by the CE Committee to review and approve an application. The standards are listed in Table 8.5. The criteria for each of the standards provide further clarification of their meaning. The com-

Table 8.4: Types of Continuing Education Activities

- Attendance at local, state and national nurse anesthesia meetings
- Participation in hospital or anesthesia department in-services
- Participation in research activities
- Attendance at college and university courses relevant to anesthesia practice
- Publication of original papers
- New clinical anesthesia experiences beyond the requirements of basic preparation
- Audiovisual media programs such as videos, audiotapes, and computerized instruction

mittee may withdraw approval status of a CE activity if the provider fails to comply with the established standards and criteria. Educational activities that are not congruent with the AANA CE program philosophy may be denied approval. An appeal mechanism exists for providers or individuals who are not satisfied with a committee decision (CE Programs, 1998).

Prior-Approved CE Activities

Prior approval is the process used to review applications and award CE credit based on predetermined criteria. Prior approval by the AANA designates that a CE activity has met specific standards and has been awarded CE credit prior to its actual presentation. In addition, it obliges the provider to assume certain responsibilities for record keeping and recording attendance. Program content must be consistent with the overall purpose and goals of the AANA's CE program. The types of activities that are eligible for prior approval include: educational programs sponsored by associations and organizations at the local, state, regional, or national level; in-service programs; provider-directed independent study; self-directed independent study; and research in anesthesia-related fields.

To obtain prior approval, the provider must submit the completed application form to the CE Committee in advance of the CE activity. Additional materials required include the application fee, evaluation form, and certificate of attendance. Notification of approval is furnished in

Table 8.5: Standards for Continuing Education Programs

1. Official application for providers	7. Teaching methods
2. Purpose	8. Faculty
3. Planning	9. Physical facilities/resources
4. Needs assessment	10. Record keeping
5. Learner objectives	11. Verification of attendance
6. Content	12. Evaluation

Note. From *Continuing Education Program of the American Association of Nurse Anesthetists 1978-1998*, pp. 5-8. AANA. Park Ridge, IL. Copyright 1998 by the American Association of Nurse Anesthetists. Reprinted with permission.

writing within 30 days of receipt of the application. If additional information is required for prior approval, the provider must submit it before the presentation of the CE activity or approval will not be granted. A code number is assigned to the CE activity and must appear on promotional activities, certificates of attendance, attendance records, and correspondence sent to the CE Department. The record-keeping process involves submission of an official AANA attendance record with the names, AANA numbers, and CE credits for each participant within 30 days after completion of the program. The provider must issue a certificate of attendance to all participants (CE Programs, 1998).

Nonprior-Approved CE Activities

The nonprior approval process is used to award CE credit to individuals for attendance at or participation in learning activities that have not been prior-approved by the AANA but were approved by a recognized approval or accrediting organization prior to the presentation. This approval mechanism is initiated by the individual who submits the application. CE credit is not considered until an application and all required documentation have been submitted. Applications for nonprior approval should be submitted within 60 days after conclusion of the activity. Examples of activities that are eligible for nonprior approval include programs that have received approval or accreditation for CE credit from another recognized professional organization. Also eligible for credit are college or university courses, publication of an original manuscript, new clinical anesthesia experiences, and research in anesthesia-related fields. The individual or group requesting the CE credit must complete the appropriate application and provide the required documentation. Written notification of approval or denial of CE credit is sent after review of the application. The committee ensures that the nonprior-approved program meets the standards and criteria for the AANA CE program (CE Programs, 1998).

Record Keeping

The AANA CE Department maintains records of CE credits earned by its members and will contract this service for nonmembers. At the end of the recertification period, this documentation is forwarded to the Council on Recertification. The CE credits are recorded during each year from August 1 through July 31 to coincide with the recertification period. AANA members can use the AANA Web site or the AANA CE interactive voice response system (CTACS) to access their CE credits 24 hours a day. They may also obtain a transcript of their CE activities by way of CTACS.

EXTERNAL AGENCIES

There are external agencies that have regulatory standards related to nurse anesthesia professional practice in addition to those of the Councils on Certification and Recertification. Often these regulations speak to the credentialing requirements for CRNAs. These agencies include the Joint Commission on Accreditation of Healthcare Organizations (JCAHO), the Accreditation Association for Ambulatory Health Care, Inc. (AAAHC) and the American Association for Accreditation of Ambulatory Surgery Facilities (AAAASF). In general, these voluntary programs are marketed to provide the public with recognition of those facilities that provide quality and safe patient care in accordance with national standards.

External agency accreditation usually requires that recognized facilities and/or credentialed individual providers submit documented evidence of compliance with each standard, including on-site observation (site visit) and interviews with

Table 8.6: Comparison of Accreditation Standards for Anesthesia Services

Joint Commission on Accreditation of Healthcare Organizations (JCAHO)	Accreditation Association for Ambulatory Health Care, Inc. (AAAHC)	American Association for Accreditation of Ambulatory Surgery Facilities (AAAASF)
PE 1.7 - 1.74 Patient is determined to be a candidate for anesthesia. A licensed independent practitioner (LIP)* makes the determination.	Chapter 9 Adequate supervision of anesthesia services is the responsibility of a physician or dentist.	RG 800.2 CRNA, who is under the supervision of the operating practitioner or an anesthesiologist, who is immediately available if needed.
When the CRNA performs the preanesthesia assessment, an LIP concurs with the planned choice of anesthesia. LIPs with appropriate clinical privileges determine whether the patient is an appropriate candidate for anesthesia based on preanesthesia assessment.	A physician, dentist or a physician-supervised qualified* individual approved by the governing body has examined the patient to evaluate the risks of anesthesia.	A physician must examine the patient immediately before surgery to evaluate the risk of anesthesia and the procedure.
Post-operative discharge by LIP or established criteria.	Discharge by a physician, dentist, or physician-supervised qualified individual.	Postoperative progress is recorded. A physician must be physically present until all patients are discharged.
*LIP definition: any individual permitted by law and by the organization to provide patient care and services without direction and supervision, within the scope of the individual's licensure and consistent with individually granted clinical privileges.	*Supervised qualified individual definition: An individual who is qualified by virtue of education, experience, competence, applicable professional licensure and privileges.	

Note. Adapted from Sandra Tunajek, CRNA, MSN. *Report to AANA Board of Directors.* September, 1999.

accreditation visitors, an exit conference with review of findings, opportunity for institution response, and assignment of accreditation status. The critical nature of these types of accreditation or recognition from external agencies is usually related to eligibility for reimbursement to institutions and providers. A comparison of accreditation standards for anesthesia services is listed in Table 8.6.

AAAHC

The purpose of the AAAHC is to organize and operate a peer-based assessment, education and accreditation program for ambulatory healthcare organizations as a means of assisting them in providing the highest achievable level of care for recipients that is efficient and economically sound. Examples of ambulatory organizations accredited by AAAHC include ambulatory surgery centers, college and university health services, endoscopy centers, office surgery centers and practices, and podiatrists' offices (AAAHC, 1999). The AAAHC corporation is organized to:

- Conduct a survey and accreditation program that will promote and identify high-quality, cost-effective ambulatory healthcare programs and services.
- Establish standards for accreditation of ambulatory healthcare organizations and services.
- Recognize compliance with standards by issuance of certificates of accreditation.
- Conduct programs of education and research that will further other purposes of the corporation, to publish the results thereof, and to accept grants and gifts, bequests and devices in support of the purposes of the corporation.
- Provide programs that will facilitate communication, sharing of expertise and consultation among ambulatory healthcare organizations and services.
- Assume such other responsibilities and conduct such other activities as are comparable with such survey, standard setting, accreditation, and communication programs. (AAAHC, 1999)

AAAASF

The AAAASF is an accreditation program certifying to the medical community and lay community at large that a surgical facility meets nationally recognized standards. The accreditation program is operated by surgeons who set and evaluate the standards, under the direction of the board of directors (AAAASF, 1999).

JCAHO

The mission of the JCAHO is to improve the quality of care provided to the public through the provision of healthcare accreditation and related services that support performance improvement in healthcare organizations. JCAHO evaluates and accredits more than 19,500 healthcare organizations that provide home care, long-term care, behavioral healthcare, and laboratory and ambulatory care services. The commission is an independent, not-for-profit organization that was established in 1951 (JCAHO, 1999). Since its inception, JCAHO has been one of the most prominent accrediting agencies to have focused on quality of care issues and standards for providers.

SUMMARY

The professional regulation (credentialing) of CRNAs comprises the certification and recertification processes through mandatory CE and compliance with external accreditation agency requirements. This chapter has described the development and implementation of these regulatory procedures. AANA's leadership and members have supported and maintained sound regulatory practices for CRNAs which have long been noted among other provider organizations as some of the strongest and most effective standards and programs ever developed. Each individual CRNA, as a member of the specialty profession of nurse anesthesia, must remain committed to maintaining the quality of anesthesia care through contining education and demonstration of contemporary practice patterns of the highest standard.

REFERENCES

Accreditation Association for Ambulatory Health Care, Inc. (1999). *Accreditation Handbook for Ambulatory Health Care.* Skokie, IL: Author.

American Association for Accreditation of Ambulatory Surgery Facilities. (1997). *Standards and Checklist for Accreditation of Ambulatory Surgery Facilities.* Mundelein, IL: Author.

American Association of Nurse Anesthetists. (1999). Philosophy. In *Bylaws and Standing Rules of the American Association of Nurse Anesthetists.* Park Ridge, IL. Fiscal Year 2000.

American Nurses' Association. (1979). *The Study of Credentialing in Nursing: A New Approach.* Vol. I. A Report of the Committee. Washington, DC.

American Psychological Association. (1985). *Standards for Educational and Psychological Testing.* Washington, DC: Author.

Bankert, M. (1989). *Watchful Care: A History of America's Nurse Anesthetists.* New York, NY: Continuum Publishing.

Bergstrom, B.A. (1996). Computer adaptive testing for the National Certification Examination. *AANA Journal.* 64 (2), 119-124.

Bryant, S.K. (1981).Voluntary certification and the uniform guidelines on selection procedures: A potential problem for personnel managers. *Health Policy and Education.* 2:135-152.

Civil Service Commission. (1978). Uniform guidelines on employee selection procedures. *Federal Register.* 43, 166.

Continuing Education Program of the American Association of Nurse Anesthetists 1978-1998. (1998). American Association of Nurse Anesthetists. Park Ridge, IL.

Council on Certification of Nurse Anesthetists. (2000). *2000 Candidate Handbook.* American Association of Nurse Anesthetists. Park Ridge, IL.

Council on Recertification of Nurse anesthetists. (1998). *Criteria for Recertification 1978-1998.* American Association of Nurse Anesthetists. Park Ridge, IL.

Credentialing Health Manpower. (1977). U.S. Department of Health, Education, and Welfare. Washington, DC.

Henderson, J.B. (1996). Job analysis. In A.H. Browning, A.C. Bugbee, & M.A. Mullins (Eds.), *Certification: A NOCA Handbook* (p. 43). Washington, DC: NOCA Publication.

Joint Commission on Accreditation of Healthcare Organizations. (1999). *Accreditation Manual.* Oakbrook Terrace, IL.

Scofield, R. (1988). Certification: What does it mean? *Current Concepts in Nursing.* 2, 6-10.

Wright, B.D. & Masters, G. N. (1982). *Rating Scale Analysis* (pp. 1-10). Chicago, IL: MESA Press.

Wright, B.D. & Stone, M. H. (1979). *Best Test Design.* Chicago, IL: MESA Press.

Zaglaniczny, K.L. (1993). Council on Certification Professional Practice Analysis. *AANA Journal.* 61 (3), 241-255.

Zaglaniczny, K.L. & Healey, T. (1998). A report on the Council on Certification 1996 Professional Practice Analysis. *AANA Journal.* 66 (1), 43-62.

Zaglaniczny, K.L. (1996). The transition of the National Certification Examination from paper and pencil to computer adaptive testing. *AANA Journal.* 64 (1), 9-14.

KEY REFERENCES

Continuing Education Program of the American Association of Nurse Anesthetists 1978-1998. (1998). American Association of Nurse Anesthetists. Park Ridge, IL.

Council on Certification of Nurse Anesthetists. (2000). *2000 Candidate Handbook*. American Association of Nurse Anesthetists. Park Ridge, IL.

Council on Recertification of Nurse Anesthetists. (1998). *Criteria for Recertification* 1978-1998. American Association of Nurse Anesthetists. Park Ridge, IL.

STUDY QUESTIONS

1. What are the key factors that were instrumental in the development of continuing education for CRNAs?

2. What is the difference in the criteria for certification and recertification of CRNAs?

3. Compare and contrast the function and organization of the Council on Certification of Nurse Anesthetists with the Council on Recertification of Nurse Anesthetists.

4. What are the processes and procedures to obtain prior approval for a continuing education program?

5. How does a CRNA comply with external agency professional regulations such as those of the AAAHC?

CHAPTER 9

CREDENTIALING AND PRIVILEGING IN CLINICAL PRACTICE

Jeanne Learman, CRNA, MS

Director of Anesthesia
Eaton Rapids Medical Center
Eaton Rapids, MI

Director of Office Anesthesia Services
Ambulatory Surgery Consultants, Inc.
Bloomfield Hills, MI

KEY CONCEPTS

- Credentialing and privileging of Certified Registered Nurse Anesthetists (CRNAs) and others who provide healthcare with a high level of autonomy help assure the public that there is a process of self regulation to promote safe patient care.

- Credentialing includes: (1) verification that the applicant meets initial educational requirements for licensing and the profession, (2) checking current licenses and certifications for the states of practice, and (3) assessing current clinical competencies.

- CRNA credentialing may be accomplished through two different pathways: human resources, or the medical staff office as an allied health provider.

- The awarding of specific clinical privileges for CRNAs is typically part of credentialing as allied health providers. Clinical privileges should accurately reflect current competencies as a patient protection. Similar to medical staff, clinical privileges for the CRNA may be considered a "property right."

- Healthcare entities must query the National Practitioner Data Bank (NPDB) when granting and renewing privileges. The NPDB receives reports about payments made for medical malpractice, and these reports may have an impact on a healthcare facility's recredentialing decisions.

- The credentialing process may help the profession by promoting order, consistency, and control in the practice of nurse anesthesia.

- All CRNAs should maintain their own credentialing file.

Purposes of the credentialing and privileging process include: (1) Assuring the public that there is self-regulation of the medical staff and other individuals who provide healthcare with a high level of autonomy, and (2) bringing "order, consistency, and control" (Affara, 1992) to the profession. Hravnak (1997) points out that professionally imposed regulations can increase the validity of practice through peer review, ensuring public safety, and limiting practice by unqualified individuals.

Attitudes toward hospital medical staff credentialing have changed rapidly in the past few decades. Prior to 1975, hospital leaders, attorneys, third-party payers, the medical legal environment, and regulatory agencies, such as the Joint Commission on Accreditation of Hospitals (now Healthcare Organizations) were barely concerned with the issue of medical staff credentialing. In contrast, today's hospital medical staffs find themselves involved in increasing numbers of interdepartmental credentialing issues for a number of reasons: The medical legal environment has become far more invasive; the Joint Commission on Accreditation of Healthcare Organizations (JCAHO) has featured the issue of hospital credentialing prominently in the results of its surveys; and the National Committee for Quality Assurance (NCQA), which accredits HMOs, has required an active credentialing process as a prerequisite of accreditation. Additionally, examples of improper or ineffectual credentialing are often discussed in professional circles and sensationalized in the lay media.

As a result of these changes, hospital leaders are challenged to establish corporate policies and procedures that assure objectivity, consistency, and clinical competency throughout the appointment, privileges delineation, and reappointment process. Hospitals generally accomplish this through medical staff bylaws, governing board bylaws, and/or departmental rules and regulations.

Historically, CRNAs were employed with their responsibilities outlined in a job description or, in many small hospitals, were included as part of the regular medical staff. It was rare to have individual clinical privileges delineated. Clinical privileges are the procedures the clinician is qualified and permitted to perform within a healthcare facility. During the 1980s and 1990s, other nonphysician practitioners (certified nurse practitioners, nurse midwives, and physician assistants) increased in numbers and the majority of hospitals now have medical staff bylaws which define a category for allied health professionals (AHPs) that typically includes clinical psychologists, podiatrists, advanced practice nurses, physician assistants and others who the medical staff believes are necessary to offer specialized services at their institution.

This increased availability of allied health providers creates many political, legal and practical questions. Which allied health professionals may have access to the facility? Will there be a different process for employed providers and contracted providers? What is the process for initial credentialing, and the process for ongoing monitoring or renewal of privileges? The governing body must approve the categories of allied health providers who are permitted access to the facility and must define the method of evaluating current competency. Whether an allied health provider has access to a hospital or other healthcare facility depends on two factors: state law, including the state's licensing act, and the facility's governing body bylaws, rules and regulations. Hospitals may open themselves to anti-trust claims if the credentialing criteria developed are so restrictive that they exclude nonphysician practitioners from the hospital.

Hospital or healthcare facility bylaws may define whether the mid-level practitioners will be providing services independently to hospital clients or whether there will be collaboration with a member of the medical staff. The CRNA may be considered a "licensed independent practitioner" if state regulations (including the nurse practice act and hospital licensing regulations) do not require physician supervision. In reality, attempting to divide practitioners into two camps in which some function independently and others must be under supervision obscures the fact that the level of independence of individuals who deliver care, diagnostics, and supportive healthcare services is a continuum. AHPs are typically individuals with advanced degrees or training and although technically unable to function totally "independently" by law in some states, they practice with independent judgment and decision making, and in reality the degree of control or supervision exerted by others may be quite limited.

IMPLICATIONS FOR CRNAS

Currently, a multiplicity of approaches to credentialing CRNAs exists. When CRNAs are contracted by the hospital to provide services independently, they are generally required to apply and be credentialed as an allied health provider, but may be processed through regular medical staff credentialing channels. When CRNAs are hospital employees, their initial verification of credentials and experiences is documented by human resources and the anesthesia department manager. Individual clinical privileges should be delineated regardless of the contractual or employment relationship that exists within the practice setting. CRNAs are responsible for seeking clinical privileges that reflect their educational preparation, clinical experience, and level of professional competence. To establish credentials for employees, the hospital should establish an appropriate interface between the credentialing office and human resources. In the absence of a specific privileging process, the CRNA practices according to department policy. In some clinical settings, the CRNA's privileges change on a case-by-case basis according to decisions made by the anesthesiologist providing medical direction. This situation creates confusion for the CRNAs, surgeons, and operating room staff and should be avoided if possible. The patient's best interests are served when the CRNA is privileged according to education and experience, not according to departmental control issues.

The nurse anesthetist practices with various levels of autonomy in different practice settings (Table 9.1). For example, in most office settings and small hospital settings, the CRNA autonomously manages the anesthesia care from preanesthesia evaluation through discharge. Hospitals do not have to permit CRNAs to do everything they are permitted to do

Table 9.1: Key Points Regarding Level of Autonomy

- The CRNA should seek a practice setting which offers the desired level of autonomy.
- The CRNA should have the educational preparation and clinical experience to perform the privileges requested.
- The CRNA should be familiar with the level of autonomy which the practice setting allows, as defined by job description or clinical privileges.

by state statutes (Blackmond, 1997), and some hospitals do limit CRNA scope of practice. Faut-Callahan (1998) states that "it should be noted that no states have nursing rules or regulations that require that nurse anesthetists be supervised by anesthesiologists." Some nurse practice acts or state laws governing healthcare do have statements which indicate that a nurse anesthetist practices under physician supervision or direction. As Blumenreich (1997) explains in "The Nature of Supervision," it is a term which can have many interpretations, and for CRNAs practicing with surgeons, it is typically a collaborative practice with each bringing their respective skills together for the care of the patient.

When CRNAs are employees of a physician group with privileges to provide anesthesia care in the hospital, there has been more uncertainty about whether to credential the CRNAs as AHPs. Many facilities have left the responsibility of initial and ongoing credentialing to the physician group and required only evidence of current licenses, certification, and professional liability be given to the hospital. Concerns by hospitals about credentialing liability may change this process. Traditionally, hospitals were not held accountable for the errors and omissions of credentialed members of the medical staff. They were viewed as independent contractors to patients, using the hospital premises. This assumption has changed as courts have recognized how much authority healthcare entities exert in the selection and retention of members of the medical staff. Thus, liability has been imposed in situations where a healthcare entity knew or should have known that a clinician was likely to cause injury to patients. Benda and Rozovsky (1996) stated that "this direct corporate liability for the selection and credentialing of medical staff/allied health providers is likely to force the undeniable conclusion that AHPs must be credentialed." To protect themselves from claims of corporate negligence, hospitals and healthcare facilities may increase their oversight of hiring, credentialing, monitoring and supervising of AHPs. This may be true whether the AHP is employed by the healthcare facility, contracted, or employed through a physician group.

A healthcare facility must also decide how to provide due process if AHPs are denied access to the hospital or subjected to disciplinary action. JCAHO requires "hearing and appeal mechanisms" for termination of privileges for licensed independent practitioners (LIPs) defined by JCAHO as "any individual permitted by law and by the hospital to provide patient care services without direction or supervision, within the scope of the individual's license and consistent with individually granted clinical privileges." As Blumenreich (1990) explains, "Hospital privileges have been interpreted as establishing that the practitioner has a property right. This property right cannot be taken away without due process. Due process includes the right to a hearing, the right to present evidence and the right to have the decision made fairly and without prejudice." Blumenreich concludes that "it seems likely that the direction of the courts in finding that CRNAs and other non-physician healthcare providers have privileges and are entitled to the same protection as physicians will continue."

INITIAL CREDENTIALING

The credentialing process (Figures 9.1 and 9.2), while striving to meet the same goals, may differ from one facility to another. In fact, JCAHO (1997) recommendations for credentialing state that "The organization establishes hospital specific mechanisms for appointment of

Figure 9.1: Allied Health Professional Initial Credentialing Process

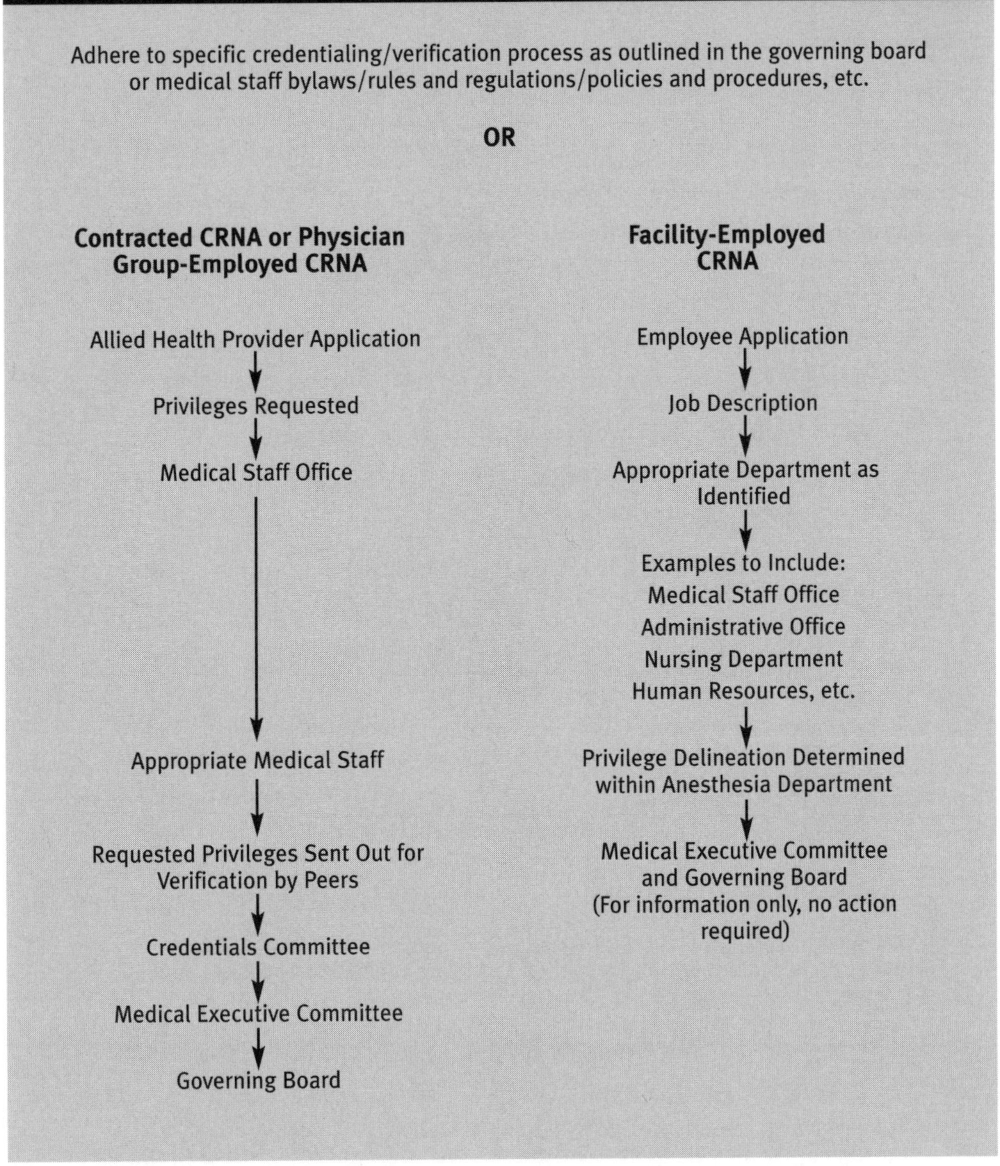

medical staff/allied medical staff members, and for granting and renewing or revising specific clinical privileges. These mechanisms may differ for medical staff members and other individuals." For the hospital-employed CRNA, the human resources department and anesthesia department determine whether initial requirements for education, licensing, certification, and experience have been met. The anesthesia department director assesses whether the CRNA has the required competencies to meet the needs of their department.

The procedures for credentialing CRNAs may follow the procedures for medical staff membership or reappointment. Ideally, the process includes an application that is specifically tailored to reflect the qualifications of a CRNA and the privileges applicable to CRNA practice (Figure 9.3); however, some hospitals

Figure 9.2: Sample Letter for Credentialing or Recredentialing a CRNA

Hospital address: ____

The following CRNA has applied for allied medical staff privileges: ________________

____

Please complete the following questionnaire:

1. Do you have direct knowledge of this applicant's current level of skill and knowledge?
   ❍ yes ❍ no

   If so, for how long? From ______ to _______.

   Please comment: ____

   Dates of affiliation with __________________ Hospital: From ________ to_________

2. In your opinion, is the applicant's current and overall competence:

   ❍ less than adequate ❍ competent ❍ above average

   If less than adequate, please explain: ______________________________

3. Would you be willing to have this applicant participate in the clinical care and management of yourself or your family? ❍ yes ❍ no

4. Does the applicant have the ability to work cooperatively in a milieu setting with all members of the interdisciplinary team? ❍ yes ❍ no

5. Are the applicant's ethical standards in conformance with the ethical standards maintained by the other members of your professional staff? ❍ yes ❍ no

6. If the answer to question 3, 4, or 5 was no, please explain:

   ____

   ____

7. Does the applicant have any mental or physical problems or disabilities that, to your knowledge, would prevent him or her from adequately performing clinical duties?
   ❍ yes ❍ no

8. Has the applicant ever been subject to any disciplinary action to your knowledge?
   ❍ yes ❍ no

9. Has the applicant, to your knowledge, ever had his/her membership, status, and/or clinical privileges revoked, suspended, reduced, or not renewed in any facility?
   ❍ yes ❍ no

10. To your knowledge, has this applicant's license and/or certification to practice in any jurisdiction ever been suspended or terminated? ❍ yes ❍ no

11. If the answer to question 7, 8, 9, or 10 was yes, please explain:________________

____

Additional comments:

____

____________________	____________________	____________________
Signature	Title	Address

Figure 9.3: Application for Clinical Privileges Form (request from AANA)

APPLICATION FOR CLINICAL PRIVILEGES

CLINICAL PRIVILEGES DELINEATION FORM

Type of Request: ☐ Initial ☐ Renewal

Category: Certified Registered Nurse Anesthetist

Soc. Sec. # ______________________________

Please check the procedures for which you are making application:

- ☐ Preanesthetic assessment
- ☐ Requesting laboratory/diagnostic studies
- ☐ Preanesthetic medication
- ☐ General anesthesia and adjuvant drugs
- ☐ Regional anesthesia techniques
  - ☐ Subarachnoid
  - ☐ Epidural
  - ☐ Caudal
  - ☐ Upper extremity
  - ☐ Lower extremity
  - ☐ Diagnostic and therapeutic nerve blocks
  - ☐ Local Infiltration
  - ☐ Topical
  - ☐ Periocular block
  - ☐ Transtracheal
  - ☐ Intracapsular
  - ☐ Intercostal
  - ☐ Other________________
- ☐ Cardiopulmonary resuscitation management
- ☐ Perianesthetic invasive and noninvasive monitoring
- ☐ Tracheal intubation/extubation
- ☐ Mechanical ventilation/oxygen therapy
- ☐ Fluid, electrolyte, acid-base management
- ☐ Blood, blood products, plasma expanders
- ☐ Peripheral intravenous/arterial catheter placement
- ☐ Central venous catheter placement
- ☐ Pulmonary artery catheter placement
- ☐ Acute and chronic pain therapy
- ☐ Post anesthesia care/discharge
- ☐ Conscious and deep sedation techniques
- ☐ Perianesthesia management of patient using accessory drugs or fluids
- ☐ Other ________________

I am mentally and physically capable of performing the privileges which I have requested:

Signature ____ Date ____________________

Name (Please print)____

The above nurse anesthetist is granted the full privileges which he/she has requested with the following exceptions and/or limitations (if none, so state).

Decision: ☐ Approval ☐ Disapproval

Signature, Chief Nurse Anesthetist ______________________________________

Signature, Medical Director ____

Signature, Director, Medical/Professional Staff Office____________________________

Date Practitioner Notified: ____

These privileges are granted initially for one calendar year following approval and must be renewed on a biennial basis. The applicant may request to have privileges changed as required during this period.

Note. From *Guidelines for Clinical Privileges*, p. 6. Copyright 1996 by American Association of Nurse Anesthetists. Park Ridge, IL.

prefer the use of a uniform credentialing application for all medical and AHPs.

CLINICAL PRIVILEGES

The American Association of Nurse Anesthetists (AANA) has developed a document titled "Guidelines for Clinical Privileges" (1996). This document continues to be a valuable guide to hospitals establishing allied medical staff privileges for CRNAs as it includes a CRNA-specific application form and a listing of specific anesthesia privileges. It is included in the *Professional Practice Manual for the Certified Registered Nurse Anesthetist.* Accomplishing an effective privileges delineation system involves classifying all major diagnostic and treatment procedures the hospital or healthcare organization permits within its walls or renders under its auspices into meaningful categories—what JCAHO calls "accurate, detailed, and specific" categories (MS 5.14, intent). The privileging of physicians in hospitals is relatively standardized, however the privileging of AHPs is far from standardized. Although healthcare organizations have the advantage of having more leeway in privileging AHPs compared to privileging physicians, they also have the disadvantage of having little guidance or tradition. CRNAs are most knowledgeable about the educational requirements and clinical practices of their profession and should take a leadership role in developing the experience requirements and definitions of privileges for their profession.

Privileges should be appropriate to the scope and complexity of care provided by CRNAs and should not be overly specific or restrictive (Table 9.2). Clinical privileging should be so defined as to permit the CRNA to provide selected procedures under specific conditions with or without supervision. The clinical privileging process includes: the qualifications of the provider; the actual practice privileges requested and granted; the conditions or limits of practice; and the process for evaluation and renewal of privileges.

PRIMARY SOURCE VERIFICATION

The medical staff credentialing and privileging path is more complex and includes requirements that are not in the human resources path. An example is that medical staff standards require primary source verification of education and training (JCAHO, 1997, MS 5.4, 3.1). "For initial granting of clinical privileges, the hospital verifies information about the applicants' licenses, specific training, experience, and current competence... with information from the primary source(s) when feasible." Primary sources are the organizations which issue the credentials (i.e., anesthesia program, board of nursing) or, to verify experience, the hospital or facility in which one obtained experience. This requirement for primary source verification was instituted by JCAHO in 1988 and eliminated the physician or allied health provider as the intermediary to transmit the credentials, documents, or experience.

The purpose of primary source verification is to reduce the possibility of forgery or falsification of credentials. Hospitals cannot accept material in the possession of medical staff applicants as sufficient evidence of credentials. Thus, credentials committees will require original letters of reference, request transcripts directly from colleges, and call the state board of nursing instead of accepting photocopies. Hospitals may still request photocopies of licenses, diplomas, etc., as helpful in the credentialing verification process. In an effort to establish that they have used "due diligence" to verify an applicant's experience, many hospitals contact all past employers and/or practice settings for the past three to five years. Because of this need for pri-

Table 9.2: Recommended Clinical Privileges

CRNA privileges and responsibilities must be consistent with law and may without limitation include the following:

Preanesthetic Preparation and Evaluation

- Obtaining an appropriate health history
- Conducting an appropriate physical screening assessment
- Recommending or requesting and evaluating pertinent diagnostic studies
- Selecting, obtaining, ordering, and administering preanesthetic medications
- Documenting the preanesthetic evaluation and obtaining informed consent for anesthesia, anesthesia induction, maintenance and emergence

Intraoperative Care

- Obtaining, preparing, and using all equipment, monitors, supplies and drugs used for the administration of anesthesia; performing and ordering safety checks as needed
- Selecting, obtaining or administering the anesthetics, adjuvant drugs, accessory drugs, fluids and blood products necessary to manage the anesthetic
- Performing all aspects of airway management
- Performing and managing regional anesthetic techniques including, but not limited to: subarachnoid, epidural and caudal blocks: plexus, major and peripheral nerve blocks; intravenous regional anesthesia; transtracheal, topical and local infiltration blocks; intracapsular, peribulbar, intercostal and retrobulbar blocks
- Providing appropriate invasive and noninvasive monitoring modalities utilizing current standards and techniques
- Recognizing abnormal patient response during anesthesia, selecting and implementing corrective action, and requesting consultation whenever necessary
- Evaluating patient response during emergence from anesthesia and instituting pharmacological or supportive treatment to insure patient stability during transfer

Postanesthesia Care

- Providing postanesthesia follow-up and evaluation of the patient's response to anesthesia and surgical experience, taking appropriate corrective actions and requesting consultation when indicated
- Initiating and administering respiratory support to ensure adequate ventilation and oxygenation in the postanesthesia period
- Initiating and administering pharmacological or fluid support of the cardiovascular system during the postanesthesia period to prevent morbidity and mortality
- Discharging patients from a postanesthesia care area

Clinical Support Functions

- Inserting peripheral and central intravenous catheters
- Inserting pulmonary artery catheters
- Inserting arterial catheters and performing arterial puncture to obtain arterial blood samples
- Managing emergency situations, including initiating or participating in cardiopulmonary resuscitation

(continued)

Table 9.2: Recommended Clinical Privileges (continued)

- Providing consultation and implementation of respiratory and ventilatory care
- Initiating management of pain therapy utilizing drugs, regional anesthetic techniques or other accepted pain relief modalities
- Selecting and prescribing medications and treatment related to the care of the patient, using consultation when appropriate
- Accepting additional responsibilities which are within the expertise of the individual CRNA and appropriate to the practice setting

Table 9.3: Suggestions for Facilitating the Credentialing Process

- Provide complete addresses for all educational institutions and practice sites.
- List a key contact person for each practice site (department manager or former colleague).
- If your work at the hospital was through an agency, provide the agency name, address and phone.
- Call the colleagues you list as references and let them know a timely response will be appreciated.
- Sending a structured reference letter (see Figure 9.2) may encourage a more rapid reply. Enclose a stamped envelope, pre-addressed to the medical staff coordinator at the facility where you are applying for privileges.
- When selecting references, use people who are familiar with your skills and patient outcomes, such as CRNAs, anesthesiologists, surgeons, and administrators.

Table 9.4: What to Maintain in Your Own Credentials File

- Nursing and anesthesia program addresses, transcripts, and diplomas
- Resume (including employment/practice history with addresses)
- RN licenses
- Accreditation and recertification certificates
- Specialty certification (if applicable in your state)
- BCLS, ACLS documentation
- Letters of reference from colleagues who practice with you
- Transcript of continuing education hours
- Immunization status: hepatitis B
- TB test results
- Professional liability insurance
- List of appropriate clinical privileges

mary source verification there are a number of things applicants can do to help the credentialing process go faster and smoother (Table 9.3). With the recent attention to credentialing and increased numbers of HMOs and hospital mergers, requirements of the credentialing process have put additional strain on medical staff coordinators and the physicians and allied health providers who must provide ever more information (see Table 9.4). A cooperative attitude is essential. Efforts in making the credentialing process go smoothly for the medical staff coordinator will most likely be rewarded by return cooperation received when you want assistance with policy changes or educational endeavors.

NATIONAL PRACTITIONER DATA BANK

Hospitals and other credentialing bodies must query the National Practitioner Data Bank (NPDB) when granting and renewing privileges (1994). Reports are made to, and obtained from, the NPDB regarding claims of medical malpractice against healthcare practitioners. Congress voted the NPDB into existence with the federal Health Care Quality Improvement Act of 1986 with the purpose of restricting the ability of incompetent physicians and other healthcare providers to move from state to state without disclosure or discovery of the practitioner's previous damaging or incompetent performance. In operation since 1990, the NPDB receives approximately 25,000 reports of adverse actions against health providers yearly. As noted by Kremer and Faut-Callahan (1998), "A limitation of NPDB information is that malpractice payments recorded in the NPDB do not necessarily constitute a comprehensive and definitive reflection of actual health care incompetence." One loophole which may soon be closed is that currently the NPDB does not require reporting on a healthcare practitioner who was dismissed from a proceeding—only those for whom a payment was made in settlement of a claim. Also, as discussed by Metter, Granville, and Kussman (1997), the NPDB practice of using claims payment as an indicator of substandard care results in significant inaccuracies because about 30 percent of claims with substandard care are not paid and will not be reported to the NPDB. CRNAs should be aware of the reporting requirements of the NPDB, its potential impact on their ability to be credentialed, and their right to enter an explanation regarding a claim.

ASSESSMENT OF CONTINUED COMPETENCY/RECREDENTIALING

The credentialing of medical staff began in the 1970s. Prior to that, medical staff members were customarily given hospital privileges once for a lifetime of practice. This periodic re-evaluation has become necessary to satisfy JCAHO and requirements for institutional licensing. The recredentialing decision is based partly on updating qualifications, but primarily on information about performance.

Written evidence of continued competency (Figure 9.4) for the employed CRNA will generally be summarized in an annual review completed by a hospital-employed manager, or for the physician group-employed CRNA, by physicians in the group. A determination of current competencies may include: demonstrations of knowledge of cardiorespiratory resuscitation and other emergency procedures, use of anesthesia and emergency equipment, and review of specific skills, i.e., arterial line placement. Requests for renewal of specific anesthesia privileges should be based on the CRNA's education, training, experience, demonstrated ability, and judgment. Requests for new privileges may be awarded after documentation of education and observed skills

Figure 9.4: Recredentialing/Continued Competency

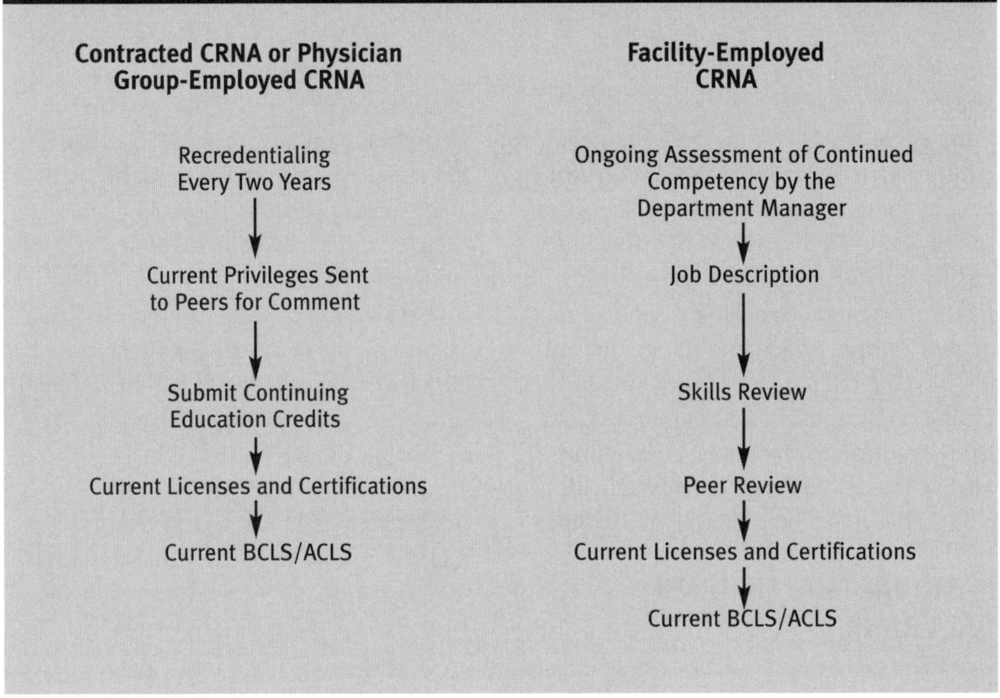

(Figure 9.5). Results of quality improvement studies should be considered. Patient satisfaction surveys can help in the recredentialing process but should not be the sole resource of measuring quality patient care.

For the contracted CRNA or physician group-employed CRNA with allied health provider status at the hospital, written evidence of continued competency will usually be assessed every two years. This privilege reappointment process may ask two or three colleagues familiar with the CRNA's work to verify the CRNA's continued qualifications for a specific list of privileges and attest to the CRNA's continued competence by completing a letter of reference similar to Figure 9.2. JCAHO standards recommend quality improvement and risk management data be considered as part of the reappointment process. Responsibility for the assessment and improvement of clinical processes and patient outcomes are characteristics of professional work, and CRNA involvement in these activities will be scrutinized. It is possible that in the future more active recredentialing will be required, i.e., skills verification by simulator testing. The American Society of Anesthesiologists determined that starting in 2000, board certification in anesthesiology is only to be granted for 10 years, after which time some type of retesting will be required to maintain board certification.

Some hospitals require a 50 percent or 60 percent attendance rate at medical staff meetings for active medical staff. This requirement rarely extends to the AHPs, but CRNAs will find time spent attending medical staff meetings to be insightful in understanding the concerns of medical staff relative to the anesthesia services. Your presence means you will help develop policies for anesthesia delivery and be able to educate the medical staff about CRNA practice. Committees

Figure 9.5: New Anesthesia Clinical Privileges Form

Anesthesia Provider: ____________________

New Privilege Requested: ____________________

Didactic Review (articles, lectures, audiotapes or videotapes):

____

____

____

____

____

____

____

Clinical Experience:	Date:	Observed by:
______	______	______
______	______	______
______	______	______
______	______	______
______	______	______
______	______	______
______	______	______

Approved by: ____________________ Date: __________

Director of Anesthesia

(e.g., CPR, infection control, conscious sedation, and obstetrics) will develop policies which have an impact on CRNA practice. CRNAs serving on these committees have found them to be an important way to influence hospital policy, provide education to nursing staff, and create positive relations for CRNAs throughout the hospital.

It is beyond the minimum requirements for credentialing and a mark of excellence to take an active part in identifying and maintaining the qualifications and competencies necessary to provide anesthesia care for your patient group. That is, if the hospital adds trauma care, open heart surgery, pain management or a labor epidural service, the professional CRNA should take an active role in establishing reliable competencies for those areas. In addition to patient care, the recredentialing process typically includes an assessment of the CRNA's documentation, teamwork, and personal accountability.

NONMEDICAL ISSUES IN CREDENTIALING

Practitioners should be evaluated on criteria which are directly related to patient care and the practitioner's ability to perform the requested privileges. If practitioners are disciplined, it will usually be because of problems which directly affect the quality of care provided. However, as Lansberg (1977) points out, both state and federal courts have upheld decisions by healthcare entities to exclude or discipline a physician for reasons not directly related to patient care. These include:

- Giving incomplete or false information on the application form.
- Unfavorable reports or references from other facilities including attitude and personality problems.
- Violation of bylaws or rules, e.g., refusing, even after warning, to follow hospital criteria for performing a particular procedure or refusing to accept every third indigent OB/GYN patient who comes to the hospital.
- Disruptive behavior or inability to work with others, e.g., dealing with hospital staff in a volatile, hostile, and uncooperative manner.
- Refusal to execute a release for a transfer of information from another hospital.
- Physician's termination for alcohol abuse.
- Criminal conduct: convicted of driving while intoxicated, second offense.
- Economic criteria: termination of radiologist's privileges based upon the refusal to sign employment contracts with the physician who was awarded an exclusive contract.
- Noncompliance with bylaws provisions: Bylaws may specify the conditions under which a medical staff member or allied healthcare provider may request a leave of absence and detail the procedure for reinstatement of privileges.

CREDENTIALS VERIFICATION ORGANIZATIONS

Although hospitals cannot accept evidence of credentials carried by applicants, they may rely on other organizations to conduct primary source verification. Credentials verification organizations (CVOs) acting as an "agent" are now common nationwide, many of them managed by hospital and physician associations. For example, Michigan Professional Credential Verification Services, Inc. was started as a joint venture of the Michigan Hospital Association and the Michigan State Medical Society. Managed care organizations (MCOs) have contributed to the growth of CVOs because a typical MCO will enroll several hundred practitioners and the burden of credentialing could be enormous. Once a CVO checks a practitioner's credentials, it does not need to check them again when another hospital requests credentialing (within a reasonable time frame). This reduces the cost and time required for credentialing and reduces the number of inquiries that agencies issuing the credentials must handle.

In 1999, a hospital typically paid about $200 per physician or allied health provider for initial credentialing and $75 for recredentialing. In an effort to reduce their costs for credentialing, some health systems are establishing an area-wide approach to credentialing with a uniform application package which, when completed, may be mailed to each healthcare facility at which you are requesting initial or renewal privileges. The NCQA certifies some CVOs. This reduces the oversight required by the healthcare facility using the CVO.

TRENDS FOR THE FUTURE

The opportunities for hospitals, healthcare systems and physician group practices to maintain quality of care and patient satisfaction while at the same time increasing the level of service and reducing costs may be maximized by utilizing allied health providers. Market forces continue to change our healthcare delivery systems, including where care is delivered (outpatient clinics and offices), and who is providing the care. Many observers of evolving healthcare market forces believe that AHPs will play an ever increasing and important role in managed care. AHPs can help accomplish the goals of the new healthcare environment to deliver health services differently, using fewer resources yet maintaining quality outcome and customer satisfaction. "You can be a victor over change or a victim of change. Set up a training program in your mind and make sure your top employee (you!) is updating his or her skills (Waitley, 1999)."

SUMMARY

The public expects and is increasingly demanding through litigation that the hospital/healthcare entity have mechanisms in place to screen the providers who care for them. Chief among those who monitor such practices is the JCAHO, which holds itself out to the public as the group that will assess whether hospitals have appropriate mechanisms to review the credentials of physicians, AHPs, and employees. Approximately 80 percent of U.S. hospitals report to their local communities that they are accountable to the public because they have met JCAHO recommendations assessed during an on-site visit (Personal communications, JCAHO Media Relations, August 29, 2000).

Hospitals are increasingly using CVOs to provide primary source verification of data required to credential medical and allied health providers. One factor prompting this change is the merger of many large hospitals and managed care systems necessitating the processing of large numbers of new medical staff simultaneously. Although JCAHO requires physician members of the medical staff to be credentialed and privileged, hospitals may choose to verify CRNA credentials through one of two mechanisms: the human resources department, or allied health providers' credentialing. Qualifications of employed CRNAs are usually processed by a human resources department at the facility. In addition, there may be allied medical staff credentialing procedures required.

The process of awarding specific clinical privileges is always part of allied health providers' credentialing and may or may not be implemented for employed CRNAs. CRNAs should be granted clinical practice privileges in the same manner as other healthcare professional staff members who are permitted by law and the facility to provide patient care services. The credentialing and privileging process should provide an objective mechanism for initial application and renewal of clinical privileges based on education, experience, legal qualifications and a practitioner's competence and ability to render quality care. There is substantial evidence that many CRNAs privileges are restricted not by initial training or experience, but by medical staff bylaws or by the employing or supervising physician anesthesiologist group.

Healthcare attorneys and risk managers are encouraging hospitals to use the AHP credentials verification process to credential all nonphysician providers, i.e., advanced practice nurses, physician assistants, physical therapists, psychologists, podiatrists, and chiropractors. They recommend that hospitals may gain some legal protection by regular recredentialing of providers who exercise a high level of independent decision making in the provision of patient care, and by providing similar due process rights as are customarily afforded medical staff. In sum, all CRNAs should be prepared for ongoing changes to the provider credentialing and privileging process by maintaining their own credential file. In doing so, they demonstrate an appreciation for the growing importance of these issues as a primary professional responsibility of the clinical practitioner.

REFERENCES

Affara, R. (1992). The fundamentals of professional regulation. *International Nursing Review.* 39(4). 113-116.

American Association of Nurse Anesthetists. (1996). Part I: Standards and Guidelines. *Professional Practice Manual for the Certified Registered Nurse Anesthetist.* Park Ridge, IL: Author.

Benda, G.D. & Rozovsky, R.A. (1996). *Managed Care and the Law: Liability and Risk Management.* Boston, MA: Little, Brown and Company.

Blackmond, B. (1997). Risk management and allied health professionals. *NAMSS Overview.* 21-24.

Blumenreich, G. (1997). The nature of supervision. *AANA Journal.* 165(3)208-211.

Blumenriech, G. (1990). Hospital privileges. *AANA Journal.* 58(1)66-68.

Faut-Callahan, M. (1998). Credentialing of CRNAs. *Advanced Practice Nursing Quarterly.* 544-62.

Health Resources Services Administration. (1994). *USDHHS National Practitioner Data Bank Guidebook.* Washington, DC: U.S. Government Printing Office.

Hravnak, M. (1997). Credentialing and privileging: Insight into the process for acute care nurse practitioners. *AACN Clinical Issues.* 8(1)108-115.

Joint Commission on Accreditation of Healthcare Organizations. (1997). *Comprehensive Accreditation Manual for Hospitals: The Official Handbook.* Oakbrook Terrace, IL: Author.

Joint Commission on Accreditation of Healthcare Organizations. (1997). Medical Staff Chapter, Standards MS, 5.4, 3.1. In *Comprehensive Accreditation Manual for Hospitals: The Official Handbook.* Oakbrook Terrace, IL: Author.

Kremer, M. J. & Faut-Callahan, M. (1998). The National Practitioners Data Bank: Implications for nurse anesthetists. *CRNA Forum.* 9(4)157-162.

Landsberg. B. (1997). Physician integrity and other non-medical issues in credentialing. Paper presented at the National Health Lawyers Association Conference.

Learman, J. & Loppnow, N. (1997). Credentialing of CRNAs: Time for a new look. *AANA Journal.* 65(3)228-234.

Metter, E. J., Granville, R. L., & Kussman, J.J. (1997). The effect of threshold amounts for reporting malpractice payments to the National Practitioners Data Bank: Analysis using the closed claims data of the office of the assistant secretary of defense (health affairs). *Military Med.* 162(4)257-261.

Waitely, D. (1999). Personal Coach. *Priorities.* 3(5)30-32.

KEY REFERENCES

American Association of Nurse Anesthetists. (1996). *Professional Practice Manual for the Certified Registered Nurse Anesthetist.* Park Ridge, IL: Author.

Blumenreich, G. (1990). Hospital privileges. *AANA Journal.* 58(1)66-68.

Faut-Callahan, M. (1998). Credentialing of CRNAs. *Advanced Practice Nursing Quarterly.* 54-62.

Learman, J. & Loppnow, N. (1997). Credentialing of CRNAs: Time for a new look. *AANA Journal.* 65(3)228-234.

STUDY QUESTIONS

1. Describe the definitions for credentialing and privileging as well as the typical process CRNAs follow in securing both as requirements for practice.

2. Discuss the reasons why credentialing and privileging are increasingly important both to the facilities that employ CRNAs as well as to a CRNA's scope of practice.

3. Discuss the intended purpose of the National Practitioner Data Bank and how CRNAs are affected by it.

4. Describe why it is important for CRNAs to maintain their own credentialing file and what should become a part of the file.

THE HEALTHCARE ENVIRONMENT

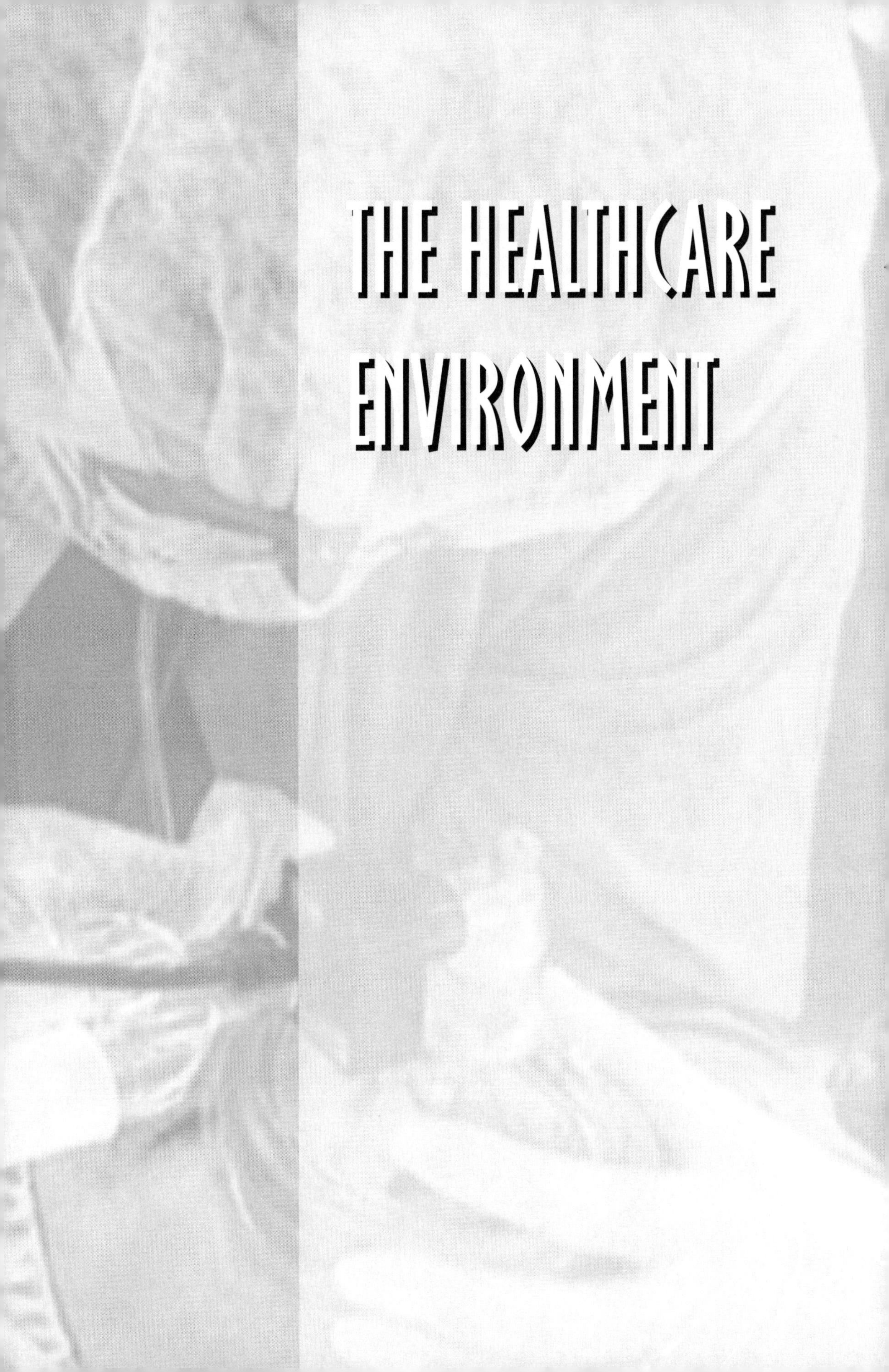

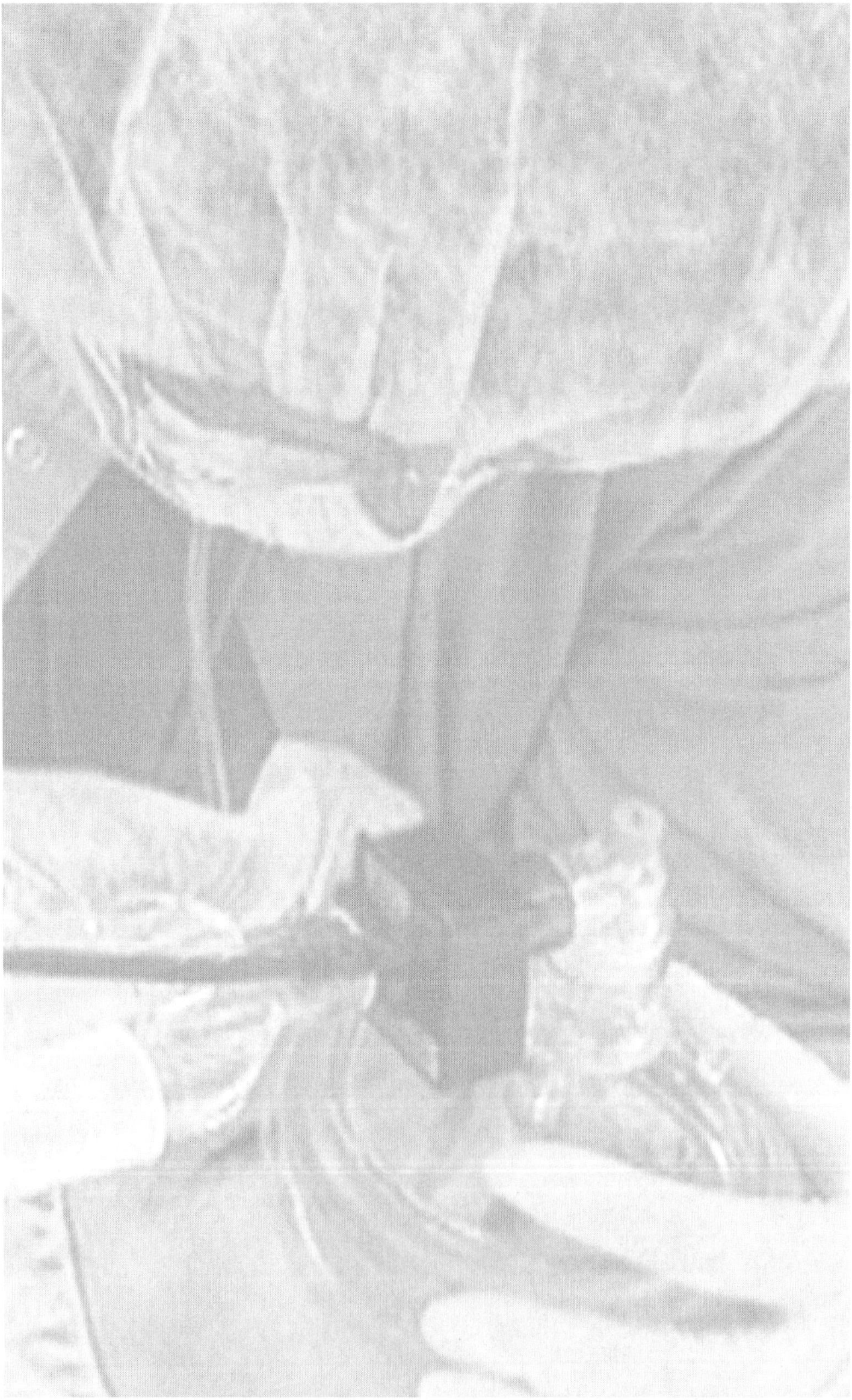

CHAPTER 10

HEALTHCARE DELIVERY IN THE UNITED STATES

Ira P. Gunn, CRNA, MLN, FAAN

Consultant
San Antonio, TX

Scot D. Foster, CRNA, PhD, FAAN

Senior Editor

Professor, Nursing
Director, Program of Nurse Anesthesia
Samuel Merritt College
Oakland, CA

KEY CONCEPTS

- The U.S. healthcare system is unique from others in the world because (1) the United States spends far more on health services than any other industrialized country, (2) segments of the U.S. health system serve as corporate, for-profit sources, and (3) there is no universal coverage for all citizens.

- The delivery system is based on social values of autonomy, free enterprise, market demand and domination by the medical community. This was achieved through restrictive licensing, credentialing and legislative protections.

- The healthcare system is composed of five basic elements or sectors: health providers (individuals and institutions or agencies); health payers (health insurers—public and private, industry, individuals); health regulators (public and private); health manufacturers (equipment, pharmaceuticals, etc.), and health clients.

- Failure of the current system is characterized by excessive costs, lack of universal access, uneven availability of service, emphasis on cure rather than prevention, and lack of attention to quality indicators.

- Wholesale reform of the national healthcare system is unlikely even though some states have adopted progressive changes to serve their local population more effectively. Ultimately change will come incrementally through legislation unless more drastic change is prompted by popular mandate or a major economic threat to business and industry.

The healthcare system in the United States differs significantly from systems in other developed countries. As such, many of its problems and features are unique. Among those distinguishing characteristics are that in 2000, health expenditures are substantially greater than in other major industrialized countries; the United States lacks a comprehensive system for paying for health services; the system is rapidly becoming a corporate profit center; and availability of care is grossly uneven among the population. However, in many cases the problems are the same: Delivery systems are overextended, too costly, egregiously slow in providing care, fail to emphasize preventative care, and don't document quality improvement efforts very well. For those with unlimited resources, the quality and scope of healthcare resources, technology and service available in the United States are still generally regarded as pre-eminent. However, it is clear that the system remains in crisis because of its failure to contain costs, protect its users from potential catastrophic financial loss for lack of coverage, or serve the basic, preventative healthcare needs of all citizens.

The configuration of the healthcare delivery system in the United States is a product of this country's founding economic tenets and the medical profession's influence on its design, as described in Paul Starr's (1982) book, *The Social Transformation of American Medicine.* Since the late 1800s, state and federal governments legislatively codified much of the structural design of the healthcare system promulgated by organized medicine. Because of these early and effective attempts at control of the system, it has taken significant effort to make any statutory or regulatory revision that would enhance system flexibility or accommodate social need.

Nearly every U.S. president since the turn of the century has attempted to influence the healthcare system to make it more available and responsive to the needs of ordinary citizens. Although there have been many notable and successful efforts at reform, such as legislating Medicare and Medicaid programs, most progress has come incrementally in the form of insurance portability, changes in reimbursement mechanisms, and more inclusive access for at-risk populations. Unfortunately, substantive progress toward a more systemized mode of delivery has been elusive, culminating in the failed attempt by the Clinton administration to implement wholesale revision of the system via the 1994 Health Care Security Act.

A more functional healthcare delivery system will most likely be built on the tenets of managed care, but it is increasingly obvious that even this paradigm is not the panacea once imagined. The public has become increasingly vocal in its concerns that managed care organizations more frequently cater to the interest of corporate profit than public good, fail to offer promised services, and ignore meaningful work that emphasizes quality of care. Institutions themselves are finding that the mega-mergers of the 1990s too often failed to save money by streamlining services, that teamwork with physicians was increasingly costly and difficult, and that governmental regulations appeared to increase in direct proportion to the decreases in third-party reimbursements. Providers also became disenchanted with erosion of their traditional decision-making authority and practice autonomy, not to mention the continuing squeeze by the government on reimbursement schedules.

Features of our healthcare delivery system today remain based largely on early social tenets from which this country grew, including concepts of free market enterprise, autonomy, entrepreneurial models, and pre-eminence of the doctor/patient relationship. Attempts to modify these factors in ways that make the system more responsive have been only marginally successful. Clearly, the U.S. system of care is still in need of fixing, but will apparently follow a more incremental approach.

Where will we go from here? Has managed care proven to be a failure? Will managed care transform into managed competition or some other related permutation and how will that affect the patient? Finally, will our system ultimately revert to a single-payer system sponsored by the federal government? Clearly, most agree that future changes must be substantial and systematic, requiring Certified Registered Nurse Anesthetists (CRNAs) to be at the locus of planning and debate. This chapter and the next consider the historical evolution of healthcare delivery in the United States, its current status, issues under study, and details of the managed care system itself.

HISTORICAL OVERVIEW

While there were a variety of types of physicians in the United States in the late 1800s, the allopathic physicians ultimately won control of the health delivery system. The early design of the system made physicians gatekeepers to healthcare and assured that persons seeking care would initially have to be seen by a physician. This was accomplished largely by passage of the medical practice acts that licensed physicians in each of the states, beginning in 1873. While some practice acts were enacted in the late 17th and 18th century, most were repealed by 1850 due to the chaotic state of medical education and wide variations in the quality of physician providers.

Some of the early practice acts were aimed at setting reimbursement rates for physicians based on their varying levels of competence and education. While some physicians were university educated, others had been trained in apprenticeship programs. It was another quarter-century before the medical education system was sufficiently stable to allow phsicians to publicly endorse a monopoly over the whole of healthcare. Bullough (1983), Safreit (1991) and Hadley (1989) state that medicine claimed the whole of healthcare for itself since no other health providers were licensed at the time, including nurses. In the intervening decades, nonphysician health providers have had to work diligently to reclaim their areas of practice through the legislative process. The South Carolina Medical Practice Act (1976) provides an apt example of the pervasiveness of this controlling influence by medicine. It states "that Medical Practice includes any person who shall diagnose, cure, relieve in any degree or profess or attempt to diagnose, cure or relieve any human disease, ailment, defect, abnormality, or complaint, whether of a physical or mental origin, by attendance or advice, by prescribing, using or furnishing any drug, appliance, manipulation, adjustment or [other] method or by any therapeutic agent whatsoever."

Licensing acts not only placed the physician in a position to control the care provided to patients but essentially extended that control over other health providers. Consequently, their economic control of the healthcare dollar was assured. Certainly, physicians had more education than other health workers at the time, so it was not difficult for them to achieve dominance. Further, they were organized to achieve that purpose, while organization of other health providers came much later. It should be noted, however, that neither the economic stature nor economic rewards for physicians at the turn of the century compare with what they are today. The U.S. population was mostly rural, and the distances patients and their doctors had to travel to see one another took a significant portion of their time. Consequently, the number of patients serviced was much smaller than is common today. Pay took the form of a dozen eggs, a couple of chickens, and in some instances, money.

There were only a few services that early physicians could provide, as medical knowledge was still ill-defined and poorly understood. Many of those responsibilities today fall within the nature and practice of nursing. Few rural areas had hospitals, and therefore patients were cared for in their homes. Thus, physicians did not rely extensively on nurses or other health professionals. In fact, except for nurses and pharmacists, many allied health professionals and technicians did not exist. The physicians' greatest competitors at the turn of the century were the so-called nostrum makers, that is, makers and sellers of patented medicines. It was not until the passage of the Federal Pure Food and Drug Act in 1906 that the American Medical Association (AMA) began to gain some control over pharmaceuticals and prescription (Starr, 1982), again by declaring it within the rightful and exclusive domain of medicine.

While nursing, or nurturing, existed even in prehistoric times, as did elements of medicine, formalized nursing in the United States did not appear until physicians were well into the process of seeking licensure. In 1873, there were three schools of nursing. By 1900, there were 432 (ANA, 1979). Many of these schools were established as a cheap source of labor for the developing hospital industry. Florence Nightingale, whose nursing philosophies and traditions influenced early American nursing, did not believe in state licensing, but felt that educational programs should be of such quality as to make graduation the sole requisite for professional credibility and recognition. However, the proliferation of nursing programs in the United States indicated that there was such variation in quality that nursing leaders eventually sought state licensure.

Unfortunately, early legislation adopted the practice of registration, wherein the title was protected, but not the practice. That is, the scope of nursing practice was not defined within a registration model as would have been the case under a licensure model. The first state to enact legislation was North Carolina. Also important and unlike other professional education disciplines in the United States, state boards of nursing were given responsibility for approving nursing education programs, in addition to registering nurses (Waddle, 1979). In 1938, the National League for Nursing Education began a private sector accreditation program for nursing education. Subsequently its name was changed to the National League for Nursing.

The urbanization of the United States began in earnest with the industrial revolution. In the early 1900s, physicians, church groups, and others began building hospitals for the care of the sick, predominantly in cities. By this time, the germ theory had been enunciated and principles of disinfection and sterilization were employed that stimulated the growth of hospitals, allowing large numbers of patients to be confined in one institution without fear of patient-to-patient contamination. Further, because of urbanization and industrialization, few families were well-equipped at home to take care of family members during serious illnesses. Through efforts of nurses and social workers, the Henry Street Settlement in New York City pioneered the public health movement and the visiting nurse concept for care of the indigent. Congress passed the Sheppard-Towner Act of 1921 to help finance public health nurses and state laws were passed to register births and license midwives. Soon statistics documented lower maternal and infant mortality and at lower cost. Predictably, opposition by organized medicine arose because these programs were not under physician control or direction. This lead inevitably to the discontinuation of the Sheppard-Towner Act (Melosh, 1982 and Diers, 1992).

Major expansion of community-based hospitals, particularly in rural areas, awaited the passage of the Hill-Burton Act by Congress in 1946. In its first 20 years, 4,678 projects were undertaken, almost half directed to communities with under 10,000 population (Stevens, 1989). Provider discrimination became a popular mechanism in many early hospitals in awarding staff membership and clinical privileges. Most often, privileges were restricted to white, male physicians. Early female physicians had to build their own hospitals if they were to benefit from this mode of practice, as did black physicians. Often a qualification for hospital staff privileges was membership in the medical society. At that time, women and blacks were not readily admitted to these societies, and were essentially forced to establish their own professional organizations (Waddle, 1979; Melosh, 1982; and Diers, 1992). This, of course, was a reflection of the social mores of the nation, at least until the civil rights legislation of the 1960s.

THE ADVENT OF HEALTH INSURANCE

Interest in health insurance actually had began in the United States by 1910. The idea put forth was for universal coverage where payment for insurance was divided between state governments, employers, and employees. In spite of early and vehement opposition by the AMA, many physicians believed its emergence was inevitable, and most eventually abandoned their traditional opposition and endorsed these early initiatives. However, World War I intervened, and compulsory insurance began to be cast in the mold of being un-American. It was often termed a "Prussianization of America." Many in the medical profession were relieved that the issue of insurance was temporarily, at least, "off the table," as it was viewed by some as a potential threat to the doctor-patient relationship, not to mention traditional methods of reimbursement.

Commercial insurance companies, physicians in New York, and a labor leader, Samuel Gompers, who preferred higher wages to fringe benefits, began to oppose universal health insurance (Numbers, 1984). In 1925, the New York State Medical Society reported that "...health insurance is a dead issue in the United States.... It is not conceivable that any serious effort will again be made to subsidize medicine as the handmaiden of the public." A medical historian stated that physicians of the time did not reckon with the great depression that was soon to come, which would threaten the financial security of both physicians and hospitals and have the effect of reopening the debate on the advisability of health insurance.

In 1929, voluntary health insurance got its start in Dallas, Texas, when teachers agreed to pay Baylor University Hospital 50 cents a month for hospital insurance. This insurance afforded each teacher 21 days of hospitalization per year. The concept was the forerunner of Blue Cross, a private, not-for-profit, hospital insurance corporation. Blue Shield, the other part of the "Blues" which covers physician payments, was not formalized until 1946.

The major impetus for the acceptance and spread of private health insurance came from the labor movement shortly after World War II, when the Supreme Court ruled that labor unions could appropriately negotiate and strike over healthcare benefits for their members. As more and more American industries offered health benefits to employees, it became almost unthinkable that major employers would someday not offer health insurance as a paid benefit. However, this benefit is now perceived by many business leaders as one central reason for their declining competitiveness in a global economy. Consequently, continued provision of health benefits is undergoing significant review and change. For example, retirees are now being eliminated from plans promised for life, coverage is being reduced or is unavailable, and beneficiaries are having to pay larger deductibles and co-payments. This may presage the inevitability of employee-paid health insurance for the future.

Essentially, as an outgrowth of American medicine's design, the healthcare delivery system became physician-controlled, acute care-centered, and hospital-based. The payment system was designed to permit physicians to be reimbursed directly by patients on a fee-for-service basis. Thus, medicine had gained through its state licensing acts exclusive privileges and a monopoly as gatekeeper to the delivery of health services in the United States.

Medicine, as a state-endorsed monopoly, has been traditionally protected from restrictive practices that in the business world would have made individuals, groups, or companies subject to federal and state antitrust laws. It was not until 1976 that the U.S. Supreme Court ruled that the nation's antitrust laws also applied to the professions (Wing, 1985). Thus, monopolization of markets, conspiring to restrain trade, and price fixing, wherein the profession did not have an exclusive legal prerogative, made physicians vulnerable to actions under both federal and state antitrust laws. A variety of antitrust allegations have been made against groups of physicians or professional societies with varying results. However, the cost of such litigation and the length of time required to finalize court decisions have reduced the number of actions taken under these laws. In some instances, either the state or federal government's antitrust operatives may seek consent decrees from persons charged with antitrust violations to correct situations in which restrictive practices and/or price fixing were alleged.

While many of the arguments the medical profession made for designing the system were based on quality concerns, there can be little question that the profession was equally concerned about its economic status. Physicians and hospitals have usually been allowed to determine the value of their own services and been given authority to charge what they believed the market would bear. Such practice is usually consistent with a capitalistic system based on the supply and demand theory of a market economy. Unfortunately, the demand for healthcare services is often significantly influenced by the principal suppliers of that system—hospitals and physicians. Some health policy analysts view the healthcare system as a traditional market, when it is really an aberration of this model, a view that constitutes a major factor in the current cost crisis in healthcare (Starr, 1982; Stevens, 1989; and Ribicoff and Danaceau, 1972).

TODAY'S HEALTHCARE SYSTEM

The basic elements of the healthcare delivery system resemble, in large measure, the early design created by organized medicine. Today's situation is certainly far more complex and more regulated, but it has been largely resistant to change. Consequently, reform measures from a variety of quarters remain at the forefront of public debate.

The major players in the healthcare delivery system today are health providers (individuals and institutions or agencies); health payers (health insurers—public and private, industry, individuals); health regulators (public and private); health manufacturers (equipment, pharmaceuticals, etc.); and health clients. In addition to physicians, hospitals have played a major role in influencing today's delivery system. Hospitals in the United States impact the delivery of health services in the following ways:

- Hospital ownership reflects the pluralism of American society itself. They are owned by the government and by private groups. Those hospitals under private ownership are usually held by various religious, racial, ethnic, and organizational groups. They may be voluntary, nonprofit, or for-profit operations, community-supported at local levels or supported by municipalities, state, or federal governments.
- Hospitals have served to define social class and race, including the poor, the wealthy, and ethnic groups. While civil rights laws eliminated overt hospital segregation of races, public and private hospitals still often segregate the poor from the wealthy in more discrete and subtle ways.
- Few American hospitals have large endowments and many depend largely on revenues generated from patient services.
- Hospitals focus on acute care, high technology, and on surgery in particular, for revenue potential.
- A symbiotic relationship exists between hospitals and physicians—the physician needs hospitals in which to admit patients, and the hospital needs physicians to fill beds and pay for its operation. Doctors are "privileged" to work in hospitals and to admit patients, and they exert a privileging control via medical staff policies to keep other providers out who might afford competition. Physician influence dominates the hospital environment, especially in policy making, often to the detriment of other health providers, including nurses, therapists, and technicians.
- Medical schools, especially those that are university-based, have undue influence on the hospital system, capitalizing virtually all resources and causing tensions related to governance and cost.

As these six characteristics are in constant interaction, hospitals are in a state of constant change. "They are affirming and defining mirrors of the culture in which we live, beaming back to us, through the scope and style of the buildings, the organizational personality of the institution and the underlying meaning of the whole enterprise, the values we impute to medicine, technology, wealth, class, and social welfare. (Stevens, 1989)."

Public Sector Roles in Healthcare

Governments, at national, state, and local levels, assume pivotal roles in healthcare. The principal roles relate to financing, delivery, and regulation, although each level of government may approach its

Table 10.1: Major Healthcare Roles of Federal, State, and Local Governments

	Financing	Delivery	Regulation
Federal	Large role through the Medicare, Medicaid, and other government-sponsored programs; subsidizes selected health professional educational programs; subsidizes much health-related research and other studies	Operates healthcare clinics and hospitals for care of military, veterans, Indians, and research subjects at the National Institutes of Health; formerly provided services at public health hospitals and clinics for seamen and patients with infectious diseases	Regulates health programs it finances through setting conditions for participation as well as qualifications, conditions and rates for reimbursement; approves drugs and devices for use in healthcare; regulates controlled substances distribution; prohibits provider discrimination in care provisions; enforces laws applicable to healthcare delivery
State	Funds Medicaid with help of federal government, including some long-term care and mental health services; provides some public health services; subsidizes health professional and occupational education	Operates mental health and mental retardation hospitals, health departments, academic health centers, prison medical facilities	Regulates health and liability insurance; licenses or otherwise credentials health institutions and personnel; defines scopes of practice; establishes health codes and standards; enforces standards
Local	Subsidizes public and teaching hospitals; funds local public health departments and clinics; subsidizes some indigent care in the absence of a municipal hospital	Operates clinics and municipal hospitals; operates public health departments	Establishes and enforces local health codes

role from a different perspective and concept of responsibility (Brecher, 1990). Secondary roles of government, which directly affect its other roles, include funding of health profession education and research. Further, each role of government, regardless of jurisdiction, is broader than is immediately apparent. Table 10.1 provides an overview of these roles at varying levels of government.

While the federal government has been a provider of healthcare services since the Revolutionary War, its role as a major financier of health services came with the enactment of Medicare and Medicaid legislation in 1965. Medicare was conceived as an earned entitlement health insurance program for the elderly paid for by Social Security taxes. The program initially afforded insurance for physician services and hospitalization. Over the years, other healthcare providers, including CRNAs, have gained direct reimbursement from Medicare for services. Many outpatient services are now covered, particularly after the enactment of the Prospective Payment System in 1983, which was devised to contain hospital costs. Because patients are now being discharged earlier as a cost-containment measure, coverage for selected home health services was added because many patients required extended or rehabilitation care.

Medicaid affords health services for the indigent, with the federal government and state governments jointly funding the program and the states operating it. Thus, eligibility for Medicaid is determined by each state, as are any restrictions on health services and reimbursement rates for providers. Unless reimbursement to selected providers is mandated by federal law, the state determines who will be directly reimbursed for covered services. It should be noted that the federal government today pays nearly half of all healthcare costs in the United States.

The Centers for Medicare & Medicaid Services (CMS; formerly the Health Care Financing Administration, or HCFA) is the major payer for the federal government, using the private insurance industry as its intermediary for reimbursing health services associated with the Medicare program. CMS is also responsible for providing the federal portion of funding to the states for their Medicaid programs. Medicaid is usually operated by the state Department of Health, using a private insurer as intermediary.

Workers' compensation programs are state-operated health programs that are designated to pay for health services and disability claims resulting from occupational injury or hazards. While administered through private insurance companies, the state may impose restrictions on services and reimbursement to healthcare providers and limit disability payments. Like all other health programs, the cost of workers' compensation programs has escalated significantly over the past few years, compounding the overall cost to business and industry for the health services of its workers.

Multiple other governmental programs assist various groups to acquire resources needed to maintain good health. These include public health services, maternal and child health programs, state rehabilitation programs for children with disabilities, and state mental health programs. Federal, state, and local governments also bear responsibility for monitoring healthcare and its delivery, including federal, state, or community services essential to the health of all citizens. Monitoring includes assessing the quality and adequacy of services, outcomes of care, adequacy and availability of health personnel and institutional resources, reportable diseases, safety of water, disposal of sewage and other hazardous wastes, environmental conditions, and food handlers and food service facilities. Another significant role of government in healthcare involves funding basic and applied research associated with disease, injury, treatment modalities, and delivery systems. In addition to establishing and funding the National Institutes of Health, including the Center for Nursing Research, many university and private research groups derive funding from government or private foundations that support healthcare services.

Finally, the government plays a major role in providing educational funding for a variety of health professionals, thus directly affecting the available supply of health manpower. The federal government maintains a Health Manpower Division and a Division of Nursing within the U.S. Department of Health and Human Services (HHS) to monitor health and human resources and to oversee disbursement of federal funds related to educational funding. Unfortunately, their effectiveness depends in part on annual congressional appropriations. Consequently, manpower issues too often become a function of the political and legislative process rather than one dependent on fact-based data demonstrating bona-fide manpower shortages. In fact, the excess of physicians projected by the end of this century reflects efforts to expand the number of medical schools and the supply of physicians, efforts which date back to the late 1960s. While federal funding for medical education has been reduced, states continue to fund increased numbers of medical schools at the behest of the powerful state medical education lobbies. At present, federal funding for health education, administered through HHS, amounts to $4.8 billion annually for medical education, while only $400 million is spent for nursing and allied health education.

The overall spending for medical education has far outstripped that portion of money allotted for nonphysician healthcare providers, both at the state and federal level. In a study performed in Texas in 1992, it was found that the average cost of preparing one physician, from the beginning of his or her premed coursework through medical school and residency, was approximately $650,000, while that of preparing a CRNA was approximately $60,000 (Gunn, 1992). The imbalance in human health resource needs, where there are shortages of nurses (including nurse anesthetists, nurse midwives, and nurse practitioners) and of allied health professionals, is in all probability a function of excess physician production when compared with other health professionals. This also includes the excess money put into medical education compared to that for other health professionals.

Although space limitations prohibit further discussion of government's role in healthcare delivery, health payers, both governmental and private, determine directly or indirectly how healthcare will be delivered, where it will be delivered, how often, and to whom it will be delivered. Nonphysician health professionals seeking more autonomy in practice and the ability to be reimbursed for services ignore at their peril the influence healthcare funding and reimbursement have on practice. The skills and capability to influence legislation and regulation are as important in configuring the environment for nurse anesthesia practice as the skills to perform intubations are to the administration of anesthesia.

Private Sector Roles in Healthcare

Private sector roles in healthcare deal largely with education, financing, delivery, research and regulation, although in the latter category this is restricted to credentialing mechanisms such as accreditation, certification, and recertification. In addition, the private sector is also involved in the research, manufacture and marketing of drugs and devices, as well as the education of health professionals who use the drugs and technology. Table 10.2 summarizes the roles of private healthcare providers, organizations, institutions, and other private sector entities in healthcare.

Other private sector groups that impact the delivery of healthcare include a variety of health provider associations, consumer health groups, and community activist organizations. While all groups have a general responsibility to their

Table 10.2: Summary of Private Sector Roles in Healthcare

	Financing	Delivery	Credentialing/ regulations
Business/ Industry	Often provides health insurance for employees; may provide health coverage utilizing HMOs or PPOs; pays for workers' compensation insurance; provides coverage for selected addiction rehabilitation	Operates occupational health clinics; may provide some health maintenance services	May regulate smoking, areas to smoke
Credentialing Bodies	Impact costs of care	Impact delivery of healthcare services; configure institutional delivery mechanisms, available resources, etc	Accredit institutional or agency providers; accredit educational programs for preparing health professionals; certify health personnel
Health Insurance	For a price, pays for health services; reimburses health professionals and institutions; performs utilization reviews and billing audits	Impacts delivery systems based on inherent incentives in insurance policies; providers and services reimbursed; conditions and levels of reimbursement	Determines qualifications for insurance coverage
Health Personnel		Provide direct health services; paid salary or on basis of charge or allowable fees	
*Health Institutions**	May have a financing function	Provide health services through organized delivery system; reimbursed by insurance or health client for most services rendered as an institution	Often provide institutional credentialing for physicians and in some instances for other nonphysician health professionals in independent practice
Professional Organizations		Recruitment of new members into the profession to assure adequacy of personnel resources for healthcare delivery; promote change, innovation in professional practice/healthcare delivery	Set educational and practice standards for the profession and its members; may participate in or provide quality assurance, risk management programs, or continuing education programs; may publish ethical code for members
Liability Insurers/ Product Liability Insurers	For a price, underwrite cost of malpractice/ product-liability claims, defense costs, and/or payments/judgments		Determine conditions for acquiring liability insurance and liability limits available; malpractice insurance may be required to obtain institutional clinical privileges

*Health institutions include hospitals, ambulatory health centers, diagnostic or treatment centers, hospices, long-term care facilities, etc.

membership, professional associations are designed to represent professions and protect the interests of their members as they relate to professional practice. Consumer health groups and community activist groups often provide monitoring services concerning healthcare and identify needs and solutions requiring public and private support to implement solutions. Other groups may be private organizations interested in publicizing the plight of patients with a particular disease, raising money for research, and educating the public concerning health matters. These groups may be national or local in scope; may be defined along racial, age, economic status, or other lines; and may, in some instances, have significant power to influence governments and the private sector. The American Association of Retired Persons, Gray Panthers, Public Citizen, and diagnosis-specific organizations are but a few of these.

HEALTH RESOURCES IN THE UNITED STATES

Service Providers

While a large number of health professionals engage in private practice, either as individuals or as groups, the healthcare delivery system today is one of the major employers in the United States. Stephan Jonas (1998) provides a succinct overview of the provider segment of the healthcare system which this author cites. In 1994, almost 10.6 million people, about 8.6 percent of all persons employed in the United States, were working in the healthcare industry. Nearly half worked in hospitals, 16 percent in nursing and personal care facilities, and over 13 percent in physicians' offices. Today there are over 700 categories of skilled health occupations, including 2.2 million nurses and over 650,000 allopathic and osteopathic physicians.

Pharmacists, dentists and optometrists account for another 400,000 professional personnel. Most surprisingly, it is estimated that in 1993 there were 16-18 other healthcare workers required to support each physician. The fact that there are 650,000 physicians today, projected to reach more than 800,000 by 2020, should give pause to policymakers as they consider the eventual impact these numbers will have economically.

Hospitals and Institutions

Hospitals, the traditional institutional health provider, are undergoing major financial stresses as government and other payers try to constrain the cost of care. In March 2000, *Modern Healthcare* reported that "even though health care will be a growth industry of the future with aging baby boomers increasing the demand for services, hospital operating margins will be thin at best." To support this observation, CMS reports that national health expenditures will grow 65 percent to almost $2.2 trillion from 2000 to 2008. Paltry profit margins, hospitals claim, stem largely from the 1997 Balanced Budget Act, which substantially reduced hospital payments, coupled with the failure of merged institutions to save costs from duplicative expenditures and increases in operating and personnel costs. Since that time, political pressures from professional organizations such as the American Hospital Association have induced the federal Congress to reinstate $16.1 billion in increased payments over five years.

Historically, congressional implementation of the Prospective Payment System as the vehicle for Medicare reimbursement of hospitals has led to shortened hospital stays and lower bed occupancy, prompting the closure or merger of many hospitals. Closures were hastened by the advent of freestanding ambulatory health clinics and surgicenters that took many of the profit-making services away from hospitals. Some hospitals have responded by establishing their own hospital-based ambulatory centers, surgicenters, and home health agencies, or by entering joint ventures with physicians as a source of patients. The changing reimbursement system for hospital care also prompted entrepreneurs to get into the field, and for-profit hospitals were born.

FUTURE CONSIDERATIONS

There is little question that the United States is the world leader in high-technology services and tertiary care. However, this nation, which often prides itself as having the best healthcare system in the world, has yet to face many challenges. In fact, Congress remains inundated with proposed legislation, some of which has languished unresolved for years, that could change the traditional face of health delivery. Current legislative proposals include:

- Basic reforms in the regulation of managed care organizations.
- Patients' bill of rights.
- Provider payment increases.
- Addition of prescription drug benefits to Medicare coverage.
- Exempting physicians from antitrust law to allow collective bargaining.
- Public access to the National Practitioner Data Bank.
- Mandating reportable medical errors as proposed by the Institute of Medicine.

These issues are only those currently under legislative consideration. Still not formally considered are the perennial problems of lack of universal coverage for all, availability of a set benefit package, child poverty and attendant health problems, and costs for services which many still cannot afford, especially for the most sophisticated or experimental treatments and services. Further, the burgeoning geriatric population will severely tax resources for the next two decades as the Baby Boomers age. For example, national expenditures on long-term care for people 65 and older are expected to increase by nearly 200 percent to more than $346 billion in today's dollars by 2040 (Bellandi, 2000), yet no legislative action is now being considered to address this challenge.

Yanklovich (1991) believes that the failure of the American public, legislators, and health policy analysts to achieve consensus with regard to the causes of the healthcare crisis is at the heart of the inability of the federal government to deal with healthcare reform. The public lays the blame on the greed of the principal players in healthcare delivery, and legislators and health policy analysts lay the blame on high technology. Many who have studied these problems believe the causes may be far more complex. Most agree, however, that any healthcare reform must meet criteria that assures broad accessibility of high-quality services to all persons at prices individuals, business, and society can afford. The extent to which we achieve these goals will largely relate to our ability to place people above politics. Jonas (1998) believes that new delivery systems will work only when they have one characteristic in common: proactive, not reactive, planning linked to financing. He further proposes that the alternatives to the current system will likely include more emphasis on "competition" among healthcare systems fueled by informed consumer/patient choice. He also notes that any new health system must "not just pay differently for things: we must pay for different things based on rational, evidenced-based data."

Other obvious issues that must be debated include the following:

- The lack of access to basic healthcare services based on geographic, social, economic, and other factors. The solutions for making healthcare accessible in rural communities are not identical to those for making healthcare accessible in the inner city or to ethnic communities within large metropolitan areas. Community-centered planning is often essential to resolve some of these problems.
- Establishing priorities in healthcare and assuring cost-effective use of high-technology services. This will require the identification of practice guidelines based on research with regard to the efficacy of high-technology services in treating patients, in addition to performing cost/benefit analyses.
- Defining more cost-effective health manpower mixes. This involves redesigning the healthcare system and pertinent statutes and regulations to assure its effective function. This will probably entail a reduced reliance on physicians; increased reliance on nonphysician providers such as nurses in advanced practice (CRNAs, certified nurse midwives, nurse practitioners, and some clinical nurse specialists); and empowering the public to take more responsibility for their own health status.
- Modification of the tort system and alternatives for compensating patients for injuries from healthcare negligence.
- Reimbursement methodologies, rates, and identification of payment recipients must be addressed. Fee-for-service medicine creates adverse incentives to cost effectiveness and is believed by many to be at the heart of escalating healthcare costs. Many believe that national health insurance with a single payer system is the only way to eliminate the administrative waste of private insurance and to avoid cost shifting.
- Ethical issues, such as the prolongation of dying and its impact on the individual, the family, and health resources needed by others more likely to benefit, need to be reviewed. Intellectual, philosophic, and scientific resources should be used to resolve these issues. In addition, other ethical issues such as those raised by the Human Genome Project to map human DNA to aid new drug development and fight inherited disease will draw substantial public attention and generate vigorous debate.

SUMMARY

Olson (2000) outlines what he believes are the eight strongest forces guiding healthcare today: (1) national health objectives, (2) the growing number of uninsured, (3) more governmental control, (4) more educated and demanding consumers, (5) a lopsided workforce with too many physicians and not enough nurses, (6) physician partnerships, (7) technology, and (8) becoming more efficient. Because everyone is affected by healthcare issues such as these, it behooves providers and consumers alike to stay abreast of this rapidly changing arena. We must continually evaluate its impact on our families, our patients, and our nation for its long-term consequences.

REFERENCES

Bellandi, D. (2000). Growth but no margins. *Modern Healthcare.* 30:12:28.

Brecher, C. (1990). The government's role in health care. In Kovner, A.R. (Ed). *Health Care Delivery in the United States* (pp. 297-323). New York, NY: Springer Publishing.

Bullough, B. (1983). Introduction to nursing practice law. In Bullough, B., Bullough, V., & Soukup, M. (Eds.). *Nursing Issues and Nursing Strategies of the Eighties* (pp. 279-291). New York, Ny: Springer Publishing.

Diers, D. (1992). Nurse-midwives and nurse anesthetists: The cutting edge in specialist practice. In Aiken, L. & Fagin, C. (Eds.). *Charting Nursing's Future: Agenda for the 1990s* (pp. 159-180). Philadelphia, PA: JB Lippincott.

Gunn, I.P. (1992). Promoting a more cost-effective health delivery system through changing the health provider mix. Unpublished manuscript.

Hadley, E.H. (1989). Nurses and prescriptive authority: A legal and economic analysis. *Am J of Law and Med.* 15:245.

Jonas, S. (1998). *An Introduction to the U.S. Health Care System* (4th ed., pp. 1-26). New York: Springer Publishing.

Melosh, B. (1982). *The Physician's Hand: Work Culture and Conflict in American Nursing* (pp. 113-158). Philadelphia, PA: Temple University Press.

Numbers, R.L. (1984). The third party: Health insurance in America. In Lee, P.R., Estes, D.L., & Ramsay, N.B. (Eds.). *The Nation's Health* (pp. 196-204). San Francisco: Boyd and Fraser.

Olson, M. (2000). Personal communications in modern healthcare. *Weekly Business News.* 30:12:28.

Ribicoff, A. & Danaceau, P. (1972). *The American Medical Machine* (pp. 135-167). New York: Harrow Books, Harper & Row.

Safreit, B. (1991). Health care dollars and regulatory sense: The role of advanced practice nursing. *Yale J Reg.* 9:417.

Starr, P. (1982). *The Social Transformation of American Medicine.* New York, NY: Basic Books.

Stevens, R. (1989). *In Sickness and in Wealth.* New York, NY: Basic Books.

Waddle, F. (1979). Licensure: Achievements and limitations. In *The Study of Credentialing in Nursing: A New Approach* (Vol. 2, pp. 126-132). Staff Working Papers, American Nurses' Association. Kansas City, MO.

Wing, K.R. (1985). *The Law and the Public's Health* (pp. 177-195). Ann Arbor, MI: Health Administration Press.

Yankelovich, D. & Immerwahr, J. (1991). A perception gap. *Health Management Q.* 3:3:11.

KEY REFERENCES

Jonas, S. (1998). *An Introduction to the U.S. Health Care System* (4th ed., pp. 1-26). New York: Springer Publishing.

Safreit, B. (1991). Health care dollars and regulatory sense: The role of advanced practice nursing. *Yale J Reg.* 9:417.

Starr, P. (1982). *The Social Transformation of American Medicine.* New York, NY: Basic Books.

STUDY QUESTIONS

1. From a historical context, discuss the ways that physicians came to exert control over healthcare delivery and services in the United States.

2. What are some of the characteristics of the healthcare system that have developed from the social tenets of the United States?

3. Early nursing leaders failed to secure nursing practice through licensure, which had substantial ramifications for practice in years to come. What are the characteristics of licensure (as opposed to recognition, registration or certification) that would have made practice for CRNAs more secure?

4. Identify the basic elements of the healthcare system and describe how each is interrelated.

5. What are some of the primary failures of today's healthcare delivery system? What do you feel the priorities for change are and why? What, if any role, do CRNAs play in those changes?

CHAPTER 11

PRINCIPLES OF MANAGED CARE: PAST, PRESENT AND FUTURE

Jeffrey C. Bauer, PhD
Russell C. Coile, Jr.

Jeffrey C. Bauer and Russell C. Coile, Jr., are senior vice presidents for Superior Consultant Company, an integrated healthcare consulting firm based in Southfield, Mich., which specializes in information systems, e-health business relationships, strategic planning, and other aspects of the digitial transformation of healthcare. Both authors are nationally recognized health futurists and widely published authors. They are currently collaborating on a new book, E-health and the Digital Transformation of Healthcare: A User's Guide to On-line Medical Markets. *This chapter is based in part on Mr. Coile's article, "Managed Care in the Millennium: New Forecast for the 'Five Stages' of Managed Care" (*Russ Coile's Health Trends. *13(1):1-12. October, 1999. By permission of Aspen Publishers.) Contact Mr. Coile by telephone at 972-403-1945 or by email at Russell_Coile@superiorconsultant.com. Dr. Bauer can be reached at 970-847-3360 or Jeff_Bauer@superiorconsultant.com.*

KEY CONCEPTS

- Managed care is based on the principles of cost control mediated through mechanisms of reduced provider payment, resource management, controlled patient access through "gatekeeping," limited panels of provider staff, and utilization of information/data that reduces redundancy and unjustified care.

- Managed care is a delivery paradigm that has had mixed success in controlling costs and is unsustainable in its present form. Evolved managed care systems of the future will most likely be based on collaborative models where risk is shared and perhaps include emphasis on new, direct relationships between provider and payers.

- Certified Registered Nurse Anesthetists (CRNAs) working in a managed care environment will need to be increasingly aware of issues relating to managing cost, documenting quality of care provided, and purposefully improving patient outcome.

- CRNAs involved in contracting situations with managed care entities should have expert legal advice to determine not only the worth, value and integrity of the contract to the provider, but that the entity itself is in good financial health.

Managed care was a defining feature of the U.S. health system for the last third of the 20th century, and its importance grew continually throughout this period. Few, if any, concepts would appear more frequently in a key word search of the era's popular press and professional literature on American medicine. Managed care attracted so much attention because it played a major role in controlling access, determining quality, redistributing income, and otherwise changing the delivery of healthcare services.

Yet, it continues to be viewed simultaneously as the solution to and the cause of the problems of our healthcare delivery system. Its proponents have become its opponents within just a few years, and sometimes vice versa. Providers who profited greatly from managed care one year could be bankrupted by it in the next. Consumer satisfaction with managed care was often very high at the same time most people seemed to be clamoring for major health plan reform. Many politicians reversed their positions on managed care from one election to the next just to get re-elected. Intense divisions on managed care issues could be found within the two major parties by the end of the 1990s.

If you are a bit confused by these contradictions, you are beginning to understand managed care. Managed care has never had a coherent or consistent meaning, despite its increasingly powerful presence over several decades. Indeed, the situation is aptly summarized by the popular quip, "If you've seen one managed care plan, you've seen one managed care plan." You certainly hadn't seen them all because plans could be substantially different from market to market at the same time, or they could change significantly in the same market from year to year.

This chapter would ideally start with a definition of managed care, but a consistent and enduring definition does not exist. As will be shown in the next section, managed care effectively encompasses several forms of reimbursement that are not traditional fee-for-service. Managed care plans generally incorporate one or more limitations (e.g., access control via a "gatekeeper," an approved drug formulary, a limited provider panel) not normally found in indemnity plans that historically allowed providers to bill without restrictions, other than their own clinical judgement. However, the differences between managed care plans can be just as great as the differences between managed care and fee-for-service. A standardized definition is inherently imprecise, potentially misleading, and probably outdated soon after it appears in print.

So what's a practitioner to do in the face of such ambiguity and uncertainty? To help answer this important question, we begin with a brief review of the history of managed care and then provide an in-depth analysis of its status at the end of the 20th century. Next, we share our thoughts about its possible evolution in the early years of the new millennium, and conclude with some practical advice for practitioners who will need to deal with managed care in the future.

A BRIEF HISTORY OF MANAGED CARE

The creation of the prepaid group practice (PPGP) delivery model in the 1920s is generally identified as the beginning of the movement that ultimately became managed care. PPGPs represented a significant change from the traditional form of reimbursement—fee-for-service—because they charged members a fixed monthly fee for a defined set of benefits. This practice was called capitation because the monthly charge was assessed *per capita,* that is, per head. The "cap" rate is also commonly designated as the premium per member per month (PMPM).

Although offering health benefits for a fixed monthly charge was not an entirely new idea at the time, the revolutionary aspect of the PPGP movement was putting providers at risk. Under the traditional fee-for-service arrangement, doctors theoretically got paid for all the care they provided. Under a capitated PPGP plan, however, doctors were obligated to provide care in accordance with the terms of the contract. They lost money on a patient if the costs of his or her actual care exceeded the PMPM. The only way to make a net profit from the arrangement was to have other patients whose care cost proportionally less. PPGPs had a financial incentive to avoid providing medical services that did not keep the patient healthy according to the terms of the contract.

Perhaps the best known PPGP was the plan organized in the late 1920s by Henry Kaiser, a very successful and socially concerned industrialist in Oakland, Calif. The Kaiser Plan identified itself as a health maintenance organization (HMO) to emphasize the proposition that keeping people healthy was a win-win situation. Preventive care, such as screening to identify diseases in early stages when treatment was less expensive, presumably maintained members' health and allowed the plan to make a fair profit. The HMOs' presumed orientation to preventive care became the key distinguishing feature of their reputation for at least 50 years, even though the research literature offers scant evidence that the theory was commonly put into practice.

Organized medicine staunchly opposed the PPGP-HMO movement from the beginning on grounds that capitation gave doctors an incentive to undertreat (i.e., to withhold care that was medically necessary). Indeed, medical associations argued that fixed reimbursement forced doctors to consider their remuneration when determining the course of treatment—a clear violation of the Hippocratic dictum that money should not influence a doctor's decisions. Due to the overall political strength of organized medicine, the early stages of managed care were effectively confined to California and a few Midwestern states for four decades.

As indemnity health insurance matured under the control of organized medicine (Bauer, 1998), the highly politicized fight against capitation diverted public attention from the countervailing proposition that fee-for-service reimbursement promoted overtreatment. Excessive care received almost no attention until the costs of Medicare and Medicaid began to "skyrocket" far beyond projected levels in the late 1960s and the early 1970s. As luck would have it, the president of the United States was a former governor of California who believed strongly in capitation and PPGP. President Richard M. Nixon successfully led the fight to base the nation's first federal health reform program on HMOs. The Health Maintenance Organization Act of 1973 gave special status to capitated health plans, legitimizing "managed care" in the process. HMOs suddenly attracted attention because they were presumably less expensive than traditional health insurance products.

The meaning of managed care became muddled almost immediately. Academic researchers and policy analysts touted HMOs for their presumed emphasis on prevention, but employers were more interested in the potential price advantage of the new alternatives to fee-for-service. (Indeed, both authors remember that discussion centered on alternative health plans, or AHPs, for most of the 1970s; managed care was not yet a common term.) Preferred provider organizations (PPO) entered the market as another alternative. PPOs reduced employers' costs of health insurance by securing discounts from medical groups and hospitals and listing them on the panel of providers authorized by the health plan.

PPOs were based almost entirely on fee-for-service arrangements and seldom put the providers at risk, but like HMOs, they attracted attention because they were an alternative to traditional insurance. The use of gatekeepers, health plan employees (often nurses) charged with the task of denying coverage for "unnecessary" services, was the only major feature shared by HMOs and PPOs. Nevertheless, with almost nothing else in common, both were lumped together under the rubric of managed care beginning in the early 1980s. By the end of the decade, managed care was firmly established as the challenger to fee-for-service health plans, even though the term itself encompassed two very different alternatives that still relied predominantly on fee-for-service arrangements below the surface.

The scope of managed care expanded even further in the early 1990s. Employee Provider Organizations (EPO), Point-of-Sale (POS) options, and other variations on the general theme added to the "alphabet soup" of managed care. Indeed, managed care's power was so strong that it became the cornerstone of President Clinton's intense but failed effort at national health reform in 1993 and 1994. The healthcare marketplace of Minneapolis-St. Paul was used widely as the model for national reform because it reportedly had the nation's lowest rate of health plan inflation and highest concentration of HMOs and PPOs. As a sign of the quick ebb and flow of managed care, the Twin Cities had some of the nation's highest premium increases and most troubled health plans just five years later. Managed care did not deliver as promised by the politicians, pundits, and policy wonks.

Managed care attracted a remarkable amount of attention over the past several decades, but did not develop a coherent definition or consistent form. The closest thing to a common trait in the evolving versions of managed care is probably the use of restrictions to prevent practitioners from making decisions free of economic constraints. The best that might be said of managed care so far is that it is an antidote for some serious problems of fee-for-service medical care. However, it has not yet proven to be a cure for the underlying economic disease of increased healthcare costs and associated ills of disparate access, sometimes dubious health outcomes, and uneven quality of care.

MANAGED CARE AT THE TURN OF THE CENTURY

The future of managed care seems less certain in the early 21st century than at any time since this alternative to traditional insurance exploded onto the national scene in the 1970s. Almost 80 million Americans, approximately 30 percent of the U.S. population, are enrolled in HMOs (Hamer, 1999a), the predominant form of managed care. Tens of millions more are covered by PPOs and other plans that "apply any discipline to an open-choice system that is based on fee-for-service financing (Kunkle, 1998)." Managed care has gained an impressive market share in just a few decades.

In spite of such success, managed care has also become a target for media criticism and government regulation. Critics far outnumber advocates, with pressure mounting to reign in managed care plans that are widely believed to favor profits over patients. A common opinion is expressed in a recent study on HMO quality by David Himmelstein, MD, of the Harvard University Medical School: "The market is destroying our health care system. We have a decade or more of policies aimed at making health care a business, and they have failed (Stolberg, 1999)."

In such circumstances, defining the practice environment of the early 21st century is difficult. Managed care in America is stalled at the turn of the century, and lacks a vision for the future. Premiums are climbing, medical care inflation is re-emerging, and its expansion seems to have slowed, especially among HMOs. Called "alternative delivery systems" only 20 years ago, managed care plans now dominate many markets, but most are losing money. Far from being models of competition and cost management, most of the large HMOs and insurers in the nation simply want to reverse their recent losses. National plans are retreating from many markets, and some of the largest players, such as Prudential, Metropolitan and Travelers, have left the business altogether. Health plans shifted their focus from growth to profitability in the late 1990s, and their provider and customer relations deteriorated at roughly the same time. Some industry observers are now writing articles with titles like the "Beginning of the End for HMOs" (Beckham, 1997, 1998).

The late 1990s situation can be summarized succinctly with data from InterStudy, a think tank based in St. Paul, Minn., which tracks the HMO industry (Hamer, 1999a):

- 78.8 million HMO enrollees.
- 652 health maintenance organizations.
- National managed care plans control 76.5 percent of the total market.
- Growth rate of only 3.3 percent in the first six months of 1998.
- Most HMOs increasing premiums by 6 percent to 8 percent for 1999 and 2000.
- HMO profitability improving for most national plans.
- Rising costs and claims, especially pharmaceuticals.
- Managed care reform endorsed by both political parties.
- Rising tide of complaints and public concern.
- Providers increasingly unwilling to assume capitated risk.

Do data such as these suggest that the managed care movement has reached its zenith? Economists like Princeton's Dr. Uwe Reinhart argue that HMOs have made their one-time impact on health costs and that health expenditures will rise sharply again without more direct intervention by government or major employers. An analysis based on the five stages of managed care market growth helps define marketplace dynamics at the turn of the century, with Stage 1 being very low market share (0 percent to 4 percent) and Stage 5 being high market share (>40 percent) (Coile, 1999). Table 11.1 demonstrates how HMOs transformed some major markets between 1994 (left number) and 1998 (right number). More recent data indicate that HMOs are still gaining ground in mid-stage markets, but in the most advanced regions, like Minneapolis-St. Paul, Minn., Miami, Fla., and Sacramento, Calif., HMO enrollment is flat or declining (Hamer, 1999b).

Data in Table 11.1 demonstrate the hazards inherent in making generalizations about managed care. Practical information aimed at practitioners in Sacramento might be meaningless to

Table 11.1: Market Stage Transitions—Five-Year (1994-1998)

	STAGE 1	STAGE 2	STAGE 3	STAGE 4	STAGE 5
Metropolitan Area	**0 - 4%**	**5 - 14%**	**15 - 24%**	**25 - 39%**	**>40%**
Boise, ID	3.7	8.3			
Erie, PA	3.1			26.7	
Merced, CA	4.8		22.4		
Charlotte, NC		7.9	23.8		
New Orleans, LA		9.2		29.7	
Indianapolis, IN		14.9	24.4		
Chicago, IL			16.6	27	
Hartford, CN			16.2	36.4	
Kansas City, MO			18.9	33.2	
Phoenix, AZ			23.3	34.2	
Salt Lake City, UT				32.7	41.4
Boston, MA				35.4	47.3
Los Angeles, CA				37.8	51.6
Minn.-St. Paul, MN				37.6	39.9
Tucson, AZ					40.5-44.7
Sacramento, CA					51.2-64

Sources: Richard L. Hamer, "HMO Regional Market Analysis." Part III. InterStudy Competitive Edge. 5(1):1-111. April 1995. And Richard L. Hamer, "HMO Regional Market Analysis." Part III. InterStudy Competitive Edge. 9(1):1-178. June 1999.

their counterparts in Boise, Idaho. Therefore, clinicians must be cautious when evaluating advice about how to deal with managed care. Actions that are helpful in one market might be counterproductive in another where the market power of managed care is dramatically different. Likewise, practice management in the same market may need to change rather rapidly as managed care rises or falls in a relatively short period of time.

The data in Table 11.1 also demonstrate a cyclic trend in the managed care marketplace, commonly characterized as the six-year insurance cycle. Understanding the cycle helps explain what happened in the 1990s as the annual growth of HMO enrollment slumped, then soared, and fell again (Table 11.2). The model is simple: When prices fall, enrollment goes up, but profits decline. To regain profitability, health plans boost premiums, but that slows enrollment growth. The model fits the current pattern in the HMO marketplace and is likely to continue into the new millennium. According to InterStudy's Richard Hamer, "With HMOs seeking to restore financial health with increased commercial premiums and a demonstrated link between growth and price inflation, it is likely that industry enrollment growth will continue to slow (Hamer, 1999a)."

Once high-flying HMOs (e.g., Oxford, United Healthcare and Aetna/U.S. Healthcare) saw total U.S. HMO enroll-

Table 11.2: Total HMO Growth and Enrollment Rate (July 1990 to July 1998)

YEAR	ENROLLEES	% GROWTH RATE
1990	34.7M	6.8
1991	36.5M	5.2
1992	38.8M	6.3
1993	42.1M	8.5
1994	47.3M	12.4
1995	53.4M	12.9
1996	63.3M	18.5
1997	73.1M	15.5
1998	78.8M	7.9

Source: Richard L. Hamer, "HMO Industry Report." Part II. InterStudy Competitive Edge. July 1999. P. vii. And "HMO Industry Report." Part II. InterStudy Competitive Edge. 9(1):viii. June 1999.

ment rise only 7.9 percent in 1998, the lowest single-digit growth rate in more than five years. After three years of price competition and losses, most HMOs sharply boosted premiums in 1997 and 1998. Even in Minnesota, the hot-bed of HMO development, some HMOs raised premiums 15 percent to 20 percent (Hudak and Barkley, 1999). But higher premiums can mean that HMO profits are improving, which may also improve stock prices for the for-profit plans. Many of the largest national HMOs (e.g., California's Wellpoint, Indiana's Anthem and United Healthcare in Minnesota) reported strong financial performance in 1999.

However, public criticism clouds the reports of renewed success. The Himmelstein study suggested that non-profit health plans provided more preventive services and early intervention than the for-profit plans, which cover 62 percent of all patients in HMOs (Stolberg, 1999). While Himmelstein does not dispute his bias against for-profit managed care organizations, other health experts like Columbia University economist Dr. Eli Ginzberg share his views: "Let's face it, people went into the for-profit managed care business to make bucks (Ginzberg, 1999)." Hence, practitioners should generally determine whether their managed care relationships would be with for-profit or tax-exempt plans. A plan's tax status may make a difference in the types of care clinicians would be rewarded for providing. However, premiums seem to rise cyclically, regardless of a plan's tax status. Raising premiums can help stabilize operations in the short term, but does not address a number of underlying problems facing the nation's HMOs:

- Inability to control medical loss ratio (percentage of premium paid to medical services).
- Rise of pharmaceutical costs by 11 percent to 12 percent yearly.
- Increasing resistance from organized providers to HMO discounts.
- Limited application of disease management programs.
- Computer problems in many plans.

- Short-term orientation regarding prevention, screening, wellness.
- High administrative expenses, averaging 15 percent even in large plans.
- Spotty performance records in quality, patient satisfaction.

Clinicians who are dealing with managed care in the early years of the 21st century should carefully evaluate their involvement with prospective health plans on their performance in these areas. Plans that have not made desired improvements will likely pose problems for patients and providers, particularly in instances where operating deficits and falling stock prices (for for-profit plans) threaten a plan's financial viability. Many managed care plans went bankrupt in the 1990s, and the outcome was dismal for all concerned. Clinicians should think twice before linking their own financial future to a health plan that is itself unhealthy and showing no signs of improvement.

Perhaps the most significant trend at the end of the 1990s was the development of a shift toward "managed care lite" health plans that intentionally tried to look less like pure HMOs. In particular, PPOs eclipsed HMOs as the most popular choice among managed care plans. PPO enrollment reached 90 million, skyrocketing 60 percent in the previous four years, according to the annual employer survey of 4,200 firms by William M. Mercer, a national health benefits consulting company (Rauber, 1999). Consumers liked the freedom of choice, flexibility, and cost control offered by PPOs. In some markets, HMOs and PPOs were competing closely on price, and many consumers chose to spend-up by $10 per month to purchase a PPO over a narrow-network HMO product. About one in 10 PPO enrollees was a member of a provider-sponsored organization, indicating some provider activity in the move toward "managed care lite."

Riding this wave of consumer popularity, PPOs were expanding nationally at the end of the 1990s. MultiPlan of New York purchased local PPOs in 10 states in two years and was looking for more acquisitions. Regional PPOs were being targeted for consolidation, and early market leaders like California's Capp Care began merging with the largest plans (in this case, Beech Street).

PPOs have also been leaders in network diversification, responding rapidly to consumer demands for choice (Robinson, 1999). Providers generally like PPOs, which typically pay doctors on a fee-for-service base and hospitals by per-diems. PPOs generally impose prior authorization hurdles for specialty referrals and expensive treatments, but they offer a broader network of provider choices.

MANAGED MEDICARE AND MEDICAID

Government is still encouraging government program beneficiaries to switch to managed care, but both managed Medicare and Medicaid capitation programs began to lose momentum in the late 1990s. Congress provided some reasons for this reversal by putting new managed care provisions in the Balanced Budget Act of 1997. To help reduce federal outlays for Medicare by $115 billion over five years, Congress slashed the Medicare HMO payment annual update to less than 2 percent. Washington did not anticipate that the 267 Medicare HMOs would respond by exiting low-payment markets, impacting 400,000 Medicare HMO enrollees, and that 43 HMOs would drop out of the program (Rovner, 1998). Congress also enacted "Medicare + Choice," an expanded set of managed care options for seniors. A new alternative for doctors and hospitals, Provider-Sponsored Organizations (PSO), was created, but it attracted little interest because of uncertainty about Medicare HMO payments. Only one PSO, a rural network in New Mexico, had been certified by the Health Care Financing Administration (HCFA; now Centers for Medicare & Medicaid Services, or CMS) a year after the program was introduced (Terry, 1999). Medicare PPOs and medical savings plans were also authorized, but they attracted relatively little interest.

In Medicaid capitation, HCFA granted "Section 1115" waivers to 19 states, authorizing them to launch Medicaid managed care programs (*Modern Healthcare*, 1999). Some conversions were expected to affect millions of Medicaid patients (Table 11.3). Over 9 million Medicaid enrollees and over 30 percent of all Medicaid eligibles signed up for managed care plans (Hamer, 1999a) under this authority, representing a huge increase from the 1.1 million members in Medicaid managed care plans in 1990. However, many observers express concern that managed Medicaid still was not bridging the gap to mainstream medicine for Medicaid patients. Over half of all Medicaid HMOs were not affiliated with national HMOs at the end of the decade, and only 39 percent of the Medicaid HMOs were federally certified.

Arizona was the pioneering state in managed Medicaid, creating its plan in 1982. Most of the HCFA waivers were granted much more recently, in the last half of the 1990s, when the largest states began converting their costly Medicaid health programs to managed care. In New York, for example, all of the state's 2.1 million Medicaid beneficiaries were being shifted to managed care, a move which attracted some vocal opposition because of its adverse impact on the income of many New York hospitals and physicians. Tennessee's "TennCare" program, covering 1.3 million Medicaid patients, stumbled in its early years due to limited planning and administrative snafus. However, by 1999, the Tennessee program was becoming a victim of its own success. Having signed up so many of the state's medically uninsured, TennCare was running short of funds and experiencing many administrative problems.

Again, the clear lesson from these experiences was that managed care did not result in the simple panacea expected in the early 1990s. Some successes were achieved, but overall, problems outnumbered successes by the end of the decade. Also, state-to-state differences were substantial because federal law did not standardize managed Medicaid programs. Clinicians who learned to operate within the rules of Medicaid managed care in one state might find that they had to start learning all over again if they moved to (or accepted patients from) another state. To rephrase an earlier statement, "If you've seen one state's managed Medicaid plan, you've seen one state's managed Medicaid plan." Many different approaches were being tried yet none afforded the desired solution to the problem of rising Medicaid expenditures.

CONSOLIDATION MEANS BIGGER IS BIGGER

Falling profits and rising expenses generated a new round of consolidation in the managed care industry in the late 1990s. The largest national firms acquired second-tier and regional plans in an attempt to expand marketshare and reduce administrative expenses. Aetna U.S. Healthcare's purchase of New York Life's NYLCare and Prudential's health insurance plans made it one of the largest managed care companies in the nation. United Healthcare's attempt to merge with Humana fell apart in 1998, but both companies continued to

Table 11.3: HCFA Waivers to States for Managed Medicaid Programs

STATE	DATE AWARDED	ENROLLMENT AS OF 1/1/99
Alabama	12/6/96	40,000
Arizona	7/13/82	380,000
Arkansas	8/19/97	39,000
Delaware	5/17/95	71,000
Hawaii	7/16/93	129,000
Illinois	7/12/96	Implementation pending
Kentucky	12/9/93	159,000
Maryland	10/30/96	315,000
Massachusetts	4/24/95	757,000
Missouri	4/29/98	233,000
New Jersey	2/13/98	Implementation pending
New York	7/15/97	2.1 million
Ohio	7/17/95	332,000
Oklahoma	10/12/95	47,000
Oregon	3/19/93	243,000
Rhode Island	11/1/93	80,000
Tennessee	11/18/93	1.3 million
Vermont	7/28/95	16,000

Source: Health Care Financing Administration, cited in "By the Numbers: Insurers and Managed Care." *Modern Healthcare*. July 19, 1999. P. 77.

look for growth through acquisition. Blue Cross consolidators like Anthem in Indianapolis, Ind., the Regence Group in the Northwest, and Virginia-based Trigon were providing capital and management to other Blue Cross and Blue Shield associations (Cochrane, 1998). Kaiser-Permanente sold several unprofitable plans after losing more than $500 million at the close of the 1990s, and some provider-sponsored HMOs were sold or put on the market.

The rising popularity of PPOs also fueled mergers in this field and was expected in 1999 to reduce the 1,035 PPOs operating across the nation, which were actually owned by about 400 companies (Rauber, 1999). Of these, only 100 were of significant size, and fewer than a dozen PPOs had more than 1 million members (Table 11.4). Hence, the PPO industry remained open to new players at the turn of the century. In 1999, Beyond Benefits, based in Irvine, Calif., made a huge acquisition of 4 million PPO members, purchasing the Preferred Health Network from Foundation Health Systems, a large managed care company in Woodland Hills, Calif. Beyond Benefits had venture capital backing for additional acquisitions and could double or triple in size, according to its president, George Bregante.

Table 11.4: 10 Largest PPOs in America in 1999

PREFERRED PROVIDER ORGANIZATION	1999 ENROLLMENT (MILLIONS)
CCN	31.9
MultiPlan	23.0
Beech Street	16.0
First Health Network	14.8
CorVel Corp	6.5
Private Healthcare Systems	5.6
National Preferred Provider Network	5.1
Aetna U.S. Healthcare	4.0
Beyond Benefits	4.0
Cigna Healthcare	3.1

Source: Chris Rauber, "PPOs Riding a Wave of Popularity." *Modern Healthcare*. June 7, 1999. P. 50.

MANAGED CARE REFORM DRIVES MORE GOVERNMENT REGULATION

Not surprisingly, a wave of state and federal regulation was sweeping the managed care industry by the end of the 1990s. Both Republicans and Democrats battled in Washington, backing their own versions of managed care reform, with President Bill Clinton threatening to veto any version of a "Patients' Bill of Rights" which did not include a patient's right to sue his or her managed care plan. In Congressional testimony, California internist Mark Smith, president of the California HealthCare Foundation, surprised no one when he told senators that he hoped the term "managed care" would disappear in 10 years (Pretzer, 1999). What began as a politician's dream issue became a political nightmare in the course of a decade.

At the state level, legislatures were not waiting for Washington to resolve its interparty and intraparty gridlock over health reform. Under a barrage of criticism from providers, consumers, and the media, almost half of the states enacted their own versions of a Patients' Bill of Rights in 1998 and 1999. Responding to complaints from hospitals and doctors, 26 states enacted "prompt payment" regulations which required health plans to pay clean claims within a specified period (*Modern Healthcare*, 1999).

Differences in governmental approaches and ongoing economic reorganization in the marketplace will undoubtedly cause managed care to change and diversify even more over the coming years. Stabilization around anything approximating a universal model or uniform nomenclature is highly unlikely. Therefore, practitioners will likely have to continue evaluating their managed care options on a case-by-case basis over time. The good news is that progress is being made. While the development of new options will not necessarily reduce the confusion that is associated with managed care at this writing, problems may be easier to avoid in the future. Managed care still has a good chance to evolve in desirable directions (Bauer, 1999).

REINVENTING MANAGED CARE ON A COLLABORATIVE MODEL

The managed care revolution of the 1980s and 1990s is over. Critics of for-profit managed care have claimed that HMOs will never succeed as long as health plans maintain their enterprise model. As consumers have become more sophisticated and skeptical, they are switching to less coercive health plan products, such as PPOs and open-access HMOs. Economist J.D. Kleinke, author of *Bleeding Edge: The Business of Health Care in the New Century,* argued that managed care was a transitional mechanism. The profitability that gave rise to the big, national, for-profit managed care companies was a temporary phenomenon designed to shake up the entire medical financing and delivery system (Rauber 1998). He and other critics contend that the market will not support a model in which so much of the premium, up to 25 percent, is siphoned off the top by HMO administrative costs and profit.

Managed care must now reinvent its basic principles and business model. The fundamental problems facing the nation's HMOs are that medical costs are rising and that managed care does not have effective systems to control them. Boosting premiums is not a sustainable business model for HMOs under these circumstances. The list of challenges facing managed care is formidable:

- Providers are demanding higher fees and consolidating in order to increase their power to negotiate with the plans.
- Consumers want plans which give patients more freedom to seek specialists and access to brand-name pharmaceuticals.
- The industry has not invested enough in information technology to effectively manage care, according to managed care author Peter Boland of Boland Healthcare, based in Berkeley, Calif. (Rauber 1998).
- Reacting negatively to HMO price increases, some employers are exploring direct contracting with providers and pharmacy benefit management companies.
- Alternative products, such as PPOs, have become more price-competitive as HMOs boost premium levels.

One of the greatest uncertainties of the millennium is who will hold and manage risk, the economic challenge of satisfying consumer expectations under health plans with prospectively defined premiums. Who will accept the challenge: plans or providers? Billions of dollars and the future of the American healthcare delivery system may be at stake relative to this issue. HMOs have been accused of managing the premium for profit, not managing care for effectiveness. Capitation-ready, provider-sponsored networks exist in virtually every market. Could providers do a better job if they had control of the premium? Could health plans and provider-sponsored networks collaboratively share the premium? The answers to these questions may well lie in the development of a collaborative model of care delivery (Coile, 2000).

Consequently, nurse anesthetists and other clinicians entering practice in the early 21st century will need to examine their prospective managed care relationships with respect to structures that have not yet been developed. The specific arrangements of these new relationships will almost certainly develop around new mechanisms for sharing risk because assuming risk has some corresponding incentives:

- Controlling allocation of the premium.

- Managing patients across the continuum of care in most appropriate settings.
- Achieving savings from more efficient care processes.
- Linking data on costs and treatments with outcomes.
- Providing incentives for desired performance.
- Producing additional savings through enrollee management.
- Educating consumers to reduce risks and improve health.

Asuming risk is risky business. Future practitioners will continually need to balance expected gains and possible losses before aligning themselves with managed care plans in the early 21st century. More than two in three HMOs lost money in the late 1990s, even while the plans had the potential ability to control resources and utilization. Pharmacy costs rose 11 percent to 12 percent per year during this period, and some plans experienced 15 percent to 17 percent increases in drug costs despite the widespread application of pharmacy benefit management programs (Grandinetti, 1999). Managed care enrollees were learning how to work the system at the same time, and providers have figured out how to be paid for their services despite HMO hassles.

Most providers have developed an infrastructure for dealing with managed care, but would they be any better at managing costs of care themselves? Past battles have made both plans and providers more suspicious of each other. By the end of the decade, Nate Kaufman, a San Diego-based managed care expert with Superior Consultant, was advising providers to get out of capitation arrangements and return to fee-for-service unless rates were very favorable and the provider organization was tightly organized to manage care and costs. Few providers can meet Kaufman's seven stringent requirements for assuming risk (Kaufman, 1999), but they are based on years of first-hand involvement in the evolution of managed care.

THOUGHTS ON THE FUTURE OF MANAGED CARE

The new millennium opened with promising signs that plan-provider cooperation—focused on health improvement of the patient, not just costs and profitability—may be possible. Minnesota's UnitedHealth, one of the nation's five largest HMOs, announced in late 1999 that it would stop second-guessing doctors in prior review of treatments. United found it was spending more to staff a medical management program with 1,200 nurses than it was saving with a review of every physician's decision. Providers heartily endorsed the end of United's prior-authorization program, and hailed it as the opening of a new dialogue with health plans about how to improve patients' health status as a cost-efficient strategy.

Aetna U.S. Healthcare, based in Pennsylvania, also announced that it was easing controls over doctors, although Aetna planned to continue reviewing some high-cost and high-volume procedures, especially in regions where utilization was higher than company benchmarks. United and other health insurers announced plans to give physicians comparative performance profiles for education purposes on a periodic basis. The success of these is not yet established or assured, but clearly, managed health plans are changing direction. A new patient-focused collaboration model may result, which would positively reinforce the patient education and care management roles of advanced practice nurses in the millennium.

One aspect of the future of healthcare is fairly certain: It will be data-driven. The quality and availability of information will increasingly separate the winners from the losers. The promise of managed care in the 1970s was an implicit assumption that it could reduce or eliminate care that did not improve a patient's health. The restrictions that would distinguish managed care from fee-for-service were presumably based on information about the effectiveness of proposed treatments. Unfortunately, managed care plans did not have the data to fulfill this expectation, which left them open to charges that cost, not care, was what they were managing. Fortunately, with the advent of telemedicine and networked information systems at the end of the 20th century, the information for cost-effective management of care is now available (Bauer and Ringel, 1999).

If the many lessons and meanings of managed care were to be distilled to a single concept that ought to be retained in every student's and practitioner's mind, it would probably be accountability. Managed care grew so fast in the 1980s and early 1990s because it appeared to hold providers accountable in terms of both cost and quality for their decisions. Whether actual performance matched this appearance is debatable, but one cannot question the intensity of purchasers' desires to link hospitals and doctors directly to the consequences of their care. The enduring legacy of 20th century managed care may well be the continuing development of explicit incentives and disincentives that cause clinicians and delivery organizations to rise or fall with the overall success of the healthcare delivery system. This highly desirable outcome will most likely be achieved if it is pursued collaboratively.

However, given providers' and patients' growing resentment toward managed care, the environment is not necessarily ripe for collaboration, but it may be the best opportunity available as managed care is forced to redefine itself. In the next five to 10 years, providers may step forward to assume risk in partnership with health plans and demonstrate successful collaborative care management models that put primary emphasis on patients. If this collaboration does not occur and healthcare costs continue to climb by double-digit levels amidst a rising volume of consumer and provider complaints, then the managed care era will probably end.

In this situation, a possible scenario for U.S. healthcare in the third millennium could be a single-payer model administered by the federal government, thus ending the American experiment with enterprise-managed healthcare. Fortunately, the authors believe that a value-based, consumer-focused system can still be created by visionary leaders in the private sector. Time will tell. The only certainty is that managed care will continue to change, and caregivers will have to change with it. Whether they lead or follow the changes is the key to their future.

PRACTICAL ADVICE FOR PRACTITIONERS

Given the historical fluidity and the uncertain future of managed care, preparing students to deal with it after graduation is an extremely difficult task. The opportunities and problems that await them when starting practice will vary with each graduate's particular circumstances. Advice that might be sound for one new practitioner could be self-defeating for another with respect to both time and place. However, a few general words of advice can be drawn from experiences of the recent past.

First, every practitioner who contemplates an independent practice work arrangement should read every managed care contract carefully before signing it. Being part of managed care is a choice, and the conditions of a practitioner's participation in a managed care plan are defined in a contract. The contract should define what is expected of each party, including obligations to provide care under the contract. If a careful reading of the contract suggests the plan will have unreasonable power to dictate the clinician's practice patterns or to refuse payment for care after it has been delivered, the practitioner should demand desired changes or refuse to join the plan. A careful reading should also look for any terms, called gag clauses, that prevent a practitioner from telling a patient about desirable but uncovered care. Experienced legal counsel should review all contracts and the provider should consult with peers who have already experienced contract negotiations as they can usually provide valuable insights.

Second, a practitioner should never sign a contract he or she does not understand. Some managed care contracts are poorly written, full of errors and omissions, or otherwise likely to create serious differences of interpretation in the event of disagreement between practitioner and plan. Ambiguity will almost always come back to haunt the practitioner because contracts are written by the managed care plan. Sadly, experience shows that the plan will almost always prevail in situations where interpretation is not crystal clear to all concerned. To add insult to injury, litigation to resolve misunderstandings is frightfully expensive, and the plans tend to have enough money ("deep pockets," in legal parlance) to outlast the practitioner even when justice would ultimately prevail on the practitioner's side.

Third, practitioners should avoid contracts that reimburse care below the costs of providing it efficiently (including a normal profit). Many practitioners have signed participation agreements out of fear that they would lose patients if they did not join the plan. Others have agreed to participate with the assumption that they could make money on volume, even though the reimbursement per patient was unprofitable. Another potential problem is an all-products clause requiring a practitioner to provide care under all contracts underwritten by a managed care plan, even though the practitioner has signed a participation agreement under only one plan. In other words, practitioners must remember that a loss leader is still a loss. Providing more care under an economically bad contract only compounds losses, and providing less care can lead to potential problems with malpractice.

Fourth, the practitioner should have clearly defined protections and rights that prevent the plan from arbitrary and unjustifiable actions. The terms of dispute resolution are particularly important because many managed care plans have terminated practitioners without clear cause or prior notification. Consequently, clear and reasonable performance criteria should be specified in the contract, along with workable mechanisms to deal with discrepancies between expected and actual performance. The right to appeal a plan's decisions, including termination, is a particularly important right that should be included in a contract. The contract should address economic credentialing, the practice of removing practitioners who have practiced outside the guidelines. Economic criteria are not bad *per se* because they are part of the theory and practice of managed care, but the criteria should be clearly stated and clinically sound. Plans that retain the right to terminate participating practitioners without clear criteria and due cause are to be avoided.

Last, but not least, clinicians about to enter practice need to become thoroughly familiar with the current and evolving realities of managed care in the market where they intend to work. Generalizations based on experiences in other times or places could lead to problems. Professional societies and specialty organizations can be particularly helpful in this regard, particularly state and local chapters that present regular continuing education programs to educate their members on the evolution of managed care. Active membership in professional associations also provides an opportunity for networking with experienced practitioners, who will often be the best source of market-specific information about managed care.

SUMMARY

It should be clear to the reader that the concept of managed care is dynamic and evolving. Nevertheless, there are certain principles which underly the process about which CRNAs need to be attentive. Notions of cost efficiency, control of resources, meaningful quality measures and evidence-based outcomes remain paramount, regardless of the iteration of managed care structure. The reader may also find valuable information on evaluating managed care contracts in chapters 15 and 16, in addition to that found in this chapter. Although some repetition may be noted, the obvious importance of contractual issues can only benefit from comparative perspectives.

REFERENCES

Beckham, J.D. (1997). The beginning of the end for HMOs. Part 1: The awakening market. *Healthc Forum J.* 40(6), 44-7.

Beckham, J.D. (1998). The beginning of the end for HMOs. Part 2: Providers have more clout than they think. *Healthc Forum J.*, Jan-Feb:41(1):52-5.

Bauer, J.C. (1998). *Not What the Doctor Ordered: How to End the Medical Monopoly in Pursuit of Managed Care.* New York, NY: McGraw-Hill.

Bauer, J.C. (1999). The future of managed care: Diagnosis, prognosis, and treatment plan. *Managed Care Practice.* 4(5), 1-13.

Cochrane, J.D. (1998). Is managed care going into a stall? *Integr Healthc Rep.* 5(11), 1-11.

Coile, R.C., Jr. (1999). Managed care in the millennium: New forecasts for the five stages of managed care. *Russ Coile's Health Trends.* 11(12).

Editors. (1999). By the numbers: Insurers and managed care. *Mod Healthc.* Suppl:70-2, 74, 76-9.

Ginzberg, E. (1999). The uncertain future of managed care. *N Engl J Med.* 340(2), 144-6.

Goldsmith, J. (1998). Are HMOs really a dying breed? *Healthc Forum J.* 41(6), 52-53.

Grandinetti, D.A. (1999). Managed care 1999. Drug costs could come out of your pocket. *Med Econ.* 76(7), 178, 183-6, 189-90.

Hudak, R.P. & Barkley, W.N. (1999). Trends in managed care organizations: Implications for the physician executive. *Physician Exec.* 25(1), 22-27.

Kleinke, J.D. (1998). *Bleeding Edge: The Business of Health Care in the New Century.* Gaithersburg, MD: Aspen Publishers.

Kunkle, C. (1998). Promoting the purchasers' point of view. A conversation with Catherine Kunkle. *Manag Care.* 7(1), 41-42, 44, 47-8.

Pretzer, M. (1999). The future of managed care: Whose prediction should you believe? *Med Econ.* 8:76(5), 43, 46, 49.

Rauber, C. (1999). Evolution or extinction? Experts say HMOs must reinvent themselves if they are to survive. *Mod Healthc.* 28(42), 36-38, 40.

Robinson, J.C. (1999). The future of managed care organizations. *Health Affairs.* 18(2), 7-24.

Rovner, J. (1998). The Medicare HMO disappearing act. *Bus Health:* 16(12), 25-7.

Terry, K. (1999). Managed care 1999. Hang on—the ride's going to get rougher. *Med Econ.* 76(7), 176-178.

KEY REFERENCES

Bauer, J.C. (1999). The future of managed care: Diagnosis, prognosis and treatment plan. *Managed Care Practice*. 4(5), 1-13.

Bauer, J.C. (1999). *Telemedicine and the Reinvention of Healthcare: The Seventh Revolution in Medicine*. New York, NY: McGraw-Hill.

Kleinke, J.D. (1998). *Bleeding Edge: The Business of Health Care in the New Century.* Gaithersburg, MD: Aspen Publishers.

Robinson, J.C. (1999). The future of managed care organizations. *Health Affairs*. 18(2), 7-24.

STUDY QUESTIONS

1. What are some of the distinguishing characteristics of managed care that are different from the traditional fee-for-service paradigm of healthcare delivery?

2. In what ways are provider payment issues (or mechanisms) different in managed care than fee-for-service?

3. Managed care has failed to universally control healthcare costs. What are some reasons that may be contributing to this continuing problem?

4. Discuss the various ways in which fee-for-service payment arrangements are included in managed care plans.

5. Practitioners in the future will undoubtedly either be signing managed care contracts themselves or working for an employer who maintains a variety of these contracts. What are some of the professional responsibilities CRNAs of any employment type will need to incorporate into their clinical practice under managed care?

CHAPTER 12

ADMINISTRATIVE MANAGEMENT

Christine S. Zambricki, CRNA, MS, FAAN

Administrative Director
William Beaumont Hospital
Royal Oak, MI

KEY CONCEPTS

- More Certified Registered Nurse Anesthetists (CRNAs) are becoming administrators and managers in hospitals because of their clinical expertise, graduate degree preparation and knowledge of standards of care in the perioperative environment.

- The key to administrative success is the ability of the CRNA manager to effectively communicate with a variety of personnel, create an environment of productivity and creativity in which to solve problems, and maintain the global needs and mission of the healthcare facility.

- Chief among the talents required of a CRNA manager is an understanding of key quality indicators in anesthesia, how to measure them, how to change practice to conform with them, and how to encourage providers to document their compliance with them.

- Many CRNA managers will have the primary responsibility of financial analysis of their department's performance. This will require that they understand the mechanics of reading and interpreting statements of operation, financial transaction details, financial performance reviews, and budget formulation including operational and capital budgets.

- As the demand for highly skilled and expensive operating room personnel such as CRNAs increases, recruitment and retention programs will become a primary responsibility of the CRNA manager.

- In large service departments, nearly 80 percent of total expenditures will be accounted for by personnel costs. This requires exquisite and detailed budgeting skills for personnel costs that can be supported by revenue projections in addition to maintaining adequate profit margins for the facility.

To a significant degree, much of what is done in an administrative or service department depends on leadership. Many Certified Registered Nurse Anesthetists (CRNAs), at some point in their careers, will be called on to assume administrative positions as leaders within their own institutions and, in turn, as leaders within the anesthesia community. The purpose of this chapter is to provide some salient insight into those responsibilities as healthcare moves more aggressively into integrated, managed care systems.

The total perioperative domain is a vital and consequential component of the hospital organization as a whole. This area not only represents between 50 percent and 70 percent of most hospitals' net operating income, it is critical to physician and patient relationships and satisfaction. There are few departments in the hospital that have such a profound impact on the institution and span multiple service areas. Due to the special characteristics of the surgical services environment, leaders in the operating room (OR) are some of the most visible and critical administrators within the organization.

EVOLUTION OF THE CRNA ADMINISTRATOR

CRNAs are not new to administrative management responsibilities. It has been common practice for CRNAs to direct departments of anesthesia or other related service areas. As hospitals move toward clinical integration according to service lines, CRNAs are assuming broader administrative responsibilities including intensive care units, nursing surgical units, and pharmacy and emergency room departments. Since the role of the CRNA director is no longer limited to anesthesia departments, it is more important than ever that the CRNA obtain knowledge and expertise in fields common to any hospital administrator, which most likely were not part of the CRNA's original education or subsequent clinical experience.

There are several reasons why CRNAs are broadening their leadership role, many of which have to do with external forces promoting integration of leadership within the institution as a whole. The Joint Commission on Accreditation of Healthcare Organizations (JCAHO) started this trend with the consolidation of operating room and anesthesia chapters within the Comprehensive Accreditation Manual for Hospitals in the late 1980s. It was after this change that more hospitals chose to consolidate management responsibilities for the entire surgical services area. In this way, one person became accountable for compliance with integrated standards and regulations.

From an internal perspective, there are two driving forces within hospital organizations that have supported the development of an integrated governance structure for operating rooms and anesthesia. First, the need for quality improvement has led to a service line approach in many hospitals. The service line movement coordinates activities across department lines for the good of a single population of patients. For the surgical-services service line, this often leads to consolidation of leadership for the anesthesia and perioperative areas. Second, as facility reimbursement from public payers decreases, hospitals are seeking to maintain an effective management structure that focuses on broad spans of authority, and thus reduce redundant administrative positions.

Leadership Characteristics

By virtue of their educational and experiential background, CRNAs bring certain skills to a leadership role and have learned to work closely with physicians—both anesthesiologists and surgeons—while delivering anesthesia care to patients in the OR. This experience is extremely useful in developing physician-staff relationships, an essential skill for effectiveness as a surgical services leader.

CRNAs are often chosen for leadership positions because they are operating room-based nurse specialists with post-graduate education. Graduate level degrees are becoming a desired or required characteristic for director-level positions in hospitals. With a strong background in critical care nursing, CRNAs have the clinical expertise to evaluate practice in the areas of anesthesia, pain management and surgery. This background, coupled with the individual capacity for interpersonal relations and leadership, has created many opportunities for CRNAs who wish to focus their professional careers on hospital administration.

There is increasing awareness among hospital executives that CRNA directors or managers can significantly impact the bottom line. There also are increasing challenges for individuals with this role and responsibility. CRNA directors must not only perform to higher clinical, financial and service standards, they must accommodate new pressures in their jobs not present in previous decades. A broadened span of control is one such pressure. As with all of nursing, a typical director now oversees an average of 50-60 full-time equivalents (FTEs) (Altaffer, 1998). This is a significant departure from the smaller staffing complements of the 1980s.

CRNA directors are also confronted with increased responsibility for aligning clinical, financial and service strategies within the institution. There may be responsibility for coordination of care with numerous out-of-hospital enterprises such as freestanding surgical centers, doctor's offices and pain clinics. They may be negotiating contracts for a variety of programs such as private practice contracts, perfusion services or instrument cleaning. The CRNA director must allocate capital and labor expenses in a highly cost-sensitive environment, while managing growing staff shortages. Despite a significant increase in responsibility, there are reduced resources in the sense of time, money and staff assistance. Meanwhile, the CRNA must schedule adequate presence in the operating room and provide clinical leadership. Increases in managerial and peripheral responsibilities significantly reduce the time available for this very important role; however, its importance cannot be underestimated in the overall scope of administrative activities.

The transition from clinical expert to administrative manager presents many challenges. The CRNA must adopt the leadership role within the context of the corporate culture within which he or she works. It is more important than ever to demonstrate consistent execution with business results, rather than focusing only on clinical results. The CRNA administrative manager may find himself or herself caught in organizational upheaval, as environmental changes drive healthcare change and the entire industry moves into the information age of the 21st century.

Quality and depth of administrative leadership is reflected in relationships with key constituencies, including other perioperative managers, CRNAs, nurses, surgeons, anesthesiologists and hospital administrators. This is a major transition for the CRNA practitioner, whose anesthesia practice has been characterized by independence and one-on-one patient relationships. Reinvention is a lifelong and continuing learning process, and in this case, the CRNA may benefit from additional education focused on management, choosing a mentor and establishing a solid support system.

Beyond the more formal aspects of preparing for the role of administrator, such as graduate education and experience, are the skills required to bring people together for a common cause or purpose. It is the job of the leader or administrator to visualize, manage, and promote the institutional mission. That goal can only be brought about by a skillful administrator who understands concepts of interdisciplinary collaboration and the importance of personal-social interactions, and who demonstrates effective communication skills.

INTERDISCIPLINARY COLLABORATION

Effective interprofessional relationships in the operating room are the foundation of excellent patient care (Fargason, 1992). Several studies reinforce the importance of these interactions in improving the quality of patient care and reducing health costs (Baggs, 1989, 1990). The American Association of Critical Care Nurses (AACCN) developed a demonstration project to link costs and patient care effectiveness to organizational attributes (Mitchell, 1989). Nurse-physician collaboration was endorsed by the AACCN as a key attribute of interprofessional relationships. This study showed conclusively that desirable clinical outcomes—that is, low mortality rates and high patient satisfaction—occurred in a critical care unit characterized by a perceived high level of nurse-physician collaboration.

Knaus and Draper (1986) evaluated outcomes using actual and predicted mortality rates for 5,030 patients in the intensive care units of 13 hospitals that ranged from 280 to 1,092 beds. Predicted mortality rates for each hospital were developed from a severity-of-disease classification system and were compared with the hospital's actual mortality rates. Results demonstrated that some hospitals had significantly more deaths than predicted, while others had significantly fewer. Researchers found that the discriminating factor in these disparate mortality rates was the level of interaction and coordination among ICU staff. The low-mortality hospitals had systems that were carefully designed to ensure communication and effective interprofessional interactions.

Four primary causes for conflict in the OR emerge from the literature: unclear work procedures, unique characteristics of the OR, diversity of values among the professions, and lack of good communication skills.

Clarification of Work Processes and Procedures

In the surgical environment, work procedures and roles may be unclear, ineffective or inconsistently applied, increasing the likelihood that conflict will occur. There may be no system in place to give people guidance on how to work together effectively. White and Charns (1980) found that organizational and managerial factors were much more important than personal factors in predicting the degree of collaboration between nurses and physicians. A collection of sensible policies, procedures, protocols and training systems will eliminate major sources of interdisciplinary conflict.

For example, the process for patient transfer following surgery involves several groups: CRNAs, anesthesiologists, surgeons, circulating and postanesthesia care unit nurses, surgical technologists, residents, anesthesia technicians, housekeepers, and operating room clerks. If this process is poorly designed, the affected parties will frequently be in conflict because a procedure that would meet everyone's needs has not been worked out. In developing effective processes, each step and each participant's involvement must be carefully analyzed. Then the process can be redesigned so that roles are clarified and wasted effort eliminated.

Traditionally, hospitals have been organized according to functional areas or disciplines (i.e., nursing, medicine), and a hierarchical decision model moves issues up the ladder for resolution. This approach will not work in the operating room, where multiple disciplines work in close, sometimes overlapping roles to achieve a goal. Because a smoothly functioning OR requires efficient patient flow, problem resolution must cut across disciplines and be supported by collaborative efforts at resolution that satisfy the legitimate concerns of all participants and clarify the work processes.

Understanding the Unique Characteristics of the Operating Room

Members of the perioperative team, as with any other team, recognize that they form a unique unit and want to be a valued member of it. Consequently, most departments value their cohesiveness as a functional group. Groups distinguish themselves in many ways. For the perioperative team, the most visible way is the group uniform—scrubs—which is recognized throughout the institution. This group is also brought together by their sensibilities to the acuity of their patients and the pace of the environment. Anesthesia and operating room professionals also possess specific tools, techniques and even reimbursement methods that separate them from others in the hospital, yet serve to make them a cohesive, functional unit.

Other factors, however, work against this sense of connectedness. In the operating room, the combination of surgeon, anesthesiologist, CRNA, circulating nurse and technologist changes constantly, particularly in large departments. In this setting, the team has little time to establish itself as an entity before the day begins and all focus centers on the patient.

Several strategies can work to promote a team ethos in the OR environment. First and simplest is proximity. Placing people physically close together in settings such as lounges and locker rooms encourages a sense of unity. In contrast, people who are isolated from one another will find it more difficult to mesh their activities, plan collaboratively and help one another. Through mutual effort and interdependence, members of the OR staff can consider colleagues to be partners with a common goal rather than competitors striving toward separate ends.

Although the concept of proximity as a building block to cohesive group functioning is widely accepted in business and education, areas separating physicians from nonphysicians remain bastions of the operating room environment. This physical separation is a vestige of an outdated hierarchical model wherein all personnel knew their place in the hierarchy. Arguments for preserving distance, such as the need for discussions about patients or business, are superficial when weighed against the mutual interdependence of today's healthcare providers. Incorporating shared spaces for team activities when contemplating institutional construction or remodeling is an investment in future team relations.

There are other unique features of the OR that, if not managed correctly and efficiently, can lead to conflict. CRNA administrative directors often find themselves involved in the more pragmatic issues of operating room management, specifically developing policies that allow for efficient functioning of the entire area. One common example would be the development of policies and procedures that determine accurate scheduling of surgical cases.

To recognize the role that different perspectives bring to conflict in the OR, one need only consider the process of surgical scheduling. Case scheduling, with urgent, emergent, elective and add-on cases all vying for priority, is potentially one of the most inflammatory issues in the OR, especially an OR that is understaffed. Control issues can dominate case scheduling. Ideally, scheduling should be predicated on policies derived through mutual agreement, effective communication and common sense.

Case duration must be estimated accurately in order to reduce the amount of overtime paid to CRNAs and other operating room personnel. Customer satisfaction, both surgeon and patient, are jeopardized when time is inaccurately allocated and preceding cases run too long. Several authors have suggested increasing OR utilization via computer-based information systems (Macario, 1999; Dexter, 1998, 1999; Skula, 1990). These systems collect large amounts of data based on a particular surgeon's previously scheduled procedures, and the mean duration of cases is used to estimate the duration of subsequent cases.

Information systems alone cannot create a flawless schedule. The surgeon may be allowed to adjust the scheduled time by a predetermined percentage in order to individualize time estimates to patient characteristics, complexity of procedure, and other factors not reflected by case type. As a further check, the OR and nurse anesthesia managers should review the schedule subjectively to determine whether the schedule appears workable.

Special problems arise with the scheduling of add-on cases. Throughout the day, judgments must be made to determine whether an add-on case will fit into the OR schedule. Poor management of additional cases can result in high cancellation rates, excessive overtime costs, loss of revenue, and poor utilization of OR time. Several algorithms exist for assigning add-on cases (Zhou, 1998 and Dexter, 1999). One method suggests that add-on elective cases should first be sorted based on scheduled duration from longest to shortest. The longest add-on cases are assigned to an OR first. Cases are assigned to rooms with sufficient additional time for the new case and the least amount of additional time available. If no OR has sufficient time for the case, a 15-minute adjustment may be made to accommodate the case. This method has been shown to increase the number of add-ons that can be accommodated in a given day; however, it does require that add-on cases are batched together and scheduled simultaneously, requiring a cut-off time for submission of add-ons. These decisions cannot be made lightly, as the implications for "bumping" a subsequent surgeon and creating an unreasonable wait for the patient present a significant customer service challenge. Regardless of what system is used, the estimate must be unbiased and precise.

Recognition of Different Values and Perspectives

Conflict may occur when people fail to understand others' rationale and motive. In many respects, professionals working in the operating room environment have similar values. All profess to be motivated by a dedication to patient care and a commitment to values of hard work and education. These joint values can form a foundation for the development of effective interpersonal relationships.

However, perspectives among professionals may differ in some areas. In many hospitals, physicians work in a private practice model, while other staff are employed on an hourly wage or salary. The economic necessity in private practice is to do more cases, whereas the motivation for employees may be to finish the day and go home. This difference can lead to conflict when physicians press to add additional cases to the schedule. Understanding the motivation for a specific behavior often makes collaboration easier, even if one does not personally benefit from the behavior.

Another common, potential point of conflict exits in many operating rooms. Because physicians are not salaried staff members, meeting time for committee work represents potentially lost income. Physicians may not want to attend meetings during the day and the director may not want to attend meetings at night. As a result, physicians may favor quick deliberations and rapid adoption of their solution to a problem rather than spending time on in-depth analysis. This approach may frustrate salaried employees who feel the need for further discussions or longer time periods for problem solving. It is inevitable that for important issues, meetings must be scheduled at a time that will not interfere with office practice or operating room time. Flexibility in scheduling will help the CRNA director build trusting relationships by sending the message that the input of all members of the team is worthwhile and necessary.

Importance of Communication Skills

Healthcare professionals tend to be very good at communicating with patients, but spend little time communicating effectively as a team. Indeed, some physicians and nurses may lack good communication skills altogether, interfering with their ability to deal with one another. Conflict usually occurs because people have not learned how to communicate with others in ways that empower rather than irritate. Because the operating room is an intensely interactive environment, good communication skills are essential. These include knowing how to listen effectively, how to be assertive without being aggressive, and how to use nonverbal communication. Good communicators also understand what types of situations produce problems, so that they can be anticipated and pitfalls avoided.

Effective communication conveys mutual respect. In too many conversations, participants are intent upon making their point, listening only for a pause in which to interject their opinion. Patronizing colleagues in the operating room is another destructive communication style. Operating rooms are very public places, with all activities and conversations "on stage" for team members to observe and hear. This physical proximity, from which one cannot easily leave, underscores the need for professional communication among colleagues.

Triangulating is an illustration of dysfunctional communication that occurs regularly in a director's position. When tension between two people increases, the process of triangulation adds a third person, usually the CRNA director. For example, when a disagreement occurs between two employees, either of them might take the dispute to the CRNA director, who is expected to resolve the issue. Triangles of communication are nonproductive because they prevent resolution of problems in the two-person system. When tension is relieved by sharing the problem with a third person, problems are ignored or never discussed between those directly involved. For the good of the long-term relationship, the two individuals should come to a mutually agreeable way to resolve their differences whenever possible.

Interprofessional communication can be enhanced in a number of ways. For example:

- Ensure that both parties in a conflict have the opportunity to be heard without regard to status. Judgment should be reserved until this occurs. Personal attacks invariably worsen the problem. In some cases, the relationship may become so contentious, involving verbal or physical harassment, that the CRNA director must intervene.
- The ambiance of the operating room always benefits from keeping one's dignity intact with a calm demeanor and a low voice. Always select words carefully before discussing sensitive issues. Keep one-to-one discussions as private as possible. In the event of a conflict in the operating room, arrange to discuss matters later when patient care responsibilities are completed.
- Differences among professionals in the operating room environment are unavoidable, and common reasons for subsequent conflicts are based on predictable factors inherent in the operating room environment such as lack of appropriate systems and procedures, differences in perspective and values, and poorly developed communication skills.
- One of the keys to solving relationship problems is to avoid personalizing the problem. Disagreement is not always undesirable, however, as different perspectives to solving patient care and systems problems can be helpful. Disagreement that improves the environment should not be discouraged. On the other hand, conflict can also be destructive and lead to poor decisions, needless stress and performance deficits. Relationships characterized by this type of conflict put all parties at risk, and efforts should be channeled toward effective conflict resolution.

WORKING WITHIN THE HOSPITAL'S ADMINISTRATIVE STRUCTURE

In orienting to a new administrative position, the CRNA director must understand clearly the governance of the organization, the major players involved, and the locus and method by which decisions are made. This can be done through observation, talking to peers, and reviewing files for approval documents and memos. New relationships with critical stakeholders, both internal and external to the organization, must be forged or renewed. The director will need to develop a relationship with the chief financial officer as well as major vendors. Within six months of assuming the position, the director should meet with all critical stakeholders in order to understand what working relationship is required and to gain perspective on the stakeholders' view of the director's role and responsibility within the organization.

There are some obvious things that the director can do to work productively within the hospital's administrative structure. It is important that the CRNA director engage in activities that support the hospital in its entirety. In these activities, the director functions in a complimentary role to the hospital mission and makes a contribution beyond his/her own parochial interests, thus increasing the director's inherent value to the organization.

One example of broadening work activity is in the arena of hospital committees. Many types of committees can be found in healthcare organizations. At the least, there will be department committees, hospital administrative committees (interdepartmental) and medical staff committees (interdepartmental). One way to get a better understanding of the needs of departments outside the operating room is to be a member of a committee in another department. For example, the intensive care unit may have a quality improvement committee. This would be an interesting and appropriate committee for a member of the anesthesia department, given the interdepartmental synergies and the clinical knowledge base required to evaluate care in this setting, particularly as it relates to the airway. Other committees of the medical or administrative staff suitable for CRNA director involvement include the pharmacy and therapeutics committee, operating room committee, medical quality committee, and library committee. Through involvement on medical and administrative committees, the director will develop relationships with many key leaders and physicians throughout the organization. These relationships will lay the groundwork for a positive working environment in the future.

Another important contribution that the CRNA director can make to the hospital organization is to exhibit a willingness to take on additional responsibility. As administrative positions vacate due to attrition, more and more chief executive officers (CEOs) are choosing to reassign duties rather than fill the positions. The director may receive additional areas of responsibility not related to nurse anesthesia or even the OR, such as heading up a service line initiative, JCAHO preparation or a new educational program. The director may not be asked whether he/she wishes to have additional responsibility; rather, it is assumed that the director will gracefully respond with the best effort to accomplish the objectives of the organization.

A CRNA administrator or manager must observe the corporate culture and develop an understanding and respect for the conventions of administrative behavior at the institution. This must not be taken lightly. Corporate culture encompasses many different elements of hospital life. Clothing is a one part of corporate culture; so is the style and format of presentations made to upper-level administrators. Respecting corporate culture does not exclude the ability to display some individualism, but to be part of the culture means embracing the major tenets and functioning within them. Some will be obvious on the first day or at the first meeting, and others may be more subtle and appreciated only over time.

A CRNA administrator must develop the ability to think outside of the context of the operating room. Due to the high degree of specialization and the physical detachment inherent in their location, operating rooms and anesthesia departments risk becoming isolated and self-centered in their thinking. The director will have a responsibility to advocate for the area; moreover, this will be expected of the director at meetings and other venues for decision making.

Beyond advocacy, the director must also keep a balanced view and an open mind regarding the needs of all patients and the overall obligations of the hospital. It is inevitable that competing priorities will arise over resources such as capital dollars, space, and patient beds. If the CRNA director is always focused solely on his/her area of responsibility, then the director will be viewed as narrow minded and lacking global perspective. Worse yet, this myopia may result in poor decisions for the hospital as a whole. With the challenges of today's healthcare, the chief executive officer needs every member of the leadership team to be working for organizational benefit, not for self-interest.

In addition to developing broad vision within the organization, the director must become knowledgeable about the healthcare industry in general. This can be accomplished by reading industry publications such as *Hospitals and Health Care Networks*, *Health Affairs,* and *Modern*

HealthCare. Another important source of information is the lay press. With increasing frequency major newspapers and news magazines cover in-depth stories on the healthcare industry and the plight of hospitals as well as medical advances and futuristic projections. The Internet is an ever-changing source of information. Extensive knowledge about national healthcare issues will provide insight into the pressures the institution is facing from the outside. The CRNA director can anticipate changes that will impact reimbursement or services offered. Knowledge of trends in healthcare provides a common language and understanding which is expected of individuals at the director level regardless of their administrative assignment.

Contemporary Administrative Challenges

A common challenge facing hospital directors today is the increasing organizational complexity of hospitals. With mergers, acquisitions, multiple business lines, contradictory payment schemes and reengineered operations, the environment is ever changing. Internally the environment is becoming increasingly complex. Regulations impacting the hospital are extensive. Technology becomes obsolete in five years. Reimbursement is being reduced and competition among healthcare facilities in the community is increasing. Complex systems such as large hospitals are networks of multiple connections and relationships. The CRNA director will not be able to focus on only one aspect of the department's function and ignore the reality of complex issues which characterize the entire organization or network of facilities.

In a more stable healthcare environment, a leader could be seen as a visionary, divining the future. This model no longer works. Leaders in healthcare must be willing to tolerate ambiguity and to act even when the future is unclear (Fogg, 1999; Peterson, 2000). Being effective in this state of uncertainty requires stamina. It is not enough to adapt to change; rather, the director must embrace change and enjoy the challenge it brings. Crisis and renewal are integral parts of healthcare industry development and hospital administrators must always invent new ways of doing things in response to unexpected challenges.

Alignment with Organizational Goals

Every hospital develops an organizational mission and values, goals and objectives by which the organization defines itself and its strategic direction. Despite the diversity of healthcare organizations throughout the United States, these organizational goals are surprisingly consistent throughout the industry. The CRNA director, functioning in a leadership position, is responsible for the alignment of departmental goals with those of the organization. This is important for two reasons. First, the relevance of departmental or service entities in a hospital will be measured in large part by the extent to which their productivity contributes to the global goals of the hospital. Second, budget allocations within the system are often determined according to the extent to which departmental activities contribute in meaningful ways to the institutional mission. In short, no relevance or productivity, no money.

Clinical Quality

The essence of a hospital is the care that is delivered to patients within the institution. As clinical departments, the operating room and the anesthesia department have many opportunities to support this goal. First, the department should have an action plan in place to achieve full accreditation status by required regulatory bodies. At a minimum, the CRNA director should be familiar with the JCAHO standards, Medicare guidelines for participation, and state health codes.

Development of a research initiative and the publication of scientific papers are other ways to promote the achievement of quality in the department. One approach to developing a research agenda involves drawing upon experience within the department. Are there common clinical questions that arise? Are there research studies being done in surgery that the nurse anesthesia department can link to? Do the pharmaceutical companies have clinical trials that the hospital may become involved in? One of the most effective methods to introduce research into a clinical department involves establishment of a multi-disciplinary research committee. The goal of the committee can be to complete a clinical study and submit it for publication. Another approach is to involve clinical faculty, including physicians, CRNAs and nurses, in the research projects of graduate students and residents. Some departments may find funding for a CRNA researcher position dedicated to staffing the research committee, preparing documents for the institutional review boards, and collecting data. Perhaps the most important reason to establish a research committee is to have a mechanism for solving clinical problems that arise in the perioperative environment.

In all cases, the department should strive for a reputation of exceeding performance minimums. Clinical excellence can be achieved through a comprehensive professional education program, supporting new techniques and technologies, and adherence to strict quality improvement initiatives (Shortell, 1992). For instance, the CRNA director may initiate a "scripted" approach to adverse events in the operating room, in which every employee knows the steps that must be taken in the event of a bad outcome. Following an adverse event, a root cause analysis must be conducted in which the culpable elements of the event, whether human error or systems problems, are exposed and changed. The practice must then be measured again over time to assess the effectiveness of change. The JCAHO requires a root-cause analysis be conducted whenever a sentinel event occurs.

Another way that the CRNA director can contribute toward the goals of clinical excellence in the institution is through improvements in patient satisfaction (Richins, 1998). The department should be measuring patient satisfaction through postoperative telephone interviews, written surveys or personal conversation. Satisfaction can be measured with a representative sample or a comprehensive method of evaluating every service, seven days per week, 24 hours per day. Letters of commendation or complaint should be shared with the staff and managers while maintaining confidentiality. Patient satisfaction may also be evaluated using standardized tools in the hospital industry such as national benchmarking patient surveys. These standardized survey instruments offer the advantage of benchmarking against like hospitals; however, the disadvantage lies in the fact that they are standardized and not specific for the special needs of a particular institution. Regardless of the method used, the CRNA director must be able to demonstrate that patient satisfaction is measured, that results are analyzed, and that change is directed toward improving weaknesses that contribute to overall improvement.

Skilled Employees

Every hospital will espouse a goal relating to employee education and satisfaction. Attracting and retaining the best employees is essential to the success of the CRNA director and involvement in employee training programs offers many advantages. First, a training program within the department will attract and retain a high caliber practicing professional and nonprofessional staff drawn by the unique characteristics of the department or institution. Departments themselves can design and implement training programs that serve as a hospital-wide resource on topics such as airway management, sterile draping, IV insertion or specimen collection. If students are involved in the department, they can be a resource to other services or public relations efforts of the institution such as CPR instruction or blood pressure screening. The CRNA director should always make certain that statistics regarding participants served, employees retained, and graduates hired as a result of these programs are maintained to justify the value of the program to the hospital, especially when the activity may not generate revenue directly.

Retention is key once recruitment efforts are successful. The CRNA director must employ departure risk management techniques to retain good employees. Frequent, informal "sensing" interviews can take place while making rounds. Performance appraisals should include time for the employee to provide feedback on their job satisfaction and make suggestions for change. The CRNA director may be held accountable for retention in his or her own performance reviews. Successful enterprises in business and industry identify key employees and develop formal processes by which outstanding employees are identified and placed on a track for retention and promotion. These employees are assigned mentors to guide them with development opportunities in the department and organization. The CRNA director and the key employee should work together to create an individual development plan to meet the individual's professional goals and objectives.

An important aspect of employee retention is conducting a comprehensive offer comparison to assure that the organization is on par with the external market. Although the human resource department can provide assistance, the onus falls on the CRNA director to pursue professional contacts to secure accurate data. This comparison includes wage and salary information, intangible characteristics of the job such as rotation of assignments, flexibility in scheduling, and educational opportunities. All benefits such as retirement and healthcare should be compared. The presence of on-site childcare, exercise facilities and off-shift security are examples of other factors that may be important in recruiting and retaining staff. Once the CRNA director has completed a comprehensive offer comparison, he/she may seek adjustments in order to be competitive in the marketplace. Where competitive strategies exist, marketing materials can be developed that highlight the strengths of the institution.

Community Contributions

Most hospitals will have a goal related to improvement of the health and wellness of people in the community served. There are many ways in which the activities of the anesthesia department and operating rooms can contribute. The CRNA director can promote volunteerism and sponsorship of charitable events by members of the department individually or as a whole. For example, the director may facilitate involvement in overseas volunteer activities by allowing scheduling flexibility or donating unused supplies. Closer to home, the department can become involved in community activities such as bike safety, anesthesia information seminars, childbirth classes, or involvement in career days at the local high school. Supporting activities promoting cultural diversity in the community is another example. In general, anything the department can do to act as a healthcare resource for community needs should be considered.

Fiduciary Responsibility

Every healthcare organization has financial solvency as an objective. Indeed, it is the ultimate and fundamental goal of the institution. Without achieving financial growth, other objectives related to patient care, employees and community cannot be met. In order to contribute to this goal, the CRNA director must achieve financial targets. In addition to traditional revenue sources from patients and payers, the director may seek additional revenue through grants, university reimbursement for teaching activities, and indirect medical education dollars from Medicare. CRNA directors can also assure financial solvency by reducing expenses. Typically, decreasing the cost of supplies and pharmaceuticals achieves this goal. Materials management may assist by minimizing inventory, standardizing items, substituting less expensive items or restructuring bidding procedures or contract terms with vendors.

Labor is the largest expense of any clinical department. It is clear that eliminating overtime, instituting flexible scheduling consistent with clinical demands, and sending staff home during times of work shortage are methods to reduce labor expenses. Reduction in workforce turnover within the department will also save substantial expenditures. The components of workforce turnover costs fall into two categories. Typical cost calculations capture only 18 percent of true turnover costs. The lion's share is due to lost productivity.

Approximately 18 percent of turnover costs are out-of-pocket expenses typically associated with attrition. These include the cost of exit interviews and separation processing. Vacation payout may be expensive and some hospitals continue benefits for a period of time. Advertising for a replacement, interviewing applicants and paying a hiring bonus and relocation expenses are cash costs of the turnover. Also, the cost of orienting the replacement, which for a CRNA may take six months to one year, is an additional out-of-pocket expense. It has been estimated that highly skilled professionals such as CRNAs and operating room nurses require a 12-month learning curve. During this time, productivity of the new employee is reduced. The distribution of productivity discount is estimated to be 70 percent for nurse specialists in the first four months of employment, 40 percent in the next four months, and 10 percent in the final four months.

The majority of turnover costs are not related to out-of-pocket expenses, rather incurred as a result of lost productivity. During the time that the employee is thinking about leaving, decides to leave, and gives notice to leave, productivity is reduced. At the same time, a coworker's productivity is reduced as the coworker becomes aware of change and focus is diverted to issues surrounding the employee's resignation. The supervisor also loses productivity due to time required to handle activities related to the resignation. This may involve redoing schedules and work assignments, handling grief on the part of the remaining employees, and meeting with the employee who is leaving to work out final details of the transition.

It is helpful to estimate turnover costs in order to realize the financial contribution made by reducing staff turnover. Turnover costs are thought to exceed annual salary costs by 56 percent. Therefore, turnover costs for three employees leaving who make $100,000 per year x 1.56 x 3 = $168,000. This calculation is based on the assumption that a position can be filled within four weeks, and that the productivity discount spans a 12-month learning curve.

Supporting the CEO in Meeting Challenges

The CRNA director is pivotal in supporting interpersonal relations between physicians working in the operating room and all levels of hospital staff, such that both are working productively to meet the organizational mission. Despite efforts at forming structural entities such as physician-hospital organizations or informal efforts at integrating the medical administration and hospital administration into one administrative structure, optimizing physician relations continues to be a major and essential challenge for CEOs. Another challenge confronting CEOs is the need to establish organizational coherence within the institution. Organizational "reengineering," common in many facilities, must be achieved with maximum flexibility and order to maintain a clear strategic vision. A CRNA director must be supportive in this effort because an ineffective link between senior administration and provider staff, when downsizing, may result in declining institutional loyalty.

Most important for the CRNA director is to engage fully in the activities and challenges to the institution and to maintain a demeanor that projects the message that the director's efforts are always focused on "being part of the solution." This can be achieved by composing and maintaining a senior management team that is professional, effective and goal directed. A good administrator or manager must develop effective meeting and time-management skills. Clearly an open communication style is helpful in directing the work of professional staff. One also must have the strength to confront dissidents to not only hear concerns, but articulate the mission and expectations of the department. In sum, the director's job is to visualize, verbalize and energize colleagues toward goals in an environment that respects and supports their knowledge, skills and abilities as professionals.

FINANCIAL ANALYSIS

Every healthcare organization has its own method of displaying and evaluating financial performance. One of the key responsibilities of an administrator is to read and understand financial statements. There are commonalties present in all financial reports regardless of the format used.

Statement of Operations

A statement of operations is a general report in tabular form that displays the relationship between revenue and expense for a given period of time, generally monthly. Prior year comparisons are often shown, as are budgeted amounts. This report aids the department director in monitoring financial activity. Hospitals will use a conventional format, which is applied to hospital-wide statements as well as individual department statements. At year-end, the same statement will be used for a summary of annual financial performance.

Revenue may be divided according to class of patients. Inpatient revenue, outpatient revenue and emergency revenue are examples of revenue divided by classes of patients. Revenue describes the charges rather than the payment received. For example, inpatient revenue is the total amount of charges billed for supplies and services rendered to inpatients. This would be equal to the amount of money received if all inpatients and their insurers paid charges in full. However, this is almost never the case. The statement of operations will reconcile the difference between what is charged and what is paid in a line item which may be called contractual allowances or revenue deductions. Contractual allowances occur because payment received is less than the amount charged. Reimbursement percentages are different for various insurers; therefore, the contractual allowance will be calculated using department-specific payer mixes and payer reimbursement discounts.

At the bottom of the revenue column will be a line for gross revenue. Gross revenue will be the total charges for all categories of patients, such as inpatient, outpatient and emergency. Gross revenue is not real money; rather, it can be used as an indicator of billable activity or of how busy the department has been compared to other months. Contractual allowances are subtracted from gross revenue to arrive at net patient service revenue. Net patient service revenue is an important line to watch when changes in reimbursement take place. For example, if a third-party insurer decides to change the methodology of billing for CRNAs from hospital-based to direct reimbursement, the CRNA director must track the net patient service revenue to determine the net impact of such a change. Is the amount reimbursed on the professional side equal to or greater than the amount calculated into overall hospital reimbursement for CRNA services? If so, all other things being equal, the net patient service revenue should improve after the change. Depending on the department, a line may be added at this point for miscellaneous revenue, such as that obtained from grants, consulting fees or other sources of revenue which are not impacted by third-party payers. Once all sources of revenue are added to create gross revenue, contractual allowances are subtracted arriving at net patient revenue. Miscellaneous revenue is then added into the equation, resulting in a final revenue line representing total operating revenue for the department.

The next portion of the statement of operations describes expenses incurred. These expenses are divided into categories. For example, salary expenses refers to the total of regular, overtime, contingent and temporary salary expenses. It also includes professional fees and the Federal Insurance Contributions Act. Detailed reports are available for each general category of expense that lists a breakdown by account of the individual components, such as overtime. Salary expense is of such significance that it appears as an individual item on most statements of operations. Beyond salaries, other direct expenses are batched together in the general statement. Other direct expenses are expenses incurred by the department, which relate specifically to services it provides. The department can control direct expenses. For this reason, most physicians will be influenced by data on direct expenses rather than overall expenses. Direct expenses include supplies, pharmaceuticals, educational seminars and other operational items. These expenses also include depreciation of capital equipment, service maintenance and other less obvious costs.

Salary expense and other direct expenses are added together, resulting in a final expense line representing total direct expenses. This is a critical line for the department director, as the department has direct control over this line. Cost containment initiatives will be measured by their impact on total direct expenses.

Operating margin is a reflection of controllable department expenses (total direct expenses) compared to gross revenue. It is derived from subtracting total direct expenses from gross revenue. Operating margin is useful in evaluating department performance and in controlling direct expenses in relationship to gross revenue.

Indirect expenses are also part of the statement of operations. "Indirects," as they are called, are expenses which include such things as fringe benefits, hospital insurance and utilities. Indirect expenses pay for the overhead of doing business in a large institution. They include a prorated portion of the expenses for support departments that do not generate revenue on their own. For example, the costs of departments such as accounting, financial analysis, public relations and information services will be allocated to all departments as indirect expenses. Depreciation for hospital buildings and equipment may be allocated to departments using factors such as square footage. Individual departments have limited or no control over their allocation of indirect expenses. The methodology of allocation is often ill-defined, with seemingly higher allocations to revenue generating departments. Allocations may increase as the fiscal year comes to a close because the financial analysis department is attempting to balance the budget before the year closes.

A statement of operations will include summary information, which is extremely useful as a monitor of departmental performance. Net income is a measure of the profitability of the department. It is derived from subtracting direct expenses, indirect expenses and contractual allowances from the gross revenue.

Some portions of the statement will be expressed as a percentage reflecting the relationship between more than one variable. Net income percent is net income related to revenue received. It is calculated by dividing net income by net revenue. As reimbursement drops, net income percent will be reduced unless costs are reduced. Operating margin percent is the relationship between operating margin and gross revenue. Operating margin divided by gross revenue results in the operating margin percent.

A statement of operations may include cost accounting information regarding billable procedures done by the department. Generally the number of procedures done during a given time interval will be reported. The revenue per procedure can be calculated by dividing the gross revenue by the number of procedures, resulting in an average amount of revenue billed per procedure in a given department. Similarly, direct expense per procedure is a reflection of the average direct expense per procedure in a given department. Dividing total direct expense by procedures results in direct expense per procedure. This metric is extremely important for evaluating department performance relative to cost-containment objectives. In a managed care environment with decreasing reimbursement, operations of the department must be actively managed to reduce the direct cost per procedure without impacting quality adversely.

The statement of operations is an essential document for the CRNA director to review monthly. It is a report card of financial performance and as such will be seen throughout the organization. It contains valuable department-specific information such as direct costs, net patient revenue and net income percent, which will assist the CRNA director in planning and managing financial resources.

Financial Transaction Detail

A financial transaction detail report provides specific information for activities that occur during the time period reported. In this way, each department is informed of the content and derivation of its monthly expenses. Items such as the number of boxes of narcotic ordered or the number of phone calls made may appear on such a statement. This statement should be reviewed by an individual involved in materials handling for the department to ascertain whether any gross discrepancies exist between what has been charged to the department and what has been delivered. This report is also helpful in targeting areas for cost reduction and assessing the results of those efforts. For example, if an anesthesia department decides to implement a program of low-flow anesthesia delivery, one way of monitoring the success of such a program will be to review the financial transaction detail for reductions in the purchase of inhalation agents.

Financial Performance Review

As a companion piece to the statement of operations, some form of financial performance review will provide detail on monthly financial activity. This tool summarizes actual activity by category or account. For example, items such as office supplies, disposables, syringes, IV solutions and books will be listed. For each of these categories, expenditures for the month, amount budgeted and year to date expenditures will be listed. Year-to-date information is a cumulative total of the current month's and prior months' activity. Year-to-date information is helpful when provided for the current year and the prior year. In this way, the CRNA director can obtain a sense of performance compared to the previous year, and attempt to reconcile this with known changes in operations such as adding additional surgical hours, hiring additional staff to reduce overtime, or deciding to use less-expensive muscle relaxants.

The difference between actual expenditures and budget will be reported as a variance. The financial performance review may provide a calculation of variance percentage, which is the percentage change in costs from actual to budgeted. It is obtained by dividing the variance by the budget. Many institutions require an explanation of budget variances, either positive or negative, when they exceed a predetermined threshold of 5 percent.

This level of detail permits the CRNA director to target the most significant positive and negative budget variances for review. It also assists in planning for next year's budget. For example, there may be a significant increase in travel and seminar expenses every August because that is when CRNAs attend the Annual Meeting of the American Association of Nurse Anesthetists (AANA). This information can be used to predict the budget, spreading expenses appropriately to minimize variance.

Budget

The budget is a management tool used to plan and control the department's operations. The administrative manager makes a commitment to both revenue and expenses when the budget is completed, and this plan serves as a template for performance throughout the budget cycle, usually for a period of one year. Because performance will be measured relative to budget, rather than to the previous year's performance, it is essential that the budget be realistic and achievable. Errors in projections of revenue from perioperative areas can have significant financial implications for the institution.

The budget process usually begins with a timetable for completion. This cycle may begin three to six months prior to the beginning of the hospital's fiscal year. An early timeline is necessary because the budget must be approved by the hospital governing board prior to the beginning of that budget year. There are many components and related deadlines for the completed budget package, and the CRNA administrative manager must be mindful of completing the budget on time, as the process proceeds in a lockstep manner, with one component building on the next.

There are two types of budgets that are part of the financial planning process—the capital budget and the expense or operational budget. The processes for developing each of these budgets may proceed simultaneously as they are two separate processes with separate regulations for funding in hospitals. There is a relationship between the two, as will be discussed later in this chapter.

Capital Budget

A capital budget will address both capital equipment and capital construction dollars. Most hospitals have guidelines classifying items that fall into the capital budget. In some cases this category is reserved for items costing over a certain dollar amount. For example, one institution may determine that capital budget items are those equipment purchases which exceed $500. Capital expense may also be defined by the depreciation life of a piece of equipment. For example, a hospital may categorize as capital any equipment that has a depreciation life of five years or more. The American Hospital Association provides guidelines regarding depreciation of medical equipment.

As competition for capital dollars becomes more intense, it is prudent to prepare a strategy for capital purchases for a period of two to five years. In this way, hospital administration can be informed of potential expenditures and gain a thorough understanding of anticipated needs. Throughout the year, it is advantageous to obtain quotations and review equipment on an ongoing basis. This is necessary to avoid the last-minute rush of contacting sales representatives and securing accurate pricing. It is not unheard of for capital dollars to be reallocated at the end of the year to fund other projects; therefore, the earlier in the year a purchase can be made, the more likely the funding will be available. Another factor in timing capital purchases relates to the accounting method used by the hospital. If capital purchases are made at the end of the fiscal year, but paid for in the next fiscal year, there may be a carryover of the funds to the next year or the dollars may have to come from next year's budget.

There are many different ways to fund capital equipment purchases (Troyer, 1999). Equipment can be purchased outright, either with cash or using a payment system over time. Some manufacturers will offer a "lease-to-buy" option. The actual cost of total payments over time should be calculated and compared to the cost of cash purchase. It may not be financially advantageous to opt for the "lease-to-buy." Even then, this may be a necessary option if there is no capital budget and the purchase can be made through the expense budget. Equipment can also be rented. In the case of lasers, lithotripters and MRIs, this is frequently done when the use is sporadic or the organization wishes to determine whether the equipment is justified by volume.

Another option for procuring capital equipment is that the hospital agrees to use a given volume of disposable items in exchange for a reduction in price or for receiving the equipment outright without charge. The charge is contained within the increased price of the disposable products and the equipment may have to be returned when the agreement expires. The price of the capital equipment may be prorated based on usage of the disposables. Prior to making a decision on the method of purchase, the director should analyze all of the purchase options to determine the best approach for the department.

When a decision is made to purchase equipment, there are many factors to be considered. Services such as MD-Buyline offer national benchmarking to subscribers regarding best price paid and other options that the buyer should be able to expect. Many hospitals belong to purchasing groups, which secure special pricing agreements for member hospitals. Regardless of whether the price is individually negotiated or reduced through hospital group purchasing, it is unusual to pay the list price for capital equipment.

When a decision is made that a piece of equipment is needed, value analysis will include not only the price, but features of the equipment as well. For large or expensive pieces of equipment, required features may be articulated in a bid process, which includes giving potential suppliers information regarding the item to be purchased and requiring a written response by a certain deadline. The bid package should also specify what training will be done and whether the training will take place on-site. Bid packages should discuss the warranty, with a one-year warranty commonly included in the purchase price. Some manufacturers will offer an extended warranty at a reduced price at the time of purchase. Another factor to be considered in the value analysis is how the manufacturer will treat upgrades. Any upgrades should be available within a year of purchase at a discounted rate and installed free of charge. The issue of upgrades has become more important as computer software becomes an integral part of all equipment.

Construction Capital

Another type of capital item is construction capital. This money is used for renovation of existing areas or construction of new space (Madrid, 1999). Construction capital projections include all components of the construction or renovation process. Architecture and engineering costs are the first step in planning a construction capital project. These are estimated to be approximately 5 percent to 7 percent of the entire project, with wide variability depending on the contractor and the scope of the work. The actual construction costs can be estimated based on square footage for the purpose of budgeting. There is usually a hospital process in place by which cost estimates can be obtained. Again, it is critical not to wait until the capital budget cycle to get these estimates. During this time, estimators are inundated with requests, and the resultant product may be quickly put together and may underestimate the actual costs, or worse yet, may not be done at all due to multiple requests.

A more realistic appraisal of construction costs is obtained during the architecture and engineering process. The unique specifications for hospital and healthcare facilities will be considered at this time (American Institute of Architects, Academy of Architecture for Health, 1996, 1997; National Fire Protection Assocation, 101 Life Safety Code, 1997). Ideally, construction budgets for architecture and engineering costs should be approved first in order to obtain an accurate estimate of actual costs. A contingency fund will be added to the project for the purpose of funding cost overruns and unexpected expenses. In summary, construction capital includes costs of architecture and engineering, actual construction costs, and a contingency pool.

An economic justification for capital costs can be done which incorporates projected volumes and reimbursement related to the capital outlay, and associated expenses. The first step in developing an economic justification involves establishing certain assumptions about the project. For example, what volume of procedures will be added if space is created for an additional operating room? What type of procedures will be done in this room? Whether the patients will be inpatients or outpatients is a major determinant of reimbursement and expense. In the case of inpatients, costs for nursing staff and expense on the patient unit must be considered, as well as revenue for hospitalization in addition to the OR/anesthesia expenses. What is the reimbursement mix for this type of case? Some procedures, such as open heart, peripheral vascular surgery and cataracts, are primarily performed on patients where Medicare is the primary insurance. Other procedures, such as outpatient orthopedics and tonsillectomy, are commonly performed on patients with indemnity insurances such as Blue Cross/Blue Shield. Since payer rates can vary widely, it is essential to estimate the payer mix for a given type of case. These factors are analyzed and a recommendation made to support the project or not, based on whether the project is economically justified.

Although capital and expense budgets may be done separately, there is frequently a relationship between the two. Ideally, the capital budget should be done first or at least at the same time as the expense budget. Frequently, a capital project will have an impact on the expense budget. For example, the construction of a building addition adjacent to the operating room suite may necessitate closure of rooms. Closure for a period of time will have an impact on both staffing and revenue if surgical cases cannot be done in usual numbers. It is important to consider adjacencies when a capital construction project is planned. For example, renovations in a surgical suite located below the neonatal ICU may result in serious vibration and noise. In the worst case, the neonatal ICU may have to be moved or the construction schedule delayed, resulting in additional expense to the organization.

The CRNA administrative manager must anticipate the impact of new programs and changes in existing processes on other departments in order for the institution-wide budget to be met. For example, if the anesthesia department plans to institute an acute pain management program in the next fiscal year and will purchase syringe pumps for use postoperatively, there could be a significant impact on other departments. In this case, some logical questions would be: Do the nursing units have syringe pumps in place? If so, are they the same manufacturer and model? Will more staffing be required to assess and manage the patient's pain with this technology? Will more resources be required to gather the pumps when patients are discharged and return them to the anesthesia department?

The CRNA administrative manager who communicates plans impacting other departments will gain the respect and appreciation of professional colleagues while contributing to an accurate and realistic budget plan.

Expense Budget

The second type of budget, in addition to the capital budget, is the expense or operational budget. The expense budget will have several component parts, with a deadline for each following in logical sequence.

The first component is the revenue projections for the year. The number and type of surgical cases to be done and their associated charges will determine the revenue side of the budget. It is imperative that the CRNA administrative manager seek input from physicians, staff, hospital planners and administrators in order to arrive at realistic expectations for the coming year. The anesthesia department must coordinate their planning numbers with operating room projections, obstetrical case projections and any off-site coverage projections for areas as diverse as endoscopy, in-vitro fertilization and radiation oncology.

During this process, many components are considered, such as year-to-date performance in the present fiscal year, new programs, new surgeons, and new procedures or extended hours. It is helpful to look outside the hospital to determine whether there are community factors which may play a role in determining volumes or mix of procedures. Is a local hospital planning to close? Are new surgeons joining an existing practice? Is the OR schedule so full that surgeons are taking their high-volume, low-acuity cases to a competing surgical center and electing to bring sicker patients to the hospital? Will the ratio of inpatients and outpatients remain relatively stable? Volume projections form the backbone of revenue projections, as reimbursement case mix, contractual allowances with the various third-party payers, and inpatient/outpatient ratios are applied to the volume projections. During the revenue planning process, there is an opportunity for input regarding current charges or the generation of new charges for new services.

The charge structure for anesthesia services has two basic components. The first is a "time-activity" charge, frequently based on the relative value guide for anesthesia services. This charge addresses the professional payment of the CRNA and/or anesthesiologist, with most payers following the methodology used by the Centers for Medicare & Medicaid Services for Medicare payments. This system provides a charge schedule for time units (15-minute increments) and base units (a given number of units are assigned to every surgical procedure based on acuity). The anesthesia department charges may also include a facility charge. The anesthesia facility charge includes the use of anesthesia capital equipment and may include supplies and pharmaceuticals. Some institutions opt to charge for supplies and pharmaceuticals using a checklist approach, while others employ bar-coding technology to automate the process. Operating rooms and postanesthesia care units generally levy a basic charge for a unit of time, such as a 15-minute or 30-minute interval, with a level increment added for each additional unit of time.

The resultant revenue projections drive the remainder of the budget process, as resources sufficient to achieve the volume projections must be estimated. In the operating room, labor remains a high-budget item; however, the plethora of equipment, instruments and supplies comprise one of the highest budget items in the hospital. The operating budget can now be constructed based on cost accounting principles. That is, if additional volume is anticipated, cost-per-procedure additions should be made to the budget in proportion to volume increases.

PERSONNEL

Attracting and retaining high-quality personnel is a primary concern for CRNA directors across the country. The issue is particularly pressing during times of workforce shortages (Buerhaus, 1998). CRNAs and experienced operating room personnel are in critical demand today, and with a dearth of nurses projected in coming decades, it is likely that this challenge will be constant.

The largest component of an anesthesia department budget is labor associated with employing CRNAs, registered nurses (RNs) and anesthesia technicians. The current nursing shortage is complicated further by the increased demand on nurses to function at much higher levels of skill and proficiency. New technologies of communication, diagnosis, information usage, advanced radiology techniques, robotics and biogenetics will heavily influence the availability and role of RNs within a few short years. At the same time, forces are driving the supply of registered nurses down (Buerhaus, 1998). Most significant is the aging of the workforce, where the average age of nurses continues to rise and as RNs age, they work fewer hours. These same demographics hold true for CRNAs.

Recruitment and Retention

There are a few tips for administrators and managers that might aid their goal of recruiting and retaining professional nursing staff of all types (Fernandez-Araoz, 1999):

- When hiring, it is helpful to develop a list of key competencies and criteria for job performance prior to beginning the interview process.
- Every job description should state the minimum level of education and specific experience required for the job. It should also list key competencies in behavioral terms, usually no more than six for realistic expectations.
- Prior to beginning the interview process, it is helpful to generate a list of priorities for the job and identify the position's "critical incidents" or commonly occurring situations that the new employee will confront and must be able to master.
- Hiring will remain problematic as long as attrition is a problem within the department.
- Retention of professional staff is aided when employees actively participate in decisions related to patient care and the work environment.
- CRNAs are most profoundly motivated when allowed to practice within their full scope of practice based on training and experience.
- Administrators must allow those who report to them directly the autonomy to solve problems in their own way and to influence care through their own decision-making initiatives.
- The mentorship of a new CRNA is key in building a sense of personal connection to the department. A personal development plan for one and five years can be formulated which offers opportunities for the employee to achieve professional goals and objectives.

Training and development are of critical importance to all professionals. Translated into a retention strategy, this includes tuition reimbursement, paid travel expenses to professional meetings, and in-house educational programs to maintain "state of the art" practice. Human resource executives often cite compensation as an insignificant factor in retention. This may be true when external market differences are slight; however, in times of shortage even a hospital paying market wages will have a difficult time differentiating itself sufficiently to attract qualified staff. Compensation based on performance, or individual merit pay, is an attractive compensation model. Profit sharing or gain-sharing pay structures are rarely used in hospitals, but provide clear incentives for professional staff and are considered attractive when compared to the option of private practice.

One approach to recruitment is the payment of bonuses. Hiring bonuses may be offered to potential job candidates with a sign-on contract stipulating a commitment to work for a given period of time. The advantage of hiring bonuses includes keeping the department competitive in the external marketplace. It is extremely difficult to recruit professional staff without a hiring bonus if they are commonplace in the community. A disadvantage of paying a hiring bonus is that existing employees may feel slighted since they have dedicated years to the institution, yet new, inexperienced staff receive bonuses. For this reason, directors have developed other bonus programs to reward existing employees. One such program is a recruitment bonus paid to employees who recruit a new staff person into a given job category. The recruit may be required to work at the institution for a certain amount of time before the payment is made to the employee. A third type of bonus is a retention bonus. The payment may be prorated based on years of employment. A retention bonus may also require a commitment on the part of the employee to remain with the organization for a certain number of years.

Advertising is one of the least effective methods of recruitment. Print ads are said to be less effective than radio; however, a personal letter to potential applicants from the CRNA director is more effective than both. Hospitals may choose to sponsor a job fair for difficult-to-recruit positions such as CRNAs, OR nurses and surgical technologists. Online employment sites have become the way to get a job in many industries. One tactic that has been successful is to sponsor an open interview approach at the job fair, with interviews and job offers completed in one day.

One long-term solution to staffing shortages is to develop or participate in an educational program for CRNAs. The hospital may elect to sponsor a program or provide a clinical rotation to students enrolled in an existing educational program. Either approach results in increased exposure for the students to the facility. The opportunity to make a good impression and recruit the best students for employment is an advantage of educational involvement. An additional advantage is the degree to which educational involvement creates a learning environment that benefits existing staff by keeping them current on new developments. When recruitment of students is successful, time and resources required for orientation are diminished or eliminated.

Staffing Models

Although CRNAs may practice in a number of different employment settings, the majority of hospitals find it advantageous to employ CRNAs in order to control the delivery of anesthesia services according to the standards and expectations of the hospital. The CRNA director needs an accurate mechanism for determining required staffing levels and monitoring labor productivity on an ongoing basis. In order to accomplish these goals, a staffing analysis must be completed. It is then necessary to develop a productivity monitoring system to evaluate departmental performance.

An accurate staffing analysis is the precursor to an appropriate staffing budget. The CRNA director must consider many factors when developing a staffing budget. The principles of projecting staffing dollars are the same regardless of type of staff. For some professional staff, standards exist which direct staffing requirements for a given service. For example, the AANA states that a minimum of one CRNA must be assigned to care for one anesthetized patient. Similarly, the Association of periOperative Registered Nurses recommends that a minimum of two staff members is required for each case. The American Society of PeriAnesthesia Nurses has developed staffing standards for perioperative areas. In this case study, the example of developing a CRNA staffing plan will be used.

The first step in developing a staffing model for CRNAs is to determine what the anticipated requirements are for coverage. Hospital A has 10 operating rooms running from 7 a.m. to 3 p.m. There are three nonoperative locations that require anesthesia coverage each day. These include the MRI, CT scan, endoscopy, radiation oncology and ECT departments. The off-site schedule is done through a centralized appointment office, with no more than three locations scheduled on a daily basis. If emergency cases need to be added for off-site services, the appointment office must call the CRNA coordinator to determine if staffing is available. CRNAs respond to all code calls in the institution as well as other requests for intubation or starting invasive lines. Two CRNA staff are assigned to OB on a daily basis. Between one and two C-section rooms may be running at a time. The epidural service is busy with 80 percent of the 3,500 deliveries per year requiring epidural catheter placement.

One CRNA is assigned to complete postoperative rounds and make postoperative phone calls per day. They also are responsible for quality assurance monitoring activities for the department. This function is rotated among staff members. One CRNA is scheduled daily to coordinate the schedule throughout the day. Off-shift coverage is provided by one CRNA in house on afternoon and evening shifts. There is no elective schedule beyond 3 p.m. One CRNA is on call on afternoon and evening shifts. Historically they are called in about 10 hours per week and paid straight salary when called in. Weekends are covered with one CRNA in house on all shifts. A second CRNA is on call all shifts. They are called in about eight hours per weekend. CRNAs are paid 20 percent of base salary for on-call hours. This continues even when they are called in. The department has no scheduled overtime; however, incremental overtime is sometimes required as cases exceed scheduled times. Historically the department pays for 500 hours of overtime per year at time-and-a-half. Another factor to consider is holiday coverage. On the four approved holidays, only two operating rooms and OB is covered. Based on this example, how should the staffing budget be calculated?

The common denominator in calculating staffing is the metric of FTEs. One FTE represents hours per week for one year or 52 weeks. One FTE represents an individual who works 40 hours per week out of a total possible of 40 hours. An FTE equals 2,080 hours per year, not including benefit time. A part-time employee will be designated as a portion of an FTE based on the ratio of approved time to a 40-hour week. For example, a part-time employee who is designated as a .6 FTE is approved to work 24 hours per week. The ratio of 24 to 40 hours results in the .6 FTE.

The concept of FTEs is the basis for calculating staffing in the above example. First, committed FTEs must be calculated based on the service demand that exists.

Coverage of ORs, OB, offsite on day shift	15 FTEs
Management (QA and coordinator role)	2 FTEs
Off-shift coverage (80/40 hours/week)	2 FTEs
Weekend coverage (48/40 hours/week)	1.2 FTEs
On-call hours worked (18/40 hours/week)	.45 FTEs
TOTAL	20.65 FTEs

Next, coverage for breaks and lunches must be calculated. In this example, each employee receives a half hour for lunch and two 15-minute breaks. On the day shift, additional staff must cover these. On the off-shift and weekends, the pace of the OR allows for self-coverage; therefore, only weekdays will be counted. Management personnel schedule their own lunches and breaks. The 15 employees on day shift require 15 hours/day (75/40 hours/week) to cover this time or approximately two FTEs. Another consideration is the hours that the cafeteria is open. In this case, it is open from 11 a.m. until 2 p.m. Therefore, two people will have to do a total of 15 lunches plus their own which is a total of 17 lunches. This is not possible considering the time for report when intraoperative care is transferred, as well as the hours of operation for the cafeteria. Only five to six lunches can be completed by each person, leaving five uncovered. In this case, judgment can be used to add .5 FTE for the additional lunch coverage. The example also describes coverage for code calls and intubations, as well as emergency add-on cases at off-site locations. This .5 position, in addition to the management CRNAs, provides additional coverage for these responsibilities.

Factoring Benefit Time

The combined time off for CRNAs is calculated next. There is now a total of 20.7 CRNA FTEs as a basis for this calculation, 20.2 from coverage and .5 for breaks/lunches. The call-in FTEs are not used for calculating benefit time since this on-call is covered by the same 20.2 FTEs. The call-in FTEs will be added when the calculation is completed to project budget dollars required. In this example, every CRNA gets four weeks vacation, one week personal time, four holidays time and one week of professional development time. Historically, CRNAs average four sick days/year. This equals 38 total days of benefit time per CRNA (38 x 20.7 = 7,866 days or 6,293 hours/year). Recall that one FTE equals 2,080 hours; therefore, 6,293/2,080 = 3.025, so an additional three FTEs are required for replacement of staff members due to benefit time. This brings the total staff CRNAs to be hired to 23.7.

How should the budget dollars for CRNAs be calculated? In addition to the 23.7 FTEs, the coverage for on-call call-ins must be added, which is .45 for a total of 24.15 FTEs. Given a salary of $50/hour, the total for regular salaries will be 24.15 x 2,080 x 50 = $2,511,600. Dollars for on-call coverage must be added. On call is paid at $10/hour. A total of 16 shifts are covered per week times eight hours/shift for a total of 128 hours/week; 128 hours/week x 52 weeks/year = 6,656 hours/year. Multiplied by the on-call rate of $10/hour, $66,560 must be added to salary dollars. Overtime dollars must also be added which equal 500 hours times $75/hour for $37,500. The difference in coverage for the four holidays should be subtracted from overall salary dollars. Normally 19.5 CRNAs are covering the clinical service on day shift. Since only four CRNAs are needed for coverage on the holidays, in the final analysis 15.5 CRNAs times eight hours times four holidays must be subtracted from the calculation. This equals 498 hours or $24,880. The final step in computing salary dollars results in the following budget requirement: regular salaries ($2,511,600) + on-call dollars ($66,560) + overtime dollars ($37,500) – holiday coverage reduction ($24,880) = $2,590,780.

This process projects salary costs based on current practice. Strategic planning involves forecasting changes in the environment, many of which will have an impact on staffing. For example, if an additional procedure room is slated to open six months into the year, the calculation must be revised to include the orientation time and the addition of a new CRNA for six months. This may add to the benefit coverage/lunch and break coverage by only a small percent; however, when calculating staffing it is important to continue to add those small percents. Otherwise the coverage will be inadequate when multiple changes occur over time. Although the CRNA director may not choose or be able to hire an additional .1 FTE, eventually these small increments will add up to a part-time or full-time person. The basis for calculating CRNA staffing requirements is the workload volume at a given point in time. A productivity monitoring system can then be put into place to monitor monthly productivity of staff in relation to fluctuating workload volumes.

As a first step, tasks performed by CRNA staff are identified and categorized as either variable or constant based on the following definitions. Variable tasks are those performed more or less frequently in direct relation with changing workload volume. In the example, CRNAs covering operating rooms could be considered variable FTEs. That is, if there are fewer cases theoretically fewer CRNAs should be paid. In reality, these CRNAs are not truly variable. Commitments have been made to the medical staff that the facility will run 10 operating rooms daily. If one room is not scheduled for any cases on a given day, the CRNA director would be adverse to giving the CRNA the day off since the surgeons know that 10 rooms are allowed and additional cases may be added. There is a variable component to these CRNAs that manifests itself in a stair-step fashion. If, for example, the hospital experienced significant competition and a reduction in surgical case volume to the extent that predictably nine rooms rather than 10 could meet the needs of the community, then CRNA coverage could be reduced. Note that it is a management decision that is critical in applying the variable standard in this case.

It can be an advantage to classify CRNA salaries as variable costs. During times of great expansion and increasing volume, variable costs will be adjusted upward in relationship to volume using standard cost accounting methods. On the other hand, salary dollars for variable positions may also be adjusted downward if volumes decrease.

Constant or fixed tasks are those performed at the same frequency regardless of changing workload volume. In the case study described, the afternoon and midnight coverage is a constant or fixed coverage component. Regardless of whether there are any cases, one case, or four cases, a CRNA must be in house and available for coverage. Again, there is a stair-step element to this coverage. If the number of emergencies in a community increases substantially, a management decision may be made to cover two operating rooms in house rather than one. Ultimately, all fixed positions, even the administrative ones, can undergo extremes of volume of work, which result in them being variable. The advantage of classifying salary dollars as constant is that the budget is more predictable and will not be affected by increases or decreases that really aren't substantial enough to justify an addition or deletion of an FTE. The disadvantage is found in institutions experiencing rapid growth. If all of the employees are classified as constant, no additional money will be added to the budget to accommodate coverage as volume increases.

A productivity monitoring system can be set up by a management engineer or business manager. The development of such a system is beyond the scope of this chapter; however, there are several conventions used in setting up such a system that are worth mentioning. For each task, a time standard is set through the use of time studies, CRNA staff logs or estimates. Each time standard is adjusted upward to reflect the amount of personal time, fatigue or delay that was not captured. The fatigue factors represent the impact of physical fatigue on the time it takes to perform a task. If a task is studied throughout an entire shift, this factor does not need to be applied because the impact is included within the standard. If data collection takes place only during the early part of the day, the standard should be adjusted upward by a maximum of 5 percent. Delay factors represent the common delays that occur in every work environment, adding to the time required to perform a given task. Tasks and time standards will vary among institutions, depending on the types of activities. For example, CRNAs may cover obstetrics, code calls, IV starts or off-site cases which need to be included in order to accurately predict the staffing complement.

SUMMARY

The operating room, and therefore the management of this unit, is subject to scrutiny unknown in other parts of the hospital. Explosive change has descended on the healthcare industry and its impact is already felt in hospitals and operating rooms. The CRNA director must respond to a wide range of internal and external influences that characterize the healthcare industry. Key managerial aspects of the role include working within the administrative structure of the organization, conducting financial planning and analysis, and securing appropriate staffing. The CRNA director must be well-prepared, remain flexible, support inquiry and, most of all, view responsibility as a challenge and opportunity for productive change.

REFERENCES

Altaffer, A. (1998). First-line managers: Measuring their span of control. *Nursing Management.* 6-39.

American Institute of Architects Academy of Architecture for Health. (1996-1997). *Guidelines for design and construction of hospital and health care facilities.* Washington, DC: The American Institute of Architects Press.

Baggs, J. G. (1989). Intensive care unit use and collaboration between nurses and physicians. *Heart Lung*, 18(4), 332-338.

Baggs, J. G., & Ryan, S. A. (1990). ICU nurse-physician collaboration, nursing satisfaction. *Nursing Economics*, 18(6), 386-392.

Buerhaus, P. I. (1998). Is another RN shortage looming? *Nursing Outlook.* 46, 103-108.

Dexter, F., & Lubarsky, D. A. (1998). Managing with information: Using surgical services information systems to increase operating room utilization. *ASA Newsletter.* 62, 6-8.

Dexter, F., Macario, A., & Traub, R. (1999). Which algorithm for scheduling add-on elective cases maximizes operating room utilization? *Anesthesiology.* 91, 1491-1500.

Dexter, F., Traub, R. D., & Qian, F. (1999). Comparison of statistical methods to predict the time to complete a series of surgical cases. *Journal of Clinical Monitoring and Computing.* 15, 45-51

Fargason, C., & Haddach, C. (1992). Cross-functional, integrative team decision making: Essential for effective QI in health care. *Quality Review Bulletin.* 157-165.

Fernandex-Araoz, C. (1999). Hiring without firing. *Harvard Business Review.* July-August, 109-120.

Fogg, D. (1999). Clinical issues. *AORN Journal.* 69, 272-276.

JCAHO, CAMH Comprehensive Accreditation Manual for Hospitals. (2000). *The Official Handbook.*

Knaus, W. A., & Draper, E. A. (1986). An evaluation of outcomes for intensive care in major medical centers. *Annals of Internal Medicine.* 104(3), 410-418

Macario, A., & Dexter, F. (1999). Estimating the duration of a case when the surgeon has not recently scheduled the procedure at the surgical suite. *Anesthesia and Analgesia.* 89, 1241-5.

Mitchell, P. H., Armstrong, S., Simpson, T. F., & Lentz, M. (1989). American Association of Critical Care Nurses Demonstration Project profile of excellence in critical care nursing. *Heart Lung.* 18(4), 332-338.

National Fire Protection Association (1997). NFPA 101 *Life Safety Code.* Quincy, MA: National Fire Protection Association.

Peterson, M. (2000). Issues for the future: A summary of the surgical services summit. *Surgical Services Management.* 6, 38-42.

Skula, R. K., Ketchan, J.S., & Ozcan, Y.A. (1990). Comparison of subjective versus data base approaches for improving efficiency of operating room scheduling. *Health Service Research.* 3, 74-81.

Troyer, J. (1999). Planning capital equipment purchases for renovation: A practical guide. *Seminars in Perioperative Nursing.* 8, 193-203.

White, S., & Charns, M. (1980). Collaboration benefits critically ill patients. *Focus on Critical Care.* 16(4). 325-236.

Zhou, J., & Dexter, F. (1998). Method to assist in the scheduling of add-on surgical cases: Upper prediction bounds for surgical case durations based on the log normal distribution. *Anesthesiology.* 89, 1228-32.

Study Questions

1. Discuss key features of a CRNA manager's role and some of the attendant challenges, given the state of the healthcare delivery system in general and specifically the demands of managed care.

2. Discuss some of the ways that you, as a current or potential employee, would fashion an effective and meaningful employee recruitment and retention program. What are some of the hidden costs hospitals must assume in maintaining an adequate workforce, in addition to issues of salary?

3. Devise a personnel budget for a clinical site with which you are familiar. What were some of the challenges to this exercise?

4. Many employees claim at one time or another that their managers don't understand the specific needs of employees. Should you eventually be in their position someday, what would you do to change the environment to a more productive one—one that is characterized by more effective communication and more emphasis on employee value?

5. Valuable employees are those who not only meet the needs of their patients, but meet the needs of others around them. What could you do as a hospital employee to increase your intrinsic value to the institution by supporting the global needs of the hospital as defined in its mission statement?

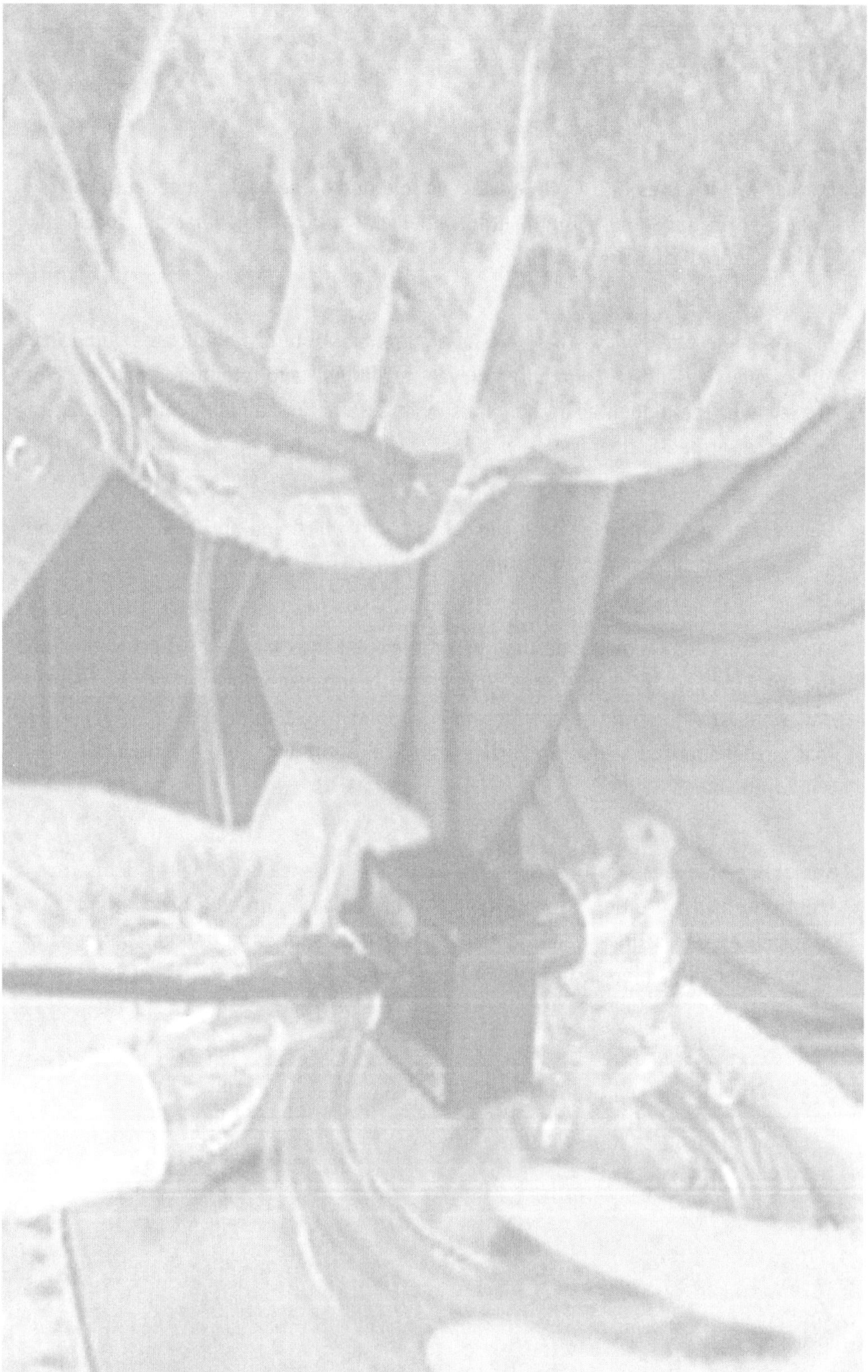

CHAPTER 13

ASSESSING AND SELECTING PRACTICE SETTINGS AND EMPLOYMENT OPTIONS

Michael J. Kremer, CRNA, DNSc

Assistant Professor
Rush University College of Nursing
Chicago, IL

KEY CONCEPTS

- Choice of employment settings should be made based on a detailed personal inventory of clinical practice preferences, desired scope of practice, type and complexity of cases sought, and required characteristics of professional working relationships with other health team members.
- Developing a solid resumé is a necessary professional skill. A good resumé focuses on prioritized information, eliminates information that does not relate directly to the job, and is devoid of florid design elements and family and personal history.
- Interviews should include a careful assessment of the quality of working relationships among personnel; consequently, one should seek perspective from a wide variety of professionals familiar with the work environment.
- Certified Registered Nurse Anesthetists (CRNAs) should familiarize themselves with general employment practices and features of employment law within the state they are seeking employment in order to clarify their rights as employees.
- Once a decision has been made, careful attention should be given to requirements of the state regulatory agency that licenses CRNAs, to determine specific and often additional requirements for CRNAs to practice legally in the state. Requirements vary substantially from state to state.

When assessing and selecting a practice setting, one must consider a myriad of factors, all of which collectively determine the probability of a successful and satisfying professional career. These factors relate both to the individual clinical role of the Certified Registered Nurse Anesthetist (CRNA) and to the CRNA's role as a member of the greater healthcare community and society at large. Among the more critical issues CRNAs must be concerned with are state statutory and regulatory requirements affecting practice, personal practice philosophies, the allowable scope of practice at a particular site, clinical policies of the institution, and personal practice or lifestyle preferences. This chapter deals with the more pragmatic issues of assessing the options of potential work environments from the perspective of either the graduating student or the CRNA already in practice.

CRNAs can choose from many different employment settings, including profit and not-for-profit hospitals or medical centers, ambulatory care centers, managed care organizations, Veterans Administration facilities, the armed forces, academic institutions, or affiliated industries, such as anesthesia pharmaceutical and equipment companies. Increasingly CRNAs are moving to office settings reflective of the trends toward outpatient surgery prompted by managed care. Regardless of site, careful consideration should be given to all potential ramifications of any particular choice as each setting has its own unique set of advantages and disadvantages.

Before embarking on a more detailed discussion of relevant points related to employment, some general observations should be made. Historically, CRNAs have had very little difficulty finding employment in the place or situation they desire and once there, tend to stay. In fact, fewer than 3 percent of CRNAs change jobs on an annual basis prompted by decisions of the employer, and fewer than 8 percent change voluntarily. In addition, there is virtually no unemployment reported by American Association of Nurse Anesthetists (AANA) members. Although there have been small swings in provider demand from time to time, they are usually a result of temporary (a matter of months) adjustments made in the healthcare delivery system. For instance, trepidation by employers about the ultimate effect of managed care on institutional solvency in the mid-1990s prompted short, temporary downturns in employment opportunities for both CRNAs and anesthesiologists. More often the demand for CRNA services is extremely high, as we are currently experiencing.

THE COMMUNITY

From a global perspective, simple geography and demographics generally head the list of primary considerations. For many new CRNAs, graduation provides the opportunity to explore all geographical regions of the country. Considerations should be given first to broad issues, including the financial feasibility of moving, attendant changes in social or cultural norms inherent to new areas, employment distribution and opportunities available (Fallacaro, 1998), likely differences in clinical practice patterns and roles, changes in regional compensation structures, and community amenities. All considerations should be made within the context of a realistic assessment of personal goals and needs.

There are many questions to be explored and answered about the region or communities that have potential for selection as a site of employment.

Spouses who are also professionals may be interested in employment opportunities in the area. CRNAs with school-age children will want to assess the local school system. The state of the local economy and prevailing political and religious attitudes are also important to consider. Assessment of neighborhood and housing opportunities should be examined thoroughly before employment commitments are made. Consultation with a local Realtor is advisable early in the search. Healthcare resources need to be identified to determine types and quality of care available, especially in more isolated or rural communities. If CRNAs have special interests, hobbies, or activities, it is important to determine if those activities are available nearby.

Clearly, no one area will provide an ideal situation, and CRNAs will have to trade off different options based on geographic concerns. For instance, highly desirable urban areas may offer less lucrative financial packages due to an abundant provider supply. Depending on regional job availability, the "ideal" job may not be immediately or geographically available; however, as market demand continues to increase (Jaffee & Revak, 1998), it is highly likely that new positions will be created. To help assess geographic needs, national professional placement agencies are available to help graduating or experienced CRNAs identify employment opportunities. These agencies typically advertise in professional journals or bulletins. As with other employment services, a finder's fee is charged by the agency to the employer. That fee can range from 5 percent to 20 percent of the annual compensation for the position to be filled.

PROFESSIONAL CONSIDERATIONS

Beyond use of placement agencies, many CRNAs make employment decisions based on their prior experience as students in a particular site, word of mouth from other CRNAs employed at the site, or family or financial constraints that limit choices to particular areas. Depending on market demand at the time, the wholesale distribution of resumés to a cross section of potential employers is a time-consuming and largely unproductive effort. Employers generally are much more interested in a "known product" and are not willing to take a chance on a candidate about whom they know little, if anything. CRNAs contemplating a move need to direct focused attention to potential employers only after they have conducted a personal needs assessment and an informed search of the area.

Once general geographic, demographic, and logistic questions have been answered, the interview process can yield specific information about the nature and function of the employment setting. During the interview process, applicants should determine key elements of a prospective practice position, such as the types of cases CRNAs are assigned, departmental equipment and resources, technician support or lack thereof, and the quality of personal and professional interactions with potential colleagues. For some practitioners, case mix and scope of practice issues will be more important than considerations such as flexible scheduling. It is important to verify what clinical privileges CRNAs have and whether they are involved in areas such as cardiothoracic or neurosurgical anesthesia, if the facility offers these services. Clinical privileges, such as the opportunities to place invasive monitoring lines or perform regional anesthesia, may be more important to some candidates than others.

Professional relationships, degree of practice autonomy, and role need to be assessed specifically and directly, as they can vary considerably among settings. One should always speak to staff CRNAs in the facility to determine if the employment setting allows the level of autonomy or collaboration desired. In turn, an applicant should direct similar questions to anesthesiologists, specifically what their expectations are of CRNA work, including level of independence, their interpretation of the anesthesia care team approach, and how the issues of medical direction and supervision relate to that philosophy. In terms of role, some groups may use the nurse anesthetist as an extra set of hands, while others will expect the nurse anesthetist to practice a full scope independently with physicians serving as consultants when needed. CRNAs may be expected to make preoperative and postoperative rounds, order appropriate preoperative medications and tests, and manage immediate postanesthesia care. Other practice settings may require the CRNA to seek consultation before making changes in anesthesia management or even exclude CRNAs from some segments of the perioperative course, most often, preoperative, postoperative, or regional block management. Before signing an employment contract, the CRNA should be comfortable with these practice arrangements. Perhaps most important, the CRNA should assess the quality of working relationships among CRNAs, anesthesiologists, surgeons, supervisors, and administrators by asking during the interview for examples of how interpretations of these relationships are manifested in the work setting.

LICENSURE AND STATE REGULATORY ACTIVITIES

The amount of time and documentation required to obtain licensure for employment (e.g., RN, state certification as a CRNA) can vary significantly by state. Subsequently, any CRNA applicant should be mindful of the time it takes, such that proper documents are obtained well before the actual employment date. The American Nurses Association Web site, www.nursingworld.org, provides a link with an index to state boards of nursing where specific professional and advanced practice nursing (APN) licensure information can be obtained. Up to six months may be required in some states for processing nursing and APN licensure and certification applications. In addition, some states may require master's degrees for nurse anesthetists and other APN designations (see chapter 7). Requirements by state for graduate degrees (Conover & Tobin, 1998) and other statutory and regulatory requirements for APNs (Pearson, 1998) are reviewed in the references cited at the end of this chapter. The reader should also refer to chapter 9 for discussions about institutional credentialing and privileging requirements that offer a comprehensive and critical view of how these issues affect a CRNA's ability to practice clinically.

BUSINESS CONSIDERATIONS

Although the majority of CRNAs will be employed by another entity, it is important that all CRNAs, regardless of employment arrangement, know and understand the "business" side of practice, if for no other reason than to be able to assess their professional worth to their employers. At the very least CRNAs must be able to calculate their financial worth to a practice setting in terms of billable revenue, to ensure that they are compensated accordingly. Whether CRNAs are employed by institutions or groups, they must become conversant with basic principles of economic theory, negotiation, and reimbursement. Without these basic tools, there is high probability that

CRNAs will suffer professionally and financially at some point in their career as others may take advantage of their position as high-income earners with substantial clinical expertise. With the expansive growth of managed care and trends in the general working population for contractual employment, there has never been a more critical time for CRNAs to assess their potential and desire for structuring and managing their own practice settings. In many cases, this may be the only option available for some CRNAs to remain employed in the area they desire. The AANA Web site, www.aana.com, provides links to information on how to start and manage private business arrangements, such as *The Business of Anesthesia: Practice Options for Nurse Anesthetists* (1994).

THE VARIETY OF PRACTICE SETTINGS

It has been well documented that CRNAs work in every practice setting imaginable, from tertiary care hospitals and medical centers (and specialty areas within them such as trauma and obstetrical units) to the smallest physician's or dentist's office. They also work in freestanding surgical centers small and intermediate-sized community hospitals, and a variety of managed care organizations such as health maintenance organizations (HMOs), preferred provider organizations, and independent practice organizations. It should be noted that due to dramatic changes in reimbursement rules of the past five years, many of the nearly 30 million surgical cases annually are done on an outpatient basis.

The important issue for CRNAs to explore in selecting a practice setting is a careful inventory of personal and professional needs and an assessment of how any potential setting would or would not meet those needs. Part of this process involves making a thoughtful analysis and assessment of accumulated work skills that addresses actual levels of clinical mastery and breadth of skills in a variety of general and specialty practice areas. Some of these clinical mastery areas might be related to case complexity, skills of invasive monitoring, regional anesthesia, or pain management. Clearly a setting should be selected that will broaden one's clinical skill base and sharpen skills of critical thinking, resourceful action, and clinical judgments.

For CRNAs entering practice, a larger facility and formalized anesthesia department may provide the security of collegial support, exposure to a wide variety of cases to maximize clinical skills, and multiple role models to aid the process of professional socialization. Furthermore, a large medical center would focus the majority of a novice's time on clinical activities and away from issues of finances, departmental management, and external departmental relationships. For the more established CRNA, a large practice could incorporate more opportunity for specialty practice and potential benefits of seniority or opportunities for experiences in departmental management, teaching, or research within the institution. A smaller hospital usually provides more independence in practice, perhaps a somewhat less frenetic pace, a less acute case mix of patients, and greater opportunity for extradepartmental activities that augment the anesthesia service.

It is noteworthy that the primary reason CRNAs give for choosing a particular employment setting has to do with geographic, family, and global financial considerations rather than any particular affinity to workplace philosophy, potential salary, or operating room demographics. This is also true with recent graduates of programs. Few tend to leave the geographic area in which they received training, probably in part because of the sense of community they have developed, as well as their familiarity with hospitals where they received clinical experience as a student.

Solo Practice

Although this setting is most often characterized by the degree of practice autonomy it provides, equally important is the increased responsibility for patient care it entails. In essence, solo practice means that a single CRNA is a sole anesthesia provider and as such must be prepared to handle all activities of the perioperative course. Functional support is limited to staff such as nurses, therapists or physician consultants. In some cases a solo practitioner may work under contract for a group of anesthesia practitioners or a hospital where some of the comprehensive, perioperative responsibilities of the single provider are shared with other anesthesia personnel.

Primary motivations for establishing a solo practice usually involve "being your own boss," establishing one's own salary structure, and establishing preferred work schedules without the need to consider partners or other groups of providers. If the CRNA is considering solo practice, there are essential professionals to consult (refer to chapter 16). The first is another CRNA who is experienced in solo practice who can provide advice about potential locations and act as an advisor for business, management, and clinical issues. A certified public accountant (CPA) should also be identified who can provide advice in the areas of billing, record keeping, and tax management strategies. Finally, an attorney experienced with the business of anesthesia can help with important issues such as contracts. Legal expertise should be retained in the planning stages of a solo practice, not after it is established. (Hamelink, et al, 1994; Mannino, 1994).

Often a solo CRNA will practice in rural areas where there are few, if any, other anesthesia providers. Because of the critical nature of their services, these CRNAs must necessarily be active in the governance of the facility or facilities where they practice. They must also serve as regular members of the medical staff, so that their voice as the single anesthesia expert is taken into consideration on policy questions. CRNAs practicing in these situations must be totally self-reliant and resourceful, as their job security, income, benefits, insurance, and retirement depend on it. The solo practitioner may have 24-hour clinical responsibilities, and relief services for vacation and meeting time are often prohibitively expensive. Solo CRNAs are more immediately impacted by the economics of anesthesia practice due to the vagaries of private billing, third-party insurance decisions, and a potentially disadvantageous patient case mix. Finally, it is important to remember that those who practice as solo providers must be as facile in the political arena as they are clinically. For all the potential advantages of this working arrangement, there is no substitute for careful thought, proven clinical expertise, and advanced planning and consultation in preparation for this new role.

Group Practice

Clinical practice in a group arrangement of anesthesia providers usually offers less autonomy than does solo practice; however, there is often a commensurate decrease in responsibility and required availability. Considerable organizational variation exists among groups. Practices incorporating CRNA and anesthesiologist shareholders or partners are becoming increasingly popular, but are still less common than groups involving only one or the other as shareholders or partners.

A shareholder or partner enjoys much more control of the group than does an employee, who routinely has little control of the group's management or practice policies. Group practices offer varying degrees of autonomy depending on the size and makeup of the group and its geographic locale. In groups with minimum supervision or medical direction requirements and a low physician/CRNA provider mix, the level of autonomy can approach that of the solo practitioner. In others, high supervisory ratios and a high physician/CRNA mix usually indicate tight control over practice prerogatives and little decision-making opportunity for the employee. For an employee of a group, there are relatively few decisions to be made (with the exception, perhaps, in clinical work) regarding details of salary, benefits, schedules, work agreements/contracts, policies, and procedures that are prescribed either by medical staff bylaws or by the corporate shareholders of the group. The extent to which a CRNA may be involved in administrative activities is usually within a management role or committee membership that facilitates the work of the group at large.

There are decided advantages to working in a group practice. First the hours are relatively stable and predictable, as are routines. In this configuration income is also predictable, and usually generous employee-benefit packages obviate the need to secure those same benefits privately. Ultimate responsibility for group performance generally remains with the shareholders.

There are also disadvantages to working in a group practice. As an employee, one disadvantage may be a lack of decision-making authority, depending on the nature and traditions of the work group. There is the issue of losing some economic autonomy; however, the ability to share clinical responsibilities and have immediate access to other providers on a consultation basis are decided advantages.

Group practice from the view of a shareholder or corporate partner entails an entirely different set of considerations and issues, most beyond the scope of this chapter. CRNAs interested in exploring such a practice arrangement should consult professionals in the area including an attorney, CPA and others who provide group management expertise. Many of those resources may be identified through the AANA. Interestingly, as managed care imposes increased financial constraints on the healthcare system, more and more CRNAs alone or CRNAs and physicians together are forming working groups to meet the challenges of changing reimbursement schedules. Clearly, contractual arrangements, whether temporary or permanent, are emerging as a predominate mode of work across healthcare disciplines and among businesses and industries of all types. Benefited employment, as we have known it previously, is thought by some experts in the field of labor, anthropology, and sociology to be a thing of the past.

Institutional Employment

CRNAs often work in large organizations, such as hospitals and medical centers, clinics, or HMOs. According to the Fiscal Year 2001 AANA Member Survey data, 33 percent of respondents were hospital employed. This type of experience and the support of a large anesthesia department can make a traditional hospital setting a comfortable first practice experience. In addition, the large group or hospital setting offers the CRNA other advantages: reasonably stable employment, opportunities for professional growth through participation in hospital-sponsored education programs, opportunities for teaching and learning, and exposure to more complex anesthesia cases. Larger hospitals frequently have the newest equipment and encourage the use of cutting-edge technologies in practice.

All practice settings are impacted to a greater or lesser extent by the general economic climate and reimbursement issues. Institutional employment is no different. Some CRNAs have been affected by the recent downturn in hospital reimbursements from Medicare that has resulted in shifting CRNA employees to hospital-contracted anesthesiologist groups. Although this practice has appeared to stabilize, potential institutional employees should be mindful of how reimbursement and other policy changes at the federal level can have a direct and compelling affect on practice.

It is important to note that most group- and institutional-employed CRNAs are considered "at-will" employees who do not have the employment security associated with contract stipulations or collective bargaining units. Under at-will employment, CRNAs can be terminated without cause unless departmental or institutional policy requires written warning protocols, benefit of hearing, and appeal. This termination prerogative can be problematic for CRNAs in geographic areas with limited employment opportunities. CRNAs should review employment policies to determine their rights in these situations prior to signing an employment agreement or contract.

Other Practice Categories

Many CRNAs serve in the military, either on active duty or as reservists. While a specific time commitment is required of those who join, there are generous programs of educational reimbursement for student tuition and living costs and additional salary compensation and retirement benefits for CRNAs. Potential disadvantages in the military are lack of control over one's career and time commitments, remote and potentially undesirable active duty requirements, and vulnerability related to combat situations. CRNAs in the armed forces have traditionally enjoyed significant autonomy in their practice settings and have contributed much to the expansion of nurse anesthesia practice over the decades. There is currently substantial demand in the armed services for CRNA services.

A teaching career for qualified CRNAs offers expanded rewards and challenges in academia that may or may not incorporate a traditional clinical career. Currently there are some 2,000 CRNAs who hold some type of academic/clinical appointment from an accredited program of nurse anesthesia and sponsoring or affiliated college or university. General qualifications for CRNAs employed by colleges and universities are a minimum of a master's degree and increasingly a preference for doctoral preparation. Advancement in the field is based on traditional promotion criteria of service (clinical or professional), teaching, and research. Professorial appointments provide CRNAs substantial work flexibility and a variety of professional experiences including teaching, grant writing, research and scholarly publications, committee work, and program administration. Fewer than 1 percent of CRNAs are doctorally prepared, and the current shortage of CRNAs nationally further exacerbates the need for more CRNAs with advanced degrees to teach nurse anesthetists and others at the graduate level.

Locum tenens can be a full-time or part-time practice option for CRNAs. Essentially, these providers offer contract services for a set interval of time, generally to fill a temporary employer need. Locum tenens coverage is frequently used in all types of settings, including urban and rural. Numerous professional placement agencies coordinate placement of the locum tenens provider, although it may be accomplished privately. The CRNA must supply necessary documents such as proof of education, credentials, and letters of recommendation to the agency that frequently oversees credentialing of their contractor and supplies the provider contract as well as the facility contract. Fees are generally forwarded from the facility to the agency and from there to the provider, each at a contracted rate.

Locum tenens employment provides significant opportunity for clinicians to work when and where they choose. They need to be maximally flexible, however, to work in a variety of settings with various qualities and availability of equipment, not to mention personnel. The downside of such employment is that work can be cyclical: more work is typically available in the summer and close to major holidays. CRNAs in this type of employment arrangement need to be attentive to their tax liabilities, since federal taxes are not withheld. One should also be mindful that in spite of the high earning potential, the typical benefits enjoyed by most employed CRNAs will probably be paid by the CRNA and not assumed by either the agency or facility.

Each type of practice setting has advantages and disadvantages. There are no ideal employment situations; however, there are limitless opportunities for CRNAs in the settings discussed, or hybrids of these models. CRNAs are in the enviable position of having myriad practice opportunities and combinations that can incorporate many of their preferences.

COMPENSATION

According to the Fiscal Year 2001 AANA Member Survey, the median CRNA salary for calendar year 1999 was approximately $100,000 nationwide, encompassing all income from anesthesia including call, overtime, and bonuses. Hospital-employed CRNAs reported median incomes of $104,000 while self-employed CRNAs earned $108,000 per annum. Many CRNAs work as employees of multiple groups or hospitals as independent contractors for additional income. Compensation in a contracted situation ranges from $50 to $80 per hour for an eight-hour day. Liability insurance may or may not be included, and there are usually no other benefits provided. There is wide variation in rates of compensation depending on market demand and geographic location. Actual terms of these employment agreements are usually spelled out in a formal contract or work agreement.

New graduates should be particularly vigilant when it comes to salary. Sometimes employers will "low ball" a typical salary of a new graduate with the justification that they are not yet certified. This is an unacceptable and unethical practice as the graduate is being used as any other employee relative to services provided, given that the graduate has received privileges commensurate with certified or recertified colleagues. For other employed CRNAs, salaries are often set by scale. Make certain that human resources personnel or others in the position of salary decision-making authority have the most up-to-date comparative regional and national salary information available.

In sum, CRNAs should be aware of the trend toward salary-based models of compensation; that is, a smaller portion of income is coming from call pay, overtime, bonus, and other nonsalary compensation. This trend demonstrates the move away from compensation structures associated with the traditional trades that compensate for work effort over 40 hours per week, toward a professional package that requires all necessary work be done, regardless of hours, for a set salary.

BENEFIT PACKAGES

This discussion is focused on the typical employed CRNA rather than a CRNA contemplating joining a group as a shareholder or partner. In that case, contract negotiations relative to salary and benefits assume greater urgency, as more of the components are usually negotiable. A CRNA should engage a CPA to analyze and customize a constellation of benefits in relationship to salary and do so within the context of the CRNA's personal requirements and goals. For an employed CRNA, benefit packages are usually uniform or a matter of institutional policy. There is little room for modification with the exception of those facilities utilizing "cafeteria benefit selection options" open to all employees. A benefit package typically amounts to 5 percent to 40 percent of annual cash compensation. Consequently, CRNAs should determine as closely as possible the value of these benefits unique to their situation in order to determine the equity of base salary offered. For example, a single anesthetist without children may receive substantially fewer benefits than a married CRNA with a family, potentially justifying an increase in base pay.

Benefits for employed CRNAs generally consist of employer-paid liability, life, health, and disability insurance; holiday, sick time, professional, or personal days (one to two days per year); and perhaps some allowance, time and financial assistance for continuing education (usually one week per year). There are often options available to the employee, after meeting a certain minimum employment interval, to receive or access matched retirement savings plans and other optional tax-sheltered savings opportunities. Because of the decided tax advantage and long-term savings growth potential of these programs, CRNAs should, if at all possible, maximize deposits to these types of retirement vehicles early in their careers. It is becoming less frequent that employers are paying for fees related to credentialing, membership in professional organizations, or professional journals. Although the value of each selected benefit will vary substantially among CRNAs, it is critically important for CRNAs to assess the extent and quality of coverage in their health and disability insurance, regardless of age. For the CRNA nearing retirement, new long-term care plans should be considered as a vital part of a benefit package, if such options are available.

RESUMÉS AND INTERVIEW TECHNIQUES

Although employment opportunities for nurse anesthetists are excellent, it is imperative that CRNAs market themselves in a professional, organized, and informed manner. Often the first chance to make a good impression is with a well-constructed, printed resume, and the last chance is during an interview. Working from this premise, CRNAs must market their educational and professional investments knowledgably and efficiently.

Drafting a Resumé

First make a personal, informal inventory of your education, clinical skills, prior experiences in employment and professional activities, clinical strengths, and employment goals, preferably in writing. Second, attempt to match those attributes with what you know about the facility to which you are applying. The resumé and interview process are, in fact, attempts on your part and the part of your potential employer to match these lists, in essence to assess the appropriateness of "fit" between you and the employer or facility. This exercise will help clarify your reasoning and intent to apply for a particular job. It will also help answer the question so many interviewers pose, "Why should I hire you?"

A resumé is not an autobiographical or lengthy account of life accomplishments; rather, it is a salient promotion of facts about your educational and work history that would prompt a potential employer to invite you for a personal interview. There are three basic formats for resumés: chronological, functional, and a combination of the two.

The chronological resumé is the most widely accepted and most familiar format. It is true to its name. First list employment and education history in reverse chronological order, beginning with the last job held and latest educational achievement. Chronological resumés are easy to write and read. They are particularly good for people with an excellent work history without gaps in employment.

A functional resumé downplays gaps in employment or frequent job changes. This format simply lists the years of employment (e.g., "1965 to present") with a brief description of what has been done during that time, emphasizing certain skills or titles held. This section is followed by an educational history only inclusive of the schools, degrees, and years degrees were granted. A combination resumé combines both the chronological and the functional formats. The only variation is that the resumé includes a reverse chronological listing of places of employment.

It is important to do several drafts when compiling a resumé. This allows opportunity to critique what has been written and assess it for clarity and relevance. Even accomplished professionals should be able to limit a resumé to two or three pages. Retain only information pertinent to employment and omit the traditional "career objective" preface, excessive or informal narrative, hobbies, church affiliations, personal family information, and formatted figures, and avoid embellished typescript and page borders. List references on the resumé. To suggest that "references are available on request" usually has no valid rationale and promotes a rather arrogant tone. Make the resumé simple, formal, and easy to read, with a clear and prioritized message. Under no circumstances should there be spelling errors or a sloppy, inconsistent format. Figure 13.1 demonstrates a resumé format that can be used successfully by most anesthesia providers. For CRNAs applying for a professorial appointment, the curriculum vitae will be more highly structured and include sections on professional service, teaching and advising, publication and grant listings, invited lectures, and other activities related to service, teaching, and research.

Once satisfied with the resumé, a cover letter is written to accompany it that personalizes and directs the resumé to the interviewer. The letter should provide a brief statement of the applicant's purpose in forwarding the resumé to that particular institution and acts as an introduction to the potential employee. It is important to arrange the letter in an appropriate business style and avoid typographical or grammatical errors. If guidance is required, reference texts on writing business correspondence are available.

Interviewing

Interviewing is an essential skill for a professional. However, there is some preparation that needs to take place prior to the meeting. It is advisable to learn as much as possible about the work setting and employer prior to the interview. This information helps establish and focus questions or concerns in more detail so they can be addressed specifically during the interview. There are many sources available for this information. Most hospitals have public relations information available describing the facility, its size,

Figure 13.1: Sample Resumé

JANE SMITH, CRNA, MSN

1005 Appian Way
Nashville, TN 93842
Ph: 324-567-4938
Fax: 324-344-6881

Education:

1991 - MSN Nurse Anesthesia, Rush University, Chicago, IL

1987 - BS Nursing, University of Michigan, Ann Arbor, MI

1985 - Non-degree seeking student, Belmont College, Scranton, PA

Employment:

1994 - Current: Full-time locum tenens.

1991 - CRNA staff in private CRNA/physician group practice in Nashville at a level I trauma center. Worked full-time, including twice weekly in-house calls. Expertise in all ASA classifications and age groups, including vascular, neurologic, obstetric, and pediatric cases. Administered over 300 regional blocks including spinal, epidural, Bier, and axillary techniques.

1987 - Went from staff nurse to nurse manager in critical and postanesthesia care.

Professional Experience:

Anesthesia research assistant: Collected data for clinical research project sponsored by Aztec Pharmaceuticals. Research findings published in the April/May issue of the *AANA Journal*, 1995.

Journal Club instructor: Facilitated Journal Club meetings once a week for 20 students from a local school for two semesters during the 1992-1993 school year.

Advisor: Obstetric Advisory Committee, Hoboken Program of Nurse Anesthesia.

Professional Membership:

American Association of Nurse Anesthetists

Tennessee Association of Nurse Anesthetists

American Nurses Association

AANA Education Committee, 1995

References:

John Doe, CRNA, MSN
Chief CRNA, Regional Medical Center
Nashville, TN 93842

Lisa Wright, CRNA, MSN
President, Placements Inc.
Conway, TX 39482

organization, philosophy, mission, services, and financial performance record. If the interview is in a different community, obtain information about it through the local chamber of commerce, small business association, or visitors bureau. Set aside time to experience the community and use every resource available to assess your potential satisfaction with it. The potential employee can establish himself or herself as someone who is sincerely interested in the particular employment situation by demonstrating initiative in preparation. Prior research will help avoid spending too much time in the interview detailing facts and information that could be obtained otherwise, allowing you to focus on work-related issues.

The success of an interview usually hinges on the rapport each participant establishes with the other. This obviously requires highly refined skills of interpersonal communication. Consequently, your verbal facility, professional demeanor, questions asked, attitude projected, and body language will figure significantly in your success. Important also is your standard of dress, which is a very powerful, nonverbal statement of self-esteem and familiarity with proper business and professional etiquette. Let the interviewer lead, but be prepared to pose questions and issues. Do not allow an interview to be dominated by the interviewer who glosses over questions critical to your success and satisfaction. It is likely the behavior you experience from the employer during the interview will be the same after you are employed.

Bring to the interview another copy of your resumé and a quick reference list of questions you need to have answered. Ask if you can meet other personnel, especially CRNAs, and spend time in the operating room assessing the general work environment and resources available. At the appropriate time, ask for a written description of benefits and a sample of the clinical work schedule that professional personnel follow. It will also be helpful to review a personnel policy manual. Let the interviewer introduce the issue of salary. Most often in large work groups of CRNAs, salary schedules are clearly delineated and usually nonnegotiable; however, you need to have firmly in mind an estimate of your professional worth to evaluate the offer. After the interview, follow up with a written letter of thanks and indicate, if appropriate, your continued interest in the position.

SUMMARY

The most important decisions you will make in your professional life are those related to choice of employment. This process, although at times arduous, must necessarily involve prior research of the geographic area, review of demographics, study of the philosophy of clinical practice operative in the work group, identification of resources available, and assessment of the quality of professional relationships at the facilities you are considering. These issues must be answered within the context of a careful inventory of personal desires, motivations, work habits, and professional goals, such that your maximum potential as a CRNA is realized.

REFERENCES

Conover, J. & Tobin, M. H. (1998). State master's degree requirements for nurse anesthetists. *AANA Journal*. 66 (4), 351-357.

Fallacaro, M. (1998). An inefficient mix: A comparative analysis of nurse and physician anesthesia providers across New York state. *Journal of the New York State Nurses' Association*. 29 (2), 4-8.

American Association of Nurse Anesthetists. (2001). Fiscal Year 2001 AANA Member Survey. Park Ridge, IL

Hamelink, M., McKibban, T., Staver, P., & Walker, K. (1994). Assessing and selecting practice settings and employment options. In S. Foster & L. Jordan (Eds.), *Professional Aspects of Nurse Anesthesia Practice* (pp. 175-200). Philadelphia, PA: F.A. Davis.

Jaffe, J. & Revak, G. (1998). CRNA manpower recruitment to retirement. Presented study. AANA Fall Assembly of States, Colorado Springs, CO. November 13.

Mannino, M. (1994). *The Business of Anesthesia: Practice Options for Nurse Anesthetists*. Park Ridge, IL: AANA Publishing, Inc.

Pearson, L. (1998). Annual update of how each state stands on legislative issues affecting advanced nursing practice. *Nurse Practitioner*. 23, (1), 14-16.

KEY REFERENCES

Conover, J. & Tobin, M. H. (1998). State master's degree requirements for nurse anesthetists. *AANA Journal*. 66 (4), 351-357.

American Association of Nurse Anesthetists. (2001). Fiscal Year 2001 AANA Member Survey. Park Ridge, IL

Mannino, M. (1994). *The Business of Anesthesia: Practice Options for Nurse Anesthetists*. Park Ridge, IL: AANA Publishing, Inc.

Study Questions

1. List key factors to evaluate in any potential employer.
2. Describe the ramifications of not having regular, voting membership on the medical staff of a facility and how it relates directly to your practice.
3. Explain the advantages and disadvantages of solo practice, group practice, and hospital employment relative to your personal inventory of requirements for an employment setting.
4. What is "at-will" employment, and what does this mean in terms of employment rights?

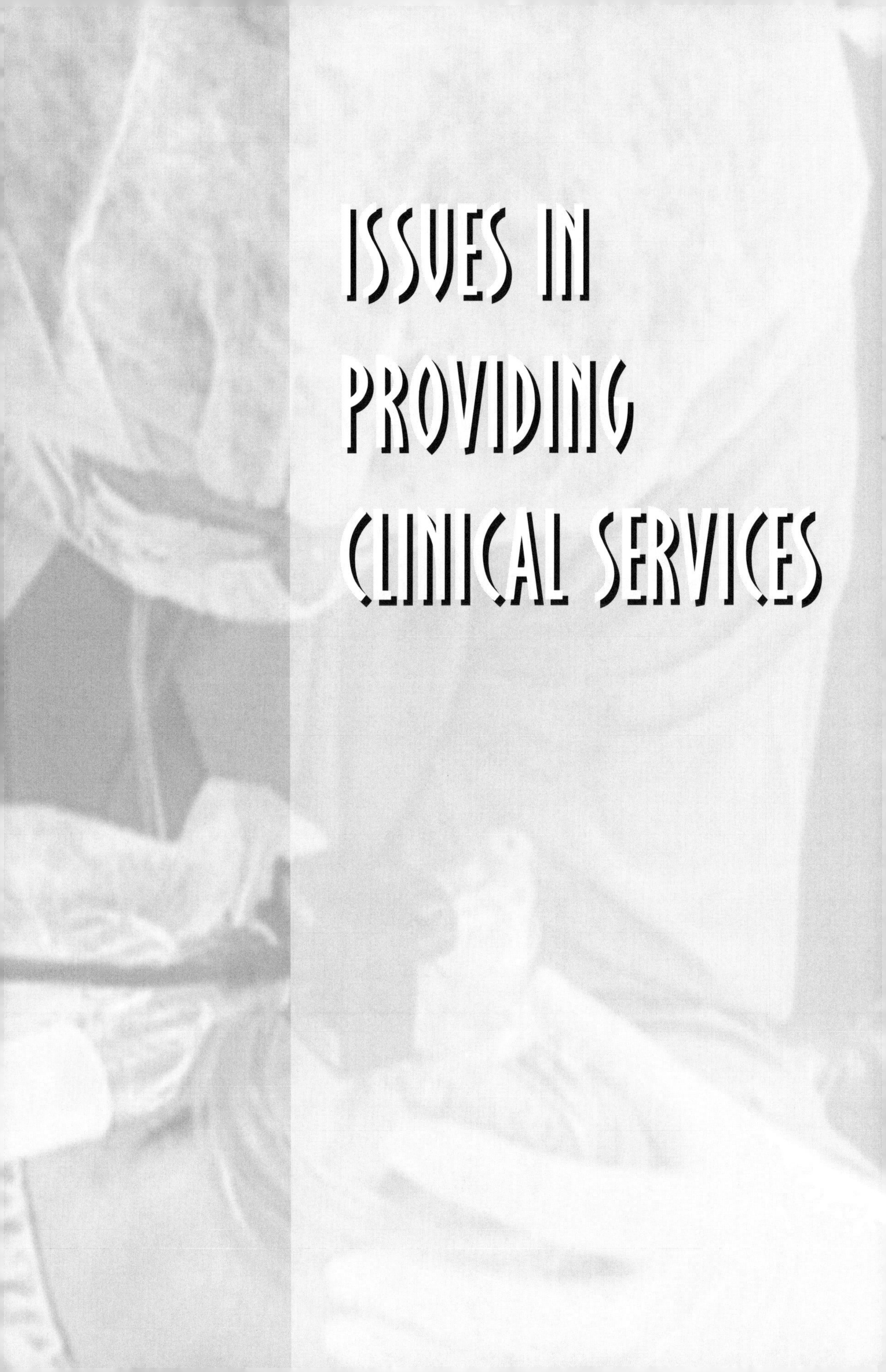

ISSUES IN PROVIDING CLINICAL SERVICES

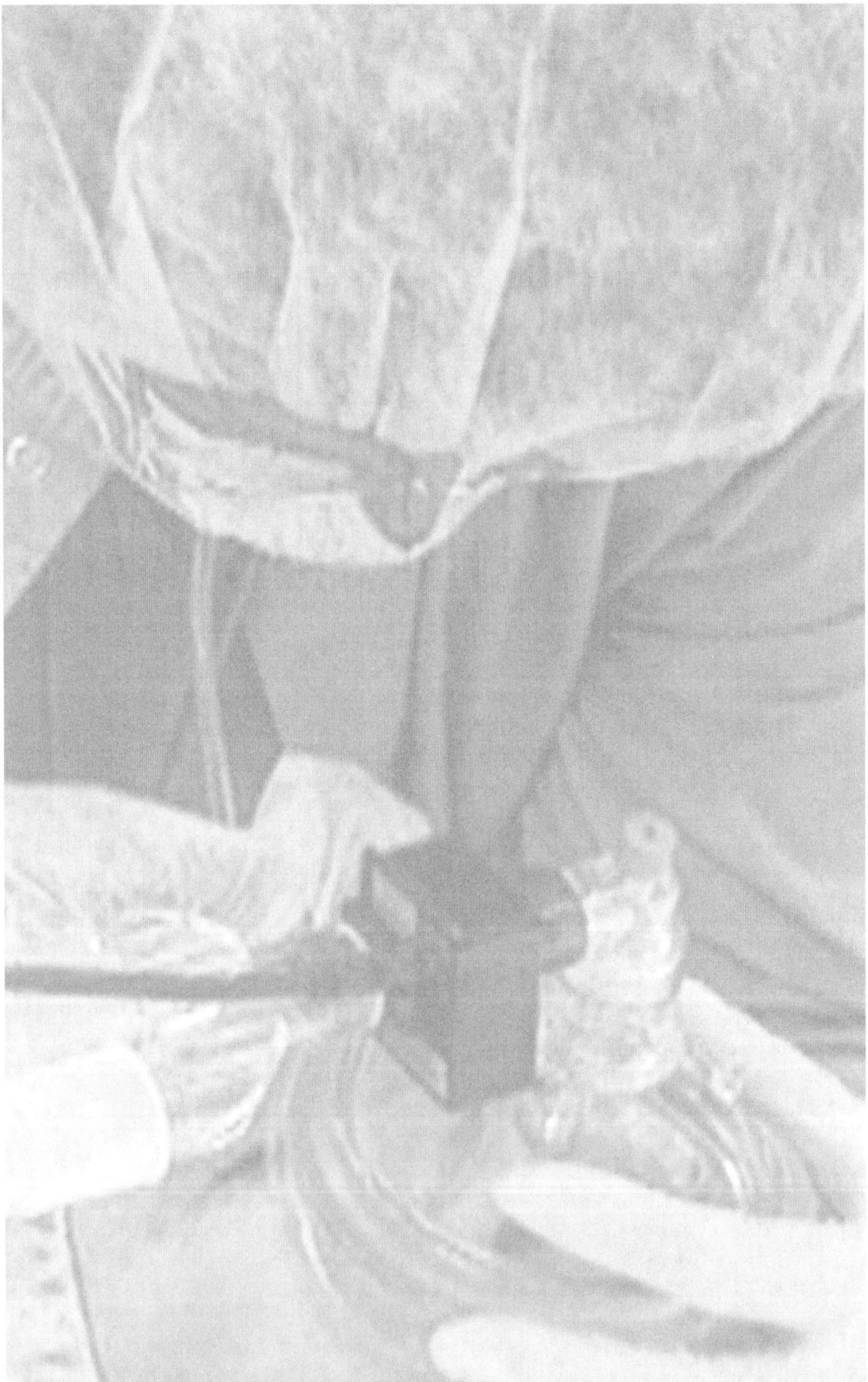

CHAPTER 14

STANDARDS OF CARE IN ANESTHESIA PRACTICE

Sandra K. Tunajek, CRNA, MSN

Director of Practice
American Association of Nurse Anesthetists
Park Ridge, IL

KEY CONCEPTS

- Professional standards contribute to and influence nurse anesthesia clinical practice.
- There is a growing demand for evidence-based outcomes in clinical anesthesia practice.
- Clinical practice guidelines have had a substantial impact on anesthesia care.
- Professional organizations have a key role in promulgation of standards, clinical practice guidelines, and position statements.
- To be useful, new standards must be effectively disseminated.

Integrity, accountability, competence and commitment to quality practice: This philosophy of self-regulation has been an inherent goal of the nurse anesthesia profession since 1931 when the National Association of Nurse Anesthetists, now the American Association of Nurse Anesthetists (AANA), set the objective "to develop educational standards and techniques in the administration of anesthetic drugs" (Bankert, 1989).

Central to professional recognition is the public's demand for professional accountability—accountability that insists upon the development of standards that promote an acceptable level of patient care and the criteria by which a practitioner can be measured.

The perception upon which a Certified Registered Nurse Anesthetist (CRNA) will be considered competent is based on the method in which he or she assimilates quality of care into interactions with patients and peers. Quality of care is most often defined as that activity involving patient and provider behavior and communication that is based on solidly defined standards of practice. Quality underlies the integrity of a nurse anesthetist's practice.

This section discusses comparative information as it relates to the establishment of quality anesthesia care, including clinical practice standards, clinical practice guidelines, and position statements. Although each is distinctly different, they are often used interchangeably with each providing a necessary component in determining quality of care. Figure 14.1 provides a conceptual graphic to describe the relationship of these three terms. This chapter will also introduce relatively new terms related to quality of care issues: benchmarking and evidence-based outcome measures

Practice standards are the highest mandate for clinical behavior. Aker & Rupp (1994) stated "a standard represents behaviors that must be exercised by the prudent nurse anesthetist in similar circumstances. Standards allow for little variation in performance behavior that cannot be justified by clear and compelling rationale."

Practice guidelines are guides to provider behavior and critical decision making that are commonly accepted within the discipline of the anesthesia profession. Practice guidelines are not mandated recommendations.

Position statements have less forceful criteria than either practice guidelines or standards. They usually represent emerging trends on a given topic or address economically driven practice modalities, or they discuss procedural policies, both clinical and nonclinical. Frequently, they evolve as the result of an identified clinical practice issue or concerns related to patient safety. Either practice guidelines or position statements may ultimately evolve into standards, given time, appropriate testing, discussion, and review. An example of such a transition is the recently adopted *AANA Standards for Office Based Anesthesia Practice.*

The AANA Board of Directors and the Practice Committee initiated data collection on this emerging practice trend in June 1997. In response to a perceived lack of oversight for patient care in the office outpatient setting, the AANA first introduced a position statement, then guidelines and finally adopted, in February 1999, the office-based standards. The standards are intended to assist anesthesia practitioners seeking guidance and support for patient safety in this setting. The standards evolved from frequently asked clinical and administrative questions and are based upon the concept that the "standard of care" is the same regardless of the practice setting. The

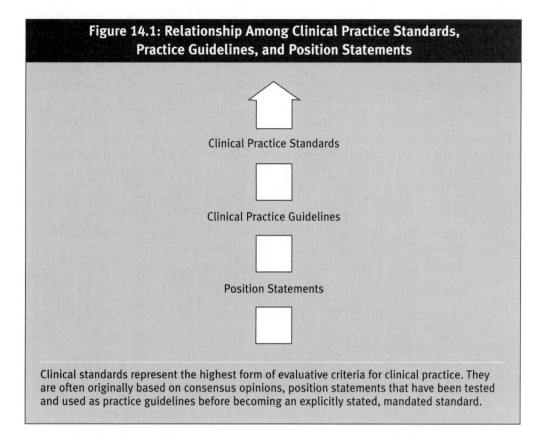

Figure 14.1: Relationship Among Clinical Practice Standards, Practice Guidelines, and Position Statements

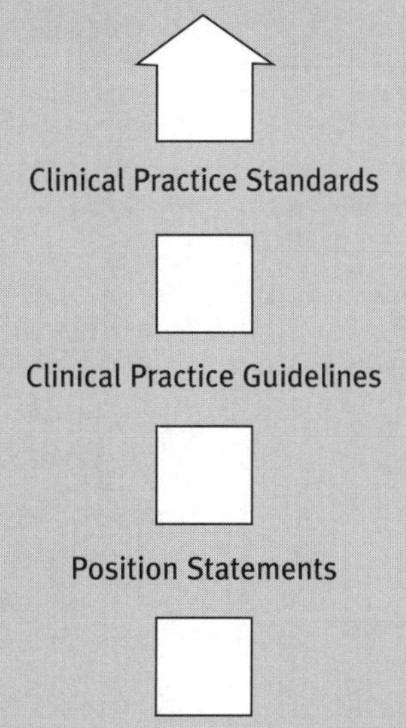

Clinical standards represent the highest form of evaluative criteria for clinical practice. They are often originally based on consensus opinions, position statements that have been tested and used as practice guidelines before becoming an explicitly stated, mandated standard.

AANA is the first organization to adopt such stringent recommendations for this setting. The standards emphasize the advocacy role of the CRNA (Table 14.1).

With the current rapidly changing healthcare delivery environment, and largely in response to public and private concerns relating to patient care, practice guidelines and practice standards have received renewed attention. Healthcare practitioners are being asked to further define, justify, improve, and document their quality of care. In short, the public, government agencies, business, and industry are demanding accountability from healthcare providers—accountability that requires entities to publicly disseminate, maintain, and enforce appropriate standards of care.

It is the inherent responsibility of a professional association to develop, disseminate, and assist in the implementation of practice guidelines and standards of practice. Additionally, the profession must hold members accountable for using the standards and must protect the public from practitioners who have not acquired sufficient expertise or have chosen not to follow professional standards. The professional organization must educate the public and regulatory agencies relative to the standards and must be responsible for disseminating new standards to the public and to practitioners.

The AANA has accepted and maintained this responsibility to the public by promulgating standards and defining the accepted level of anesthesia care provided by its members. This activity is largely the responsibility of the AANA Practice Committee which, with the input and consent of the membership and the Board of Directors, tracks emerging trends and issues and develops recommendations for practice.

The AANA Board of Directors first

Table 14.1: Standards for Office Based Anesthesia Practice

Introduction

Certified Registered Nurse Anesthetists (CRNAs) have long been the predominant anesthesia practitioners and leaders in providing anesthesia services in physicians' offices. As the professional organization representing nurse anesthetists, the American Association of Nurse Anesthetists (AANA) advocates high quality, appropriate standards of care for all patients in all settings, including the office based practice setting. As in other settings, CRNAs provide anesthesia working with physicians such as anesthesiologists, surgeons and, where authorized, podiatrists, dentists and other healthcare professionals.

The AANA has been at the forefront in establishing clinical practice standards, including patient monitoring standards. The standards of care in the office based setting are congruent with the *AANA Scope and Standards of Nurse Anesthesia Practice* and are intended to:

1. Provide assistance to CRNAs and other practitioners by promoting a common base for the delivery of quality patient care in the office based setting.
2. Assist the public in understanding what to expect from the practitioner.
3. Support the basic rights of patients.

Although the standards are intended to promote high quality patient care, they cannot assure specific outcomes.

Anesthesia in the Office Setting

There are some unique and specific responsibilities that should be considered prior to administration of anesthesia in the office setting. When considering an office based practice, anesthesia practitioners should determine if there are appropriate resources to manage the various levels of anesthesia for the planned surgical procedures and the condition of the patient. Most office based practice settings are not regulated, therefore, the CRNA should consider the benefit of uniform professional standards regarding practitioner qualifications, training, equipment, facilities and policies that ensure the safety of the patient during operative and anesthesia procedures in the office setting.

At a minimum, the CRNA shall determine that there are policies to address:

a. patient selection criteria
b. monitoring equipment with a backup electrical source
c. adequate numbers of well-trained personnel to support the planned surgery and anesthesia
d. the treatment of foreseeable complications
e. patient transfer to other healthcare facilities
f. infection control practices, including Occuptional Safety and Health Administration (OSHA) requirements
g. minimal pre-operative testing, including required consultations
h. ancillary services (e.g., laboratory, pharmacy, consultation with outside specialists)
i. equipment maintenance
j. response to fire and other catastrophic events
h. recovery and discharge of patients
i. procedures for follow-up care

The CRNA shall comply with all applicable state and federal rules and regulations relating to licensure, certification, and accreditation of an office practice.

(continued)

Table 14.1: Standards for Office Based Anesthesia Practice (continued)

SECTION I

Standard 1

Perform a thorough and complete preanesthesia assessment.

Interpretation: The responsibility for the care of the patient begins with the preanesthetic assessment. Except in emergency situations, the CRNA has an obligation to complete a thorough evaluation and determine that relevant tests have been obtained and reviewed.

Application to Office Practice:

Preanesthesia assessment of the patient undergoing office based surgery should include documentation of at least:

a. assigned physical status
b. airway assessment
c. previous history
d. allergies
e. fasting status
f. history and physical

Standard 2

Obtain informed consent for the planned anesthetic intervention from the patient or legal guardian.

Interpretation:

The CRNA shall obtain or verify that an informed consent has been obtained by a qualified provider. Discuss anesthetic options and risks with the patient and/or legal guardian in language the patient and/or legal guardian can understand. Document in the patient's medical record that informed consent was obtained.

Application to Office Practice:

The CRNA shall confirm that consent has been given for the planned surgical or diagnostic procedure and that the patient understands and accepts the plans and inherent risks for anesthesia in the office setting.

Standard 3

Formulate a patient-specific plan for anesthesia care.

Interpretation:

The plan of care developed by the CRNA is based upon comprehensive patient assessment, problem analysis, anticipated surgical or therapeutic procedure, patient and surgeon preferences, and current anesthesia principles.

Application to Office Practice:

A patient-specific plan of care is based on patient assessment and the anticipation of potential problems in this unique setting. The operating practitioner concurs that the patient is cleared for the planned anesthetic.

Standard 4

Implement and adjust the anesthesia care plan based on the patient's physiological response.

Interpretation:

The CRNA shall induce and maintain anesthesia at required levels. The CRNA shall continuously assess the patient's response to the anesthetic and/or surgical intervention and intervene as required to maintain the patient in a satisfactory physiologic condition.

Application to Office Practice:

The CRNA shall continuously assess and monitor the patient's response to the anesthetic. Prior to administration of anesthesia the CRNA shall verify a means to deliver positive pressure ventilation and to treat emergency situations including the availability of necessary

(continued)

Table 14.1: Standards for Office Based Anesthesia Practice (continued)

emergency equipment and drugs. If "triggering agents" associated with malignant hyperthermia are used, adequate dosages of dantrolene should be immediately accessible. (See AANA Position Statement 2.5, *Preparedness for Treatment of Malignant Hyperthermia*, on p. 275.)

Standard 5

Monitor the patient's physiologic condition as appropriate for the type of anesthesia and specific patient needs.

A. *Monitor ventilation continuously.* Verify intubation of the trachea by auscultation, chest excursion, and confirmation of carbon dioxide in the expired gas. Continuously monitor end-tidal carbon dioxide during controlled or assisted ventilation. Use spirometry and ventilatory pressure monitors.

B. *Monitor oxygenation continuously* by clinical observation, pulse oximetry, and if indicated, arterial blood gas analysis.

C. *Monitor cardiovascular status continuously* via electrocardiogram and heart sounds. Record blood pressure and heart rate at least every five minutes.

D. *Monitor body temperature continuously* on all pediatric patients receiving general anesthesia and, when indicated, on all other patients.

E. *Monitor neuromuscular function and status* when neuromuscular blocking agents are administered.

F. *Monitor and assess patient positioning* and protective measures at frequent intervals.

Interpretation:

Continuous clinical observation and vigilance are the basis of safe anesthesia care. The standard applies to all patients receiving anesthesia care and may be exceeded at any time at the discretion of the CRNA. Unless otherwise stipulated in the standards, a means to monitor and evaluate the patient's status shall be immediately available for all patients. As new patient safety technologies evolve, integration into the current anesthesia practice shall be considered. The omission of any monitoring standards shall be documented and the reason stated on the patient's anesthesia record. The CRNA shall be in constant attendance of the patient until the responsibility for care has been accepted by another qualified healthcare provider.

Application to Office Practice:

Minimum monitors in the office based setting include: pulse oximetry, ECG, blood pressure, O_2 analyzer and end-tidal CO_2 analyzer when administering general anesthesia, body temperature for the pediatric patient, an esophageal or precordial stethoscope, and peripheral nerve stimulator as indicated.

Standard 6

There shall be complete, accurate, and timely documentation of pertinent information on the patient's medical record.

Interpretation:

Document all anesthetic interventions and patient responses. Accurate documentation facilitates comprehensive patient care, provides information for retrospective review and research data, and establishes a medical-legal record.

Application to Office Practice:

The CRNA confirms there is a plan for accurate record keeping and documentation of the following:

a. informed consent
b. preanesthesia and postanesthesia evaluations
c. course of the anesthesia including monitoring modalities and drug administration, dosages, and wastage
d. discharge follow-up

(continued)

Table 14.1: Standards for Office Based Anesthesia Practice (continued)

The CRNA shall confirm that there is a systematic mechanism for documentation of compliance with U. S. Drug Enforcement Agency rules, Board of Pharmacy regulations, Food and Drug Administration requirements, and U. S. Department of Transportation regulations for accountability and appropriate storage.

Documentation of provider licensure and credentials, facility licensure, and continued competence is recommended.

Standard 7

Transfer the responsibility for care of the patient to other qualified providers in a manner that assures continuity of care and patient safety.

Interpretation:

The CRNA shall assess the patient's status and determine when it is safe to transfer the responsibility of care to other qualified providers. The CRNA shall accurately report the patient's condition and all essential information to the provider assuming responsibility for the patient.

Application to Office Practice:

Postanesthesia care is consistent with other practice settings in that there is a designated area staffed with appropriately trained personnel. At least one qualified provider: a surgeon, anesthesia practitioner, or a registered nurse who is certified in advanced cardiac life support, remains in the facility until all patients are discharged. An accurate postanesthesia record is documented.

Standard 8

Adhere to appropriate safety precautions, as established within the institution, to minimize the risks of fire, explosion, electrical shock and equipment malfunction. Document on the patient's medical record that the anesthesia machine and equipment were checked.

Interpretation:

Prior to use, the CRNA shall inspect the anesthesia machine and monitors according to established guidelines. The CRNA shall check the readiness, availability, cleanliness, and working condition of all equipment to be utilized in the administration of the anesthesia care. When the patient is ventilated by an automatic mechanical ventilator, monitor the integrity of the breathing system with a device capable of detecting a disconnection by emitting an audible alarm. Monitor oxygen concentration continuously with an oxygen supply failure alarm system.

Application to Office Practice:

The CRNA confirms equipment is routinely maintained by appropriately trained professionals. Prior to use, equipment is inspected for risk of malfunction and electrical/fire hazards.

Standard 9

Precautions shall be taken to minimize the risk of infection to the patient, the CRNA, and other healthcare providers.

Interpretation:

Written policies and procedures in infection control shall be developed for personnel and equipment.

Application to Office Practice:

The CRNA shall confirm that policies are in place and a process exists to document compliance with Occupational Safety and Healthcare Administration (OSHA) standards relating to blood borne pathogens, medical waste, and hazardous materials, including personal protection devices, disposal of needles and syringes, and contaminated supplies.

Standard 10

Anesthesia care shall be assessed to assure its quality and contribution to positive patient outcomes.

(continued)

Table 14.1: Standards for Office Based Anesthesia Practice (continued)

Interpretation:
The CRNA shall participate in the ongoing review and evaluation of the quality and appropriateness of anesthesia care. Evaluation shall be performed based upon appropriate outcome criteria and reviewed on an ongoing basis. The CRNA shall participate in a continual process of self-evaluation and strive to incorporate new techniques and knowledge into practice.

Application to Office Practice:
Prior to administration of any anesthetic in an office facility, the CRNA shall review the AANA minimal elements (Section II) and evaluate compliance and applicability to the setting. The CRNA shall participate in assessment and review of appropriateness of anesthesia care provided in the office setting. There should be a process to document patient satisfaction and outcomes.

Standard 11
The CRNA shall respect and maintain the basic rights of patients.

Interpretation:
The CRNA shall support and preserve the rights of patients to personal dignity and ethical norms of practice.

Application to Office Practice:
The CRNA shall act as the patient advocate. The patient has the right to dignity, respect and consideration of legitimate concerns in the office setting. Patients should be involved with all aspects of their care.

SECTION II (Supplemental Resources)

Minimum Elements for Providing Anesthesia Services in the Office Based Practice Setting Assessment Checklist

PRACTITIONERS

CRNA
- ❍ Will the Board of Nursing and state laws allow the CRNA to work with this physician type?
- ❍ Will your liability insurance cover office anesthesia?
- ❍ Does the state have rules/regulations specific to the office based anesthesia?
- ❍ What classes of patients, types of surgical procedures, and anesthesia will be performed?

Operating Physician
- ❍ Does the physician have liability coverage, current licensure/Drug Enforcement Agency (DEA) number?
- ❍ Does the physician have hospital privileges for procedures?
- ❍ Does the physician have admitting privileges at the nearest hospital?

FACILITY
- ❍ Is the facility licensed?
  - ❍ By whom? Indicate name: ____________________
- ❍ Is the facility accredited?
  - ❍ By whom? Indicate name: ____________________
- ❍ Operating Room (OR) size, recovery room, preoperative area adequate for anesthesia and surgical procedures?
- ❍ Is there a transfer agreement?
- ❍ Does the facility have an emergency service agreement?
- ❍ Telephone numbers accessible and posted? Emergency Medical Services (EMS), Malignant Hyperthermia (MH) hotline, hospital, etc.

(continued)

Table 14.1: Standards for Office Based Anesthesia Practice (continued)

EQUIPMENT

Local, Intravenous Sedation, Regional and General Anesthesia

- ❍ Monitors include pulse oximeter, electrocardiogram, blood pressure monitor.
- ❍ Oxygen supplies. A minimum of two oxygen sources must be available with regulators attached.
- ❍ Positive pressure ventilation sources including an ambu bag and a mouth-to-mask unit.
- ❍ Defibrillator (charged).
- ❍ Suction machine, tubing, suction catheters, and Yankaur suctions.
- ❍ Anesthesia cart to provide for organization of supplies including endotracheal equipment, masks, airways, syringes, needles, intravenous catheters, intravenous fluids and tubing, alcohol, stethoscopes, and appropriate medications.
- ❍ Emergency medication to include at a minimum, atropine, epinephrine, ephedrine, lidocaine, diphenhydramine, cortisone, and a bronchial dilator inhaler.

For General Anesthesia

- ❍ An authorized factory technician or qualified service personnel has checked out anesthesia machine(s).

  The following items are available as an integral part of the anesthesia machine:
  - ❍ O_2 Fail-safe system
  - ❍ Oxygen analyzer
  - ❍ Waste gas exhaust system
  - ❍ End-tidal CO_2 Analyzer
  - ❍ Vaporizers—calibration and exclusion system
  - ❍ Alarm system
  - ❍ Pulse oximeter, electrocardiogram, blood pressure monitors

Emergencies

- ❍ Emergency equipment
  - ❍ Basic airway equipment (adult and pediatric)
    - ❍ Nasal and oral airway
    - ❍ Face mask (appropriate for patient)
    - ❍ Laryngoscopes, endotracheal tubes (adult and pediatric)
    - ❍ Ambu Bag
  - ❍ Difficult Airway Equipment (laryngeal mask airway, light wand, cricothyrotomy kit)
  - ❍ Defibrillator
  - ❍ Supplemental O_2
  - ❍ Emergency drugs
  - ❍ Compression board
  - ❍ Suction equipment (suction catheter, Yankaur type)
  - ❍ Drugs and equipment to treat MH on site
- ❍ Back-up power

Pharmaceutical Accountability

- ❍ Is there an appropriate mechanism for documenting and tracking use of pharmaceuticals including controlled substances?
  - ❍ Lock box
  - ❍ DEA 222 forms
  - ❍ Count sheets
  - ❍ Waste policy
  - ❍ Expiration checklist or policy

Policies/Procedures and Protocols

- ❍ Are there policies/protocols regarding:
  - ❍ Preoperative lab requirements
  - ❍ Patient selection
  - ❍ Nothing by mouth (NPO) status
  - ❍ Discharge criteria

(continued)

Table 14.1: Standards for Office Based Anesthesia Practice (continued)

Policies/Procedures and Protocols (continued)
- ❍ Case cancellations
- ❍ Advanced Cardiac Life Support (ACLS) algorithms
- ❍ MH protocols
- ❍ Latex allergy protocols
- ❍ Pediatric drug dosages
- ❍ Emergency
  - ❍ Cardiopulmonary
  - ❍ Chemical spill
  - ❍ Fire
  - ❍ Building evacuation
  - ❍ Bomb threat
- ❍ Reporting adverse reactions
- ❍ Infection control in adherence to OSHA rules for control of medical waste, disposal of sharps and personal protection

Record Keeping
- ❍ Is there a system for record keeping for patients and providers?
- ❍ Anesthesia record
- ❍ Consent forms
- ❍ Credentials
- ❍ Q/A mechanism
- ❍ Patient satisfaction/follow-up
- ❍ Preanesthesia equipment and supplies
- ❍ Purchasing agreements

PERSONNEL

OR	❍ RN	❍ LPN	❍ OR Technician	
PACU	❍ RN	❍ LPN	❍ Anesthetist/Surgeon	
ACLS Certified	❍ Surgeon		❍ Anesthetist	❍ RN
BCLS Certified	❍ RN	❍ LPN	❍ Others	

Anesthesia Equipment and Supplies Checklist *(To be kept in log book)*

Date	Checked-out by	Location

A. ❍ Oxygen pipeline pressure or primary source _____ pounds per square inch
❍ Oxygen tank pressure (second source) _____ pounds per square inch
B. ❍ Back-up power
C. ❍ Defibrillator and crash cart available
D. ❍ Anesthesia cart supplies checked, i.e., intravenous equipment, anesthetics, stethoscope
E. ❍ Suction equipment tested
F. ❍ Ambu bag tested
G. ❍ Electrocardiogram (ECG) operational
H. ❍ Pulse oximeter operational
I. ❍ Blood pressure monitor
❍ Back-up blood pressure cuff
J. ❍ Atropine
❍ Epinephrine
❍ Ephedrine
❍ Lidocaine
❍ Other emergency medications as indicated

(continued)

Table 14.1: Standards for Office Based Anesthesia Practice (continued)

K. ❍ Endotracheal equipment, airways

If general anesthesia is planned: Anesthesia machine no.____________

L. ❍ Leak test performed and other tests as indicated
M. ❍ Oxygen analyzer is ON
N. ❍ Capnometer connected
O. ❍ Temperature monitor available
P. ❍ Emergency airways available, i.e., laryngeal mask airway, combitube, or cricothyrotomy kit
Q. ❍ Succinylcholine
❍ Dantrolene
❍ Other anesthesia medications as indicated

Note (if problem):____

____

____

Follow-up (who, what):____

____

____

adopted standards of practice in 1980 with the publication of the *Guidelines for Nurse Anesthesia Practice.* Subsequent revisions followed in 1983, 1989, and 1992. A 1996 revision incorporated the "Patient Monitoring Standards" into Standard V of the newly titled *Scope and Standards for Nurse Anesthesia Practice* (Table 14.2).

The initial guidelines clarified the scope of nurse anesthesia practice to the public, outlined the responsibilities for anesthesia care, and provided a structured framework for accountability of the practitioner to the public and to the individual patient. Currently, a comprehensive collection of standards, guidelines, and position and consideration statements titled *Professional Practice Manual for the Certified Registered Nurse Anesthetist* (AANA, 1999) is available. The manual is divided into the sections listed in Table 14.3 and is updated on a regular basis.

STANDARDS OF PRACTICE

Standards are rules or minimum requirements for the clinical practice of a professional. Standards represent generally accepted principles of patient care and determine the expectations against which current and future performance can be measured. Standards evolve through a process of consensus and consideration of scientific evidence and are based on the concept that if a practitioner adheres to the standards, outcomes will be positive.

Standards have been used to evaluate nurse anesthesia care in a number of ways. They serve to provide direction and a framework for the evaluation of practice. Standards describe a profession's accountability to the public and the performance outcomes for which a nurse anesthetist is responsible. Standards also establish an expected level of patient care and enable the measurement of a nurse anesthetist's competency. Standards have been used to ensure quality and in managing individual and institutional risk.

Standards are classified as regulatory, voluntary, and involuntary. Regulatory standards are usually based on govern-

Table 14.2: Scope and Standards for Nurse Anesthesia Practice

The AANA Scope and Standards for Nurse Anesthesia Practice offer guidance for Certified Registered Nurse Anesthetists (CRNAs) and health care institutions regarding the scope of nurse anesthesia practice. The scope of practice of the Certified Registered Nurse Anesthetist addresses the responsibilities associated with anesthesia practice and is performed in collaboration with other qualified health care providers. Collaboration is a process which involves two or more parties working together, each contributing his or her respective area of expertise. CRNAs are responsible for the quality of services they render.

Scope of Practice

The practice of anesthesia is a recognized specialty in both nursing and medicine. Anesthesiology is the art and science of rendering a patient insensible to pain by the administration of anesthetic agents and related drugs and procedures. Anesthesia and anesthesia-related care represents those services which anesthesia professionals provide upon request, assignment, and referral by the patient's physician or other health care provider authorized by law, most often to facilitate diagnostic, therapeutic and surgical procedures. In other instances, the referral or request for consultation or assistance may be for management of pain associated with obstetrical labor and delivery, management of acute and chronic ventilatory problems, or the management of acute and chronic pain through the performance of selected diagnostic and therapeutic blocks or other forms of pain management. CRNA s practice according to their expertise, state statutes and regulations, and institutional policy.

CRNA scope of practice includes, but is not limited to the following:

1. Performing and documenting a preanesthetic assessment and evaluation of the patient, including requesting consultations and diagnostic studies; selecting, obtaining, ordering, and administering preanesthetic medications and fluids; and obtaining informed consent for anesthesia.
2. Developing and implementing an anesthetic plan.
3. Initiating the anesthetic technique which may include: general, regional, local, and sedation.
4. Selecting, applying, and inserting appropriate non-invasive and invasive monitoring modalities for continuous evaluation of the patient's physical status.
5. Selecting, obtaining, and administering the anesthetics, adjuvant and accessory drugs, and fluids necessary to manage the anesthetic.
6. Managing a patient's airway and pulmonary status using current practice modalities.
7. Facilitating emergence and recovery from anesthesia by selecting, obtaining, ordering and administering medications, fluids, and ventilatory support.
8. Discharging the patient from a postanesthesia care area and providing postanesthesia follow-up evaluation and care.
9. Implementing acute and chronic pain management modalities.
10. Responding to emergency situations by providing airway management, administration of emergency fluids and drugs, and using basic or advanced cardiac life support techniques.

Additional nurse anesthesia responsibilities which are within the expertise of the individual CRNA include:

1. Administration/management: scheduling, material and supply management, supervision of staff, students or ancillary personnel, development of policies and procedures, fiscal management, performance evaluations, preventative maintenance, billing and data management.
2. Quality assessment: data collection, reporting mechanism, trending, compliance, committee meetings, departmental review, problem focused studies, problem solving, interventions, documents and process oversight.

(continued)

Table 14.2: Scope and Standards for Nurse Anesthesia Practice (continued)

3. Educational: clinical and didactic teaching, BCLS/ ACLS instruction, inservice commitment, EMT training, supervision of residents, and facility continuing education.
4. Research: conducting and participating in departmental, hospital-wide, and university-sponsored research projects.
5. Committee appointments: assignment to committees, committee responsibilities, and coordination of committee activities.
6. Interdepartmental liaison: interface with other departments such as nursing, surgery, obstetrics, postanesthesia care units (PACU), outpatient surgery, admissions, administration, laboratory, pharmacy, etc.
7. Clinical/administrative oversight of other departments: respiratory therapy, PACU, operating room, surgical intensive care unit (SICU), pain clinics, etc.

The functions listed above are a summary of CRNA clinical practice and are not intended to be all-inclusive. A more specific list of CRNA functions and practice parameters is detailed in the AANA Guidelines for Clinical Privileges.

CRNAs strive for professional excellence by demonstrating competence and commitment to the clinical, educational, consultative, research, and administrative practice in the specialty of anesthesia. CRNAs should actively participate in the development of departmental policies and guidelines, performance appraisals, peer reviews, clinical and administrative conferences, and serve on health care facility committees. In addition to these activities, CRNAs should assume a leadership role in the evaluation of the quality of anesthesia care provided throughout the facility and the community.

The scope of practice of the CRNA is also the scope of practice of nurse anesthetists who have graduated within the past 24 months from a nurse anesthesia educational program, accredited by the Council on Accreditation of Nurse Anesthesia Educational Programs, but have not yet passed their initial certification examination. Students enrolled in nurse anesthesia educational programs accredited by the Council on Accreditation of Nurse Anesthesia Educational Programs practice pursuant to the Council's Standards and Guidelines.

Standards for Nurse Anesthesia Practice

Introduction

These standards are intended to:

1. Assist the profession in evaluating the quality of care provided by its practitioners.
2. Provide a common base for practitioners to use in their development of a quality practice.
3. Assist the public in understanding what to expect from the practitioner.
4. Support and preserve the basic rights of the patient.

These standards apply to all anesthetizing locations. While the standards are intended to encourage high quality patient care, they cannot assure specific outcomes.

Standard I

Perform a thorough and complete preanesthesia assessment.

Interpretation:

The responsibility for the care of the patient begins with the preanesthetic assessment. Except in emergency situations, the CRNA has an obligation to complete a thorough evaluation and determine that relevant tests have been obtained and reviewed.

Standard II

Obtain informed consent for the planned anesthetic intervention from the patient or legal guardian.

(continued)

Table 14.2: Scope and Standards for Nurse Anesthesia Practice (continued)

Interpretation:

The CRNA shall obtain or verify that an informed consent has been obtained by a qualified provider. Discuss anesthetic options and risks with the patient and/or legal guardian in language the patient and/or legal guardian can understand. Document in the patient's medical record that informed consent was obtained.

Standard III

Formulate a patient-specific plan for anesthesia care.

Interpretation:

The plan of care developed by the CRNA is based upon comprehensive patient assessment, problem analysis, anticipated surgical ortherapeutic procedure, patient and surgeon preferences, and current anesthesia principles.

Standard IV

Implement and adjust the anesthesia care plan based on the patient's physiological response.

Interpretation:

The CRNA shall induce and maintain anesthesia at required levels. The CRNA shall continuously assess the patient's response to the anesthetic and/or surgical intervention and intervene as required to maintain the patient in a satisfactory physiologic condition.

Standard V*

Monitor the patient's physiologic condition as appropriate for the type of anesthesia and specific patient needs.

A. Monitor ventilation continuously. Verify intubation of the trachea by auscultation, chest excursion, and confirmation of carbon dioxide in the expired gas. Continuously monitor end-tidal carbon dioxide during controlled or assisted ventilation. Use spirometry and ventilatory pressure monitors.

B. Monitor oxygenation continuously by clinical observation, pulse oximetry, and if indicated, arterial blood gas analysis.

C. Monitor cardiovascular status continuously via electrocardiogram and heart sounds. Record blood pressure and heart rate at least every five minutes.

D. Monitor body temperature continuously on all pediatric patients receiving general anesthesia and when indicated, on all other patients.

E. Monitor neuromuscular function and status when neuromuscular blocking agents are administered.

F. Monitor and assess the patient positioning and protective measures. (Effective April 6, 1998.)

Interpretation:

Continuous clinical observation and vigilance are the basis of safe anesthesia care. The standard applies to all patients receiving anesthesia care and may be exceeded at any time at the discretion of the CRNA. Unless otherwise stipulated in the standards a means to monitor and evaluate the patient's status shall be immediately available for all patients. As new patient safety technologies evolve, integration into the current anesthesia practice shall be considered. The omission of any monitoring standards shall be documented and the reason stated on the patient's anesthesia record. The CRNA shall be in constant attendance of the patient until the responsibility for care has been accepted by another qualified health care provider.

* Adopted 1989 to become effective January 1, 1990; revised 1992, 1996

(continued)

Table 14.2: Scope and Standards for Nurse Anesthesia Practice (continued)

Standard VI

There shall be complete, accurate, and timely documentation of pertinent information on the patient's medical record.

Interpretation:

Document all anesthetic interventions and patient responses. Accurate documentation facilitates comprehensive patient care, provides information for retrospective review and research data, and establishes a medical-legal record.

Standard VII

Transfer the responsibility for care of the patient to other qualified providers in a manner which assures continuity of care and patient safety.

Interpretation:

The CRNA shall assess the patient's status and determine when it is safe to transfer the responsibility of care to other qualified providers. The CRNA shall accurately report the patient's condition and all essential information to the provider assuming responsibility for the patient.

Standard VIII

Adhere to appropriate safety precautions, as established within the institution, to minimize the risks of fire, explosion, electrical shock and equipment malfunction. Document on the patient's medical record that the anesthesia machine and equipment were checked.

Interpretation:

Prior to use, the CRNA shall inspect the anesthesia machine and monitors according to established guidelines. The CRNA shall check the readiness, availability, cleanliness, and working condition of all equipment to be utilized in the administration of the anesthesia care. When the patient is ventilated by an automatic mechanical ventilator, monitor the integrity of the breathing system with a device capable of detecting a disconnection by emitting an audible alarm. Monitor oxygen concentration continuously with an oxygen supply failure alarm system.

Standard IX

Precautions shall be taken to minimize the risk of infection to the patient, the CRNA, and other health care providers.

Interpretation:

Written policies and procedures in infection control shall be developed for personnel and equipment.

Standard X

Anesthesia care shall be assessed to assure its quality and contribution to positive patient outcomes.

Interpretation:

The CRNA shall participate in the ongoing review and evaluation of the quality and appropriateness of anesthesia care. Evaluation shall be performed based upon appropriate outcome criteria and reviewed on an ongoing basis. The CRNA shall participate in a continual process of self evaluation and strive to incorporate new techniques and knowledge into practice.

Standard XI

The CRNA shall respect and maintain the basic rights of patients.

Interpretation:

The CRNA shall support and preserve the rights of patients to personal dignity and ethical norms of practice.

The scope of practice statement included herein was previously published in the 1980, 1983, 1989, and 1992 predecessors of this document which were respectively titled: The American Association of Nurse Anesthetists Guidelines for the Practice of the Certified Registered Nurse Anesthetist *(1980,1983);* Guidelines for Nurse Anesthesia Practice *(1989); and* Guidelines and Standards for Nurse Anesthesia Practice *(1992).*

Adopted 1996

Table 14.3: Practice Manual Contents

Topic Sections of the *Professional Practice Manual for the Certified Registered Nurse Anesthetist*

- Guidelines for Clinical Privileges
- Guidelines for the Management of the Obstetrical Patient for the CRNA
- Postanesthesia Care Standards for the CRNA
- Guidelines for Expert Witnesses
- Standards for Office Based Anesthesia Practice
- Qualifications and Capabilities of the CRNA
- Professional and Legal Issues of Nurse Anesthesia Practice
- Quality of Care in Anesthesia: A Synopsis of Published Information Comparing CRNA and Anesthesiologist Patient Outcomes
- Documenting the Standard of Care: The Anesthesia Record
- Informed Consent in Anesthesia
- AANA Position Statements/Considerations for Policy Development
- Code of Ethics
- Environmental Safety

ment mandates. Voluntary standards are those developed by healthcare practitioners, often the work of the professional organization. Involuntary standards are those defined by professional liability carriers. Standards may also be categorized according to the scope of influence such as national, state, local or institutional.

Standards are designed to provide guidance, but in the event of a lawsuit, such standards may be relied upon to define the standard of care. Students should note that there is a single standard for the provision of anesthesia care in this country. Standards do not vary according to type of practitioners. According to Blumenreich (1991): "Some people erroneously assume or question whether there is a dual standard of care in the anesthesia field. In fact, because of the nature of anesthesia and the fact that attention and proper monitoring of patients is the overwhelming consideration in the practice of anesthesia, there is, in fact, a single standard of care."

The nurse anesthesia profession, through the AANA, has established standards of care. These standards of care are not different from those of anesthesiologists. As Blumenreich (1991) has indicated, "There is a rather uniform quality of care between nurse anesthetists and anesthesiologists, and that is further evidence that the 'standard of care' is the same." With the emergence of new technology and knowledge and the ability to rapidly disseminate such knowledge, there is a trend for healthcare practitioners to be held to a single national standard of care. National standards, developed by professionals, may also be contained in federal legislative or regulatory language. Therefore, local policy development must be scrutinized to reflect national standards.

The standard of care should provide guidance in practice to avoid negative outcomes. Certainly, standards have not been developed for every clinical situation; nurse anesthetists need to use their own knowledge and expertise to guide their clinical practice. As professional nurses as well as nurses in advanced practice, nurse anesthetists have the responsibility to maintain competence and continually review any changes in existing standards or the introduction of any new standards.

Aker and Rupp (1994) state that: "Standards promulgated by a profession are representative models that delineate contemporary principles of practice, reflect the philosophic values and clinical priorities of the profession and provide a foundation by which clinical practice can be evaluated." Furthermore, standards furnish practitioners and the judiciary with confirmation of what constitutes the standard knowledge and skill that a practitioner should apply in the daily care of anesthetized patients. Members of the profession must be accountable to the public for adhering to all published standards.

Standards are divided into two types: *process* and *outcome.* Process standards refer to a particular behavior or the mechanism by which a specific task is performed. Process standards mandate a clinical conduct. As contained in the *Scope and Standards for Nurse Anesthesia Practice,* the completion of a preanesthesia visit and the documentation of anesthesia care are examples of process standards (procedural or "how to" standards). Standard V, which includes the patient monitoring standards, is also an example of a process standard.

There is a growing demand for objective, comparative information about practitioner performance and patient care outcomes. Outcome measures are rapidly becoming the benchmarking tool for a healthcare institution, therefore directing practitioner clinical performance. Institution-based outcome standards have been introduced as a mechanism to identify exemplary performance and best practices. For example, outcome standards focus on the requirement for a CRNA to provide data beyond the "how to" process, to tangible evidence of patient care results. Additionally, nurse anesthetist competencies are being assessed, documented, and linked to overall institutional patient care results. Standards for institutional accreditation mandate documentation of continuous quality improvement. Outcome standards provide visual signs of such improvement. In the future, such standards will most likely emphasize specific outcome criteria relating to patient care.

Outcome standards are problematic in that medicine is not an exact science. Circumstances affecting patient outcome may be beyond the control of the practitioner. Hospitals vary in the level of technology and staffing they provide. In some instances there may be pre-existing medical problems that would overshadow any chance of an improved postoperative outcome. As such, even with adherence to standards and guidelines, results cannot be guaranteed. However, these facts have not prevented outcome data from being applied as a measurement of quality of care.

The advent of expanding technology and quality of care to patient concerns, combined with increased required reporting regulations, have given rise to the use of a new term: benchmarking. Based on standards of care and outcome data, benchmarking compares institutional outcomes, presumably a measurement of quality care, with other institutions' outcomes for the same types of procedures or diagnosis. Hospitals regularly report outcome data concerning their patient population in an effort to market their services to patients, payers, and practitioners. Considerable controversy has evolved concerning the comparison of data generated by the healthcare facilities that provide care to much sicker patients and the data generated by facilities that do not. Despite the controversy, outcome standards appear to be here to stay. Consequently, it is imperative that the individual CRNA, as well as the professional organization, be involved in the collection and interpretation of outcome data that accurately reflect the high quality of care provided to patients.

CLINICAL PRACTICE GUIDELINES

Practice guidelines are official policy statements of a professional association that are developed to assist the nurse anesthesia practitioner to understand the indications for and the methods to perform clinical procedures (e.g., the administration of anesthesia to the obstetrical patient). They also may depict basic clinical management options for complications or a disease process, such as the treatment of a malignant hyperthermia crisis. Practice guidelines are not only useful in guiding practice, but they also have relevance in education, research, and the development of continuous quality improvement processes (see chapter 24). Practice guidelines provide assistance in the instruction of the student anesthetist in the administration of anesthesia for specific surgical procedures, guide the researcher in the identification and development of methods to investigate a specific clinical problem, and serve as a benchmark to measure and improve ones practice. Although they do not carry the influence of standards, practice guidelines can and have been used in malpractice litigation.

Practice guidelines are systematically developed recommendations supported by analysis of current literature and by a synthesis of expert opinion, clinical feasibility data, and consensus surveys. Evidence-based practice guideline development is an endeavor that looks at the literature available, evaluates it on the basis of scientific merits, evaluates the results, and makes recommendations as the best options for patient care.

Although based on validated research, guidelines are not intended to be standards or absolute requirements. As the Agency for Health Care Policy and Research (AHCPR, 1995) explains, "Clinical practice guidelines should be viewed as a tool, not a rule."

Practice guidelines, to be understood and implemented, should be accompanied with statements that interpret or explain the intent of the guideline. Although clinical practice guidelines may be described in many different terms, including practice parameters, practice guidelines, patient care protocols, clinical pathways, and care maps, the intent of each evidence-based guideline is to encourage practitioners to improve patient care services.

Practice guidelines also examine the quality of care provided and serve as a reminder to practitioners to practice in an acceptable, prudent, and cost-effective manner. Recently, managed care healthcare organizations have undergone intense scrutiny for their attempts to mandate the use of clinical practice guidelines that limit certain patient care treatments or services. Additionally, in an effort to control costs and misuse of services, private insurance companies are instituting polices that insist upon, or at least encourage, the use of clinical practice guidelines in the management of those individuals they insure.

Guidelines developed by national professional organizations may help individual practitioners, but strong evidence that existing guidelines are based on true science is lacking. Experience to date suggests that clinical practice guideline implementation has been modest and in many cases problematic. The primary problems appear to be related to physician practitioner acceptance, the need for extensive modification and/or education of staff, and increased cost of implementation.

A more systematic approach to the development of practice guidelines, with emphasis on specific objectives, clinical cost/benefit ratio, and research-based evidence for the intended objectives, has emerged. Additionally, information technology advances provide quick access to practice guidelines in any location from the clinical site to the practitioner's office or home. The AHCPR has published practice guidelines in several general areas that also have relevance for anesthesia practitioners (e.g., pain management, sickle-cell anemia and cataracts). These guidelines, developed to encourage standardized practice patterns and eliminate waste and excessive costs to patients, provide a template for future development of evidence-based practice guidelines.

Guidelines, such as those published by the AHCPR, evolve from a consensus of scientific evidence, expert opinions, and clinical experience. Expert opinion is vital to the process to assist in the evidence collection process, but more important, input from practitioners must be solicited to ensure that the guidelines are functional in clinical settings. For example, if a practice guideline mandated the use of transesophageal echocardiography for the detection of air embolism during neurosurgical procedures, it is unlikely that the guideline could be followed in every hospital.

Recently the Joint Commission on Accreditation of Healthcare Organizations (JCAHO) implemented standards that require the use of clinical practice guidelines in ambulatory care facilities and encourage accredited hospital facilities to consider the use of clinical practice guidelines in improving quality of care processes, a move that will most likely lead to the inclusion of mandated standards for the implementation and use of clinical practice guidelines in all JCAHO accredited facilities.

PRACTICE GUIDELINE INTERPRETATION

The intent of practice guidelines is to assist the practitioner in determining the appropriate actions needed to address specific clinical circumstances. The wording of the guideline is intentionally structured to allow for flexibility and individual patient needs. They are advisory, not intended to apply to all situations, and recommend behaviors that lead to positive outcomes. According to Aker and Rupp (1994), practice guidelines may become what is considered a functional standard of care simply by utilization, demonstrating the care that a reasonable and prudent nurse anesthetist would provide.

In 1998, the *Guidelines for the Management of the Obstetrical Patient for the Certified Registered Nurse Anesthetist* (Table 14.4), an example of practice guidelines, were adopted by the AANA Board of Directors. The guidelines, based on other organizations' existing standards for obstetrical care, include intent statements and outline mechanisms to implement the guidelines. The interpretative statements offer guidance related to practitioner decision making when confronted with simultaneous situations in obstetrical emergencies. For example, the guidelines clearly indicate that the anesthesia provider stay with the patient at all times. However, in a small rural practice with a solo practitioner, the CRNA may be required to respond to more than one obstetrical emergency. Guidelines are realistic, yet are flexible enough to allow providers to use independent clini-

Table 14.4: Guidelines for the Management of the Obstetrical Patient for the Certified Registered Nurse Anesthetist

Introduction

CRNAs have been the predominant providers of anesthesia services to obstetrical patients. CRNAs provide obstetrical anesthesia services with physicians such as anesthesiologists, obstetricians and family practitioners, and with nurses such as nurse midwives and nurse practitioners. In recognition of that role, the AANA advocates establishing clinical guidelines that promote quality patient care.

While pregnancy and childbirth are normal physiologic processes, many variables have the potential to complicate overall patient management. The American Association of Nurse Anesthetists (AANA) developed the "Guidelines for Anesthesia Management of the Obstetrical Patient" to (1) promote safe and effective anesthesia care for obstetrical patients, and (2) provide guidance for Certified Registered Nurse Anesthetists (CRNAs) and healthcare institutions.

In the context of these guidelines, anesthesia is the care provided for surgical intervention (i.e., cesarean section), and labor analgesia is the care provided for pain management (i.e., labor epidural). The AANA "Scope and Standards of Nurse Anesthesia Practice" shall apply to all patients who undergo anesthesia in the obstetrical setting.

Guideline 1

Possess the appropriate skills and credentials to initiate and/or manage regional (intrathecal, spinal, epidural or caudal epidural) labor analgesia and anesthesia and general anesthesia for the obstetric patient.

Interpretation:

The CRNA shall be able to develop and implement a plan of patient care specific to the needs and predispositions of the obstetric patient and based on current anesthesia principles.

Guideline 2

The CRNA shall be aware of fetal status prior to each analgesia/anesthesia intervention.

Interpretation:

Fetal status is monitored and documented in the patient's record.

Guideline 3

Insure that anesthesia equipment is consistent with other anesthetizing locations in the facility. Emergency airway management equipment and drugs for resuscitation of the neonate shall be available.

Interpretation:

Departmental policies should define the anesthesia equipment required to provide high quality anesthesia care to the parturient and the neonate.

Guideline 4

The CRNA shall be immediately available, as defined by institutional policy, when analgesia and anesthesia is administered.

Interpretation:

During the conduct of a continuous epidural infusion for analgesia, the CRNA must be immediately available to assess the level of analgesia and adjust the plan of care as appropriate. Following bolus epidural or intrathecal injection for analgesia, the CRNA must be immediately available to assess the level of analgesia until that level has stabilized.

Guideline 5

During the conduct of an anesthetic, a qualified healthcare provider, other than the CRNA, shall be available in the event neonatal assessment and resuscitation are required.

Interpretation:

The primary responsibility of the CRNA is to the patient receiving anesthesia for the obstetrical procedure.

(continued)

Table 14.4: Guidelines for the Management of the Obstetrical Patient for the Certified Registered Nurse Anesthetist (continued)

Guideline 6

Initiate, in the event of an emergency, anesthesia care in accordance with institutional policy.

Interpretation:

At a minimum, the policy should be congruent with the American College of Obstetrics and Gynecology (ACOG) guidelines. "Local circumstances must dictate the way in which these guidelines are best interpreted to meet the needs of the particular hospital, community or system. The nursing, anesthesia, neonatal resuscitation and obstetric personnel should be in the hospital or readily available. Readily available should be defined by each institution within the context of its resources and geographic location."

Guideline 7

Insure that postanesthesia care for the obstetrical patient is consistent with institutional policies.

Interpretation:

Departmental policies should define the resources required to provide high quality postanesthesia care to the parturient.

Adopted August 1998 to become effective January 1, 1999.

cal judgment. This illustrates the primary difference between standards and guidelines.

Guidelines are subject to change as new technology or procedures become available or are developed. As new information is communicated or specific issues and trends require an official position from a professional association, AANA will develop new guidelines and modify the existing ones.

POSITION STATEMENTS

Position statements are documents that recommend clinical practice or reflect emerging practice trends. Position statements may notify the practitioner of conduct related to clinical practice and of professional or generic issues related to anesthesia and nursing. Position statements related to clinical anesthesia practice are not published as standards by a professional organization, but may refer to a specific practice that is accepted and commonplace within the anesthesia profession. Accordingly, position statements, like practice guidelines, may form a functional standard although not labeled as such. As a functional standard, the statement would reflect the care that a reasonable and prudent anesthetist would provide to his or her patient in similar circumstances.

Tables 14.5 through 14.9 are AANA position statements related to clinical anesthesia practice. The position statement titled *Qualified Providers of Conscious Sedation,* first adopted by the AANA Board of Directors in 1991 (Table 14.5), provides guidelines for the administration of conscious sedation. The intent of the statement is the promotion of safe care to patients undergoing intravenous (IV) conscious sedation and to address questions raised by nursing organizations and healthcare facilities concerning the role of the registered nurse in conscious sedation. Table 14.6 lists specific recommendations for the treatment of malignant hyperthermia and references the Malignant Hyperthermia Association of the United States recommendations. The intent of this position statement is to increase the prac-

Table 14.5: No. 2.2, Qualified Providers of Conscious Sedation

The AANA believes the safest administration of conscious sedation is provided by a professional, educated in the specialty of anesthesia and skilled in the administration of conscious sedation, monitored anesthesia care, regional and general anesthesia, providing his or her sole attention to the patient.

Conscious sedation may easily become deep sedation or loss of consciousness because of the agents used as well as the physical status and drug sensitivities of the patient. The administration of conscious sedation requires continuous monitoring of the patient and the ability to respond immediately to any adverse reaction or complication. Conscious sedation should only be provided by an individual who is qualified to select and administer the appropriate agents and who is capable of managing all anesthetic levels and potential complications including airway management, intubation and resuscitation.

Registered nurses have become increasingly involved in assisting physicians in providing conscious sedation. The American Association of Nurse Anesthetists has developed *AANA Considerations for Policy Guidelines for the Registered Nurse Engaged in the Administration of Conscious Sedation*, to provide guidance for policy development and to promote the quality and safety of patient care when conscious sedation is administered by persons who are not qualified anesthesia providers.

Adopted by AANA Board of Directors, May 1988; revised April 1991 and June 1996

titioner's awareness of the need to be adequately prepared to treat suspected or unsuspected episodes of malignant hyperthermia. This position statement is also incorporated into the AANA standards relating to office-based anesthesia practice. Although portions of this position statement are supported by an extensive bibliography (which is not reprinted here), the statement is different from a practice guideline in that there is no procedural description for the diagnosis or treatment of malignant hyperthermia.

The position statements, *Administration of Regional Anesthesia* (Table 14.7), *Pain Management* (Table 14.8), and *Utilization of Invasive Monitoring Techniques* (Table 14.9), provide summary information of professional consensus for the CRNA to administer regional anesthesia, provide pain management modalities, and use invasive monitoring techniques. Statements such as these may assist the CRNA in the development of institutional and departmental policies regarding insertion of central venous, pulmonary artery, and arterial monitoring catheters, as well as the provision of pain management services.

CONSIDERATIONS FOR POLICY DEVELOPMENT

Anesthesia practitioners are often required to participate in policy development and interpretation. The AANA documents that relate to considerations for policy development are designed to assist CRNAs and other professional practitioners in this development process. Examples of such documents include *Considerations for Development of an Anesthesia Department Policy on Do-Not-Resuscitate Orders* (Table 14.10); *Considerations for Policy Guidelines for Registered Nurses Engaged in the Administration of Conscious Sedation,* (Table 14.11); and a minimum elements checklist for consideration in the establishment of an office-based anesthesia practice (see Table 14.1), which is now required as part of the AANA's *Standards for Office Based Anesthesia Practice* (August 2001).

Advisory statements, or practice parameters, are intended to assist in decision making in areas of patient care

Table 14.6: No 2.5, Preparedness for Treatment of Malignant Hyperthermia

Position: The American Association of Nurse Anesthetists (AANA) recommends that every anesthetizing location have a well-defined written protocol for the diagnosis and treatment of malignant hyperthermia.

The AANA recognizes the Malignant Hyperthermia Association of the United States (MHAUS) as experts in establishing protocol for the diagnosis and treatment of malignant hyperthermia and advocates that all anesthesia providers and healthcare facilities adhere to the MHAUS published recommendations.

The AANA believes that the following recommendations of MHAUS are essential practices which should be implemented by anesthesia providers and healthcare facilities:

1. All anesthesia departments and anesthesia providers should be prepared to treat a malignant hyperthermia episode. (A preoperative and intraoperative treatment protocol is available from MHAUS.)
2. All operating and recovery room personnel should be trained in the recognition and treatment of malignant hyperthermia. (Inservice materials can be provided by MHAUS.)
3. A designated cart containing dantrolene (36 vials) and the ancillary medications and equipment as recommended by MHAUS should be immediately available in the anesthetizing and recovery areas. (A listing of recommended supplies is available from MHAUS.)
4. A written treatment plan should be posted with the cart in appropriate area. (A poster is available from MHAUS.)
5. The 24-hour emergency hotline number of the MHAUS/Medical Alert Foundation should be posted on the cart and appropriate areas.

Purpose: To improve patient safety in anesthesia by increasing the awareness of the anesthesia provider of the necessity for thorough preparation to successfully manage a suspected or unsuspected occurrence of malignant hyperthermia.

Background: Malignant hyperthermia is a well-recognized syndrome which can occur in the presence of anesthesia. The morbidity of this syndrome can be quite high if it is not recognized and treated appropriately.

The American Association of Nurse Anesthetists believes that thorough preoperative screening and prevention is the first step in protecting the public. Despite the increased awareness among healthcare professionals and screening for personal and familial history of the disease, malignant hyperthermia still occurs. Because of the seriousness of this syndrome and the continued rate of occurrence, the AANA believes that measures should be taken for early detection and treatment of the disease process. With the trend toward more surgical procedures and anesthetics being performed in nontraditional settings, it is imperative that anesthesia practitioners be prepared to handle a malignant hyperthermia crisis in any and all anesthetizing locations.

NOTE: MHAUS publications referenced in this position statement can be obtained upon request from MHAUS at P.O. Box 1069, Sherburne, NY 13460-1069, (607) 674-7901. The MHAUS hotline telephone number is 1 800 MH HYPER (1-800-644-9737).

where scientific evidence is insufficient. Advisories are a synthesis of expert opinion, clinical feasibility, and consensus surveys. They are not intended to be standards of practice and may be accepted as is, modified, or rejected according to clinical needs and constraints. Parameters are intended to promote beneficial or desirable outcomes, but cannot guarantee any specific outcome. Variances in practice may be acceptable based upon the judgment of the practitioner.

SOURCES OF PROFESSIONAL STANDARDS

Standards relevant to anesthesia also orig-

Table 14.7: No. 2.6, Administration of Regional Anesthesia by Certified Registered Nurse Anesthetists

Position: Regional anesthesia can be administered by a CRNA who has received education and training in the administration of regional anesthetics.

Purpose: To recognize the current professional consensus regarding the administration of regional blocks by CRNAs.

Background: Regional anesthesia requires motor skills and can be performed safely by properly trained professionals. The scope and extent of this training is difficult to define. Didactic and clinical requirements can be set forth in a general way in the curriculum of the school, and these can be reviewed for evidence of fitness by the accrediting and credentialing bodies. Performance of a given number of the more common blocks could be made requisite to completion of the training program.

A point soon is reached, however, beyond which the identification of skill necessary to perform each blocking procedure becomes irrational. No one in anesthesia training, or in practice for that matter, performs all types of regional blocks. Certain fundamental precepts can be stated relative to the safe administration of local anesthetic drugs and to principles of asepsis, nerve localization and evaluation of the resulting analgesia. Beyond these basic principles, boundaries must be established by fiat and can prove troublesome to defend if exposed to close scrutiny. No statutory or regulatory preclusions for administration of regional anesthesia by CRNAs currently exist in the United States.

Overall, the risks related to regional anesthesia are no greater than those imposed by general anesthesia. To affirm the legitimacy of nurse anesthesia practice, and restrict the scope of practice at the same time, is to impose restraints that may be inimical to the health care of the community. The nurse anesthetist can function effectively only if all safe and satisfactory anesthetic procedures are made available and can be utilized on proper indication.

Title: Administration of Regional Anesthesia by Certified Registered Nurse Anesthetists

This position reinforces the prevailing positive attitude toward regional anesthesia performed by nurse anesthetists. Since many schools now incorporate this training as part of their programs, there would seem to be no need to belabor this position. Further, it would serve no useful purpose to draw boundaries. As the number of nurse anesthetists who administer blocks increases, the barriers will diminish. This is best developed in an atmosphere of peaceful evolution. The evidence of competent performance of blocks by nurse anesthetists is now overwhelming; the fact that this development is progressing rapidly is undeniable. Let it proceed.

Adopted by the Council on Nurse Anesthesia Practice, May 1978
Adopted by AANA Board of Directors, February 1989

inate from a number of ancillary sources. Additionally, individual practitioners often develop personal standards based on clinical habits (e.g., the use of a pericardial stethoscope or an anesthesia machine checkout list) that are repeated daily and become incorporated into the practice for that practitioner or a department of anesthesia.

Personal standards are acknowledged by Aker and Rupp (1994) as an original source of promulgated professional standards and may further evolve into consensus policies and procedures that are subsequently adopted by an anesthesia department to become "departmental standards." For example, anesthesia department policies address such issues as "nothing by mouth" policies formulated from clinical experience and scientific support of the morbidity associated with aspiration. Such policies outline the anesthesia care of the patient who is considered "at risk" for aspiration. The departmental policy is derived from the consensus of the department members who recognize that a rapid-sequence induction would be the standard of care for the

Table 14.8: No. 2.11, Position Statement on Pain Management

The management of pain is the central component of total anesthesia care. Recognizing the individual patient's right to the treatment of pain, nurse anesthetists acknowledge that it is their professional and ethical responsibility to participate in the management of pain.

By virtue of education and individual clinical experience, CRNAs possess the necessary knowledge and skills to employ therapeutic, physiological, pharmacological, and psychological modalities in the management of acute and chronic pain. CRNAs adhere to a total patient care philosophy directed at the promotion and maintenance of health and well being with special emphasis on the alleviation of pain.

Adopted by AANA Board of Directors June 1994
Revised by AANA Board of Directors June 1997

Table 14.9: No. 2.10, Certified Registered Nurse Anesthetists' Utilization of Invasive Monitoring Techniques

The practice of anesthesia requires adequate patient monitoring. Utilization of the technology assists the CRNA in observation and evaluation of the patient's condition throughout the preoperative, intraoperative and postoperative periods.

Through education and individual clinical experience, the CRNA receives the knowledge and skill to initiate and manage all aspects of invasive monitoring techniques deemed necessary to provide appropriate patient care. These techniques include, but are not limited to, the placement of arterial lines, central venous pressure lines, pulmonary artery catheters and transesophageal echo devices. CRNA capabilities to provide these services as a component of anesthesia care is an acknowledged fact as demonstrated by COA guidelines for accreditation,[1] and HCFA's[2] policy to reimburse CRNAs for providing the service. Studies indicate that CRNAs are involved and capable to perform these techniques.[3,4]

Adopted by AANA Board of Directors, June 1987
Revised by AANA Board of Directors, June 1997

Bibliography:

1. Standards for Accreditation of Nurse Anesthesia Educational Programs. Park Ridge, Illinois: Council on Accreditation of Nurse Anesthesia Educational Programs. 1994.
2. U. S. Department of Health and Human Services, Health Care Financing Administration, Baltimore, MD
3. Stein CS. A Patient Based Approach to Medical Direction Within the Anesthesia Care Team (MS Thesis, University of California, Los Angeles, 1994).
4. Fassett SL, Calmes, SH. April 1995. Perceptions by an Anesthesia Care Team on the Need for Medical Direction . *Journal of the American Association of Nurse Anesthetists* 63:No. 2:117-123

induction of general anesthesia to this patient. Additionally, the policy identifies a specified provision of care to patients and the expected practitioner behavior.

Nonprofessional sources, such as insurance companies, often introduce standards that have an impact on the administration of anesthesia. Medical malpractice insurance companies can and do mandate specific clinical behaviors, such as the use of specific monitoring devices, as requirements for insurance. The St. Paul Fire and Marine Company advised the anesthesia providers that it insured in 1986 to use pulse oximetry during each anesthesia procedure as well as encouraged the use of capnography. Currently, failure to

Table 14.10: No. 4.1, Considerations for Development of an Anesthesia Department Policy on Do-Not-Resuscitate Orders

Policy on Do-Not-Resuscitate Orders

The presence of a Do-Not-Resuscitate Order (DNR) can pose moral and ethical dilemmas for both the perioperative patient and the CRNA. Surgical intervention requiring an anesthetic may be medically indicated for a patient with a DNR order. The Patient Self Determination Act and the principle of patient autonomy establish the ethical right of a patient to make decisions about their medical care. Strict adherence to patient directives in support of their right to choose medical care can ignore the principle of professional autonomy and the integrity of the CRNA. CRNAs have obligations under the principles of beneficence and nonmaleficence which may conflict with the autonomous decisions of their patients.

The rationale for DNR orders is to acknowledge the patient's right to choose to die with dignity without prolonging his/her life by artificial means. In recognition of the fact that therapeutic interventions germane to the practice of anesthesia i.e., endotracheal intubation, controlled ventilation, administration of fluids and vasoactive drugs, might be deemed inappropriate interventions for a patient with a DNR order, the policy for a patient with a DNR order should be one of, "required reconsideration" (Cohen & Cohen). The DNR order should be discussed with the patient or, in the case of a patient no longer capable of independent decision making, his or her proxy. The conversation should be documented in the patient's chart. Documentation should include a summary of the agreed plan of care, the parties involved in the discussion and the circumstances under which the DNR order is to be restored, if suspended during the perioperative period. If the decision is made to retain the DNR order during surgery, the specific therapeutic anesthetic interventions that are to be withheld must be understood and documented in the patient's chart.

Background: Since December 1, 1992 hospitals that receive Medicare or Medicaid funds must advise patients of their right to execute advanced directives. In addition, hospitals seeking accreditation from the Joint Commission on Accreditation of Healthcare Organizations are required to have DNR policies. At one time it was deemed inappropriate for a patient with a DNR order to undergo surgery, today more and more patients present for palliative surgical procedures with DNR orders.

In many institutions the standard policy for patients undergoing surgical intervention and anesthesia in the OR is to automatically suspend the DNR order. Automatic suspension of the DNR order during the perioperative period fails to comply with the principle of patient autonomy and the patient's ethical right to make decisions about their medical care. In addition, if the patient or proxy is not informed of the automatic DNR suspension during the process of informed consent to surgery and anesthesia, then the validity of the informed consent is in question and the potential for a "wrongful life" suit is raised.

If the DNR order is retained during the perioperative period, serious moral and ethical issues are raised on behalf of the CRNA and other members of the surgical team. Automatic retention of the DNR order during perioperative anesthesia care may negate the professional autonomy of the healthcare provider to act in a manner that is consistent with their moral, ethical and professional values. The principle of beneficence requires health care providers to "do good" and the principle of non-maleficence requires them to "do no harm." These principles are violated when a patient's physiological response to the anesthetic requires therapeutic intervention by the CRNA that cannot be rendered because of a DNR order.

An either/or approach to the problem posed by a DNR order in the perioperative setting is ethically problematic. Adopting a policy statement that requires reconsideration of all DNR orders before patients undergo surgery and anesthesia demonstrates respect for patients rights, as well as respect for the CRNA's moral, ethical, and professional values. Required reconsideration provides all parties the opportunity to share information and clarify any misunderstandings about the goals of palliative surgical procedures and anesthesia care. Patients or their proxy may elect to suspend the DNR order once they realize that certain perioperative events require routine therapeutic anesthetic interventions that may be deemed inappropriate while a DNR order is in effect. Furthermore, if therapeutic anesthetic outcomes cannot be achieved or if the patient's condition deteriorates, the DNR order can be reinstated as agreed by all parties. The specific issues addressed during the conversation and the decisions reached must be

(continued)

Table 14.10: No. 4.1, Considerations for Development of an Anesthesia Department Policy on Do-Not-Resuscitate Orders (continued)
documented in the patient's record.
If the patient or proxy decides to retain the DNR order, the CRNA and other health care providers should honor the request. If the CRNA is not morally or ethically willing to honor the patient's request then the CRNA should facilitate the transfer of the patient's anesthesia care to a colleague who can abide by the patient's request.
Adopted by AANA Board of Directors, June 1994

monitor patients with pulse oximetry and capnography is considered a breach of the standard of care. Any insurance company strongly influences the development and use of standards by refusing to insure those who do not adhere to specific monitoring modalities and standards of care.

Federal agencies such as the Centers for Medicare & Medicaid Services (CMS; formerly the Health Care Financing Administration, or HCFA) continue to impact the development and use of standards. CMS has proposed broad, sweeping revisions to the hospital and ambulatory care standards, including stronger enforcement of compliance requirements.

Voluntary agencies for accreditation, such as the JCAHO, and more recently, accreditation agencies for the office ambulatory care setting, have expanded the capacity for the establishment of guidelines and standards of practice. For example, JCAHO and the American Association for Ambulatory Heath Care accreditation standards specify that a comprehensive preoperative and postoperative anesthesia assessment (a process standard) must be performed.

Equipment manufacturers and product standard organizations publish "voluntary" standards that assist practitioners in the operation, maintenance, or purchase of anesthesia-related equipment. An example is the Z-79 Committee of the American National Standards Institute. The Z-79 Committee is responsible for the development of standards for anesthesia machine construction as well as the construction and testing of endotracheal tubes, anesthesia ventilators, and oxygen analyzers. The Food and Drug Administration (FDA) is a federal agency that is responsible for published standards on anesthesia equipment. The FDA *Anesthesia Apparatus Checkout Recommendations* resulted in the development of preanesthesia checklists, which have evolved into an expected practitioner behavior in the clinical setting.

The determination of the standard of care by the judiciary also establishes new standards. As previously stated, the standard of care is expected to be the same in all settings. Anesthesia providers are generally required to meet a national standard of care. At the point in time that a judge or jury, based on testimony by an expert witness, determines this, a standard results. The testimony should convey factual information relative to the case being litigated. The opinions of these experts, if accepted by the judge or jury, assist in the establishment of new standards.

SUMMARY

Members of the profession are responsible for interpreting, disseminating, and applying practice standards and guidelines in their own institutions and individual practices. Although at present there is limited research evidence about

Table 14.11: No. 4.2, Considerations for Policy Guidelines for Registered Nurses Engaged in the Administration of Conscious Sedation

Introduction

Although the safest care for the patient receiving conscious sedation is provided by a qualified anesthesia provider, a large number of registered nurses are involved in the administration of conscious sedation. To promote safe care during conscious sedation and to address questions which have been raised by nursing organizations and health care institutions with respect to the necessary qualifications of registered nurses involved in this care, the American Association of Nurse Anesthetists suggests the following policy considerations. These considerations do not supersede or give the effect to more restrictive relevant laws, regulations, judicial and administrative decisions and interpretations, accepted standards and scopes of practice established by professional nursing organizations, or institutional policies applicable to registered nurses, which should be reviewed prior to the development of any conscious sedation policy.

Definition

Conscious sedation describes a medically controlled state of depressed consciousness that allows protective reflexes to be maintained. The patient retains the ability to independently maintain his or her airway and to respond purposefully to verbal commands and/or tactile stimulation. The American Society of Anesthesiologists (ASA) Task Force on Sedation and Analgesia has developed *Practice Guidelines for Sedation and Analgesia by Non-Anesthesiologists* which states "sedation and analgesia describes a state that allows patients to tolerate unpleasant procedures while maintaining adequate cardiorespiratory function and the ability to respond purposefully to verbal command and tactile stimulation. The Task Force decided that the term sedation and analgesia more accurately defines this therapeutic goal than does the more commonly used but imprecise term 'of conscious sedation.' Those patients whose only response is reflex withdrawal from a painful stimulus are sedated to a greater degree than encompassed by sedation/analgesia."

Conscious sedation may easily be converted to deep sedation and the loss of consciousness because of the agents used and the physical status and drug sensitivities of the individual patient. The administration of conscious sedation requires constant monitoring of the patient and ability of the administrator to respond immediately to any adverse reaction or complication. Vigilance of the administrator and the ability to recognize and intervene in the event complications or undesired outcomes arise are essential requirements for individuals administering conscious sedation.

A. Qualifications

1. The registered nurse is allowed by state law and institutional policy to administer conscious sedation.
2. The health care facility shall have in place an educational/credentialing mechanism which includes a process for evaluating and documenting the individual's competency relating to the management of patients receiving conscious sedation. Evaluation and documentation occur on a periodic basis.
3. The registered nurse managing and monitoring the care of patients receiving conscious sedation is able to:
   a. Demonstrate the acquired knowledge of anatomy, physiology, pharmacology, cardiac arrhythmia recognition and complications related to conscious sedation and medications.
   b. Assess the total patient care requirements before and during the administration of conscious sedation, including the recovery phase.
   c. Understand the principles of oxygen delivery, transport and uptake, respiratory physiology, as well as understand and use oxygen delivery devices.
   d. Recognize potential complications of conscious sedation for each type of agent being administered.

(continued)

Table 14.11: No. 4.2, Considerations for Policy Guidelines for Registered Nurses Engaged in the Administration of Conscious Sedation (continued)

e. Posses the competency to assess, diagnose, and intervene in the event of complications and institute appropriate interventions in compliance with orders or institutional protocols.

f. Demonstrate competency, through ACLS or PCLS, in airway management and resuscitation appropriate to the age of the patient.

4. The registered nurse administering conscious sedation understands the legal ramifications of providing this care and maintains appropriate liability insurance.

B. Management and Monitoring

Registered nurses who are not qualified anesthesia providers may be authorized to manage and monitor conscious sedation during therapeutic, diagnostic or surgical procedures if the following criteria are met. These criteria should be interpreted in a manner consistent with the remainder of this document.

1. Guidelines for patient monitoring, drug administration, and protocols for dealing with potential complications or emergency situations, developed in accordance with accepted standards of anesthesia practice, are available.
2. A qualified anesthesia provider or attending physician selects and orders the agents to achieve conscious sedation.
3. Registered nurses who are not qualified anesthesia providers should not administer agents classified as anesthetics, including but not limited to Ketamine, Propofol, Etomidate, Sodium Thiopental' Methohexital, Nitrous oxide and muscle relaxants.
4. The registered nurse managing and monitoring the patient receiving conscious sedation shall have no other responsibilities during the procedure.
5. Venous access shall be maintained for all patients having conscious sedation.
6. Supplemental oxygen shall be available for any patient receiving conscious sedation, and where appropriate in the post procedure period.
7. Documentation and monitoring of physiologic measurements including but not limited to blood pressure, respiratory rate, oxygen saturation, cardiac rate and rhythm, and level of consciousness should be recorded at least every 5 minutes.
8. An emergency cart must be immediately accessible to every location where conscious sedation is administered. This cart must include emergency resuscitative drugs, airway and ventilatory adjunct equipment, defibrillator, and a source for administration of 100% oxygen. A positive pressure breathing device, oxygen, suction and appropriate airways must be placed in each room where conscious sedation is administered.
9. Back-up personnel who are experts in airway management, emergency intubations, and advanced cardiopulmonary resuscitation must be available.
10. A qualified professional capable of managing complications which might arise is present in the facility and remains in the facility until the patient is stable.
11. A qualified professional authorized under institutional guidelines to discharge the patient remains in the facility to discharge the patient in accordance with established criteria of the facility.

Adopted By AANA Board of Directors, June 1996

the characteristics of how standard and guideline recommendations influence provider behavior, Grol and Grimshaw (1999) observed that there is greater acceptance if the standards and guidelines are reasonable, define expected performances clearly, and do not demand radical change. Therefore, the prudent professional association should focus on the development of standards that are tailored to the individual clinician and professional values.

CRNAs can anticipate multiple changes in the nurse anesthesia specialty. We will come under increasing pressure to deliver value-based care and to demonstrate the worth and quality of the care we deliver. To best serve the public and the nurse anesthesia profession, it is imperative that all CRNAs be aware of the practice standards, guidelines, and position statements of the professional organization. Each is a measure for the evaluation of the nurse anesthetist and a method to validate professional practice. The organization must continue its efforts to develop research-based standards of practice and practice guidelines. The profession must examine how standards and practice guidelines can be rapidly disseminated and used more effectively to enhance and promote the quality of clinical practice. The future clearly indicates increasing reliance on practice standards and guidelines with far-reaching implications for the profession's ability to maintain practice rights, reimbursement authority, and statutory and legal recognition.

REFERENCES

AHCPR. (1995). *Using Clinical Practice Guidelines to Evaluate Quality of Care*, 1. Agency for Health Care Policy and Research, 23.

Aker, J.G. & Rupp, R.R. (1994). Standards of Care in Anesthesia Practice. In S. Foster (Ed.), *Professional Aspects in Anesthesia* (pp. 89-112). Philadelphia, PA: F.A. Davis

American Association of Nurse Anesthetists. (1999). *Professional Practice Manual for Certified Registered Nurse Anesthetists.* American Association of Nurse Anesthetists. Park Ridge, IL: Author.

American Nurses' Association. (1998). *Legal Aspects of Standards and Guidelines for Clinical Nursing Practice.* Washington, DC: Author.

Bankert, M. (1989). *Watchful Care: A History of America's Nurse Anesthetists.* New York., NY: Continuum Publishing.

Blumenreich, G. (1991). The standard of care. *AANA Journal.* 55, 302.

Grol, R. & Grimshaw, J. (1999). Evidence-based implementation of evidenced-based medicine. *Journal on Quality Improvement.* 25, 503-513.

STUDY QUESTIONS

1. Discuss professional responsibility for the development of standards for patient care. Include reasons why professions would most likely develop standards.

2. Describe the implications for dissemination of new standards.

3. Practice standards and guidelines best serve the public health and the nursing profession when developed by the discipline of nursing. Why?

4. Clinical practice guidelines appear to be effective tools, in part, to ensure quality of care. Outline the main components of a clinical practice guideline. How is it different from standards?

5. Evidence-based outcomes support documentation of practitioner competency. Why is this true?

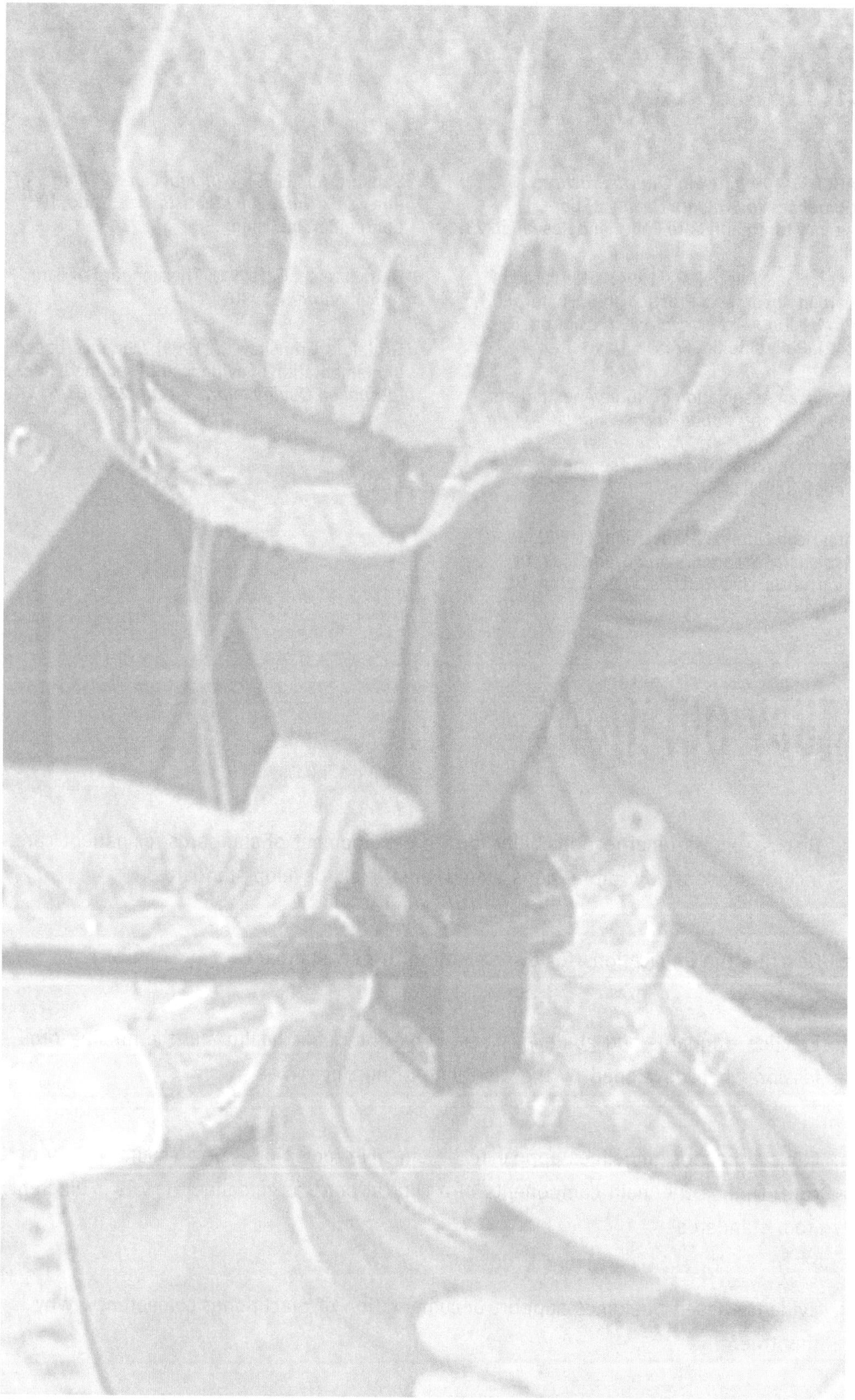

CHAPTER 15

REIMBURSEMENT FOR ANESTHESIA SERVICES

Lee S. Broadston

President and CEO
BCS, Incorporated
Waconia, MN

KEY CONCEPTS

- The reimbursement for anesthesia services is one of the most complex aspects of managing today's anesthesia practice. Unlike any other medical specialty, anesthesia reimbursement is very unique in that several case-specific components must be evaluated individually in order to determine professional fees.

- Reimbursement for anesthesia services involves the identification, utilization, and understanding of the present primary, secondary, and tertiary practice environments, a relative value charge system, gross and net revenue values, as well as a selected conversion factor.

- Detailed analysis of the practice's marketplace, case mix, and managed care penetration must also be indentified and included within the overall analysis and must incorporate potential revenue generated by today's Certified Registered Nurse Anesthetist (CRNA) in the nonoperative practice setting, which will more than likely be reimbursed under the separate resource-based relative value system.

- Achieving successful anesthesia reimbursement requires CRNAs to become aware of the numerous anesthesia reimbursement policies and procedures of their local Medicare Part A and Part B carrier and to be able to identify how these issues will impact reimbursement for anesthesia services.

- Maintaining successful anesthesia reimbursement is an ongoing process requiring routine involvement in each of the detailed avenues of anesthesia practice management. Ignoring even one aspect of these details will result in a potential revenue loss.

Understanding the numerous aspects of the reimbursement perspectives of today's anesthesia practice is an extremely important element in achieving and maintaining a successful practice. Today's practice environments demand precise clinical skills as well as equally defined practice management skills. Each of the contributing elements noted throughout this chapter must be initially identified and continually monitored throughout the life of the practice in order to maintain success.

Prior to January 1989, reimbursement for the professional services of anesthesia administration was primarily limited to the anesthesia services provided by a physician. At the federal legislative level, the enactment of the Omnibus Reconciliation Act of 1987 required the federal Medicare program to implement a separate payment within the professional services sector for the services provided by Certified Registered Nurse Anesthetists (CRNAs). This change was to become effective January 1, 1989. This sector of the Medicare program, titled Medicare Part B, would then be responsible for the reimbursement of nearly all services of CRNAs throughout the federal Medicare payer system. Up to this point, CRNA services were reimbursed to hospitals under Medicare Part A, which is the division of Medicare responsible for the hospital or institutional payment system of the program. This change in the reimbursement for CRNA services within the Medicare program was budget neutral, since the responsibility of reimbursement for CRNA services was simply being moved from the Medicare Part A program to the Medicare Part B program.

This simple change within the Medicare system triggered a much broader chain reaction throughout the healthcare reimbursement system that continues today. Now that Medicare would separately recognize the services provided by CRNAs, private health insurers and state public health plans began recognizing separate reimbursement for CRNA services as well. Although these changes have given birth to a much more even playing field with physician anesthesia providers, they have also proven to be a complex and often confusing area of the healthcare reimbursement arena. Today, reimbursement for CRNA services is many times ignored, overlooked, or assumed, all of which can result in a negative economic impact upon CRNAs within the healthcare marketplace. Today's healthcare spending is highly scrutinized; therefore, no reimbursement opportunities can be left untapped, including those present in the system for the services of CRNAs. The future of the profession relies on the ability of CRNAs to accurately understand the healthcare marketplace. CRNAs must be able to identify their worth, understand the reimbursement process, and assist their employer or secure for themselves through private practice the proper portion of today's healthcare dollar that is due for the services they provide.

ANESTHESIA PRACTICE ENVIRONMENTS

Anesthesia can be administered in a variety of settings with a varying combination of anesthesia providers and employment models. The combination of these practice elements can be classified into three subgroups: primary, secondary, and tertiary anesthesia practice environments. The primary anesthesia practice environment addresses the question of who employs the CRNAs in the practice—physician anesthesia providers, a hospital, or a CRNA group practice; the secondary anesthesia practice environment addresses the manner in which anesthesia services are delivered—physician anesthesia providers exclusively, CRNA anesthesia providers exclusively, physician anesthesia providers and CRNA anesthesia providers together without interaction, and last, physician anesthesia providers practicing with CRNA anesthesia providers, better known as the anesthesia care team (ACT). The third or tertiary anesthesia practice environment addresses and analyzes the financial and reimbursement aspect of the practice.

The Primary Anesthesia Practice Environment

There are numerous employment models in today's anesthesia services marketplace. The predominant three employment models for CRNAs are employment by a physician anesthesia provider group, a hospital, or a CRNA group practice. Each of these categories could easily have several models underneath them, such as partnership within a physician or CRNA group practice or hospital entity, true employment by the physician practice or CRNA group practice or hospital entity, or subcontractor type relationships between the physician group and/or a CRNA group or hospital entity. Each practice environment carries with it advantages and disadvantages that must be weighed to determine the best primary anesthesia practice environment for you and the practice in question.

Although some employment models have had a tendency to change quickly in the past few years, for the most part, the most secure practice environment is one of true employment by either a group practice or hospital entity. In this setting, employment benefits may be greater; however, the tradeoff will be lower salaries and more than likely some restrictions within the CRNA scope of practice. This will particularly occur within the physician group employment setting in the urban practice environment. In the more rural practice setting, CRNAs will more than likely be the primary anesthesia providers and therefore faced with a broad range of responsibilities ranging from clinical anesthesia to quality assurance data gathering and compiling, to department head responsibilities of inventory control, staff scheduling, and equipment procurement. The upside to this more rural practice environment will be greater salaries and fulfillment of the CRNA scope of practice. Smart hospital executives will evaluate and recognize that in the proper setting and under the proper practice circumstances, employment of both physicians and CRNAs will secure their facility the greatest reimbursement for these services.

Partnership with a physician or CRNA group can have several benefits along with some limitations and even legal obstructions. In many states, CRNAs and physicians cannot be true partners in certain types of corporate entities. Therefore, consultation with local legal representation is always necessary when evaluating a legal contract such as a partnership agreement. Partnerships, regardless of their legal structure, are in fact a form of self-employment. Self-employment, partnership, or even subcontracting carry with them issues that include the provision of start-up capital, cash flow development, benefits packages, and business office operations such as coding, billing, cash management, and patient accounting. Each of these issues is a piece of the partnership or self-employment pie and must be adequately addressed to ensure success. Benefits of self-employment can be greatly rewarding both clinically and financially. Oftentimes CRNAs in self-employment will generate an income far greater than their true employed colleagues (some as much as twice the current employment salaries); however, they must expect to face issues that these same colleagues do not have to deal with. Furthermore, each anesthesia practice must be evaluated for its ability or inability to support the independent level of practice. The best independent practice settings balance clinical with financial requirements to produce a positive outcome. What may appear as an excellent clinical practice may well be a poor revenue producer and subsequently would fail to support independent practice; therefore, a more traditional employment environment may be required.

The Secondary Anesthesia Practice Environment

There are four separately identifiable ways in which anesthesia services can be delivered. Each of these four delivery methods has a potential economic impact on the practice and therefore must be identified. Anesthesia administration can occur by the exclusive services of an anesthesiologist or by the exclusive services of a CRNA. Anesthesiologists and CRNAs can also practice exclusive of each other but within the same operating room system. Lastly, these two types of anesthesia providers can work together on the same surgical case in a practice arrangement referred to as the ACT.

Anesthesia Services Delivered Exclusively by Anesthesiologists

In this practice environment anesthesiologists provide 100 percent of all anesthesia services. These services would include the preanesthetic evaluation, prescribing the anesthesia plan, the full-time provision of all anesthesia administration, and postanesthesia care services, including discharge to the postanesthesia recovery area. Each anesthesiologist may be a part of a group practice or practicing independently. Although this delivery method makes up only a small percentage of the total anesthetics delivered annually to the patient population, this type of practice environment is often found in a facility that has had little history of working with CRNAs. Furthermore, the facilities where this practice environment is found have very little knowledge of the actual revenue that is generated from a private anesthesia practice. Consequently, the surgical staff at these facilities has been educated to believe that working with anesthesiologists is the best and only acceptable method of anesthesia delivery. Although the greatest percentages of anesthetics administered nationwide are done so by CRNAs, penetration into this practice environment by CRNAs is often quite difficult.

Anesthesia Services Delivered Exclusively by CRNAs

In a significant number of operating rooms across the nation, the anesthetics are administered 100 percent of the time by CRNAs without any anesthesiologists within the practice setting. Although this practice environment tends to be more rural than urban, CRNAs continue to increase their independence in the urban anesthesia marketplace as well. Under this practice environment the CRNAs can be employees of the facility in which they practice or independent contractors billing the facility for their professional services; or the CRNA group can be truly independent and operate completely autonomously of the facility, billing all patients and their subsequent third-party payers directly for all professional services. Under the true employment arrangement as well as the independent contractor arrangement, CRNAs allow the facility to bill for their professional services, while in the autonomous arrangement, the CRNA group is responsible for all aspects of billing and reimbursement. Regardless of who is performing the complex billing functions for the anesthesia services provided by the CRNAs, the CRNAs hold a moderate to significant level of responsibility in these activities, depending on their relationship with the facilities where they practice. CRNAs must understand that the only way in which their group or their employer will maximize reimbursement for their services is to be certain that the complex billing, coding, and related functions are completed in an accurate, timely, and efficient manner. Employed CRNA groups hold the fiscal responsibility to their facilities of making certain that these issues are adequately addressed as well. In today's bottom line-oriented healthcare marketplace, only those practices that are supported by maximized reimbursement will survive.

Assuming that the business office personnel of the facility understand and appropriately address the issues surrounding professional anesthesia reimbursement is a mistake. These individuals are oftentimes overworked and underpaid and focus on the larger ticket reimbursement items for the facility. It is only when a facility's administrative team goes looking for areas to reduce expenses that they frequently see a reimbursement shortfall in the area of professional anesthesia fees. By this time the CRNAs will have to put forth a much greater effort to address the problem and may not be allowed to adequately do so. The key to success in this area is for CRNAs to become educated and involved in the reimbursement process and do so early. The chief CRNA or department head should be routinely involved in all aspects surrounding the performance of the department, and reimbursement has now become a significant aspect of such performance evaluation.

Anesthesiologists and CRNAs Practicing with Limited Clinical Interaction

It is not uncommon to find anesthesia departments that are staffed with anesthesiologists and CRNAs, yet these two provider types will have no or limited clinical interaction. Both types of anesthesia providers run their own operating rooms and may call on one another for assistance in a specific time of clinical need or consultation. Under the right circumstances there is cooperation between the two provider groups, and these types of practices function quite satisfactorily. However, in the instances where these two provider groups compete heavily for the existing caseload, there are often difficulties. The realistic issues of case assignment, call coverage, and weekend coverage become stumbling blocks to a smooth operation. The oftentimes artificially created issues of surgeon liability and quality of care further complicate the situation to a point where constant friction exists between the two provider types. It has been proven best to resolve these types of issues between the two provider types without involving the facility's administrative teams; however, if the issues persist, administrative intervention may be likely. Economically, when these types of arrangements do encounter difficulties, the CRNAs typically experience a disproportionate level of call coverage, lower paying patient-payer or case-mix ratios, and problems obtaining case assignments with particular types of surgical specialists, such as orthopedists. The contractual agreement to provide coverage or the policies of the department should address these important issues. If they do not and an equitable arrangement cannot be reached between the two provider types, then administrative intervention may be required.

The Anesthesia Care Team

When an anesthesiologist chooses not to personally perform an anesthetic, but fulfills specific requirements outlined by the federal Medicare program, which include the criteria listed below, the anesthesiologist and the CRNA are considered a part of the ACT practice environment. The ACT setting is also commonly referred to as medically directing CRNAs.

Qualifying Medical Direction Criteria per the Medicare Carriers Manual Section 15018 Item C.

The anesthesiologist is deemed to have met the Medicare requirements for directing a CRNA in order to be reimbursed if the anesthesiologist does the following:

1. Performs a preanesthesia examination and evaluation.
2. Prescribes the anesthesia plan.
3. Personally participates in the most demanding aspects of the anesthesia plan if applicable, including induction and emergence.
4. Ensures that any procedures in the anesthesia plan that he or she does not perform are performed by a qualified individual.
5. Monitors the course of anesthesia administration at frequent intervals.
6. Remains physically present and available for immediate diagnosis and treatment of emergencies.
7. Provides indicated postanesthesia care.

Under current Medicare regulations, the anesthesiologist can medically direct no more than four concurrent CRNA-administered anesthetics. If at anytime the anesthesiologist is involved in more than four concurrent CRNA-administered anesthetics, then the anesthesiologist's service is termed supervising instead of medically directing. Supervising CRNAs allows only a maximum of four total procedure units with no direct relationship to case length. Through the billing process, CRNAs and anesthesiologists are required to utilize certain alphabetical code modifiers, indicating whether an anesthetic is medically directed or medically supervised by the anesthesiologist. These same Medicare regulations have come to be accepted as the general policy for the provision of anesthesia medical direction by anesthesiologists across some non-Medicare payer types, e.g., Medicaid, Blue Cross, managed care, and commercial/indemnity insurance products. It is important to note that most third-party payers do not recognize the service of medical direction or medical supervision of CRNAs and therefore do not allow payment for such medical services performed by the anesthesiologists. These limitations vary state by state, but generally speaking outside of the federal Medicare program and some state Medicaid and the Blue Cross plans, reimbursement for the medical direction services of an anesthesiologist of a CRNA are not a covered benefit. Hence, when submitted to the payer as medical direction or supervision services, these services are not payable by the third-party payer.

Identical to a CRNA practice, an anesthesiologist personally performing anesthesia services can administer as many as 1,000 anesthetics annually. This impressive potential pales in comparison with the fourfold increase many anesthesiologists can experience when working in a medical direction or ACT delivery mode instead of personally performing the anesthetic administration. The profitability of medically directing CRNAs can be artificially increased when the anesthesiologist is medically directing CRNAs who are not his/her employees. Essentially, in this scenario, the significant employment expense of the CRNA is the responsibility of the facility, and the anesthesiologist faces a relatively low practice cost. Anesthesiologists who medically direct facility-employed CRNAs often do so at the same conversion factors as their anesthesiologist counterparts who do employ CRNAs. Recognizing this low practice expense when the CRNAs are not employed by the anesthesiologist, many healthcare facilities are looking to the physician groups to take on the expense of the facility-based CRNA group by becoming their employer

The Tertiary Anesthesia Practice Environment

The tertiary anesthesia practice environment is essentially a result of the primary and secondary environments described earlier. The employment arrangement between a group of CRNAs and their facility and/or the anesthesiologist group will determine the financial viability and cost-effectiveness of the entire practice. Keep in mind that the most profitable relationship for the anesthesiologist group is not necessarily the most profitable position for either the CRNA group or the facility. It may also not be the most economical or efficient way to delivery anesthesia to the patient community. For example, in the practice environment that includes a separate anesthesiologist group medically directing a separate CRNA group, both providers or their employers are essentially seeking the same reimbursement dollar. As discussed earlier, the federal Medicare program and only a handful of other payers are willing to make a payment for anesthesia services to both the anesthesiologist group and the separate CRNA group. The remaining payers simply do not have the knowledge, understanding, or economic desire to create such an environment for anesthesia reimbursement and therefore will only make a single payment. This single payment is oftentimes made to the provider whose charge reaches the payer first. The charges from the other provider (physician, CRNA, or CRNA's employer) are routinely denied as a duplicate of the first. This sets up the paradox where both provider groups are seeking the same anesthesia reimbursement dollar. To alleviate this dilemma, alignment of the two groups needs to take place, thus achieving uniformity in the anesthesia billing process and resulting in the production of only one professional charge for both anesthesia service providers' services.

Provider Alignment Options

Anesthesiologists and CRNAs do not always make good business partners, and some states do not allow it to occur. If there is an understanding group of both anesthesiologists and CRNAs, the group may be able to be created assuming the state's business climate is conducive; however, forcing these two groups together generally results in distrust of one another and failure. A workable solution in this instance may be that the healthcare facility steps in and becomes the owner of the financial aspects of the practice. In this solution, the facility handles all aspects of patient account billing and owns the accounts receivable, thereby controlling all economic drivers within this practice environment. The healthcare facility then contracts or employs the two groups to perform their roles in the delivery of anesthesia services. This allows a harmonious relationship to exist without the economic pressures of two separate provider groups.

The facility also has the option to allow the alignment process to take place by allowing the anesthesiologist group to contract or employ the CRNA group. This alleviates the issues of two separate anesthesia provider groups seeking the same reimbursement dollar; however, it allows the economic drivers to remain within the anesthesiologist group. Furthermore, in doing so, the facility relinquishes all control over its operating room schedule and subsequent efficiency. The economic drivers of the medical direction practice environment will control the practice more than facility administration desires or patient care needs. This type of alignment has potential to result in a significant set of difficulties. For example, the anesthesiologist group will most likely not hire all of the CRNAs presently on staff, and the CRNAs of the group with the more aggressive and independent personalities may find themselves excluded from the group. The CRNAs with more at risk such as salary, retirement, and healthcare benefits will more than likely seek employment with the group in hopes of maintaining any or all of these important aspects of their employment. The final result is not necessarily inclusive of the best clinicians in the newly formed group practice, but does often contain the most controllable clinicians. This could have an adverse effect upon the quality of care and the overall performance of the group.

In the tertiary practice environment that includes a facility-employed group of CRNAs who are not medically directed by an anesthesiologist group, the facility can determine whether it wants to be in the anesthesia business at all. If the facility decides its goals and objectives include the employment of a CRNA group, then maximum anesthesia reimbursement should be achieved. Anesthesia procedure coding, charge development, reimbursement, and the billing process must be efficient and accurate. If this level of reimbursement cannot be achieved, then the facility may find it more cost-effective to simply remove itself from the anesthesia marketplace and recommend that the CRNA group become its own entity separate of the facility. In doing this the CRNA group will be responsible for all aspects of practice operation and responsible for its financial livelihood via the third-party reimbursement process. Assuming an average of 500 to 800 cases per year per CRNA are available with an average combination of payers, referred to as the practice's case mix, the practice should be able to support independence.

CRNAs should not make the decision to move into independent practice based solely on the fact that an independent practice opportunity is presented to them. The tertiary or economic practice environment must be evaluated in order to determine if the practice will support independence, if the practice will require facility financial assistance, or if independent practice cannot be economically achieved.

Identifying the tertiary practice environment simply equates to evaluating the overall economic impact of the primary and secondary practice environments. Although quality of care is the centerpiece of anesthesia delivery, the result of the economics of the practice environments will direct the overall practice organization and ultimate performance and, thus, the quality of care available to the patient community.

FEDERAL MEDICARE PART A REIMBURSEMENT FOR ANESTHESIA SERVICES

Pass-Through Costs

An essential part of any comprehensive practice evaluation is the identification and review of the presence of any regulations that may influence the practice. An example of an influencing regulation within an anesthesia practice would be the facility's participation or nonparticipation in the Medicare Part A pass-through process. In 1983, the federal Medicare program implemented the prospective payment system (PPS), which essentially produced a lump sum payment to hospitals based upon diagnosis-related groups (DRGs) for all services provided to a Medicare beneficiary. These payments came from Part A of the federal Medicare program. Without realizing it, this policy change assumed that the cost for CRNA services would come out of this DRG payment, yet the anesthesiologists would be allowed to bill Medicare directly and receive a separate payment from Medicare Part B. This created a disincentive to utilize CRNAs, since a hospital could shed itself of its CRNA staff and bring in an anesthesiologist group to provide all anesthesia services and allow this group to bill Medicare directly for their services. In doing so, the facilities not employing CRNAs could retain the same DRG payments from Medicare Part A.

The congressional response to this issue was the creation of the pass-through process. This process would allow a facility to be reimbursed for its CRNA expense from the Medicare program over and above the DRG payment of the PPS. This restored the equal playing field between anesthesiologists and CRNAs.

Under today's reimbursement system, which now allows for CRNAs or their employers to receive direct reimbursement from Medicare Part B, the pass-through process remains alive. The pass-through process is available only to smaller healthcare facilities that meet specific criteria. Generally if a hospital does not employ or contract with more than one full-time CRNA, does not employ or contract with any anesthesiologists, and performs fewer than 500 surgical procedures per year, the facility may qualify for the pass-through process. If this process is selected, the CRNA and the facility agree not to bill Medicare Part B for CRNA anesthesia services but rather include the costs of those services as they relate to the treatment of Medicare patients, in the annual Medicare Cost Report. Medicare will then return a portion of these CRNA expenses to the facility during the next calendar year.

As will be discussed in more detail later in this chapter, in evaluating a practice opportunity, the total number of surgical procedures performed per year must be identified. If this total is below 500, the CRNA should identify if the practice is operating under the pass-through process. A healthcare facility is not automatically included in the pass-through process and must elect it; therefore, a CRNA cannot make this assumption simply based upon the total number of surgical procedures performed. If the facility is using the pass-through process and the facility wants the CRNA to be independent and bill all services directly to third-party payers, the CRNA and the facility must comply with the agreement between Medicare and the facility. A facility receiving pass-through funding agrees not to submit a charge to the federal Medicare Part B program for any CRNA services provided at the facility. This includes the direct submission of any charges to the federal Medicare Part B program by the CRNA. Therefore, CRNAs evaluating this practice opportunity must realize that they will have to seek reimbursement for the services they perform for Medicare patients from the facility and not from Medicare Part B. Doing so would be a violation of the pass-through regulations and could potentially result in damage to both the CRNA and the facility. CRNAs who do work within pass-through facilities are free to negotiate whatever compensation they can with these facilities; reimbursement at the fee schedules set by Medicare may not be required.

THE RELATIVE VALUE SCALE

The terms relative value scale (RVS) and relative value guide (RVG) refer to types or methodologies of establishing a measurement of intensity for a particular anesthesia service. There are several versions of RVSs for anesthesia services known throughout the United States; however, there is only one such scale or methodology that has been adopted by the federal Medicare program. This adopted RVS is a modified version of the RVS that was developed by the American Society of Anesthesiologists (ASA), known as the ASA RVG.

An RVS is the most accurate methodology presently available to measure the intensity of the provision of anesthesia services for specific surgical and diagnostic procedures. The Medicare adopted RVS assigns various weights or units of measurement to various anatomical groups that correspond to the codes within the anesthesia section of the American Medical Association (AMA) publication, Current Procedure Terminology, Fourth Edition, more widely recognized as CPT-4. In addition to these weights of measurement or base values, as they are more commonly known, is the element of time as measured in 15-minute increments. The end result is a total number of units for the administration of a particular anesthetic. Therefore, utilizing the CPT-4 coding system coupled with the assigned weighted values produces a valid relationship between the procedure and the intensity of the anesthesia administration. It is recommended that the published RVS adopted by the federal Medicare program be utilized as the basis for establishing a measurement of the intensity of the professional aspect of anesthesia administration. The relative value method of measurement is a measurement methodology of only the intensity of a particular anesthesia service and should not be confused with a pricing methodology for professional services. Only after a conversion factor or dollar amount per unit is applied to the total number of procedure units does the adopted RVS become a basis for a professional anesthesia charge.

For example, an appendectomy with an anesthesia service duration of one hour would equate to the following under the Medicare adopted relative value scale: The *CPT-4* code 00840, "Anesthesia Services for Intraperitoneal Procedures," would be selected, which has a base value of six units. The duration of service is one hour, and when broken out into 15-minute increments, results in four time units. These two values when combined result in 10 total procedure units. Therefore, the measurement of the intensity or weight of this particular appendectomy is 10 relative value units. Only when these 10 relative value units are multiplied by a chosen conversion factor is an actual charge for anesthesia services generated. It is important to understand that if the duration of service were shorter or longer than in the example, the resulting intensity measurement and corresponding charge would also differ accordingly.

The Measurement of Anesthesia Time

The second component of the RVS is the addition of the duration of the anesthesia service in the form of 15-minute increments. Throughout the United States there are other methods of measuring the duration of an anesthetic. For example, there are measurements that reflect the exact minutes of service, 15-minute increments of service, and 10-minute increments of service. Historically, some anesthesia practices have chosen to utilize the 10-minute increments as a way of increasing their total procedure units; however, in some markets this could be interpreted as a form of up-charging. The federal Medicare program requires the reporting of exact minutes of service, while the most widely utilized measurement of the duration of service is 15-minute increments. Although a particular third-party payer may require the reporting of the duration of service in a specific way, it is extremely important that the anesthesia practice utilize the same methodology to measure time units for all services provided to all patients regardless of the payer that may be involved. In doing so the professional charge methodology remains the same for all services provided.

OBSTETRICAL ANESTHESIA SERVICES

The duration of service is often interpreted differently when anesthesia for labor and delivery is discussed. The definition of the duration of anesthesia services for labor/delivery should be equal to the face-to-face involvement of the anesthesia provider with the patient. Furthermore, this face-to-face time must be adequately documented in the patient's chart.

The customary obstetrical pain relief services, such as continuous epidural infusion and intrathecal narcotics, are services that are in addition to the anesthesia services provided to a cesarean section patient. Depending upon the type of anesthetic required for the cesarean section, the charges for these obstetrical pain services are in addition to the anesthetic required for the cesarean section itself. If a general anesthetic is administered, then the relative value for this procedure is in addition to the value established for the obstetrical pain services. However, if the cesarean section is completed under a type of anesthetic already administered as part of the obstetrical pain relief service, then the additional service charge is comprised solely of surgical time for the anesthetic administration. No base value or weight is added for the surgical procedure itself.

Healthcare facilities nationwide continue to broaden and enhance all aspects of obstetrical care. The addition of a comprehensive obstetrical pain relief service has become an integral part of these comprehensive services. More often than not, private anesthesiology practices tend to limit their involvement in providing a comprehensive 24-hour obstetrical pain service. The primary reasoning behind this limited involvement is the fact that obstetrical pain relief services are labor intensive and require the anesthesia provider to be close at hand to assist the patient for an extended period of time. Some private anesthesiology practices have lost significant contracts with healthcare facilities due to this limited stand on providing obstetrical pain relief services. When these circumstances occur, a door of opportunity opens for CRNAs. Therefore, CRNAs should be fully versed in all aspects of obstetrical pain relief services.

PAIN MANAGEMENT SERVICES

Chronic and acute pain management services are often provided by either CRNAs or anesthesiologists; such services may include single and continuous epidural injections or infusions, intrathecal injections, nerve blocks, and other regional blocks. From the third-party payer world, these services are viewed as medical services, not as anesthesia services. Recognized RVSs address pain services adequately; however, the federal Medicare program recognizes them as medical services and, therefore, subjects them to a different type of intensity measurement known as the resource-based relative value scale, more commonly referred to as RBRVS. The RBRVS is based on methodology similar to the anesthesia relative value scale; however, it has been developed to place an intensity measurement on all aspects of medical services provided to the patient community. Under either relative value measurement methodology, pain management services are based on a fixed weight or value, and time is not an element and therefore not a part of the weight or measurement. Hence, time is not normally a factor in developing a pain management service charge. Under the RBRVS system, this fixed weight is multiplied by an RBRVS conversion factor. The product is the allowable reimbursement under the RBRVS scale. The conversion factor utilized in the RBRVS calculation should not be confused with the conversion factor used in the anesthesia relative value computations. These are two separate conversion factors. For example, the federal Medicare fee schedule may calculate an anesthesia conversion factor of $16 per relative value unit, while for medical services the federal Medicare program may calculate an RBRVS conversion factor of $35.50 per RBRVS unit of measure.

Chronic and acute pain services are more frequently reimbursed under the Medicare RBRVS methodology from both Medicare and the commercial non-governmental payers. Therefore, it would be prudent for any pain management service to design its charge basis for chronic and acute pain management services around the RBRVS scale. The values assigned to all medical procedures by the federal Medicare program are available from many private organizations and also from the federal Medicare program via the Freedom of Information Act. A pain management practice should not adopt the RBRVS conversion factor or dollar amount per RBRVS unit, but rather only the weights or measurements of intensity by procedure. The conversion factor could be any amount selected by the group of providers.

ESTABLISHING A CONVERSION FACTOR FOR YOUR ANESTHESIA SERVICES

Once the decision has been made to utilize an RVS to place a measurement of intensity upon the anesthesia services provided by your practice, a conversion factor will have to be selected. A conversion factor or dollar amount per unit is the mechanism used to convert the RVS's intensity measurement into an actual charge for your services. Identifying the conversion factors of other practices within your geographical region may be difficult. A general idea of the conversion factors in the area can be used to assist in competitively selecting your conversion factor. If the factor is too great, the resulting gross charges will be too high and may reflect negatively upon your practice in the eyes of surgeons or the healthcare facility. Another method that may be used is to multiply the federal Medicare conversion factor for anesthesia services by 3.5 or 4. For example, if the local Medicare conversion factor is $15 per RVS unit, then multiplying it by 3.5 results in $52.50. This formula tends to produce a marketable rate and a place to start in considering unit conversion factors. If the local Blue Cross carrier openly publishes its contractual conversion factor for anesthesia services, this may also be a valid measurement. It is not necessary to place your conversion factor exactly at these identified local conversion factors, but a well-priced practice should not exceed the locally identified conversion factors by more than 10 percent or 12 percent. Exceeding the locally identified conversion factors for anesthesia services may result in an unrealistic accounts-receivable balance and difficulty supporting your chosen conversion factor should the issue arise.

The end result of the total procedure units multiplied by a chosen conversion factor is the gross revenue or gross charge for the services provided. In order to maintain compliance within your charge structure, this chosen conversion factor must remain the same for all patients treated within all financial classifications, e.g., Medicare, Medicaid, Blue Cross, and private pay.

The Billing Process for Anesthesia and Chronic and Acute Pain Management Services

Following the identification and evaluation of the environment encompassing your anesthesia practice, the adoption of a charge mechanism, such as an RVS, and the establishment of the practice's unit conversion factor, the practice is ready to prepare and submit charges for services provided.

The actual payers for today's healthcare services are broad and numerous. As will be discussed later in this chapter, the third-party payer world includes the federal Medicare program, the state Medicaid systems, private health maintenance organizations, preferred provider organizations, commercial and indemnity payers, and the U.S. military systems known as CHAMPUS and ChampVa. To understand the healthcare reimbursement process, you need to understand that the charges for healthcare services are divided into two basic groups, facilities/hospital charges and professional charges. Each of these two groups has its own billing and charge submission format. The charge submission format for facilities/hospitals is known as UB-92, an acronym for the Uniform Billing Act of 1982 that was revised in 1992. The charge submission format for professional charges is known as CMS-1500, an acronym for the Centers for Medicare & Medicaid Services 1500 claim format. Basically, institutional charges appear in the UB-92 format and professional services provided by independent or group providers appear on the CMS-1500 format.

The actual process of billing for anesthesia services and for chronic and acute pain management services is complex. This complexity is multiplied by the number of potential third-party payers in the reimbursement community, many of whom have their own specific requirements for the proper submission of professional charges. Unfortunately, uniformity does not exist. A claim that has all data elements completed in the correct 33-plus specific areas of the CMS-1500 format is referred to as a "clean claim." It is the goal of the healthcare provider to produce a clean claim and submit it to the correct payer the first time the claim is prepared. This will result in the most economical reimbursement for the services provided. Unfortunately, the production of a clean claim does not always guarantee prompt payment by a payer.

Generally speaking, all professional charges of healthcare providers that are submitted to Medicare, Medicaid, CHAMPUS, and nearly all third-party payers must appear on the CMS-1500. Some payers, including some state Medicaid plans, continue to have their own versions of the CMS-1500 that they require providers to utilize. This requirement further complicates the billing process. In general, these customized formats utilize data elements of the CMS-1500, however, the locations of the data are different on the actual format, and some unique data may be required. The CMS-1500 format can be presented for processing to the payer in either an electronic form known as the 1500 NSF (national standard format) or in a paper format such as the CMS-1500. The AMA adopted the use of the latest version of the format for professional services billing in August 1988, while CMS adopted the latest version in December 1990. The number of payers that continue to require providers to utilize their own versions of the 1500 claim format continues to decline; however, if you fail to utilize a payer's required claim format, your charges will be denied. The mass majority of patient accounting systems available to the healthcare community will prepare charges in the standard 1500 format; if yours does not and is not adaptable to the payer-specific CMS-1500 claim format, you will have to manually complete the form.

On the entire CMS-1500 claim format, there are 33 separate primary data elements or fields which may or may not need to be completed for the claim to be processed. The required data for these 33 fields is somewhat standardized; however, many payers have different case-specific data elements they want in certain locations on the CMS-1500 in order for the claim to be processed and paid. A payer-specific editing process by the provider should take place prior to claim submission to the payer to reduce the potential for claim denial. Several claim-editing software programs are available; some are quite sophisticated, yet few are able to be tailored to the unique specifics of any one payer. It is highly recommended that a provider not attempt to manually complete a CMS-1500.

Each of the 33 different fields on the CMS-1500 format is labeled with a number in the upper left corner of each field that signifies the field locator. These form locators can be separated into three different sections, each contributing an important piece of the overall picture of the services provided to the patient.

CMS-1500 Form Locators 1-11

This top portion of the CMS-1500 format is comprised of data regarding the patient and the responsible party or guarantor of the patient account. Items addressed include patient demographic information, the patient's primary and secondary insurance coverage and appropriate identification numbers, the patient's relationship to the insured, whether this service is the result of a work-related injury, and the patient's or responsible party's employment information. One example of the complex third-party payer requirements begins with this portion of the CMS-1500. Form locator 11 is the area where a secondary carrier would be indicated. Under Medicare Part B, a paper claim must have this field completed with the appropriate insurance information or in the case of no secondary coverage, the word "NONE" must appear in form locator 11. If this field is left blank, the paper claim will be denied and returned to the provider.

CMS-1500 Form Locators 12-13

These two sections of CMS-1500 are extremely important and often have different meanings to different payers. Form locator 12 is where the patient's signature or indication that the signature is on file with the provider must appear. The only acceptable phrase in this field other than the actual patient's signature is the phrase, "Signature on File"; if this field is left blank, the federal Medicare program will reject and return the claim to the provider. Completion of this field indicates that any medical records pertinent to the processing of these submitted charges be released by the patient to the third-party to whom the CMS-1500 has been submitted. The payer may utilize this information to determine whether the services provided were within the payer's definition of covered services. The signature itself appears on file with the facility and is obtained during the admission process. All providers should have as a part of their contractual agreement with the facilities in which they practice a phrase that allows them access to all medical records pertinent to the processing of a patient's charge. The patient's authorization to access the records for claims processing reasons has been obtained during the patient's admission to the treating facility.

Form locator 13 is where the patient's signature or indication that the signature is on file with the provider must appear. The only acceptable phrase in this field other than the actual patient's signature is the phrase, "Signature on File"; if this field is left blank, the federal Medicare program will reject and return the claim to the provider. Completion of this field indicates any benefits payable under the submitted payer will be paid directly to the provider of the services and bypass the patient. Although CRNAs are required to accept assignment from the Medicare Part B program and accept Medicare's allowance as payment in full and therefore receive direct payment from the Medicare Part B program, this form locator still must be completed. If this form locator is left blank and the claim is being submitted to a commercial payer, the payer will process any benefits due under the payer's agreement directly to the patient. This will increase the cash flow turnaround time for the provider and increase the potential for a collection problem. For all nongovernmental payers, the provider should obtain an assignment of payable benefits from the patient so that the charges can be immediately processed to the insurance carrier and payment made directly to the provider.

CMS-1500 Form Locators 14-24K

These fields provide all of the medical and procedural data related to the services being billed by the provider. These data include the date at which the illness or injury occurred, the hospitalization dates, dates the patient was unable to work, the name of the ordering or referring physician, and prior authorization indicators. This section includes critical presenting and historical diagnosis coding utilizing the *ICD-9-CM* coding system (*International Classification of Diseases, 9th Revision Clinical Modification*). Specialized coding for the place of service, the type of service (anesthesia is type of service 7), *CPT-4*, and the required modifiers relative to the services is provided. This section identifies the actual charge for the services provided, the frequency of the services provided or time involved, whether the services are related to family planning or of an emergency nature, and local payer-designated fields.

CMS-1500 Form Locators 25-30

These form locators provide data relative to identifying the provider of services; the provider's tax identification number; whether or not the claim is assigned to the provider; the total charges and amounts paid by other payers; and the balance due.

CMS-1500 Form Locators 31-33

These last three items of the CMS-1500 format are extremely critical to proper payment of the claim. These locators are frequently utilized differently by different payers. Form locator 31 states that the provider, or another qualified individual who was under his/her employ at the time the service was provided, did in fact provide the service. Form locator 32 states the name and address where the services were provided—a hospital, office, or ambulatory surgery center. Form locator 33 identifies the name of the group or entity to which the payer is to issue payment. The provider's mailing address must also appear in this section. Many payers will require a group identification number, or a payer-specific individual and/or group provider number in form locator 33. Many payers will reject a claim if the data in these fields do not

Figure 15.1: Health Insurance Claim Form

PLEASE DO NOT STAPLE IN THIS AREA

CARRIER

PICA **HEALTH INSURANCE CLAIM FORM** PICA

1. MEDICARE (Medicare #) MEDICAID (Medicaid #) CHAMPUS (Sponsor's SSN) CHAMPVA (VA File #) GROUP HEALTH PLAN (SSN or ID) FECA BLK LUNG (SSN) OTHER (ID)

1a. INSURED'S I.D. NUMBER (FOR PROGRAM IN ITEM 1)

2. PATIENT'S NAME (Last Name, First Name, Middle Initial)

3. PATIENT'S BIRTH DATE MM DD YY SEX M F

4. INSURED'S NAME (Last Name, First Name, Middle Initial)

5. PATIENT'S ADDRESS (No., Street)

6. PATIENT RELATIONSHIP TO INSURED Self Spouse Child Other

7. INSURED'S ADDRESS (No., Street)

CITY STATE

8. PATIENT STATUS Single Married Other

CITY STATE

ZIP CODE TELEPHONE (Include Area Code) ( )

Employed Full-Time Student Part-Time Student

ZIP CODE TELEPHONE (INCLUDE AREA CODE) ( )

9. OTHER INSURED'S NAME (Last Name, First Name, Middle Initial)

10. IS PATIENT'S CONDITION RELATED TO:

11. INSURED'S POLICY GROUP OR FECA NUMBER

a. OTHER INSURED'S POLICY OR GROUP NUMBER

a. EMPLOYMENT? (CURRENT OR PREVIOUS) YES NO

a. INSURED'S DATE OF BIRTH MM DD YY SEX M F

b. OTHER INSURED'S DATE OF BIRTH MM DD YY SEX M F

b. AUTO ACCIDENT? YES NO PLACE (State)

b. EMPLOYER'S NAME OR SCHOOL NAME

c. EMPLOYER'S NAME OR SCHOOL NAME

c. OTHER ACCIDENT? YES NO

c. INSURANCE PLAN NAME OR PROGRAM NAME

d. INSURANCE PLAN NAME OR PROGRAM NAME

10d. RESERVED FOR LOCAL USE

d. IS THERE ANOTHER HEALTH BENEFIT PLAN? YES NO *If yes*, return to and complete item 9 a-d.

READ BACK OF FORM BEFORE COMPLETING & SIGNING THIS FORM.

12. PATIENT'S OR AUTHORIZED PERSON'S SIGNATURE I authorize the release of any medical or other information necessary to process this claim. I also request payment of government benefits either to myself or to the party who accepts assignment below.

SIGNED ______ DATE ______

13. INSURED'S OR AUTHORIZED PERSON'S SIGNATURE I authorize payment of medical benefits to the undersigned physician or supplier for services described below.

SIGNED ______

PATIENT AND INSURED INFORMATION

14. DATE OF CURRENT: MM DD YY ILLNESS (First symptom) OR INJURY (Accident) OR PREGNANCY (LMP)

15. IF PATIENT HAS HAD SAME OR SIMILAR ILLNESS. GIVE FIRST DATE MM DD YY

16. DATES PATIENT UNABLE TO WORK IN CURRENT OCCUPATION FROM MM DD YY TO MM DD YY

17. NAME OF REFERRING PHYSICIAN OR OTHER SOURCE

17a. I.D. NUMBER OF REFERRING PHYSICIAN

18. HOSPITALIZATION DATES RELATED TO CURRENT SERVICES FROM MM DD YY TO MM DD YY

19. RESERVED FOR LOCAL USE

20. OUTSIDE LAB? YES NO $ CHARGES

21. DIAGNOSIS OR NATURE OF ILLNESS OR INJURY. (RELATE ITEMS 1,2,3 OR 4 TO ITEM 24E BY LINE)

1. ___ . ___ 3. ___ . ___

2. ___ . ___ 4. ___ . ___

22. MEDICAID RESUBMISSION CODE ORIGINAL REF. NO.

23. PRIOR AUTHORIZATION NUMBER

24. A DATE(S) OF SERVICE From MM DD YY To MM DD YY	B Place of Service	C Type of Service	D PROCEDURES, SERVICES, OR SUPPLIES (Explain Unusual Circumstances) CPT/HCPCS MODIFIER	E DIAGNOSIS CODE	F $ CHARGES	G DAYS OR UNITS	H EPSDT Family Plan	I EMG	J COB	K RESERVED FOR LOCAL USE
1										
2										
3										
4										
5										
6										

25. FEDERAL TAX I.D. NUMBER SSN EIN

26. PATIENT'S ACCOUNT NO.

27. ACCEPT ASSIGNMENT? (For govt. claims see back) YES NO

28. TOTAL CHARGE $

29. AMOUNT PAID $

30. BALANCE DUE $

31. SIGNATURE OF PHYSICIAN OR SUPPLIER INCLUDING DEGREES OR CREDENTIALS (I certify that the statements on the reverse apply to this bill and are made a part thereof.)

SIGNED DATE

32. NAME AND ADDRESS OF FACILITY WHERE SERVICES WERE RENDERED (If other than home or office)

33. PHYSICIAN'S, SUPPLIER'S BILLING NAME, ADDRESS, ZIP CODE & PHONE #

PIN# GRP#

PHYSICIAN OR SUPPLIER INFORMATION

(APPROVED BY **AMA** COUNCIL ON MEDICAL SERVICE 8/88) ***PLEASE PRINT OR TYPE*** APPROVED OMB-0938-0008 FORM HCFA-1500 (12-90), FORM RRB-1500, APPROVED OMB-1215-0055 FORM OWCP-1500, APPROVED OMB-0720-0001 (CHAMPUS)

match database information on this particular provider.

It is careless to assume that all payers require the same data in these fields. This is why the claim preparation procedure has become very complex. The ultimate result of an improperly completed CMS-1500 format—paper or electronic—is the rejection and nonpayment of a claim. Many payers have time limits within which they will accept and process claims. If a claim is rejected due to preparation errors and is not corrected and resubmitted within these time parameters, the payments for the services will be permanently denied. If this occurs with a state, federal, or contracted payer, the provider is prohibited by law or contractual commitment from holding the patient responsible for the cost of providing the services. The provider has only one choice: to absorb the cost of that service and reduce the balance on the account to zero by adjusting it off the accounts receivable.

THE *ICD-9-CM* CODING SYSTEM

International Classification of Diseases, 9th Revision, Clinical Modification

A specific alpha-numeric coding scheme has been developed to identify nearly every known medical condition. This coding document is referred to as the *International Classification of Diseases, 9th Revision, Clinical Modification,* but is more commonly referred to under the acronym *ICD-9-CM*. *ICD-9-CM* is a very technical coding process and should be done only by a certified coding individual who has completed one of the several educational and certification programs nationwide. These individuals maintain national certification through continuing education throughout their career. Every CMS-1500 format requires *ICD-9-CM* codes, and without such the claim will be rejected; therefore, coding process is very critical to correct processing and ultimate reimbursement.

The actual *ICD-9-CM* code itself can be numeric or alpha-numeric, with up to five digits, including a two-place decimal. For example, 650 and 789.06 are both valid *ICD-9-CM* codes. The greater the number of digits, the greater specificity of the code. Most payers require five-digit *ICD-9-CM* coding to ensure complete and accurate claim data. Codes that are too general are often returned for more information regarding the condition of the patient and the services provided. *ICD-9-CM* is updated annually in October, and it is important to note that as codes are changed and deleted, they should not continue to be used into the next calendar year. If a diagnosis needs to be coded from a previous year, only valid *ICD-9-CM* codes for that year should be used. *ICD-9-CM* coding should be left to those who are properly trained and accredited; however, every provider should be aware of *ICD-9-CM* and its relationship to reimbursement.

THE *CPT-4* CODING SYSTEM

Current Procedure Terminology, 4th Edition

The *CPT-4* coding system, developed by the AMA, is the nationally recognized method of identifying professional medical services provided to the patient community. Payers nationwide will require that at least one *CPT-4* code appear as part of the CMS-1500 format in order for payment processing to be completed. As noted earlier, *CPT-4* is divided into various sections such as anesthesia, surgery, medicine, and radiology. In the area of anesthesia practice management, the two sections of *CPT-4* that are used are the anesthesia and surgery sections. Certain payers will require the use of codes from one of these sections of *CPT-4*. It is the responsibility of the provider to determine which code is to be utilized for which payer. Ongoing research into payer specifics is the best method available to maintain an accurate database of which codes are required by which payers. Some payers will erroneously refer to the anesthesia section of *CPT-4* and "ASA Codes" and further confuse the issue.

The actual *CPT-4* codes are numeric codes with five places and no digits to the right of the decimal place. Examples of anesthesia *CPT-4* codes are 00142, 00840 and 00520; examples of surgical *CPT-4* codes are 52000, 59514 and 43239. *CPT-4* codes that end in a series of nines, such as 64999, are referred to as unlisted procedures and require documentation to support the services provided. Unlisted procedure codes are certain to delay reimbursement and should be used only when no other *CPT-4* code exists that best indicates the services provided. Examples of supportive documentation would include copies of operative, procedure, and/or anesthesia reports supporting the services being billed. There are also *CPT-4* codes that are very general. Using these general codes often results in return of the form for more information regarding the condition of the patient and the services provided. In either case (the 64999 code type or the general *CPT-4* code), claim processing will be delayed as the payer attempts to identify the procedures provided. *CPT-4* is updated annually in January. It is important to note that as codes are changed and deleted they should not be used into the next calendar year. If a procedure needs to be coded from a previous year, only valid *CPT-4* codes for the previous year should be used. A copy of *CPT-4* can be purchased through several publishers nationwide at a moderate cost. Coding of procedures should be left to those who are properly trained and credentialed; however, every provider should be aware of *CPT-4* and its relationship to reimbursement, and every provider should have access to a current publication.

THE THIRD-PARTY PAYER ENVIRONMENT

Public and Private Health Insurance Plans

In today's healthcare reimbursement arena, there are numerous players. These players may consist of employers, professional associations and labor unions, federal and state governmental agencies, commercial indemnity insurers, managed care entities, and physician-hospital organizations. These players are what make up the third-party payer environment. These players can be easily separated into two distinct groups, public agencies or organizations and private organizations. The public agencies tend to be highly regulated with relatively low reimbursement that is tied in some way to the federal Medicare fee schedules, while the private organizations tend to be more individual in their reimbursement strategies and tie their reimbursement more to historical regional reimbursement trends.

Public or Governmental Payers

The federal Medicare program, state Medicaid programs, and CHAMPUS, the payer for the nation's military personnel, are all examples of public or governmental third-party payers. The federal Medicare program is regulated by CMS (formerly the Health Care Financing Administration, or HCFA) and administered through specific intermediary payers throughout the country. Examples of these Medicare plan administrators or intermediary payers are specialty divisions of local Blue Cross and Blue Shield plans and commercial payers such as

Aetna and Heritage National Insurance. The federal Medicare program has numerous rules and regulations that must be followed in order to receive reimbursement and do so legally. Furthermore, if one or several of the required claim preparations are not properly completed, the Medicare program will simply reject the claim and return it to the provider for correction and resubmission. The federal Medicare program requires CRNAs and anesthesiologists to submit their claim data utilizing the anesthesia section of the current year's version of *CPT-4*. This information is coupled with the duration of anesthesia services to calculate the allowable reimbursement amount.

Although state Medicaid plans receive federal funding, they are regulated in the most part at the state level. This is particularly evident with regard to recognizing CRNAs as independent providers. The fact that CRNAs are a recognized provider by the federal Medicare program has helped in achieving state Medicaid plan recognition; however, it is not always a guarantee. Many state Medicaid plans attempt to parallel the federal Medicare plan when it comes to anesthesia reimbursement methodology, but many have dramatically lower conversion factors. Most state plans are very slow at processing claim data, are inefficient, and often produce erroneous claim payments. State Medicaid plans will vary as to which section of *CPT-4* they require for anesthesia claim processing, the anesthesia section or the surgical code section; therefore, it is important to learn the required processes for each state Medicaid plan within a particular practice. State Medicaid plans often have a strict rule for timely filing that allows them to process claims that are received only within a particular time frame following the date of service. Claims that are received outside of these tight requirements are denied and must be absorbed by the provider. Additionally, the state Medicaid plans place a heavy burden and redundancy upon all providers in requiring each provider involved in a particular Medicaid recipient's care to include pertinent medical record documentation supporting the medical need for the services provided. If these documents are not received with the claim data, the charges will be denied. In some cases, the charges cannot be resubmitted with the documentation or a corrected document since only one submission of the claim data is allowed.

The CHAMPUS program is the third-party payer for dependents of the nation's active military personnel and is administered through the Department of Defense. The CHAMPUS program will follow a traditional relative value system for anesthesia reimbursement; however, the reimbursement for anesthesia services may have maximum allowances placed upon it regardless of the duration of an anesthesia service. CHAMPUS payers, like the federal Medicare and state Medicaid plans, require all providers to have credentials with an assigned or designated provider identification number. The CHAMPUS plans contain many detailed regulations as well, and constant monitoring is required in order to maintain compliance with these regulations.

Commercial Managed Care Organizations and Private Organizations

In the private sector of the reimbursement arena, the providers may be organized into groups such as preferred provider organizations, health maintenance organizations, or physician hospital organizations. These organizations attempt to market their designated network of providers to certain employer groups throughout a region and direct the patient population into their hospital and provider networks in order to maximize utilization. Traditionally, a provider's reimbursement is governed under a form of a contractual commitment that identifies the provider's reimbursement methodology. These contractual commitments are sometimes very strict and do not allow any form of reimbursement to noncontracted providers, and others are more flexible and allow a reduced reimbursement to noncontracted providers. The goal is to direct the patient flow into the provider's networks to utilize the provider's groups of hospitals, clinics, physicians, and other healthcare providers. In some regions, these organizations are very powerful and can shift large percentages of a facility's or provider's patient base back and forth between provider networks year after year. Constant monitoring of these developing provider networks is necessary in order to maintain the practice's financial viability. It can be financially devastating to an anesthesia practice if the practice fails to be recognized by this type of plan. Research into the type of managed care plans currently in place and constant monitoring of the environment will help protect the livelihood of an anesthesia practice.

Traditional indemnity insurance plans are those that typically reimburse the provider of services without a predetermined written participation or reimbursement contract. These types of payers may represent as much as 10 percent to 20 percent of an anesthesia practice's patient case mix or as little as 2 percent to 3 percent. Since the reimbursement received from these payers will represent the greatest percentage of the whole reimbursement dollar, it is important to identify the percentage of the patient population that is represented by these types of third-party payers. Generally these payers will assess a submitted anesthesia charge by comparing it with regional and historical data from either their own claim database or data purchased from third-party vendors. They will attempt to reduce the submitted charge to whatever level their data support as usual and customary for the services provided and base their benefit payment to the provider upon this amount. A prudent practice manager will scrutinize these types of attempts to reduce reimbursement, and practices with a strong compliance program will not accept these payments as payments in full.

Managed Care Plans and Governmental Plans

Federal and state governments have adopted the perceived concept that managed healthcare can save them money. In adopting these concepts, both the federal Medicare program and many state Medicaid programs have moved from their traditional governmental administrative setting to the managed care setting with a private insurance carrier. For example, United Health Care is a large managed care organization (MCO) that operates managed care plans to replace the traditional Medicare and Medicaid plans in many states across the United States. Providers of service must be members of the MCO under a reimbursement and participation agreement and appropriately credentialed prior to being reimbursed for the services provided to the patient. Even though a provider may already have a provider identification number with the local Medicare office, the provider still must become a recognized provider with the MCO. In becoming a participating member of the MCO, the provider agrees not to bill the traditional payer, Medicare or Medicaid, but to bill the MCO for all services provided. It is possible in some markets to negotiate reimbursement that is over and above the reimbursement from the traditional Medicare and Medicaid plans. Oftentimes the contractual offerings of this type will be based on a percentage over the Medicare or Medicaid reimbursement levels. For example, an MCO may offer to reimburse providers in the Medicare/ Medicaid primary product line at 145 percent of the maximum allowable amount payable under the traditional Medicare Part B fee schedule. Beware, however, that these negotiations can have two sides. Some plans impose withholding stipulations that allow the MCO to pay the provider 145 percent of the Medicare allowable amounts but to withhold a percentage until the end of each calendar year and return it to the providers only if the plan is profitable. Additionally, many of these plans have timely filing stipulations, which clearly state that they will not pay any claims that are submitted after a specific number of days following the date of service. Frequently these timely filing stipulations are simply far too short and must be extended during the contract negotiations. If they are not extended at this time, there will be no way to alter the reimbursement contract once it is in place.

Other MCOs will attempt to limit the types of providers within their network. They may allow CRNAs into their network, but only a specific number of providers for a given population will be allowed in a particular region. Furthermore, some MCOs may attempt to limit the providers to only physician providers. Each of these types of MCOs must be approached individually, and negotiations must be separate with each one. It is not necessary to disclose specific contractual details with one competing MCO to another; just indicating that you are a provider with a competing MCO may be enough for the MCO to allow your practice to participate.

PRACTICE VALUATION AND DETERMINING YOUR WORTH

Althought it is different from practice evaluation, which may include evaluating all positive and negative aspects of a particular anesthesia staffing position, the process of practice valuation is very important as well. Practice valuation is the process by which a CRNA can attempt to place a monetary value on a particular practice. If the practice opportunity is an independent offering, the CRNA can determine if he/she can generate adequate income to support all of the providers needed to form the group. Furthermore, this same process can be used in an employment opportunity to place a monetary value on the services provided by a particular provider. The practice valuation data can then be used as a basis of discussion and comparison in negotiating salary offers. Certainly, in an employment offer the CRNA cannot expect to be compensated at a rate of 100 percent of the value of the services he/she provides to the group; however, a percentage of that value is an excellent place to begin.

By identifying specific criteria for a specific period about a specific practice opportunity or environment, a monetary valuation can be projected. The following are the minimum specific criteria that are necessary in order to make this determination:

- The period of time from which the data have been generated, e.g., monthly, quarterly, or annually.
- The primary practice environment, e.g., hospital employed, CRNA group employed, or physician employed.

- The secondary practice environment, e.g., medically directed or nonmedically directed anesthesia services.
- The total number of anesthetics administered during the period reviewed.
- The total number of relative value units generated (multiply the total number of anesthetics by the average number of relative value units per case of 10.5 units).
- The surgical case mix/payer mix breakdown, e.g., 15 percent commercial, 35 percent Medicare, 10 percent Medicaid.
- The specific reimbursement rates per relative value unit per section of the case mix/payer mix. If a specific unit rate is not available, use the selected usual and customary unit conversion factor for the group. For example, Medicare may be identified as $15 per unit, HMO Plus may be contracted at $30 per unit, and traditional commercial insurance should be calculated at the usual and customary rate of the group, which may be $40 per unit. To complete the valuation, the data outlined above are simply calculated out for each section of the case mix/payer mix.

As outlined in Table 15.1, each line or section of the case mix/payer mix is calculated at its identified conversion factors. The final sum is the financial valuation of the practice based upon the analyzed criteria.

The graphic illustration of the same data (Figure 15.2) can further illustrate the relationship between the various sections of the case mix/payer mix compo-

Table 15.1: Medprovider Scenario Matrix

BCS, Incorporated Practice Evaluation
Sample Practice Valuation
Anesthesia Gross and Net Revenue Generation

Total Gross Revenue	$1,512,000.00
Total Cases	3,600
Total Units	37,800.00
UCR Conversion	$40.00

Financial Class	Case Mix	Units	Conv. Fact	Net Revenue
Comm	15.00%	5,670.00	$40.00	$226,800.00
MGD Care	10.00%	3,780.00	$34.00	$128,520.00
Medicare	35.00%	13,230.00	$15.00	$198,450.00
Medicaid	10.00%	3,780.00	$15.00	$56,700.00
Self Pay	10.00%	3,780.00	$40.00	$151,200.00
Blue Cross	20.00%	7,560.00	$32.00	$241,920.00
Local MGD Care	.00%	.00	$.00	0
Other	.00%	.00	$.00	0
Total	**100.00%**	**37,800.00**		**$1,003,590.00**

Period of Time Covered: One Year.

Primary practice environment: CRNA group opportunity.
Secondary practice environment: Nonmedically directed CRNA group.
Total number of anesthetics for the period: 3,600.

Figure 15.2: Medprovider Scenario Matrix Charts

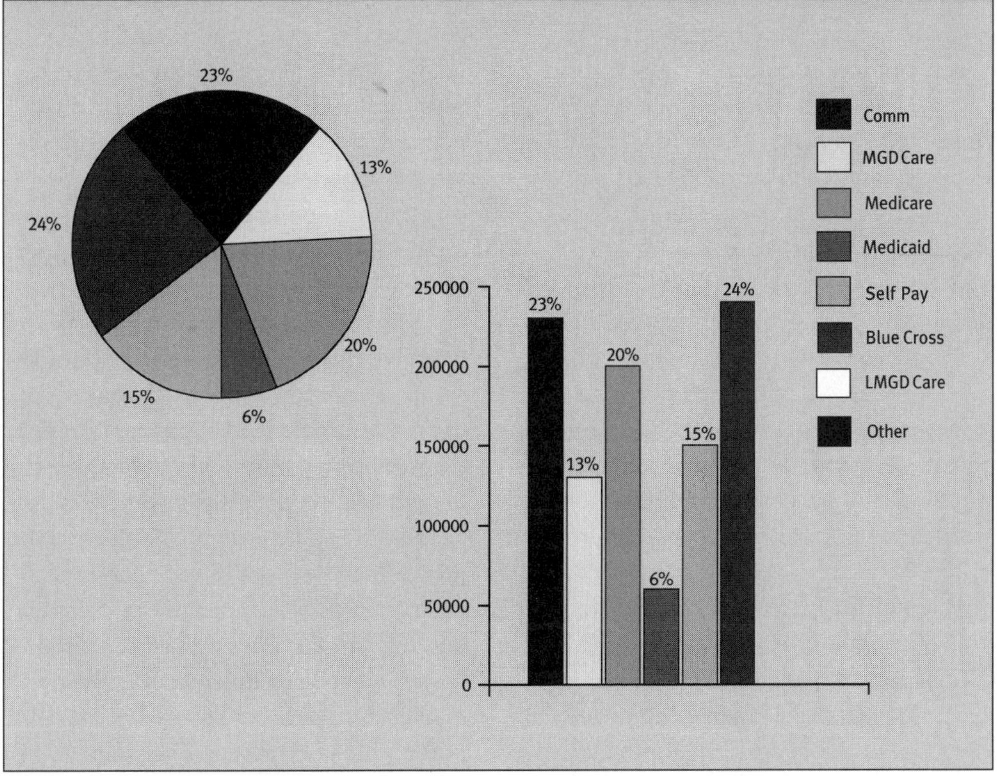

nents. For example, although the table indicates that the greatest percentage of cases are Medicare at 35 percent, the Medicare reimbursement is not the greatest contributor to the overall return to the group. In fact, the Medicare section of the case mix/payer mix results in only 24 percent of the total dollars returned to the practice. The greatest contributor to the overall return to the practice is generated from the Blue Cross section of the case mix/payer mix. This type of analysis is very important in determining the monetary generation capabilities of the practice and the impact of the various sections of the case mix/payer mix.

The results of this analysis can be quite interesting and often enlightening. It is very important, however, to realize that these estimates are simply that—a basis from which to evaluate opportunities or offerings. The estimated values of any practice are not something that should be shared outside the group of providers.

Although this practice valuation process is designed to produce only an estimate, this process is quite beneficial in determining the financial value of any of today's anesthesia practice opportunities.

SUMMARY

Understanding the numerous aspects of the reimbursement perspectives of today's anesthesia practice is an extremely important element in achieving and maintaining a successfully practice. Each of the contributing elements noted throughout this chapter not only must be initially identified, but also must be continually identified and monitored throughout the life of the practice in order to maintain success. Both the primary and secondary practice environments play key roles in correctly computing the tertiary practice environment. The impact of a correctly developed and supported charge for all anesthesia and related services is critical for practice survival and maximization of available reimbursement. Failure to properly identify and negotiate with the practice's third-party payers and to select correct procedure and diagnosis codes will further delay reimbursement and may damage the practice both politically and financially. Proper understanding of specific payer requirements within the actual billing process is essential. Furthermore, CRNAs must understand that these payer-specific requirements will change and, therefore, broad assumptions will always remain risky. The process of placing an estimated value on a practice can be quite beneficial during the overall practice evaluation process; however, the results are estimates, and a sudden change in any element within the many facets of the issues evaluated will result in a new estimated value. It is also important to understand that these estimates of practice value are developed privately and should not be readily shared among CRNA staffs or hospital/healthcare facility administrative teams. These estimates should be used for evaluation purposes only. Releasing this information inappropriately or indiscriminately may result in negative repercussions.

The services provided by CRNAs are in high demand and are an important key component in the clinical administration of anesthesia. As reimbursement pressures continue, more light is shed upon the critical role that is played by CRNAs as full-time anesthesia providers. It is the proper management of this economic pressure that determines the success or failure of an anesthesia practice; therefore, it must be evaluated correctly and managed properly to ensure the maximum return from the ever-changing reimbursement community.

REFERENCES

About ICD-9-CM. Retrieved February 25, 2002, from http://www.ahacentraloffice.org/coding/icd-9-cm_about.asp.

American Society of Anesthesiologists. (2000). *Relative Value Guide*. Park Ridge, Illinois.

Centers for Medicare & Medicaid Services ICD-9-CM Coordination and Maintenance Committee. Retrieved February 25, 2002, from http://www.hcfa.gov/medicare/icd9cm.htm.

Centers for Medicare & Medicaid Services—1500. Retrieved February 25, 2002, from http://www.hcfa.gov/pubforms/14_car/b42010.htm#_1_1.

American Medical Association. (1977). Medicare Carriers Manual. Chicago, IL.

Simonson, D. & Garde, J. F. (1994). Reimbursement for clinical services. In S. Foster & L. Jordan (Eds.), *Professional Aspects of Nurse Anesthesia Practice* (pp. 129-142). Philadelphia, PA: F.A. Davis.

MedProvider Scenario™ (1997). Anesthesia practice valuation software. BCS, Incorporated. Waconia, MN.

The Economics of Your Anesthesia Practice. (1998). Lecture series. BCS, Incorporated. Waconia, MN.

Understanding the Practice Management Jargon of Today's Anesthesia Practice. (1998). *A Glossary of Practice Management Terms*. BCS, Incorporated. Waconia, MN.

STUDY QUESTIONS

1. Define the primary, secondary, and tertiary anesthesia practice environments and indicate the significance of each environment.

2. In what ways can the practice environment of an anesthesia practice impact the success or failure of the economic performance of today's anesthesia practice?

3. Indicate three separate methods of determining a market-sensitive, usual and customary conversion factor for an anesthesia practice.

4. What economic impact, if any, on a hospital's anesthesia practice would the election of the Medicare pass-through program create?

5. What advantages or disadvantages did the shift from Medicare Part A to Medicare Part B for CRNA reimbursement create?

6. What role does the case mix/payer mix play in the determination and ongoing success of today's anesthesia practice?

7. What is the primary purpose of the coding systems commonly known as *CPT-4* and *ICD-9-CM*?

CHAPTER 16

THE ENTREPRENEURIAL SPIRIT

Larry G. Hornsby, CRNA, BS

Private Contractor
Birmingham, AL

KEY CONCEPTS

- The demand for contract employees in healthcare and other segments of the economy is increasing as a way to fill positions for highly skilled, high-demand professional personnel who can work for limited terms to meet temporary organizational needs.
- Contract personnel generally work for a higher wage than employed personnel, as their fees do not usually include typical benefit packages. They also generally work for shorter terms and are highly mobile.
- The reason Certified Registered Nurse Anesthetists (CRNAs) are reluctant to enter contracted situations is twofold. First, they usually desire the security of a full-time benefited position, and second, they are uncertain of their ability to successfully negotiate a contract.
- The key element to successful contractual employment generally involves an in-depth study and understanding of the needs the other party has and your ability to meet those needs better than anyone else. This requires a carefully detailed contractual plan to ensure all associated costs of business are included before a contract price is offered.
- In simple terms, most contracts consist of several sections, including definitions of competent parties, subject matter, legal considerations, mutuality of agreement, and mutuality of obligation. Contracts should also address issues of term, anti-competitive language, and escape or termination.

Nearly 80 percent of all Certified Registered Nurse Anesthetists (CRNAs) in the United States are employed by healthcare facilities or physician groups. In these types of employment relationships, salary and benefits are not usually delineated by formal contract, but rather in a work agreement, by professional appointment or some other type of informal arrangement that defines, at minimum, the employee's salary, benefits, and perhaps work hours. It is also usual that formal credentialing and privileging documents are part of this package. These detail the extent of the employee's ability to provide care according to the employee's education and experience. Within these arrangements, there is typically an implicit understanding by employees that they work within the policies, procedures and salary/benefit structure designed by the employer and/or medical staff. In short, there is little room for discussion or negotiation of terms involved in the work offered. Consequently, the traditional contract, per se, is rare in these work settings.

There are, however, a significant number of CRNAs who are working, not as employees, but as contracting professionals either in solo or group practice, as employees of other CRNAs or physician anesthesiologists, or as contracted employees to another independent individual, group, or agency who may, in turn, be under contract to a larger facility. These types of employment arrangements are most often described in detailed contracts between the parties involved. It is generally characteristic of these types of entrepreneureal practitioners that they provide anesthesia services for a global fee to a facility or other provider, either of which may be collecting reimbursements from public or private third-party payers or the facility or hospital with which they are contracting. Contractors work most often for a set salary and no benefits, although, of course, those details can be addressed differently in the contract. In short, contracting CRNAs work in a host of different employment arrangements for generally higher wages because they assume no claim to benefits as employees do. They do not enjoy the typical protections of due process (unless otherwise specified in the contract), and they are mobile in providing their services and are immediately available. In certain contracting situations, the wages are higher because the contractor assumes significant overhead costs (e.g., billing services, insurance, supplies, equipment).

The purpose of this chapter is to introduce the reader to alternative employment arrangements generally involving contracted services. This discussion is not comprehensive in scope or meant to constitute legal advice, but rather to provide a "flavor" for the role of what is commonly referred to as the "independent provider" or "solo practitioner." CRNAs who enter into contracted services should consider retaining the services of a professional accountant and attorney to ensure their rights and protection.

It is clear that the number of contracted, professional workers in anesthesia will likely increase in the future, parallel to trends in the U.S. workforce outside healthcare, in which highly skilled, specialized, and mobile professionals are sought to fill temporary needs. This is done in order for business and industry to remain flexible, attentive to changing market demand, and cost efficient.

WHO SEEKS THIS TYPE OF EMPLOYMENT ARRANGEMENT?

Perhaps the better question to ask is this:

What opportunities and responsibilities does this type of arrangement provide? First and foremost, it requires that a CRNA be fully confident in his or her abilities to practice independently, that is, capable of making decisions alone or with other professional consultants if they are available. It also requires that the CRNA be prepared in the full scope of practice, as CRNAs with limited skills will be of little use to a surgeon or facility. It demands that the CRNA be able to handle all risk categories of patients. The CRNA should be well acquainted with the standards of care of the profession, use good judgment in determining what is in the best interest of the patient, and always act or intervene within the boundaries of experience and qualification. Finally, CRNAs must be effective communicators, as without this skill, it is unlikely they will be able to secure productive or long-lasting contractual relationships.

CRNAs will often cite this type of work arrangement as providing them with greater latitude to select practice environments, assume a great range of responsibilities for anesthesia services, become more autonomous in decision making and, in short, exercise their full potential as anesthesia providers. There are also benefits of potentially higher wages, but with those benefits come increased responsibilities for making sure coverage is always provided and work hours are not confined to typical "shift" rotations. With new business responsibilities comes the need to find individual insurance coverage for self and family and potentially for employees. There are also numerous overhead costs associated with business management or ownership that often never occur to an employed worker. Clearly, with any great potential, there can be considerable risk. In order to enter the work of contracted employment, preparatory study, planning, and hard work in projecting potential success and roadblocks are vital first steps.

One of the most often cited barriers to CRNAs exploring entrepreneurial practice arrangements is that they feel ill at ease with their negotiating skills. Many believe that there is some well-kept secret about the true art of negotiation when, in fact, every CRNA has some ability to negotiate and many have great expertise. Think about how many times you gave something in order to gain something in return from a sibling, a parent, or a friend. Did you ever promise to do something in return for a favor or to win the opportunity to watch a particular movie or dine at a particular restaurant? So why is it the case that one could be so passionate about one of the aforementioned situations and feel so completely inept when faced with the prospect of negotiating a pay raise with the boss or a contract with a facility? Perhaps it is related to the adage of "fearing the unknown."

A PERSONAL STORY

I started my first corporation in 1993 and the first step, in fact the cornerstone of the business, hinged on my ability to convince a board of directors that I could deliver a group practice that would be advantageous for the facility over the other alternatives they might consider. To say that I experienced anxiety prior to facing that board would be a tremendous understatement. In reality, the only way that I could possibly accomplish my mission was to be successful at my "first time at bat." The important fact is that I did go to the plate to take my swing. Far too many CRNAs have the opportunity and the ability to be successful in this practice arrangement, but decide not to proceed because they fear the first step—the negotiation that could lead to that first contract. So how do you prepare for such an occasion?

Preparing to Offer a Contract

Do your homework and know the facts about your potential contracted partner. You must first know the needs of the facility and have a plan as to how you can address its needs. How do you get that information? If it is a new facility and has yet to do a case, you must learn the characteristics of the facility. How many surgeons will be utilizing your services and what are the expectations of these individuals? What specialties are represented and are you in a community that can reasonably support these procedures? If you are looking at an existing facility, then what created the potential for change that has involved you? Is the facility adding anesthesia for the first time or does it currently have anesthesia services available and want to make a change? These two scenarios present you with incredibly different informational needs and will likely result in very different expectations during the negotiations.

If the facility has been providing anesthesia services, ask for the payer mix and the surgery schedules for the past 12 months. You may then have a billing agent review the cases performed and make an estimation based on factual information that will provide you with some idea of the financial forecast for the future. This information will provide a tremendous advantage as you negotiate particular terms of the contract.

What is it that you can do that the others cannot or will not do? If you are involved in a situation where the facility is unhappy with its current provider(s), then remember to concentrate on what you do well rather than what the others do poorly. Never enter the situation with a negative position on the competition, but continue to accentuate the positive aspects of your proposal. Concentrate efforts on demonstrating, with objective criteria, how you can bring a solution to the facility's needs or problems by doing what you do well. Never expect to reach your goals by pointing out the shortcomings of the competing group.

Can you provide the services that the facility desires in a cost-effective fashion? Can you decrease it's cost while providing an equal or improved service? If the cost is too great, it is unlikely that you will get the opportunity to demonstrate what great service you can provide. No matter how wonderful the service, if you cannot manage a profit, it is unlikely that your business venture will last very long. Can you identify your competition and determine the things that you can do better? Did another group fail because it underbid the contract and experienced financial difficulty?

Formulating a Contractual Plan

When you feel confident you can meet the requirements of the facility, you are in a position to formulate a plan, determine cost, and develop a fee schedule or contract price that will become the basis for the proposal. This is a critical stage, as an error here could have long-term negative implications. Generally speaking, when formulating a plan, overestimate cost and overhead and underestimate income and profit. Formulate more than one plan in order to remain flexible in case new needs or concerns you had not anticipated are expressed by the persons involved. You must be preparing long before you reach the table, and that preparation will give you the confidence to move forward through the process. Table 16.1 provides a conceptual idea of a contractual plan, listing items that should be considered. This is not an exhaustive list, as inclusions will necessarily vary on the basis of circumstances.

Table 16.1: Elements of a Contractual Plan

Considerations for Individual Employee Contract

- Salary or hourly rate versus guaranteed daily minimum compensation
- Actual cost of liability insurance based on mature premium
- Paid vacation and cost of coverage
- Employer taxes
- Payroll expenses and accounting costs
- Pension contribution, including maintenance costs and accounting fees
- Paid sick leave and cost of coverage

Considerations for Facility Contract

- Professional staffing costs, including benefit packages
- Facility expectations for call and overtime
- Utilization of available operating rooms (multiple morning startups versus to-follow cases)
- Recruitment fees
- Legal fees
- Accounting fees
- Equipment and supplies
- Administrative costs and office space
- Department requirements (e.g., committees, continuous quality improvement work)
- Potential for earnings outside contract (e.g., pain management)

It is critical that you understand exactly what services, supplies, equipment, and staff the facility expects you to provide. Determine the number of days per week and hours per day required and any expectation of after-hours call or holiday coverage. These are areas that could greatly increase your cost and must be anticipated in the proposal. If you are preparing a proposal on a fee-for-service basis, you must have accurate information on the payer mix, total number of cases, and average time per case. It is advisable to have a reputable billing agent review the cases and apply the payer mix to provide some estimate of past revenue. Consider sharing your information with an accountant experienced with similar businesses to evaluate staffing costs and state, county, and city fees. Proceed only after you have sufficient information to prepare a written proposal.

Submitting the Proposal

The proposal should be delivered along with a biographical sketch of your business and the individuals involved in providing the service. These descriptions should be concise and provide information to demonstrate that you can deliver the service that you are proposing. Do not underestimate the importance of this contract feature, as you could easily be in a situation of having a financial position very similar to a competing proposal, and the scales may be tipped in your favor based on your qualifications and a well-executed biographical sketch. Once submitted, you should make a follow-up phone call and send a letter thanking the business for the opportunity to submit your proposal and offer to answer any questions that may arise. It would also be appropriate to ask what time frame to expect for the interview process.

At this point, you must wait to see if you are invited for an interview. Eventually, you will be notified that your proposal was rejected, accepted as submitted or, most likely, that you are being invited for a personal meeting with the administrator. If your proposal was rejected, be very professional. Submit a follow-up letter, thank the person for the opportunity, and offer to be of assistance in the future. If your offer was accepted as written, you can assume that yours was the only proposal on the table, that you were superior to the competitors, or that you were less expensive. The latter would be a cause for concern and should make you question whether you missed something critical in calculating cost. It would be most unlikely that any proposal would be accepted without a face-to-face meeting with the decision-making authorities of the facility. The most likely scenario would be that the person (or group representative) submitting the top two, three, or four proposals would be called in for an interview.

This is the part of the process that seems to be the most difficult for many. It is the time that you must be prepared to defend your position and still be flexible, to a point. Again, ask some questions and do your homework. When you are scheduling your appointment, take this opportunity to collect data. Ask who you will be meeting with. If it is a group of people, find out how many so you can provide them with any additional information that you think is necessary or important. Offer to send each of them an individual copy of the proposal and take that as an opportunity to provide a personalized cover letter to each. You should ask how many proposals are being considered and ask who they are from. You may not be given that much information, but it will not hurt to ask. If you can determine the competition, take the opportunity to learn all that you can about them and any personal connections that they might have with those who will make the decision. You may find the going a little difficult if your competition is the brother-in-law of the administrator.

Once you have obtained all information possible, review the financial data that was the basis for your original proposal and formulate your final plan for the meeting. I strongly suggest that you establish firm goals and write them down. List all of the issues that are important to you, and then prioritize the list. It is unusual for the final decision to be based only on cost. The true nature of most negotiated settlements will involve two, three, or four issues that are central to one or more of the parties involved. This concept will separate the negotiator from the one who haggles over price. Know your goals, and perhaps more important, know your limitations and always understand that all business is not good business. Be willing to walk away if you cannot reach a settlement that offers some advantage to you or would place you in a situation of delivering substandard services. Your reputation as a provider of quality anesthesia care is of far greater value than any contract and should never be subject to question.

Once the meeting is over, attempt to determine the time period for the final decision, submit a follow-up letter of thanks, and go on with the activities of your business. If you are notified that you were not selected, attempt to determine why. Was it cost or was it something that you could not deliver? This is important information that can help you in your next attempt. If your offer was accepted, then begin preparation for the next important step.

The Contract

Before discussing various aspects of a typical contract, be reminded that this narrative does not constitute legal advice. That should come from an attorney familiar with contract law. I am frequently asked by other anesthetists if it is necessary to have a written contract. I have worked in several situations without a written agreement, but I do not encourage it and do not believe it is in either party's best interest to proceed without a signed agreement, even if it is a very simple document. The negotiating process described above can be very labor intensive, and you may spend months or years negotiating, working toward an agreement with a facility. After that much effort, it is not a sound business decision to begin service without a written agreement that will specifically address all of the issues that were of such great importance during the negotiation.

In simple terms, a contract is an agreement between two or more persons that creates an obligation to do or not to do particular things. Its essentials are competent parties, subject matter, legal considerations, mutuality of agreement, and mutuality of obligation. It is essential that you know who has the authority to enter into a contractual agreement as early in the process as possible, so that you do not reach an agreement with one individual only to learn that he or she is not the final decision maker. You will find it common practice to negotiate with an administrator, CEO, or even an office manager, when ultimately the contract will need approval by a board of directors, partners, or owners whom you may have never met.

After the agreement is reached, you should meet again to address specifics of the contract. I would make a point of insisting that the decision-makers be present for this meeting, if at all possible. Also, this may be a meeting at which you would consider having your attorney present to be certain all key issues are included. My personal preference is to have my corporate attorney prepare the contract, even if it is at my expense, as it provides me with some degree of confidence that there is nothing problematic hidden in the legal terminology. After the document is completed, both parties should have their own legal review performed, and only then should either consider signing the document. Never allow anyone to rush you to sign. If you are uncomfortable about a clause, say so and state that you must have legal counsel before proceeding. Never attempt to rush the other party. Allow time for adequate review and always understand that legal concerns could result in further negotiations that may alter the original agreement or make the entire document void and result in starting the entire process over again. This is literally the last opportunity to correct a problem that you may otherwise be forced to live with for the duration of the contractual period. Use the time wisely, and take this opportunity seriously.

Other Contractual Considerations

If you are an independent contractor and enter into an agreement with a group that is sending you to practice at different facilities, it is likely that you will sign a document with strong anticompetitive language. Any anticompete clause should have a reasonably well-defined geographical radius and a set time limitation. This clause offers protection to the employer that you will not go into "their" facility and negotiate an arrangement that would displace them, resulting in loss of revenue for them. If you are working for an agency, it is also likely that the agency will have a clause in the contract with the facility that would require the facility to pay a fee should the facility employ any individual who has worked at the facility as an agency employee.

Another specific part of the contractual relationship that should be discussed is the escape or termination clause. This should be included as a part of the contract in any of the relationships identified previously. This offers a degree of protection to both entities that the contract can be terminated by specifying a time when notice must be given before either party can end the relationship. For example, I entered into a contractual agreement with a hospital several years ago, and the termination clause was written such that termination for any reason was not possible for the first year, and after that either party could terminate the relationship with 90 days' written notification. Most agree that 30 days would be a minimum and honestly offers little protection for the employer in a market where providers are difficult to find. Termination clauses can require as much as 180-day notification, but the 90-day period usually allows either party to make arrangements for the transition without prolonging a potentially uncomfortable situation.

Finally, the term of the contract should be specified. The most common term is for a one-year period with a clause that will automatically renew the contract unless either party chooses to renegotiate some portion at the date of renewal. Usually one party will be required to notify the other within a specified time period to make a change. If neither party wishes to change the agreement, it will simply continue as written for the next 12-month period. It is also possible to have a specified time period until the contract terminates when parties meet and discuss terms. Examine this carefully and determine what you are comfortable with based on the circumstances. For example, a three- to a five-year arrangement is advisable in most situations, as there is so much effort required to start up and staff a new point of service. A potential problem could occur should this location be one in which you are agreeing on a fixed contract price and the cost of labor suddenly rises during this period. Suddenly, the arrangement becomes unprofitable before the end of the contractual relationship. The only relief is offered by a well-written escape clause.

Make certain that the contract clearly defines the services that you are agreeing to provide, as well as those not provided. Some situations may be specific to the hours per day and the days per week, while others may specify only that anesthesia services be provided during normal business hours, leaving those hours to be defined by the facility. Another important consideration would be any additional services that might be outside of the contracted fee, such as pain management; after-hours, on-call services; and certainly any equipment or supplies that either party would be expected to provide. A good example would be a surgeon who has decided to open a surgical area and requires anesthesia services. You may enter into an agreement to provide the service and then learn that the physician's understanding was that you would also provide the equipment, supplies, and pharmaceuticals necessary. Again, it is best to have all of this spelled out in the initial agreement so that there is no misunderstanding when the service is implemented. It is always much easier to agree going into a situation than to settle a dispute after a problem has occurred.

It is not possible to cover every situation that could create a dispute in the written contract. I would not suggest that you attempt to accomplish this, nor do I believe it necessary. The contract should not be considered a replacement for ethical and honest business practice, but more of a "road map" that establishes the major points of the agreement and establishes boundaries for both parties to work within. Many continue to work with a verbal agreement and a handshake, believing that a written contract is only for those you do not trust. I would suggest that a contract is a necessary agreement between professionals and point out that it is unlikely that you will have any legal recourse should a problem occur unless you have a written contractual relationship.

SUMMARY

As in any work or employment relationship, all parties should concentrate first on delivering the finest anesthesia care available. Surround yourself with good people, and seek advice from an attorney and accountant when necessary. Never go into a meeting unprepared, and never surrender opportunity for security. Prepare yourself today to grasp tomorrow's possibilities in a 21st-century marketplace.

STUDY QUESTIONS

1. Discuss among peers your perceptions of how the roles and responsibilities of employed CRNAs may be different from those of contracted CRNAs.

2. What are some of the considerations you would have to make in planning a contract price for services? In other words, what associated business costs must be considered in proposing a fee structure that would be inclusive of all potential costs?

3. What are the elements of a typical contract for services? What is the basic role of each, and why would it be important for defining your relationship with the other contracted party?

4. What are some of the basic "rules of thumb" one should remember in negotiating a contract? What "values" should never be compromised?

THE POLITICS OF HEALTHCARE

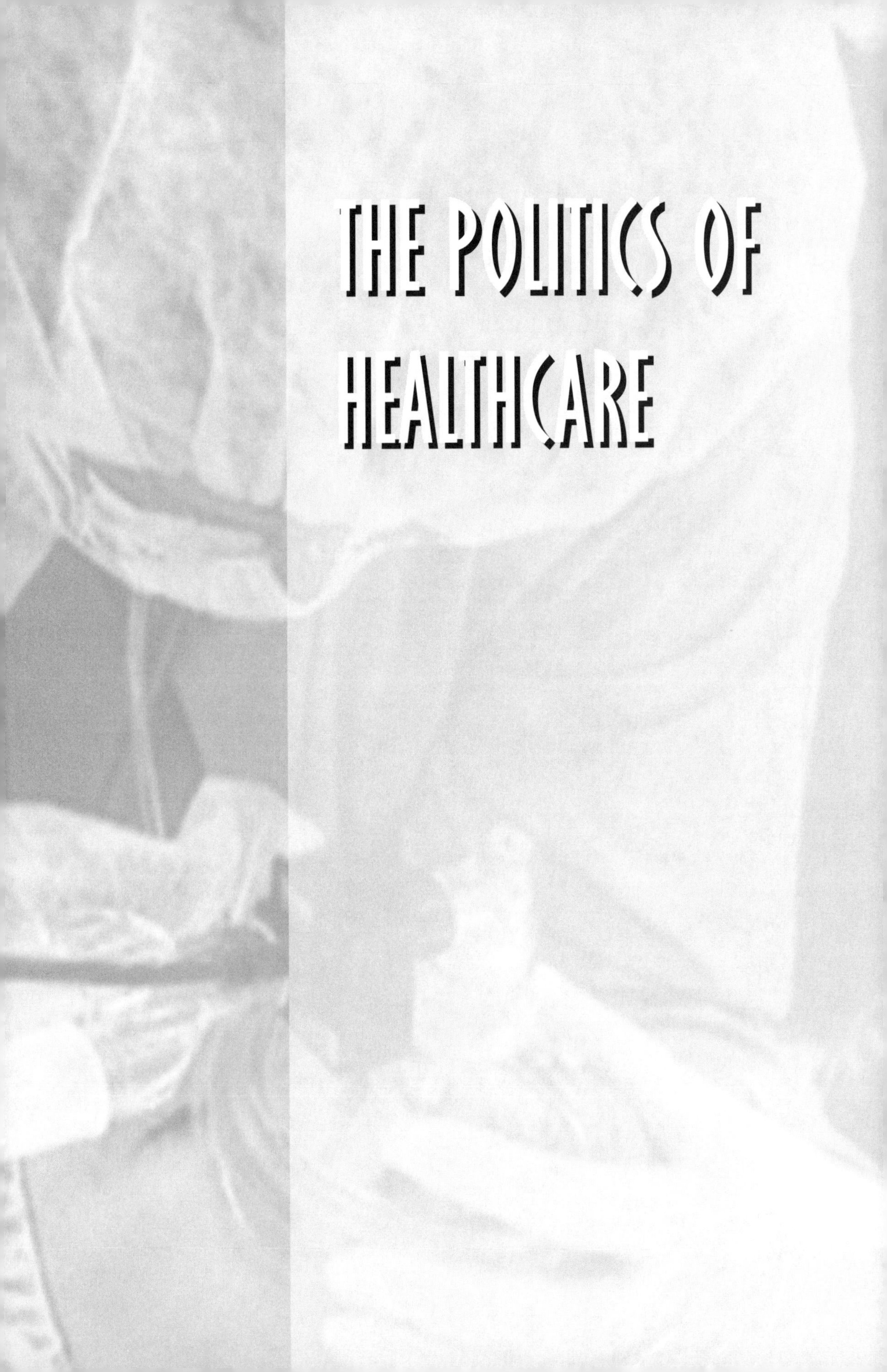

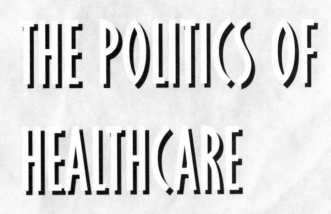

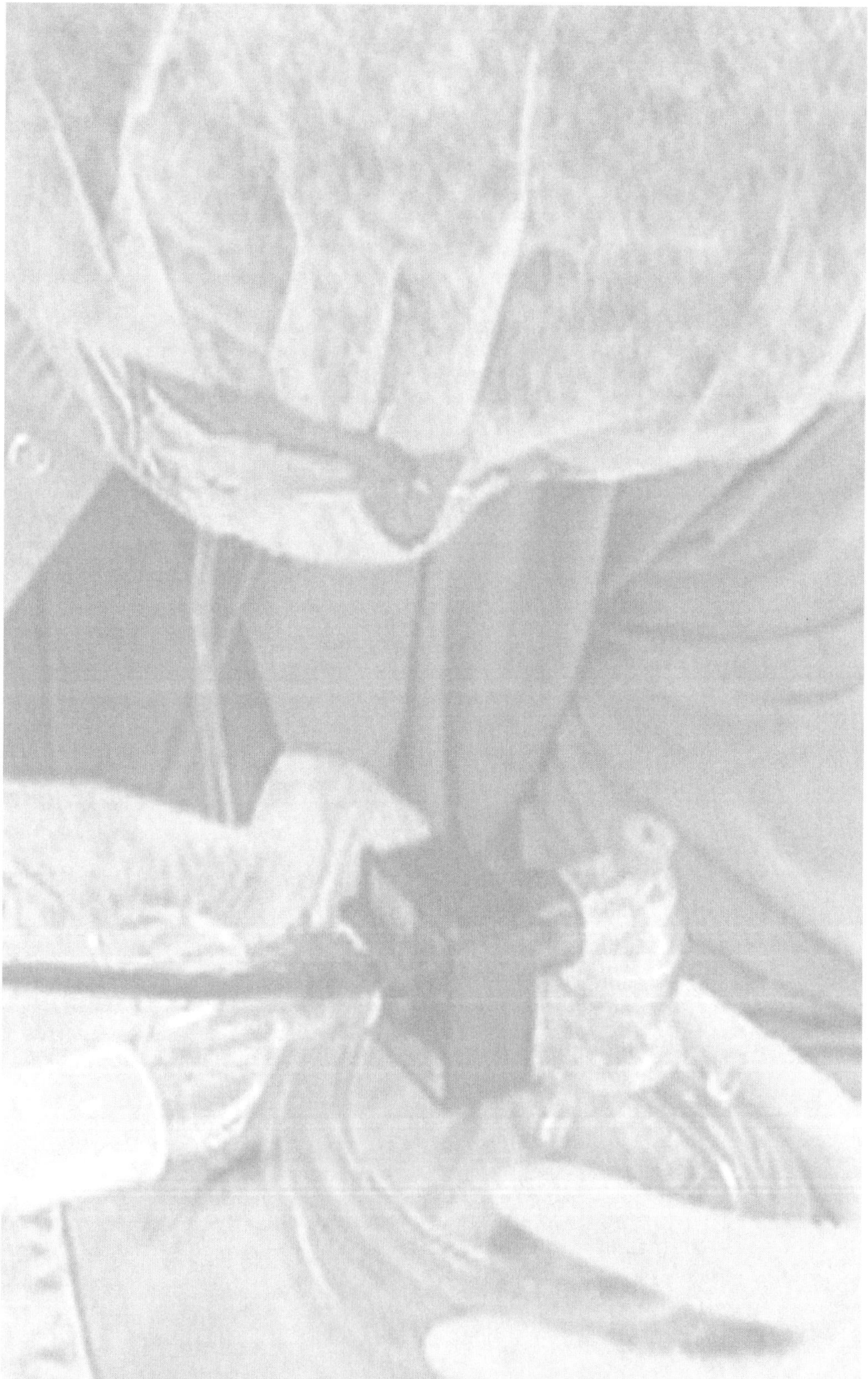

CHAPTER 17

ASSERTING INFLUENCE IN HEALTHCARE POLICY

David E. Hebert, JD

Director of Federal Government Affairs
American Association of Nurse Anesthetists
Washington, DC

KEY CONCEPTS

- Virtually all issues affecting clinical practice are influenced in some manner by the legislative process.
- It is a key responsibility of all Certified Registered Nurse Anesthetists (CRNAs) to know at least one legislator in their district or state to the degree that the legislator views the CRNA as a valued and primary source of information about the profession of nurse anesthesia.
- It is of paramount importance for CRNAs to understand that the legislative agenda of the American Association of Nurse Anesthetists cannot be accomplished without the active involvement of CRNAs at the local level. Legislators want to hear from the voters. The association serves to implement your message. Only you can bring the message.
- Contact with your legislator, regardless of the method, must be rehearsed and well organized. It must be delivered with the attitude that CRNAs are attempting to be "part of the solution," and that they appreciate the global implications of their requests and the needs of the legislator's other constituents.
- Legislative contact is effective only when there is follow-up by phone, letter or personal contact. Fax and emails are substantially less effective.

Democracy means the rule of the people—including you. State and federal legislators can only represent and serve you well if you educate them on health issues through legislative and political involvement. The purpose of this chapter is to provide information on how the American Association of Nurse Anesthetists (AANA) is involved in the political and legislative arenas, how one can become politically active, how state and federal governments determine health policy, and how state and federal legislative processes can be influenced.

AANA INVOLVEMENT IN NATIONAL POLITICS AND LEGISLATION

Political Activity

The AANA registered the AANA Separate Segregated Fund, its political action arm, with the Federal Elections Commission in 1983. In addition, the AANA volunteer structure includes an eight-person political action committee (CRNA-PAC). The purpose of the CRNA-PAC is to promote and facilitate the accumulation of voluntary contributions from members of the AANA or others who may legally be solicited into the fund. Distributions from the fund are made by the committee to support candidates in elections that have national importance. The committee directs distributions from the fund to support candidates who have taken responsible positions on quality healthcare.

Legislative and Regulatory Activity

Through membership in the AANA, Certified Registered Nurse Anesthetist (CRNA) interests are represented before federal legislative and regulatory officials. The voice of the AANA is strong because it represents 95 percent of the CRNAs and student nurse anesthetists in the anesthesia profession.

Policy Formation

The legislative positions that AANA lobbyists champion come from the policies adopted by the AANA Board of Directors. Recommendations to the Board come from individual CRNAs, state associations, and resolutions passed at the AANA Annual Meeting. As effective as the association is at representing your views, however, it still requires your personal communication with legislators to enhance the credibility of the association message.

AANA OFFICE OF FEDERAL AFFAIRS

The AANA Office of Federal Government Affairs, in Washington, D.C., was opened in July 1990. Its role is to monitor federal government activities and analyze their impact on the nurse anesthesia profession. In addition, it develops draft position papers and statements for approval by the AANA Board of Directors. Information on federal government affairs is shared with the AANA membership in four ways: (1) a weekly "government affairs hotline" of current events; (2) a column in the *AANA NewsBulletin* that describes the political, legislative, and regulatory activities of the association; (3) a bimonthly column in the *AANA Journal* that presents an in-depth analysis of a particular federal health topic; and (4) a written update for the AANA Board of Directors and participants at each AANA Assembly and Annual Meeting.

The Washington office has a professional staff of five people, which includes a director of federal government affairs, two associate directors, a political affairs coordinator, and a support staffer. The office monitors the following issues:

- Medicare reimbursement issues in Congress and the Centers for Medicare & Medicaid Services (CMS; formerly the Health Care

Financing Administration, or HCFA)

- Federal Employees Health Benefits plan (reimbursement)
- Civilian Health and Medical Program of the Uniformed Services, or CHAMPUS (reimbursement)
- Senate Finance Committee (reimbursement)
- House Ways and Means Committee (reimbursement)
- House Commerce Committee (reimbursement)
- House Education and the Workforce Committee (Employee Retirement Income Security Act)
- Medical liability/tort reform
- Drug Enforcement Administration
- National Practitioner Data Bank
- General Accounting Office/Office of Management and Budget/ Congressional Budget Office
- CRNA-PAC/Federal Elections Commission
- House and Senate Appropriations committees
- House and Senate Budget committees
- Reauthorization of the Nurse Education Act
- Reauthorization of the Higher Education Act
- Reauthorization of the National Health Services Corps
- Division of Nursing nurse anesthesia educational programs
- Office of Rural Health
- Military pay and promotions
- Veterans Administration pay and promotions
- Indian Health Service pay and promotions
- House Energy and Commerce Committee (health programs)
- Senate Health, Education, Labor and Pensions (HELP)
- Agency for Health Care Policy and Research (AHCPR) practice guidelines, including pain management, cataracts, and acquired immune deficiency syndrome (AIDS)
- AHCPR research
- National Center for Nursing Research
- AIDS, both congressional and Centers for Disease Control and Prevention
- Access to healthcare legislation
- Food and Drug Administration
- Trauma and Advisory Council

FEDERAL POLITICAL DIRECTOR PROGRAM

Many individual CRNAs have a close legislative and political relationship with their members of Congress. The AANA has formalized that relationship with the development of the legislative contact network. The purpose of the network is to provide CRNA legislative contacts with timely information about legislation of interest that the AANA would like members of Congress to support in some fashion. Examples include introduction of legislation, cosponsorship of legislation, voting for legislation, or amending legislation to include an AANA-endorsed provision. In addition, when appropriate, CRNA legislative contacts may be asked to attend local fundraisers for their member of Congress when the CRNA-PAC has decided to contribute to that member's campaign.

The AANA Federal Political Director (FPD) program provides valuable resources for the Washington office. In each state, an FPD is appointed by the state president to be the federal political "eyes and ears" for CRNAs, as well as the liaison to AANA's Washington office. When the AANA needs help getting CRNAs to contact Capitol Hill, it is the job of the FPD to spring into action and generate as many telephone calls, letters, or telegrams as possible to federal offices. The FPD may also be asked to provide guidance to CRNA-PAC about whom to support in congressional races. In addition, the FPD often will work with other CRNAs in the state to get them more involved in campaigns. The FPD does not take the place of the key contact. The "key contact" is the individual whom the FPD recruits to be the political contact to a particular senator or representative. This key contact needs to develop a strong working relationship with the member of Congress and his or her staff. This is generally accomplished by telephone and visits to the district office and/or trips to Capitol Hill during the AANA Mid-Year Assembly. While on some occasions the FPD may be the key contact, particularly in a small state where there may not be enough CRNA volunteers, it is important to note that whenever possible the FPD is essentially the "coordinator" for grassroots activities, while making every effort to find key contacts for the various members of that state's congressional delegation. CRNAs will be contacted throughout the year and asked to contact their members of Congress to cosponsor a bill, oppose a bill, sponsor an amendment, oppose an amendment, speak to the association, or write a letter to CMS or other federal agencies on behalf of AANA.

WAYS TO GET POLITICALLY INVOLVED

To be a player in the game of politics, the first thing that one should do is get on the playing field. Do not make the common mistake of thinking that you have to make a major time commitment to some type of political activity to make a difference. Any effort to which you can contribute will make a difference. Start by determining a reasonable time commitment, one that can be realistically followed and completed. The following are suggestions of ways to become politically involved.

- Join your state and/or national associations and participate in their government relations or political action committees.
- Become active in the League of Women Voters, which often is involved in voter registration drives and "get out the vote" campaigns during elections.
- Join your state Democratic or Republican party so that you can pay your "political dues" to the party structure. This is important if you ever want to run for political office.
- Make a generous financial contribution to your state and/or national association's political action committee.
- Approach local talk show hosts about healthcare issues that you care about or call in to talk to health guests on shows.
- Volunteer to be a speaker on healthcare issues before local senior and consumer organizations.
- Build a coalition of individuals like yourself, so that you have the additional power of a collective voice. Then use the coalition as a legislative network for lobbying on issues.
- Participate in professional research, because the database that research provides is key to the shaping of healthcare policy.
- Run for elective office.
- Campaign to get appointed to a

board, commission, or other decision-making body that will influence health policy.

- Invite key decision makers to visit your place of work. There is no more effective way to teach decision makers about the importance of the job you do than by showing them firsthand.
- Write an article on a healthcare issue for your local newspaper.
- If a legislator or other decision-maker does something important on a healthcare issue of concern to you (such as successfully championing your bill through the legislative process), arrange a media "photo opportunity" at which the decision maker is given an award by your state or national association for his or her efforts.
- Participate in a formal or informal legislative/political internship or fellowship. At the local level, contact your city councilperson's office or mayor's office about any volunteer positions. At the state level, call your state association or the offices of your state representative and senator to find out if there are any programs. At the federal level, contact the AANA or the offices of your member of the House of Representatives and your two members of the Senate.
- Host a candidate's night at a meeting of your local or state association to discuss health policy issues.
- Participate in a candidate's election campaign.

Prior to Election Day

- Stuff envelopes with the candidate's campaign literature.
- Put up yard signs in favor of your candidate.
- Distribute campaign literature door to door.
- Canvas door to door to determine voter opinions.
- Staff phone banks to urge voters to vote for your candidate.
- Chauffeur the candidate to functions (this is an especially good time to talk about healthcare with candidates because you literally have a captive audience).
- Write policy papers for the candidate to use.
- Participate in mass mailing efforts to registered voters or a targeted audience.
- Serve as the candidate's representative at functions.
- Build a base of your colleagues so, for example, you can have a "Tuesday CRNA night" at the campaign headquarters during which CRNAs do all the necessary tasks, such as answering the phones, stuffing envelopes, and answering mail.
- Host a "meet and greet" function for the candidate in your home.
- Hold a fundraiser for the candidate in your home.
- Make a generous financial contribution to the candidate.

On Election Day

- Staff phone banks to remind voters to vote on election day.
- Distribute your candidate's campaign literature at polling places (contingent on election laws).
- Provide transportation and babysitting services to voters.
- Watch the polls (to ensure that the voting process is carried out according to the election laws).
- Host a victory party for your winning candidate.

NETWORKING

It is very rare for a single group alone to promote a piece of legislation, especially a controversial one, through Congress. American society is too complex and diversified for there to be easy consensus on most issues. Therefore, you may need to form coalitions with other groups that have a mutual interest in a given public policy. While alliances may be necessary, approach them with caution because there is usually a price to be paid in terms of needing to compromise or to accommodate the needs of the other groups in the coalition. It is a political call whether the benefits of a coalition outweigh the inherent negatives.

There are areas you should consider before formally associating with other groups. You should make sure that there will be an even division of responsibility. You also want to make sure that you can trust the judgment of your partners. There is nothing worse than finding out that you are associated with a campaign that is unethical or irresponsible. By the same token, you do not want to join every coalition. There are limits to how much your organization can do. You should also be concerned about appearing to be active on too many fronts. Being overextended can damage your credibility in the legislative arena as much as being inactive can. Specific parameters should be set when you join a coalition. At a minimum, the coalition ought to be restricted to a specific issue, event, or period. If no such limitations are established, you may find yourself in a situation you cannot easily escape later.

Steps for a Successful Coalition

1. Define and agree on the goal—why is this legislation necessary?
2. Establish guidelines and rules for the coalition. All groups are free to act for themselves, except when they use the name of the coalition.
3. Define tasks.
4. Establish a coordinating committee.
5. Organize resources to complete the necessary elements of the campaign.
6. Keep everyone together and focused on the one area of agreement. Do not let areas of difference or other issues cause infighting.
7. Keep jealous feelings to a minimum. Make sure everyone feels involved and assure all that their individual interests are well represented.
8. Watch legislators' attitudes toward your group to ensure that they are positive.
9. Establish effective communication methods for educating the public. It is important that the coalition speak with one voice.
10. Try to meet at least once a month to keep apprised of activities.
11. Keep members informed with a regular update.
12. Investigate any legal requirements that may apply to your coalition, such as lobbying requirements.

POTENTIAL LEGISLATIVE BENEFITS OF POLITICAL ACTIVITY

Political activity and legislative activity are the flip sides of the same coin. Therefore, always keep in mind that politics may help you achieve your healthcare policy objectives because the political arena provides access to decision makers. Your relationship with key decision makers may help influence their decisions on vital health policy issues. Your political activity on behalf of a candidate will not always result in the elected candidate voting the way you want, but it does give you the opportunity to eloquently make your case to the candidate. The following are lists of dos and don'ts regarding political activity.

Do

- Build a professional image.
- Work on developing your writing and speaking skills.
- Learn all you can about a candidate's positions before you volunteer to work in his or her campaign.
- Make realistic time commitments about what you can offer a campaign.
- Follow through on your commitments in a responsible manner.
- Have business cards with you at all times for networking.
- Work to expand your network by recruiting other volunteers.
- Vote and encourage others to vote.

Don't

- Be afraid to volunteer for a low-level task.
- Neglect traditional political organizations.
- Forget to get very clear directions about what the campaign's expectations are of you regarding job responsibilities and time commitments.
- Be discouraged if it takes time to work up to more senior roles in a campaign.
- Put off getting involved until the timing is perfect—it never will be.
- Forget to take fair credit for the work that you have done.

HOW STATE AND FEDERAL GOVERNMENTS DETERMINE HEALTH POLICY

Typical State Legislative Process

As state legislatures take greater initiative in determining health policy, many organizations are taking their first steps into state government affairs. With the exception of Nebraska, state legislatures consist of two houses: the senate (commonly referred to as the upper house) and, depending on the state, either the house or assembly (commonly referred to as the lower house). Bills are identified by state, house of origin, and number: for instance, California Senate Bill 1 (casl); Nebraska Legislative Bill 3 (ne13); and New York Assembly Bill 3695 (nya3695).

State legislatures adopt resolutions and bills. Some resolutions are adopted by only one house; others are adopted by both houses. The substance of resolutions varies; some are used to express legislative concern about a specific issue, and some are simply congratulatory. Most states do not require action by the governor for resolutions to become officially adopted.

Although each legislature has its own unique set of rules and procedures, most bills follow the same general path—introduction, consideration by the first house, consideration by the second house, and consideration by the governor.

Bill Introduction

The state legislative process begins when a bill is introduced. In most states, bills may be introduced only by members or committees of the legislature. In about half the states, bills may not be introduced until the legislature convenes. The remaining states allow the introduction of bills prior to the official convening date for presession study. This practice is called prefiling.

Committee Referral and Action

After introduction, bills are referred to a committee for public hearing. The number, structure, and operating procedures of committees are unique to each state. Some states use a joint committee system to review bills, but most states have separate committees in each house dealing with specific subjects, such as health.

Committees usually have the authority to recommend that bills be passed as introduced, passed as amended, substituted by the committee, or killed. Often, bills that would cost money or have some other financial consequence are reviewed by two committees; a policy committee reviews the substance of the bill, while the fiscal committee reviews the financial aspects of the bill.

Floor Action

Many bills do not receive committee approval and thus proceed no further. The bills that are approved by committees (either as introduced, amended, or substituted) proceed to the floor for consideration by the entire chamber. The chamber may pass the bill in the form recommended by the committee(s), amend the bill and pass it, or kill it.

Second Chamber

When a bill is passed by the chamber of origin, it is sent to the second chamber and the procedure is repeated: committee referral, committee action, and floor action in the second chamber. As in the chamber of origin, bills may be approved, amended, substituted, or killed in committee or on the floor.

Concurrence and Conference Actions

Bills that are amended in the second chamber return to the chamber of origin for concurrence. If the chamber of origin concurs with the amended version of the bill passed by the second chamber, the bill is eligible to be sent to the governor for signature. If the chamber of origin does not concur, the second chamber may withdraw the amendments. If the second chamber does not withdraw the amendments, a conference committee is appointed to resolve the differences between the chambers. The report of the conference committee must be approved by both chambers for the bill to move on to the governor.

Governor's Actions

When a bill is approved and passed by the legislature, it is sent to the governor. In most states, the governor may sign a bill into law; veto all or part of the bill (line item veto); or, depending on whether the legislature is in session or adjourned, let the bill die without signature or let it become law without signature. North Carolina is the only state in which the governor does not have veto power.

Vetoed bills are returned to the chamber in which they were introduced. The legislature may pass bills that have been vetoed by the governor if a specified majority of both chambers (usually two thirds) votes to override the veto. Figure 17.1 provides a flow chart of a typical state legislative process.

FEDERAL LEGISLATIVE PROCESS

Nowhere are policy and process more intertwined than in the Congress of the United States. Skillful legislators use the legislative process to advance their policy goals. Sponsors often amend the wording of a bill to keep it from being referred to a hostile committee. For instance, an antiabortion amendment may be added to a House appropriations bill and may be germane because it restricts federal funding for abortions. Procedural techniques and policy interact at many stages of the legislative process. "Legislation is like a chess game more than anything else," Representative John D. Dingell (D-MI) has said. "It is a seemingly endless series of moves, until ultimately someone prevails through exhaustion, or brillance, or because of overwhelming public sentiment for their side."

By the mid-1980s, the federal budget deficit and the complex special budget process that Congress devised for dealing with it resulted in the increased use of omnibus bills. Rather than separate bills going all the way through the normal legislative process, many often unrelated proposals were packaged in a single, large piece of legislation. These so-called omnibus budget reconciliation bills contained literally hundreds of provisions that were supposedly necessary to develop an overall budget plan for the year. The opportunities to debate and amend these bills are often severely limited. Consequently, omnibus bills allow measures that would not normally be approved as separate bills to get adopted. Sometimes this global approach contains provisions that benefit CRNAs, and sometimes it contains provisions that harm CRNAs. A positive example is the authority for CRNAs to receive direct Medicare reimbursement, included in the Omnibus Budget Reconciliation Act of 1986.

Figure 17.1: Typical State Legislative Process

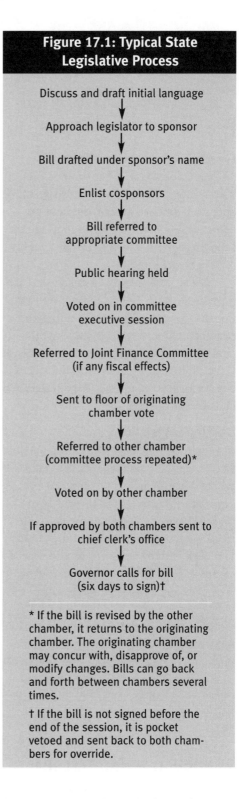

Discuss and draft initial language
↓
Approach legislator to sponsor
↓
Bill drafted under sponsor's name
↓
Enlist cosponsors
↓
Bill referred to appropriate committee
↓
Public hearing held
↓
Voted on in committee executive session
↓
Referred to Joint Finance Committee (if any fiscal effects)
↓
Sent to floor of originating chamber vote
↓
Referred to other chamber (committee process repeated)*
↓
Voted on by other chamber
↓
If approved by both chambers sent to chief clerk's office
↓
Governor calls for bill (six days to sign)†

* If the bill is revised by the other chamber, it returns to the originating chamber. The originating chamber may concur with, disapprove of, or modify changes. Bills can go back and forth between chambers several times.

† If the bill is not signed before the end of the session, it is pocket vetoed and sent back to both chambers for override.

LEGISLATIVE VEHICLES

There are four basic forms in which a legislative proposal may be introduced: bills, joint resolutions, current resolutions, and simple resolutions.

Bills are the most common form. They are prefaced by "H.R." in the House and "S." in the Senate, followed by a number assigned based on the order of its introduction during a congressional session.

Joint resolutions may originate in either the House or Senate and are labeled "H. J. Res." or "S. J. Res." followed by a sequential number. The most common usage is to continue an existing law. It is subject to the same procedure as bills, unless it is proposing an amendment to the Constitution. If it is the latter, then it must be approved by a two-thirds vote of each chamber and be sent directly to the administrator of general services for submission to the states for ratification. Constitutional amendments are not presented to the president for his signature.

Concurrent resolutions are designated by "H. Con. Res." or "S. Con. Res." They must be approved by both the House and Senate before they can become effective. A concurrent resolution does not require the president's signature and does not have the force of law. It expresses the opinion of Congress and is used for matters affecting the operations of both chambers.

Simple resolutions are designated "H. Res." or "S. Res." They are used for a matter concerning the operation of only one chamber and are adopted only by that chamber. They may also be used to create a special investigating committee, change chamber rules, or express the sense of the chamber on specific issues.

Drafting Legislation

Legislation can be drafted by congressional staff or legislative counsels at the request of individual members or committees. Legislation is also drafted by executive branch departments and agencies, as well as by interest groups. Much of the legislation dealt with by Congress in any year is comprised of bills reauthorizing expiring laws, bills appropriating money to run the federal government, and bills submitted by the president and the executive branch to implement the administration's programs. Pursuant to the Constitution, revenue legislation originates in the House. By custom, appropriations legislation also originates in the House. All other bills may originate in either chamber.

INTRODUCTION AND REFERRAL OF BILLS

Members of the House of Representatives are elected for two-year terms, and senators are elected for six-year terms. The length of each Congress mirrors the length of a House term—two years. Each Congress conducts its business in two regular sessions that begin in January of successive years. For example, the first session of the 107th Congress convened in January 2001; the second session of the 107th Congress convened in January 2002. Any bill that has not received final congressional approval when Congress adjourns automatically dies and must be reintroduced in the next Congress and begin the entire process again.

To become law, proposed legislation must be approved in identical form in both the House and the Senate. The bill is subject to delay, defeat, or substantial modification. "It is very easy to defeat a bill in Congress," President John F. Kennedy once observed. "It is much more difficult to pass one."

Any bill or resolution must be introduced by a representative or senator when Congress is in session. There is no limit to the number of bills a member may introduce. The legislative leader of a proposal is the key to its survival. The fact that a bill has a high-ranking sponsor automatically escalates its importance as a piece of legislation.

A House member may introduce a bill or resolution by handing it to the clerk of the House or placing it in a box at the front of the House chamber, called the "hopper." Senators usually submit their proposals and accompanying statements to clerks in the Senate chamber or may introduce their bills from the Senate floor. If objection to the introduction of the bill is offered by any senator, introduction of the bill is postponed until the next day. It is not uncommon for a representative and a senator to sponsor "companion" (identical) bills, each introducing his or her version simultaneously in their respective chambers. This is done to encourage both chambers to consider the measure simultaneously to dramatize the importance or urgency of the bill and to show broad support for it.

The House or Senate bill is then numbered, referred to the appropriate committee(s), labeled with the sponsor's name, and sent to the Government Printing Office for copies to be made. A representative or senator who is interested in actively promoting legislation often will seek cosponsors. This allows other legislators to jointly introduce the bill and indicate their support for it. Bipartisan sponsorship can be very important, as can endorsement by members of the committee to which the bill will be referred. There is no limit on the number of cosponsors that can be added to a House or Senate bill or resolution. A bill written in the executive branch and proposed as an administration measure usually is introduced by the chair of the committee that has jurisdiction over the bill's subject matter.

COMMITTEES AND SUBCOMMITTEES

Structure

Committees are the heart of the legislative process. They have existed in the House and the Senate since 1789 and have allowed for a division of work and orderly consideration of legislation. The size of the Senate (100 members) and the House (435 members) makes it extremely difficult for all members to consider each piece of legislation. Consequently, each chamber has established its own committees to study and consider legislation. In turn, committees have established subcommittees to allow even further division of work.

Both the House and Senate have standing (permanent) committees and special (select) committees. There are 19 standing committees in the House and 18 in the Senate. Each standing committee has jurisdiction over certain subject areas of legislation, and all legislation that would affect that particular area of law is referred to that committee of jurisdiction. The number of select committees changes. The select committees are usually investigative in nature, convene for the duration of the matter under investigation, reach a decision or make recommendations, and are then dissolved.

The real nuts and bolts of the legislative process take place in committees and subcommittees, including research, investigation, and public hearings. This is the time to contact your elected legislator and let him or her know your stand on the bill. It is at this stage that you have the most ability to influence the movement of a bill. If legislators receive numerous letters in support of a bill, they will relay that to the subcommittee or committee chair, and that often expedites action on the bill. Conversely, if the legislator receives numerous letters opposing the bill, that will be conveyed to the subcommittee or committee chair, and the bill may die in committee without any action being taken.

Membership ratios on committees between the majority and minority parties are determined at the beginning of each Congress and are generally based on the ratio that exists for the entire membership of each chamber plus the political judgment of the majority party. Individuals are assigned to committees by caucus of the respective parties, and these assignments are confirmed by a floor vote. A member usually seeks election to the committee that has jurisdiction over a field in which he or she is most qualified and interested.

Subcommittees and committees are responsible to their parent bodies. However, because of the complexity of their assignments, they have substantial independence and autonomy. The chair of a committee or subcommittee is a dominant figure in the legislative process because he or she can set the agenda for committee meetings, set up the hearings, and hire the staff. When a bill is referred to a committee, the chair can either guide it through his or her committee or sit on the bill and effectively kill it.

In Congress, seniority is power. Members rank in seniority on the committee in accordance with their appointment to the committee. The majority member having the most years of service in Congress is usually designated chair. The most senior member of the minority party is ordinarily designated as "ranking minority member." Better committee assignments and bigger committee staffs usually go hand in hand with tenure on Capitol Hill.

Subcommittee seniority is generally assigned in a similar way, with the full committee determining subcommittee membership and maintaining the same majority/minority ratios. In general, senators may serve on two major legislative committees and one lower-ranking committee. In the House, a representative usually serves on two committees.

Committee Jurisdiction

Formally, a bill is to be referred to the appropriate committee by the speaker of the House or the presiding officer of the Senate. Informally, the parliamentarians of the two chambers act on behalf of the speaker and the Senate presiding officer and actually refer the bills to committees. Bill sponsors may indicate their preferences for referral, although custom, chamber rules, and committee jurisdiction generally govern.

In turn, the chair of the committee will refer the bill to one of its subcommittees unless the chair decides to have the full committee act on the proposal. It is important to note that the 1970s witnessed a reform of the seniority system, resulting in restraints on committee chairs and a diffusion of power from committee chairs to subcommittees. Each committee has its own method of determining where the predominant policy role and power are exercised, at the full committee or the subcommittee level.

When a bill contains language that cuts across the jurisdiction of two or more committees, it may get a referral to multiple committees. In the Senate, multiple referrals are implemented by unanimous consent agreements. In the House, referral authority remains with the speaker. There are three types of multiple referrals. First, there is "sequential referral," the most common form, which allows one committee to take action first and then refer the bill on to the second committee. Second is "joint referral," where a bill is referred, within specific time limits, successively to one committee and then to another. An example of joint referral would be bills that deal with Medicare Part B, for which both the House Energy and Commerce Committee and the House Ways and Means Committee share jurisdiction. Third, there is "split referral," where a bill is referred to several committees, each having jurisdiction over specific parts of the bill. Multiple referrals often can kill legislation since several committees are unlikely to agree on a version of the bill or even to report the bill at approximately the same time, if at all. On the other hand, when several committees report a multiple-referred bill, the chances of that bill's passage can be greatly enhanced.

Failure of a committee to act on a bill is equivalent to killing it; the measure can be withdrawn from the committee's purview only by a discharge petition signed by a majority of the House membership on House bills or by adoption of a special resolution in the Senate.

Discharge attempts rarely succeed. The full House and Senate seldom question a decision of one of their committees not to report a bill.

Referral to Subcommittee

The first committee action taken on a bill usually is a request for comment by interested agencies of the government, such as the Department of Health and Human Services on health bills. This gives the committee a preliminary indication if it should have the relevant subcommittee hold hearings on a bill. The committee chair may then refer the bill to a subcommittee for study and hearings, or it may be considered by the full committee. Subcommittee hearings provide the opportunity for members of Congress, executive branch staff, and representatives of industry, interest groups, and academia, to formally present their views and positions on the legislative topic. An increasing trend is to have celebrities testify on particular issues, such as Robert Redford on environmental issues or Elizabeth Taylor on funding for AIDS research. Panels of witnesses are often scheduled together to hear similar perspectives at the same time or to probe the conflicting points of view of the panelists. Witnesses usually give prepared comments and then answer questions from the subcommittee members. The time that each subcommittee member has to ask questions is usually limited by the chair. Verbatim transcripts of hearings are recorded and generally printed for committee and public use.

Depending on the nature of the bill, hearings may be conducted for a few hours, for several days, or for weeks. The timing and duration of subcommittee hearings depend largely on the discretion of the subcommittee chair. Most hearings are held in open session. More frequently, the subcommittee chair will limit the number and type of individuals and organizations that may testify. This is done either to expedite the subcommittee's deliberations or to create a particular attitude at the hearings; for example, only those in favor of a chair's bill are asked to testify. There has also been an increase in recent years in the number of field hearings that are held in the subcommittee chair's district or state.

On completion of the hearings the subcommittee "marks up" the bill, which means amends the bill. During this step, a member may offer amendments that he or she supports. As a rule, informal votes are taken on each amendment to obtain a consensus. Because of the political trade-offs and controversies that occur during markups, they are often closed to the public. The subcommittee has several options regarding actions it may take on the bill. It can

- Fail to take action or complete action on a bill.
- Report it favorably without amendments.
- Report it favorably with amendments.
- Reject the bill.
- Report it unfavorably or without recommendation.
- Report favorably on a "clean bill." If amendments are adopted that are substantial, the subcommittee may order a clean bill introduced, incorporating all amendments in new bill language. The original bill then is put aside and the clean bill is then reintroduced, assigned a new number, and referred to the full committee.

Full Committee Action

After a subcommittee approves a bill, the full committee can choose from the same options for action that the subcommittee had to choose from.

Although the full committee can duplicate the subcommittee's procedures by holding hearings and markup sessions, it seldom does so. Committee discussion is more general, and although amendments may be offered, they are normally fewer than those considered in subcommittee. Committees generally rely on and accept the conclusions of the subcommittee. The full committee then votes on its recommendation to the full House or Senate. This procedure is called "ordering a bill reported." Occasionally a committee may order a bill reported unfavorably, but most of the time a report calls for favorable action because the committee can effectively kill a bill simply by failing to take any action.

When a committee sends a bill to the chamber floor, it explains its reasons in a written statement called a "report," which accompanies the bill. Often, committee members opposing a bill issue dissenting minority statements that are included in the back section of the report. The points made in the dissent section typically signal where the areas of contention are that will arise on the House or Senate floor. The rules of the House and Senate specify some aspects of the contents of reports; for example, they must show changes in existing law. These reports may also include an analysis of the legislative language and a statement of the committee's reasons or intent for passing the bill. In addition, the written statements from government agencies are ordinarily included in the report.

After a bill becomes law, there may be confusion or disagreement about the meaning of the actual legislative language. The committee report is often used to try to determine the "legislative intent" of the bill. For example, when the executive branch writes regulations or the courts rule on legislation, they will often rely on the report background if the law itself is not clear. Each report is given a number; for example, House Report 107-1 designates the first House committee report of the 107th Congress. Report language is often used by lobbyists to protect their association's interests. For example, the annual health appropriations bill lists only how much money is to be spent for nurse anesthesia educational programs. The accompanying report contains directives to the federal agency that implements the law on how the money is to be spent.

Floor Action

When the full committee has approved a bill, it is reported back to the chamber where it originated. Accounts of floor debate and action taken in each chamber are published daily in the *Congressional Record*. The differences between House and Senate floor procedures are largely the result of the fact that the Senate is smaller, which allows greater opportunity for informal arrangements. The larger, more complex House emphasizes rules and precedents. In the House, the completed committee bill is sent to the House Rules Committee to establish the length of time for debate and to determine whether floor amendments will be allowed.

Because debate is restricted and the amending process frequently limited, the House is able to dispose of legislation more quickly than the Senate. The Senate, although it has rules and procedures, more often operates by unanimous consent. Each Senate member, even the most junior, is offered a deference rarely seen in the House. The privileges of engaging in unlimited debate, the filibuster, and offering nongermane amendments are highly cherished traditions in the Senate that are not permitted under House rules. Given these conditions, it is not surprising that the Senate may spend days considering a measure that the House has debated and passed in a single afternoon.

Except for the House Rules Committee review, procedures are generally similar in the House and Senate. The bill is placed on a calendar for a vote. When, and sometimes whether, a bill is brought to the floor depends on many factors, including what other legislation is awaiting action, how controversial the measure is, and whether the leadership judges its chances for passage to be improved by immediate action. For example, the leadership may decide to delay taking up a controversial bill until its proponents can gather sufficient support to guarantee its passage. A bill is brought to floor debate by varying procedures. If it is a routine bill, it may await the call of the calendar. If it is urgent or important, it can be taken up in the Senate either by unanimous consent or by a majority vote. The policy committee of the majority party in the Senate schedules the bills that it wants taken up for debate. In the House, debate precedence is granted if a special rule is obtained from the Rules Committee.

House debate is limited by the rule under which the bill is considered. Senate debate is usually unlimited. It can be halted only by unanimous consent or by a "cloture" vote, which requires a three-fifths majority of the entire Senate. Cloture limits senators to one hour of debate.

Voting on bills may occur repeatedly before they are finally approved or rejected. The full House or Senate must approve, alter, or reject the committee amendments before the bill itself can be put to a vote. In addition, floor amendments may be offered to further certain objectives. First, members may offer floor amendments to dramatize their stands on issues, even if there is little chance that their amendments may be adopted. Second, some amendments are introduced at the request of the executive branch, a member's constituents, or special interests. Third, some are tactical tools for gauging sentiment for or against a bill. Fourth, others are used to stall action on a bill. Finally, some amendments may be designed to defeat the legislation. One common strategy is to try to load a bill up with so many unattractive amendments that it will eventually collapse under its own weight. Another strategy is to offer a "killer" amendment that if adopted would cause members who initially supported the bill to vote against it on final passage. Conversely, amendments known as "sweeteners" may be offered to attract broader support for the underlying measure.

The Senate has three different methods of voting: voice vote, a standing vote (called a division), and a recorded roll call vote to which members answer "yea" or "nay" when their names are called. The House uses voice and standing votes but has replaced the time-consuming roll calls with an electronic voting device to record the "yeas" and "nays." Another method of voting, used in the House only, is the teller vote. This is where members file up the center aisle past counters; only vote totals are announced. The teller vote is rarely used now, however. The most common method of voting in both the House and Senate is by voice vote.

The House votes on the rule for the bill, various amendments, and then the bill itself. The Senate votes on various amendments and then the bill. Final approval of a bill requires a majority vote of the members present.

Action in the Second Chamber

After a bill is passed in one chamber, it is sent to the other chamber for action. This body may take one of several steps. First, it may pass the bill as is. Second, it may send the bill to its committee of jurisdiction for study or alteration. Third, it may reject the entire bill and advise the other chamber of that fact. Finally, it may simply ignore the bill while it continues work on its own version of the same legislation. Frequently, one chamber may approve a version of a bill that is greatly at variance with the version already passed by the other chamber and then substitute its amendments for the language of the original bill. This retains, in effect, only the other chamber's bill designation, without the original substance.

Often the second chamber makes only minor changes in the first chamber's bill. If these changes are agreed to by the first chamber, then the bill is sent to the president for signature. However, if the first chamber does not agree to the second chamber's changes, then the bill is sent to a conference committee to reconcile the differences in the two chambers' versions. The chamber that physically possesses the bill requests a conference. If the other chamber does not agree to a conference, then the bill dies.

Conference Committee

Sometimes known as the "third house of Congress," the conference committee usually consists of senior members (conferees) from the committees that have reported the bills. However, designated sponsors of major amendments to the bills also may be appointed to the conference committee. Conferees are appointed by the presiding officer of the Senate and the speaker of the House. The number of conferees may vary, the range usually being from three to nine members from each chamber, depending on the complexity of the bill involved. There does not have to be an equal number of conferees representing each chamber because a majority vote controls the action of each group, so that a large representation on one side does not give that chamber an advantage.

Theoretically, conferees are not allowed to write new legislation when reconciling the two versions before them, but this curb is sometimes bypassed. Many bills have been put into acceptable compromise form only after new language was approved by the conferees. Some of the hardest bargaining in the entire legislative process takes place in the conference committee, and the ironing out of differences may go on for days, weeks, or even months. The real constraining factor for conferees is that the chambers they represent must accept the compromises. When the conferees have reached agreement, they prepare a conference report embodying their recommendations to each chamber.

The conference report must be approved by each chamber. Consequently, approval of the report is approval of the compromise bill. If no agreement is reached by the conferees, or should either chamber not accept the conference report, the bill dies.

Presidential Action

After a bill has been passed by both the House and the Senate in identical form, it is sent to the White House for action. The president has four options. First, the president may sign the bill, date it, and write the word "approved" on the document. The Constitution requires only the president's signature. The president may allow the bill to become law without signature. This occurs if the president takes no action for 10 days (Sundays excepted) when Congress is in session. Third, the president may "pocket veto" the bill. This occurs if Congress passes a bill and then adjourns before the president has had the 10-day option to return the bill with a veto. In this instance, the bill will not automatically become law. Fourth, the president may veto the bill within the 10-day option and return it to Congress with a message stating the reasons for the veto. The message is sent to the chamber that originated the bill. If no action is taken there on the veto message, the bill dies. However, Congress

Figure 17.2: Federal Legislative Process

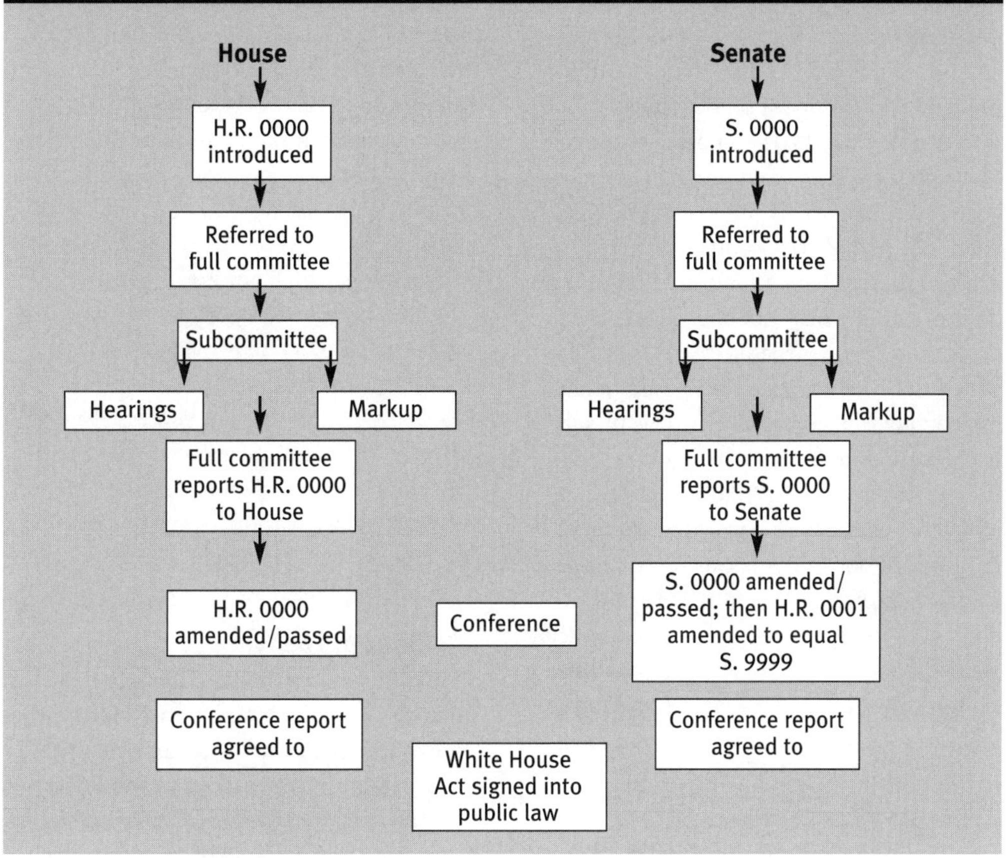

can attempt to override the president's veto and enact the bill. The overriding of a veto in each chamber requires a two-thirds vote of those present, who must number a quorum and vote by roll call. If the president's veto is overridden, the bill becomes law, otherwise it dies.

When bills are passed and signed, or passed over a veto, they are given public law numbers in numeric order. They are identified by the Congress that passed them and by the law number, for example, Public Law 107-802 means the 802nd public law passed by the 107th Congress. Figure 17.2 designates the flow of legislation through the House and Senate.

FEDERAL REGULATORY PROCESS

All rules start with Congress passing, and the president signing, a public law creating a federal program. The law defines the goals of regulatory programs, identifies the agency responsible for achieving them, and contains substantive and procedural guidance as to how the agency is to conduct its work. Rules fill in the details of legislation, with Congress retaining an oversight function. The law usually authorizes the agency to formulate rules to carry out the purposes of the law. For example, within the Department of Health and Human Services, Medicare and Medicaid rules are handled by CMS.

The agency of jurisdiction prepares draft rules, which are published in the *Federal Register* each federal working day. The Administrative Procedures Act establishes a two-step procedure that an agency ordinarily uses for rule making.

First, an agency must publish in the

Federal Register a notice of proposed rule making, which contains the text of the proposed rules or a description of the subjects and issues involved and an invitation for the public to comment on the rules. Concerned individuals and organizations may submit written comments on the proposed rule, usually within a 30- or 60-day comment period. The comments help bring to the agency's attention information that the agency may not have taken into account in drafting the proposed rule. The content of the final rule may be influenced by the views presented during this period.

Second, an agency carefully considers the public's comments and, if the agency still believes a rule is necessary, adopts a final rule. Prior to the issuance of a final rule, however, further internal review is done at all levels of the agency and by the White House's Office of Management and Budget. The final rule, with a statement of its basis and purpose, is usually published in the *Federal Register* at least 30 days before its effective date.

Increasingly, rules and rule making play a pivotal role in the policy process by transforming legislative provisions into a blueprint for regulatory program operations. More often than not, the rule-making process is transformed into a battleground of contending interests, where major political and policy issues deferred during the legislative process are resolved, at least until the rules that emerge are themselves challenged. It is not unusual for rule making by an agency to stimulate interest groups to demand new legislation.

HOW YOU CAN INFLUENCE THE LEGISLATIVE PROCESS

The following information references the federal level, but it is usually applicable to the state level as well.

What Is Lobbying?

Lobbying is trying to persuade decision makers to enact measures, such as legislation, favorable to your cause. Alternatively, you may want legislation defeated or repealed that is unfavorable to your cause. You are an expert on healthcare; typically your legislator is not. Your lobbying efforts involve sharing information with a legislator that he or she would not normally have easy access to. Table 17.1 outlines useful information for lobbying.

The normal place to get the answers to the questions cited in Table 17.1 is from your professional organization. Normally, whoever asks you to lobby will provide you with these facts, along with the call for action. You should never be asked to lobby without being armed with the necessary facts. Table 17.2 gives general tips for lobbying.

Methods of Lobbying

The different methods of lobbying include scheduling a personal visit with the legislator or the legislator's health staff person in the district or the legislator's state or federal office, calling the legislator or the health staff person, corresponding with the legislator or the health staff person, and testifying at hearings.

How to Make an Appointment for a Personal Visit

Call the legislator's office directly, or call the U.S. Capitol Switchboard, which can connect you to the legislator's office. The numbers for the U.S. Capitol Switchboard are (202) 224-3121 (Senate) and (202) 225-3121 (House). When you connect with the legislator's office, first ask for the legislative assistant (LA) for health. Tell the LA that you are a CRNA constituent of the legislator and that you want to meet with the legislator for 15 minutes on a specific date to discuss a particular health issue. The health LA may make the appointment for you with the legislator's scheduler or may refer you directly to the scheduler. Make sure you write down the name of the LA

Table 17.1: What Do You have to Know to Lobby?

To lobby effectively, you have to know your issue and your legislator. You will typically need to know the following things about the bill that deals with your issue:

- What is the number of the bill?
- What is the status of the bill?
- What is the substance of the bill?
- Why is this important to the legislator's constituents?
- What will happen if the bill passes?
- What will happen if it does not pass?
- What is the fiscal estimate on the bill?
- What other groups support the bill?
- What other groups oppose the bill?

Typical questions about your legislator include

- What are his or her past votes on the issue?
- What are his or her positions on health issues generally?
- What political party does he or she belong to?
- What is his or her profession?
- What are his or her legislative interests?
- What are his or her key committee memberships or leadership positions?
- What legislation has he or she introduced?
- What is his or her voting record?
- How long has he or she served in the legislature?
- When is he or she up for reelection?
- Does he or she have an opponent in his or her reelection campaign?

and the scheduler, and get a specific time, meeting room number, and building, for example, 10 a.m. in Room 205 in the Hart Senate Office Building. Leave your name and phone number where you can be reached if the legislator needs to cancel the meeting. If you request it in advance, the legislator's office can usually arrange for a photographer to be present to take your picture with the legislator. An autographed picture is always a nice memento of your visit, and most offices will be happy to send it to you when developed. If a picture is being taken, request 20 minutes for your visit. Table 17.3 provides many useful tips for personal visits with legislators.

Telephoning

When time is short on an issue, a telephone call may be necessary. Call the legislator later at an appropriate time in his or her office. If the legislator is not available, then ask to speak to the health LA. Clearly state your name, that you are a CRNA constituent, the bill number, and what action you want the legislator to take, for example, "I am Jane Doe, a CRNA constituent of the senator's. I'm calling about S.1, the

Table 17.2: General Lobbying Tips

The following basic lobbying tips apply regardless of what type of interaction you have with the legislator.

- Call your state legislative hotline, if they have one, to find out the status of bills; at the federal level the legislative update number is (202) 225-1772.
- Get to know your legislator and his or her staff before you need help on an issue.
- Identify yourself as a voter from a specific congressional district or state. Identify any personal or professional relationships that will add weight and credibility to your position on the issue; for example, "I am the county campaign manager for the legislator" or "I am a member of the (your state) Association of Nurse Anesthetists."
- Clearly identify the bill that concerns you by number and subject matter, for example, S. 1, the reauthorization of the Nurse Education Act. Indicate precisely what action you want the legislator to take (e.g., introduce, cosponsor, support, amend, or oppose the bill).
- State what your position is on this issue and why. Personalize your position by telling the legislator how the issue affects his or her constituency.
- Respect the right of the legislator to disagree with you because of the merits or politics of the situation.
- Ask for a commitment—but do not expect a commitment before all the facts are in.
- Make periodic contact with the legislator. One visit, letter, or phone call will not establish a relationship. Continue to contact the legislator as the issue moves through the process for example, on introduction to cosponsor, to vote in favor at the subcommittee level, to vote in favor at the committee level, to vote in favor on the House or Senate floor, to support your version of the bill in conference committee, to vote for a presidential override.
- Always thank the legislator when he or she has taken positive action on your request.
- Work in conjunction with your state and national association lobbyists on issues, as well as networking with other groups.
- Invite legislators to your nursing meetings and community events; politicians love crowds and cameras.
- Furnish the legislator with your address and telephone number.
- Understand the positions of your association before you lobby.
- Report all contacts to your state or national legislative staff so that appropriate district and national follow-up can occur. This is also valuable for planning future strategy.
- Never leave a legislator out on a political limb by changing your position after the legislator has publicly stated support for a position that you urged him or her to take.
- Do not threaten the legislator with political reprisals.
- Remember that you need the legislator's vote on issues, and he or she needs your vote at election time.
- Invite your legislator to come and see how you practice.

reauthorization of the Nurse Education Act, which I support. I would like him to vote in favor of the bill when it comes up for committee action tomorrow. Thank you."

Corresponding with the Legislator

Letter writing techniques are provided in Tables 17.4, 17.5, and 17.6.

Email

Increasingly, email is becoming an effective way to communicate with elected officials. Email addresses can be obtained through a legislator's office or Web site.

Table 17.3: Dos and Don'ts Regarding Personal Visits with Legislators

DO:

- Give as much notice in scheduling your appointment as possible (at least two weeks).
- Make an appointment rather than dropping by, because it will greatly increase your chances of seeing the legislator; schedule the specific amount of time that you need—15 minutes is normally sufficient. Tell the appointments person what you want to talk about so the legislator may ask his or her staff person who handles that topic to sit in on the meeting.
- If the legislator is unavailable when you want to meet, it is definitely worthwhile to meet with the health LA. He or she can become your best friend in the office. Rest assured that if you try to circumvent or ignore staff, you will find it difficult to get staff cooperation in the future.
- Before making your appointment, find out if other nurses have already made appointments. Team lobbying is more effective. If you are in a group, select a spokesperson to lead the discussion.
- Be punctual.
- Be professional in your appearance and approach. Carry business cards with you so that you can network at all times.
- Address legislators by "Representative" or "Senator" until they tell you to call them something different.
- Identify yourself immediately as a constituent and a CRNA when you meet with the legislator; public officials meet too many people to remember everyone.
- Assume that legislators do not understand your issue; if they do they will tell you, if they do not you have saved them from looking foolish.
- Have an outline of the points that you want to make.
- If you cannot answer a question knowledgeably, tell the legislator that you or your association will send him or her the information as soon as possible and then do so.
- Do not take up the entire 15 minutes with your presentation; allow at least 5 minutes for the legislator to ask questions.
- Listen carefully to the legislator's view on your issue.
- Ask the legislator to help promote support with his or her colleagues on your issue.
- Ask for your legislator's advice on ways to lobby your issue.
- Ask the legislator what the opposition says about your issue; rebut the arguments if you can.
- Ask your legislator to keep an open mind on your issue even if he or she states that he or she currently opposes your position. Remember that controversial legislation and regulation usually result in compromise. Be ready with alternatives or solutions as well as criticisms.
- Leave your legislator with a one-page fact sheet on the issue, your position, and exactly what you want him or her to do. Provide articles or data that back up your view, if possible.
- Keep the door open for further discussion even if the legislator's attitude appears to be negative. Leave on a positive note.
- Follow up with a thank-you letter for the visit and again include a summary of the points that you made.

DON'T:

- Be angry if the legislator cannot meet with you when it is convenient for you. Make another appointment or meet with the health LA.
- Visit your legislator at home without an invitation.
- Call your legislator off the chamber floor unless it is truly an emergency.
- Visit the legislator more than once on an issue unless you have something new to say.
- Expect an on-the-spot endorsement of your bill or issue.

(continued)

Table 17.3: Dos and Don'ts Regarding Personal Visits with Legislators (continued)
• Portray your personal opinion on an issue as that of the association; if your personal position differs from the association, make that clear to the legislator.
• Let a legislator sidetrack you on another issue for the entire meeting so he or she does not have to address your issue.
• "Cry wolf" on every issue; overreaching diminishes credibility.
• Forget that the impression that you leave is as important as the substance of your discussion.
• Repeat off-the-record comments of one legislator to another—keep them confidential.
• Criticize your legislator for introducing a bill that you dislike, without finding out if the legislator is serious about pushing the bill.

Table 17.4: Address the Letter Properly	
House member:	The Honorable ____________________ U.S. House of Representatives Washington, DC 20515
Senate member:	The Honorable ____________________ U.S. Senate Washington, DC 20510
President:	The Honorable ____________________ President of the United States Washington, DC 20500

Table 17.5: Sample Letter to Senators

The Honorable (name of Senator)

Address

Washington, D.C. 20510

Dear Senator____________________:

I am writing to express my strong support for S.1, the bill to reauthorize the Nurse Education Act. I would like you to cosponsor this important bill because it provides funds for nurse anesthesia educational programs, student traineeships, and faculty development.

The education of Certified Registered Nurse Anesthetists (CRNAs) is especially important now because of the severe shortage of anesthesia providers in this country. The CRNA shortage has affected your district as evidenced by________________.

I appreciate your consideration of this critical piece of legislation and hope you will cosponsor it. I would appreciate hearing from you regarding your position on this issue.

Sincerely,

Table 17.6: Dos and Don'ts of Letter Writing

DO:

- Contact your own representative and two senators. As a constituent, you have a better chance of influencing their actions than you would by writing to the entire Senate and House of Representatives.
- Consider the factor of timing. Try to write when the bill is still in committee and awaiting action.
- Address the letter properly.
- Write legibly or type your letter for easiest reading.
- Use your personal stationery unless you have been asked to write on your association's or employer's letterhead.
- Sign your full name and address to the letter so you can be contacted. Envelopes are sometimes lost. Be sure the address that you give is within the legislator's district.
- Write to your legislator at his or her office rather than at home, so that your correspondence is filed to receive a response and for future reference.
- Mention the fact that you have a personal connection with the legislator (if indeed you do) because the staffer reading the letter will be more inclined to forward it directly to the legislator.
- Stick to one subject per letter and limit the letter to one page, if possible. If you need to include copies of articles or research data, attach them to the letter.
- Identify the bill number and popular name, if possible; for example: S. 1, the reauthorization of the Nurse Education Act.
- Clearly state your position and why you have taken that position in the first paragraph.
- Personalize the effect of the bill on you, your family, your practice, your community, your state. Form letters and petitions are not considered as valuable as personal letters.
- Request the legislator to communicate his or her position on the bill to you.
- Write to say thank you for a favorable vote to let your legislator know that you appreciate a job well done. Make sure to mention helpful staff in your thank-you letter.
- Send copies of your correspondence with legislators and their responses to the AANA Washington office.

DON'T:

- Become a "pen pal" and write on every issue being considered.
- Apologize for taking up the legislator's time—it is what they are elected for.
- Send a copy to a senator when you have written to a representative or vice versa.
- Be insulted if you receive a form letter in reply—legislators receive thousands of letters. After a few letters have been received regarding a particular issue, a standard form letter is written by a staff member and approved by the legislator. This form letter is then sent as a reply to all people writing about that issue.
- Send form letters or petitions, unless it is the only way a contact will be made.
- Forget to write and say thank you when legislators do something you approve of.
- Postpone writing; there is never a truly convenient time.

Overnight/Second Day Delivery

United Parcel Service, Federal Express, and the U.S. Postal Service all provide overnight and two-day delivery service.

TESTIFYING AT PUBLIC HEARINGS

An effective presentation by a CRNA at a health hearing could have a great impact on the ultimate fate of a bill. During hearings on legislation, representatives from professional associations, special interest groups, the executive branch, academia, and interested members of Congress are invited to speak. Your audience can be expected to be members of Congress, members of the press, congressional staff members, and lobbyists for organizations interested in the bill. The number of people in the audience will depend on the controversial nature of the legislation. At the federal level, hearings are usually scheduled in the morning because the House and Senate normally go into session around noon. Once Congress is in session, there is always a chance that a floor vote will require committee members to leave to go vote, which has a disruptive effect on the hearing.

The twofold objective of association testimony is to inform and persuade. What you have to say is important, but how well you say it is just as important. Your presentation can be very effective because you will be speaking as one directly affected by the proposal being considered, because you have special knowledge of the subject, or because you represent the viewpoint of many CRNAs. Your appearance increases the likelihood that your association will be consulted on other issues. A hearing can be instrumental in establishing permanent lines of communication with legislators.

Scope of Testimony

Every piece of testimony should include the following:

1. Identification of individuals appearing.
    a. Name, title, and place of work.
    b. Background to establish credibility as a witness.
    c. Identity of organization and constituency you are representing.
2. Identification of legislation or issue.
    a. Specify bill by number, issue by title.
    b. State your position briefly and early.
    c. Paraphase your understanding of the intent or purpose of the legislation or issue.
3. Areas under consideration.
    a. Define them.
    b. If supportive, explain why.
    c. If opposed, state why and give alternatives if any exist.
4. Lengthier explanation of your position and your rationale.
5. Summation, including what you would like to see accomplished
6. Thanks for being allowed to present your views.

Tables 17.7 and 17.8 provide more useful information for testifying.

The importance of individual congressional committees to health issues varies with changing circumstances, such as committee jurisdiction, the personality and political strength of individual committee chairs, and the current prominence of an individual health issue during a session of Congress. For the most part, however, the most influential committees are those that deal with the funding of discretionary health programs such as the Nurse Education Act (appropriation and budget committees) and those that deal with the financing of entitlement programs such as Medicare and Medicaid (authorization committees). Following are descriptions of the health-related committees of the Senate and the House of Representatives that have jurisdiction over the issues that are of greatest concern to CRNAs. Their juris-

Table 17.7: Preliminary Information Necessary before Testifying

Before you testify on a bill, you should have been provided with the following information by your staff person:

- What are the key provisions in the legislation?
- What are the arguments on both sides of the issue?
- Who are its supporters and opponents?
- What is the bill's impact on your practice?
- Has there been any prior hearing on this topic before the panel? Can you get copies of those earlier testimonies?
- What other interest groups and associations are testifying and what are their concerns with the legislation?
- What are the concerns of the individual committee members?
- Will the legislation have a significant impact on any of the constituents of the committee members?
- Does the chair have a special interest in the bill?
- What amendments are expected to be offered during the markup process? Will the amendments alter your association's position? Do you need to propose any amendments?
- What arguments will be used to oppose your association's position? Your testimony should counter those arguments.
- What are the committee's rules of procedure?
- What districts are represented by the committee members?
- Has your staff suggested "friendly questions" to the committee members that they may ask you to help you expand on your testimony?

dictions and important subcommittees are detailed, as well as how to contact these committees.

HEALTH-RELATED COMMITTEES OF THE U.S. SENATE

Appropriations

S-128 Capitol Building, Washington, D.C. 20510-6025; phone (202) 224-3471.

Jurisdiction: All discretionary funding for federal programs.

Key subcommittee: Labor, Health and Human Services, Education, and Related Agencies. SD-186 Dirksen Senate Office Building, Washington, D.C. 20510; phone (202) 224-7230.

Subcommittee jurisdiction: Nurse anesthesia education funding, National Center for Nursing Research, AIDS funding.

Armed Services

SR-228 Russell Senate Office Building, Washington, D.C. 20510-6050; phone (202) 224-3871.

Jurisdiction: Military funding, including CHAMPUS.

Key subcommittee: Manpower and Personnel (same address as full committee).

Subcommittee jurisdiction: Military incentive special pay.

Budget

SD-624 Dirksen Senate Office Building, Washington, D.C. 20510-6100; phone (202) 224-0642.

Jurisdiction: Total health funding and financing ceiling.

Governmental Affairs

Majority is SD-340 Dirksen Senate Office Building, Washington, D.C. 20510-6250; phone (202) 224-2627. Minority is SH-605 Senate Hart Office Building, Washington, D.C. 20510-6250; phone (202) 224-4751.

Table 17.8: Dos and Don'ts of Testifying

DO:

- Arrive promptly. Witnesses will usually be allowed to enter a hearing room first, before the public. When you arrive, inform committee staff that you are there.
- At the state level, you may need to fill out a witness registration slip, where you indicate whether you are for or against the bill. Persons who wish to speak indicate so on the registration slip. At the state level, if you have traveled some distance to appear and will be returning home that day, note that fact on the registration slip. The committee chair will often call such witnesses early in the hearing to allow for their travel home.
- Be prepared to wait. There may be other bills heard before yours. It is also difficult to judge how long each speaker will take. Do not be surprised if you have to wait for some time before being called.
- If possible, bring a copy of the bill with you. This will allow you to refer to specific sections in your presentation or when answering questions.
- Providing copies of written testimony to the committee is advised even for those who present oral testimony. At the federal level the committee staff will inform you of how many copies of testimony are necessary for the committee.
- A longer written testimony will usually be submitted for the record. You will usually be presenting 5- or 10-minute remarks that are a brief summary of the lengthier text. Rehearse your presentation thoroughly and time it. Do not exceed your time limit under any circumstances. In fact, some committee rooms have green, yellow, and red lights to let you know how you are managing your time. Regardless of where you are in your prepared remarks, when the red light goes on you should finish your sentence, and say thank you.
- Usually the message in a piece of testimony is so vital that a script is essential for complete accuracy; however, do not use the script as a crutch, burying your eyes in it.
- Tailor the text delivery and style of your testimony to fit your own personality. It should be simple, focused, and natural. The end result should be like a conversation between you and someone you like.
- Work with the staff person who is drafting your testimony so that you are comfortable with the way the ideas are expressed. A good use of your familiar expressions and real-life examples in the testimony will make you feel better and make the testimony seem more genuine.
- Be prepared to answer questions. The association staff should go over anticipated questions that you may receive from the committee and provide you with possible answers. Hearing tough questions in advance is much better than encountering them for the first time at a hearing.
- If you are testifying on a controversial topic, be prepared for media at the hearing. Work with your staff person on how to handle a media interview if requested.
- Your staff will not sit at the witness table with you, but they can sit right behind you in case you need some help.
- If neither you nor your staff person know an answer to a question, admit it and offer to supply the information later for the record.

DON'T:

- Assume that all committee members are familiar with all aspects of the bill: That is the purpose of the hearing. Review the specific provisions of the bill that are of concern.
- Repeat at length the points made by a previous speaker. If you have something to add to what was said, by all means do so. If not, simply note your agreement with the earlier speaker and move on to the rest of your presentation. To be effective, your presentation must be somewhat flexible. Pay attention to what other speakers are saying.
- Attempt to answer questions for which you do not have answers or facts. If you are requested to appear by a staff member of a trade association, ask the committee chair if that staff member can respond with better facts or experience than you might have. You may also offer to provide additional information after the hearing.

(continued)

Table 17.8: Dos and Don'ts of Testifying (continued)

- Be disappointed if only one or two legislators show up for the hearing. That does not diminish your testimony—often legislators have two or more hearings scheduled for the same time. Be comforted that everything you say is going into the hearing record and will be closely studied by the committee staff.

Jurisdiction: Total health funding and financing ceiling.

Finance

SD-219 Dirksen Senate Office Building, Washington, D.C. 20510-6200; phone (202) 224-4515.

Jurisdiction: Taxes, Medicare, and Medicaid.

Key subcommittees: Health (same address as full committee); Medicare and long-term care (same address as full committee).

Health, Education, Labor and Pensions Committee

SD-428 Dirksen Senate Office Building, Washington, D.C. 20510-6300; phone (202) 224-5375.

Jurisdiction: Health authorizations and reauthorizations, including nurse anesthesia education funding.

HEALTH-RELATED COMMITTEES OF THE U.S. HOUSE OF REPRESENTATIVES

Appropriations

H-218 Capitol Building, Washington, D.C. 20515-6015; phone (202) 225-2771.

Jurisdiction: All discretionary funding for federal programs.

Key subcommittee: Labor, Health and Human Services, Education. 2358 Rayburn House Office Building, Washington, D.C. 20515; phone (202) 225-3508.

Subcommittee jurisdiction: Nurse anesthesia education funding, National Center for Nursing Research, AIDS funding.

Armed Services

2120 Rayburn House Office Building, Washington, D.C. 20515-6035; phone (202) 225-4151.

Jurisdiction: Military funding, including CHAMPUS.

Key subcommittee: Military Personnel. 2340 Rayburn House Office Building, Washington, DC 20515; phone (202) 225-7560.

Subcommittee jurisdiction: Military incentive special pay.

Budget

309 Cannon House Office Building, Washington, D.C. 20515-6065; phone (202) 226-7270.

Jurisdiction: Total health funding and financing ceiling.

Commerce

2125 Rayburn House Office Building, Washington, D.C. 20515-6115; phone (202) 225-2927.

Jurisdiction: Public health and health facilities.

Key subcommittee: Health and the Environment. 2125 Rayburn House Office Building, Washington, D.C. 20515; phone (202) 225-2125.

Subcommittee jurisdiction: Health authorizations and reauthorizations, including nurse anesthesia education funding, Medicaid, and shared jurisdiction with Ways and Means Committee over Medicare Part B.

Ways and Means

1102 Longworth House Office Building, Washington, D.C. 20515-6348; phone (202) 225-3625.

Jurisdiction: Taxes and Medicare.

Key subcommittee: Health. 1136 Longworth House Office Building, Washington, D.C. 20515; phone (202) 225-3943.

Subcommittee jurisdiction: Medicare Part A and shared jurisdiction with Energy and Commerce Committee over Medicare Part B.

HOW TO OBTAIN CONGRESSIONAL DOCUMENTS

Bills, Reports, and Public Laws

One copy of six different items (bills, reports, public laws) may be requested in writing daily from the Senate Document Room; phone orders are not accepted. One copy of 12 different items may be requested in writing daily from the House Document Room; phone orders of up to six items are accepted. Multiple copies of one item are not available. Please enclose a self-addressed, gummed label to facilitate the return mailing.

Senate Document Room
B-04 Hart Building
Washington, D.C. 20510

Hearing Documents

A free copy of a House or Senate committee print or hearing record can be requested by sending a self-addressed label to the publications clerk of the committee from which the document was issued. Mail requests for prints and records may also be sent to:

Superintendent of Documents
Government Printing Office
Congressional Sales Office
Washington, D.C. 20402-9315

Single copies of Government Printing Office documents are free; additional copies may require a fee. Hearing records are generally available two months after the close of hearings.

SUMMARY

It is hoped that the information provided in this chapter, on how the AANA is involved in the political and legislative arenas, will provide you with the impetus to assert your own influence in healthcare policy. Educating yourself on the political process will give you the power to have input on the issues that will ultimately affect you. This input will allow you to educate legislators on health issues and put the democratic process in motion.

GLOSSARY

Act: Term for legislation that has passed both chambers of Congress and has been signed by the president or passed by a two-thirds majority in a presidential veto override, thus becoming law.

Amendment: A proposal of a legislator to change the language or content in a bill.

Bill: Legislative proposal originating in either chamber of Congress and designated "H.R." in the House and "S." in the Senate. The bill number is usually assigned in the order in which legislation is introduced from the beginning of each two-year congressional term.

Calendar: The agenda or list of pending business before either chamber of Congress or before a committee.

Chamber: Meeting place for the total membership of the House or Senate, as opposed to committee rooms.

Cloture: Process by which debate (or filibuster) can be limited in the Senate, other than by unanimous consent. Requires the vote of 60 senators present and voting. Under cloture, each senator is limited to one hour of debate.

Conference committee: The more controversial a bill may be, the more likely it will pass the Senate and House in different forms. Unless either body is willing to accept the changes of the other, the two versions must go to a conference committee. This means that a committee (the number is not fixed), chosen from the originating Senate and House committees, is appointed to work out a compromise. An agreement, if reached, is known as a "conference report." It must then be approved by both the Senate and the House.

Congressional Record: Daily printed account of the proceedings of both the House and Senate chambers, with debate, statements, and so on, reported verbatim.

Executive session: Meeting of a committee at which only the committee's members, and no public or press, are allowed to attend.

Federal Register: Daily printed account of the activities of federal agencies, including rule making.

Filibuster: A device, used only in the Senate, to delay or prevent a vote by time-consuming talk. This tactic is often used by a minority in an effort to prevent a vote on a bill that would probably pass if brought to a vote. It can be stopped only by a 60-member vote of the senators present and voting.

Law: An act of Congress that has been signed by the president or passed over the president's veto by Congress.

Markup: After public hearings, a subcommittee will go into executive (either closed or open) session to start the markup of a bill; that is, to write amendments into it, delete sections, or revise the language. Views of both sides are stated in detail, and at the conclusion of deliberation, a vote is taken to determine subcommittee action. It may decide to report the bill favorably to the full committee, with or without amendments, or suggest that the bill be tabled. Each member of the subcommittee has one vote.

Omnibus bill: A legislative proposal concerning several separate but related items.

Quorum: Number of members whose presence is needed to conduct business. This would be a majority of the members, or 51 in the Senate and 218 in the House. Any member may object to the conduct of business without a quorum and thus force a roll call to bring in absentees. Roll calls are frequently used as a delaying tactic. Much legislation is passed without a quorum because it is noncontroversial. If a point of order is made that quorum is not present, the only business that can be done is either a motion to adjourn or a motion to direct the sergeant-at-arms to request the attendance of absentees.

Roll call vote: Members vote as their names are called by the clerk of the chamber.

Rule of germaneness: Used to knock out language that does not pertain to the purpose of the bill. Also used to kill an appropriation where the expenditure has not been previously authorized by a separate bill. The Senate may impose the rule on itself under a unanimous consent agreement to limit debate on a pending matter. A two-thirds vote is necessary to retain the language.

Standing vote: An unrecorded vote taken when all members in favor of a proposal stand and are counted and then all members opposed stand and are counted.

Veto: Action taken by the president rejecting a bill presented by Congress for signature. When Congress is in session, the president has 10 days, excluding Sundays, to veto a bill, or it automatically becomes law.

Voice vote: The presiding officer of either chamber calls for "yeas" and "nays" to determine the results.

REFERENCES

Mason, D.J. & Talbott, S.W. (1985). *Political Action Handbook for Nurses.* Menlo Park, CA: Addison-Wesley.

Lederer, J.C. (1987). Legislate success: Learn to lobby. *ASAE Association Management.* December, 29-32.

From Idea to Law: The State Legislative Process. (1989). State Net, Sacramento, CA.

Pressures in Congress. (1983). *The Washington Post.* A14, June 26.

Oleszek, W.J. (1989). *Congressional Procedures and the Policy Process* (3rd ed.). Washington, DC: CQ Press.

Davies, J. (1986). *Legislative Law and Process* (2nd ed.). St. Paul, MN: West Publishing.

Congress and Health. (1989). National Health Council, New York.

How Congress Works (2nd ed.). (1991). Washington, DC: Congressional Quarterly.

Gwyn, K.H. (1992). Presenting testimony before a congressional committee. *ASAE Government Relations.* 2:1-10.

Testifying with Impact, rev. ed. (1983). Chamber of Commerce of the United States, Washington, DC.

KEY REFERENCES

Bacchus, W.I. (1983). *Inside the Legislative Process.* Boulder, CO: Westview Press.

Bryner, G. (1987). *Bureaucratic Discretion: Laws and Policy in Federal Regulatory Agencies.* New York, NY: Pergamon Press.

Congress A to Z: CQ's Ready Reference Encyclopedia. (1988). Washington, DC: Congressional Quarterly.

Davidson, R.H. & Olezsek, W.J. (1990). *Congress and Its Members* (3rd ed.). Washington, DC: CQ Press.

Dodd, L.C. & Oppenheimer, B.I. (Eds.). (1990). *Congress Reconsidered* (4th ed.). Washington, DC: CQ Press.

Froman, L.A., Jr. (1967). *The Congressional Process: Strategies, Rules, and Procedures.* Boston, MA: Little, Brown.

Meier, K. (1985). *Regulation: Politics, Bureaucracy and Economics.* New York, NY: St. Martin's Press.

Smith, S. (1989). *Call to Order: Floor Politics in the House and Senate.* Washington, DC: Brookings Institution.

STUDY QUESTIONS

1. What is the function of a Political Action Committee and what role does it play in advancing the legislative agenda of the association?

2. Describe the process of how legislation is passed into law at the federal level, including requirements for review by various committees.

3. List some of the primary methods that CRNAs can use to communicate effectively with their legislators.

4. Role play with your colleagues the presentation of a particular issue that you might present to a legislator. Pretend that you have 10 minutes to make your case. What will you say and what will you prepare to leave with him or her as pertinent reference material?

5. Discuss the ways in which your involvement in the political/legislative process has had a direct effect on your clinical practice.

6. Devise some innovative strategies on how you can teach your CRNA colleagues necessary skills of political involvement/action.

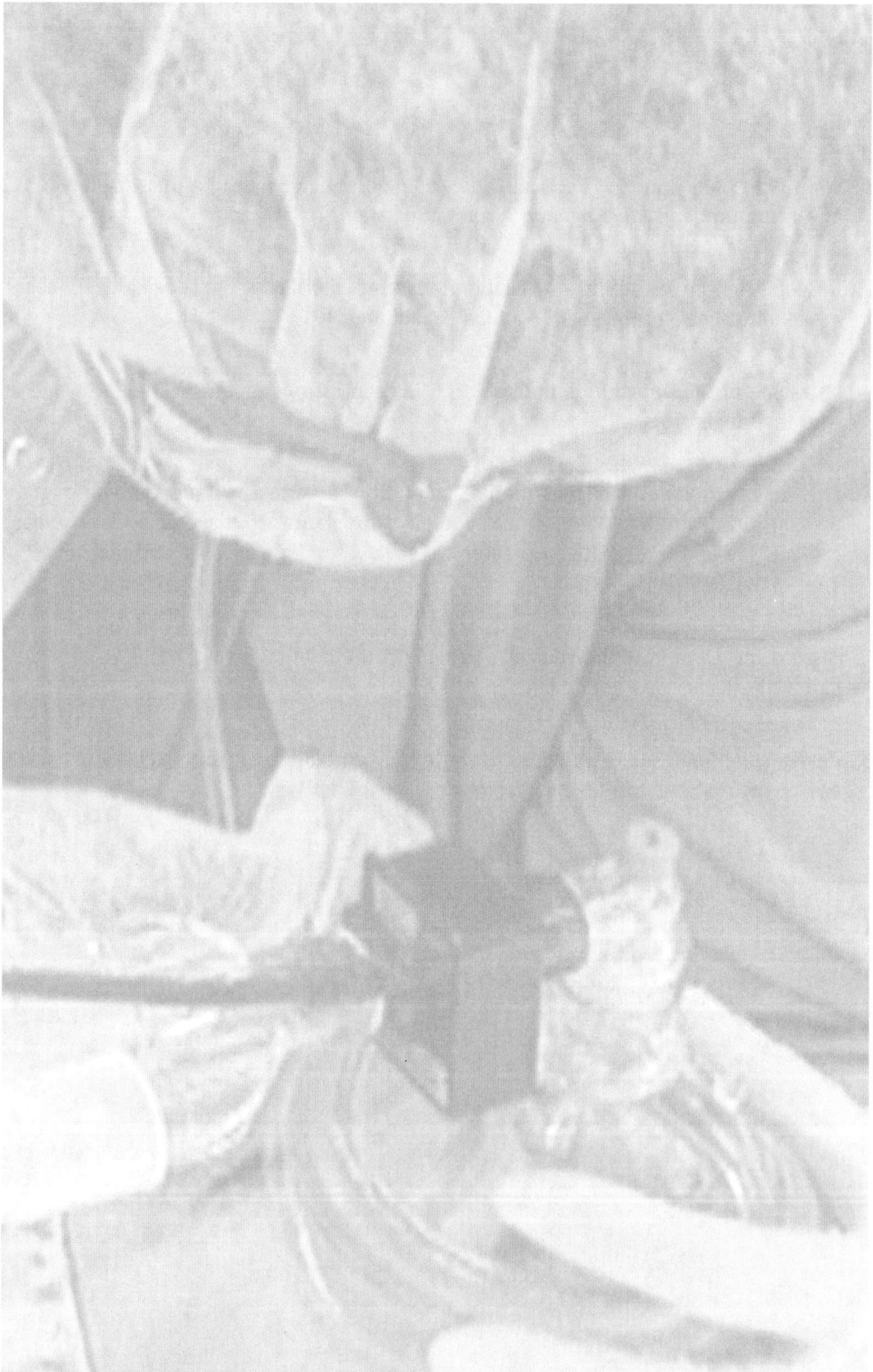

CHAPTER 18

FEDERAL HEALTHCARE POLICY: HOW AANA ADVOCATES FOR THE PROFESSION

Nancy Bruton-Maree, CRNA, MS

Program Director
Raleigh School of Nurse Anesthesia/University of North Carolina at Greensboro
Raleigh, NC

Rita M. Rupp, RN, MA

Special Assistant
Office of the Executive Director
American Association of Nurse Anesthetists
Park Ridge, IL

KEY CONCEPTS

- Research supports the position of the American Association of Nurse Anestthtists (AANA) that changes in the Tax Equity and Fiscal Responsibility Act rules favoring less restrictive conditions for payment would allow flexible allocation of anesthesia personnel and provide a more efficient service to consumers.

- Deferring to state law in reference to physician supervision of nurse anesthesia in the proposed rules and regulations for hospital reimbursement from Medicare would be consistent with language used by the Centers for Medicare & Medicaid Services for other healthcare practitioners.

- AANA has actively lobbied for changes in Medicare reimbursement rules and regulations that would promote the profession of nurse anesthesia while maintaining patient safety and a quality standard of care.

- Since the inception of healthcare reform, AANA has taken a proactive position in support of legislation that ensures consumers a choice of provider and accountability in healthcare.

- AANA has guarded the ability of Certified Registered Nurse Anesthetists (CRNAs) to compete in the healthcare marketplace through supporting antitrust and antidiscrimination legislation.

- More than 75 percent of all graduates of anesthesia programs over the last decade have received federal money as either direct student aid, or indirectly through new program start-up funds or faculty-assistance plans.

A number of federal initiatives in the 1980s and 1990s had a significant impact on the nurse anesthesia profession. Sponsored legislation and regulatory advocacy were most often brought to the attention of policy makers by the American Association of Nurse Anesthetists (AANA) or state organizations in the form of annual legislative agendas. Issues most often dealt with related to equity issues in reimbursement, regulatory recognition, quality of care, insurance, antitrust and antidiscrimination. This chapter will address the advocacy role of the AANA in a select number of these federal healthcare initiatives. Before discussing each of these areas in detail, the authors have provided some contextual background on the Medicare program as it relates to the issues of supervision and medical direction of Certified Registered Nurse Anesthetists (CRNAs).

UNDERSTANDING THE MEDICARE PROGRAM

The Medicare program is divided into three major sections, which are commonly referred to as Medicare Part A, Medicare Part B, and Medicare Part C. Medicare Part A outlines the rules and regulations by which hospitals and ambulatory care facilities are reimbursed for services, supplies, drugs, and equipment provided to Medicare patients. Medicare Part A does not include any reimbursement that goes directly to anesthesiologists, nurse anesthetists, or anesthesiologist assistants (AAs). As of this writing, the Medicare Part A regulations require physician supervision of CRNAs as a condition for hospital, ambulatory surgical centers (ASC), and critical access hospitals (CAH) to be eligible to participate and receive reimbursement from Medicare (51 *F.R.* 22010, June 17, 1986; 57 *F.R.* 33878, July 31, 1992; 47 *F.R.* 34082, August 5, 1982; 57 *F.R.* 33878, July 31, 1992; 60 *F.R.* 45851, September 1, 1995; and 62 *F.R.* 46037, August 29, 1997).

Medicare Part B sets forth the payment regulations for healthcare professionals who are eligible to receive direct reimbursement through the Medicare program. The requirements that must be met to receive reimbursement from Medicare Part B are distinct and separate from Medicare Part A. Currently there are two types of reimbursement provisions for anesthesiologists under Medicare Part B related to their working with CRNAs. These provisions include payment for medical direction and medical supervision of anesthesia services (63 *F.R.* 58921, November 2, 1998; 48 *F.R.* 8928, March 2, 1983).

If Medicare is billed for medically directed anesthesia services by an anesthesiologist, he/she must be directing no more than four concurrent procedures involving residents, CRNAs, or anesthesia assistants. The seven conditions of payment enacted as a result of the Tax Equity and Fiscal Responsibility Act of 1982 (TEFRA) must be followed (Table 18.1). In these medically directed cases, the anesthesiologist receives 50 percent of the payment for each case that he/she is medically directing, and a medically directed CRNA administering the anesthesia receives the other 50 percent.

Medicare Part B also includes a provision for payment to anesthesiologists for medical supervision of nurse anesthetists who are administering anesthesia. While current Medicare statutes define the conditions for medical direction, there is no specific definition for medical supervision. Medical supervision is indirectly defined in the Medicare Carrier's Manual section §15018, subpart D, which states that in cases where the "physician leaves the immediate area of the operating suite for other than short durations or devotes extensive time to an emergency case or is otherwise not available to respond to the

Table 18.1: Department of Health and Human Services, Centers for Medicare & Medicaid Services
Medicare Program Conditions for Physician Payment of Medically Directed Anesthesia Services

Original Rules	***Proposed Rules***	***Current Rules***
42CFR §405.552 Conditions for payment of charges: Concurrent anesthesiology services.	**42CFR §415.110 Conditions for payment: Medically directed anesthesia services.**	**42CFR §415.110 Conditions for payment: Medically directed anesthesia services.**
(Source: As adopted 48 *F.R.* 8938, March 2, 1983; effective October 1, 1983)	(Source: As proposed 63 *F.R.* 30884, June 5, 1998)	(Source: As adopted 63 *F.R.* 58912, November 2, 1998; effective January 1, 1999)
(a) (1) For each patient, the physician:	(a) (1) For each patient, the physician:	(a) (1) For each patient, the physician:
(i) Performs a preanesthetic examination and evaluation;	(i) Performs a preanesthetic examination and evaluation, or reviews one performed by another qualified individual permitted by the state to administer anesthetics;	(i) Performs a preanesthetic examination and evaluation;
(ii) Prescribes the anesthesia plan;	(ii) Participates in the development of the anesthesia plan and gives final approval of the proposed plan;	(ii) Prescribes the anesthesia plan;
(iii) Personally participates in the most demanding procedures in the anesthesia plan, including induction and emergence;	(iii) Personally participates in the most demanding procedures of the anesthesia plan;	(iii) Personally participates in the most demanding aspects of the anesthesia plan including, if applicable, induction and emergence;
(iv) Ensures that any procedures in the anesthesia plan that he or she does not perform are performed by a qualified individual as defined in program operating instructions;	(iv) Ensures that any aspect of the anesthesia plan not performed by the anesthesiologist is performed by a qualified individual as specified in operating instructions;	(iv) Ensures that any procedures in the anesthesia plan that he or she does not perform are performed by a qualified individual as defined in operating instructions.
(v) Monitors the course of anesthesia at frequent intervals;	(v) Monitors the course of anesthesia at intervals medically indicated by the nature of the procedure and the patient's condition;	(v) Monitors the course of anesthesia administration at frequent intervals;
(vi) Remains physically present and available for immediate diagnosis and treatment of emergencies; and	(vi) Remains physically present and available for immediate diagnosis and treatment of emergencies; and	(vi) Remains physically present and available for immediate diagnosis and treatment of emergencies; and
(vii) Provides indicated postanesthesia care.	(vii) Provides indicated postanesthesia care or ensures that it is done by a qualified individual as described in paragraph (a) (1) (iv) of this section.	(vii) Provides indicated postanesthesia care.
		* Note: Documentation requirements for the above conditions were revised on January 1, 1999. (See note at bottom.)

* The medical documentation rules adopted by the Health Care Financing Administration (now the Centers for Medicare & Medicaid Services) as published in the November 2, 1998, *Federal Register* and effective January 1, 1999, are as follows: (b) *Medical documentation.* The physician alone inclusively documents in the patient's medical record that the conditions set forth in paragraph (a) (1) of this section have been satisfied, specifically documenting that he or she performed the preanesthetic exam and evaluation, provided the indicated postanesthesia care, and was present during the most demanding procedures, including induction and emergence where applicable.

immediate needs of the surgical patients, the physician's services to the surgical patients are supervisory in nature..."

The other reference to supervision refers to situations where a physician is involved in furnishing more than four procedures concurrently, or is performing other services while directing the concurrent procedures. Clearly, the current statutes recognize the level of involvement required for a physician to be medically directing a case, and situations wherein the physician is providing supervisory services.

The current payment methodology for medically supervised anesthesia cases is:

1. Physician anesthesiologists are paid at a base of three units (with an additional one unit if they were present during induction). This represents payment for physician involvement in the presurgical anesthesia services. [42C *F.R.* §414.46]

2. CRNAs and AAs are reimbursed at 50 percent of the total fee if a physician is involved in the medical supervision/direction of the case.

The requirement for a CRNA to be reimbursed through Medicare Part B is that he/she must meet the state licensure requirements in the state in which he/she practices and meet the requirements of the Council on Certification of Nurse Anesthetists and Council on Recertification of Nurse Anesthetists. Also, graduate nurse anesthetists must be certified within 24 months of graduation to continue receiving Medicare Part B reimbursement.

NURSE ANESTHESIA REIMBURSEMENT

In 1983, the Prospective Payment System (PPS) legislation was passed in an effort to control hospital costs to the Medicare program (Gunn, 1997). The law provided that all services by providers other than those reimbursed through Medicare Part B would be bundled into a hospital diagnosis-related group payment. The caveats for CRNAs in this law were several: (1) it would be impossible for the anesthesia component of payment to cover the full cost of hospital-employed CRNAs; (2) unbundling of services and payment was prohibited; and (3) anesthesiologists who had been billing for CRNA services under Part B by considering them a physician service could no longer bill through this mechanism (Gunn, 1997). Simply put, CRNA services were, for all practical purposes, nonreimbursable.

Because of the potential negative impact of the PPS legislation on nurse anesthetists, AANA advocated the following legislative changes (Gunn, 1997):

1. A provision allowing a temporary pass-through of hospitals' CRNA costs for a three-year period, which would assure hospitals would not lose money on CRNA services;

2. A single exception to the unbundling provisions of the law for anesthesiologist-employed CRNAs, because it was questionable if anesthesiologists could bill for CRNA services under the new provision; and

3. Inclusion of direct reimbursement for CRNAs in the Omnibus Reconciliation Act (OBRA) of 1986, to become effective January 1, 1989, with the two temporary provisions being extended to the effective date of the legislation. Two payment schedules were incorporated in the law—one for CRNAs not medically directed by anesthesiologists and the other for CRNAs working under anesthesiologist medical direction.

As a part of OBRA 1989, Congress mandated a study of reimbursement mechanisms that would not serve as disincentives for using CRNAs.

TAX EQUITY AND FISCAL RESPONSIBILITY ACT OF 1982

TEFRA was enacted into federal law as a means to control escalating Medicare costs for hospital-based services which included anesthesiology, pathology, and radiology. Among the many cost concerns that TEFRA addressed was a need to ensure that an anesthesiologist demonstrated that he or she provided certain services as part of a given anesthetic to qualify for payment for medical direction of a CRNA. Prior to the enactment of TEFRA, anesthesiologists could bill for their services in conjunction with medical direction of hospital-employed CRNAs without demonstrating that they provided specific services to qualify for such payment. While the 1976 Medicare manual (4-76, 2050.2, Rev. 3-512, 2.21) did require that the "physician be close by and available to provide immediate and personal assistance and direction," the Medicare manual stated that availability by telephone did not constitute direct, personal and continuous service. Because some anesthesiologists failed to comply with Medicare rules and because the number of anesthetics administered by CRNAs that could be supervised and billed by anesthesiologists had no limit, some private payers began refusing to reimburse for more than two concurrent procedures. In addition, Medicare's Inspector General's Office expanded its search for fraudulent practices for anesthesia billing.

In 1983, the Health Care Financing Administration (HCFA; now the Centers for Medicare and Medicaid Services, or CMS) published the final rules implementing TEFRA relative to payment for anesthesiology physician services (U.S. Department of Health and Human Services [HHS], 48 *F.R.*, March 2, 1983). In instituting the rules, HCFA chose a 4:1 ratio of medical direction, limiting payment to anesthesiologists to no more than four concurrent procedures administered by CRNAs. The rules implemented seven conditions that an anesthesiologist must satisfy if he or she was to obtain reimbursement for the medical direction of CRNAs. These original conditions are listed in Table 18.1.

In its comments on the proposed TEFRA rules, AANA expressed concern that the limitation of concurrent procedures reimbursable on a charge basis not be linked to presumptions about the quality of anesthesia services furnished by CRNAs under a physician's general supervision. HCFA's published response was as follows: "The distinctions we are making is [sic] between physician services to providers and individuals, not between good and bad anesthesia services. Anesthesia administered by non-physician anesthetist is a covered service, reimbursable on a reasonable cost basis. Therefore the criteria for 'medical direction' should not be interpreted as standards of practice or standards of quality, but rather as a description of those elements of common medical practice that are expected to be present when a physician has significant involvement with an individual patient (HHS, 48 *F.R.*, March 2, 1983)."

Even though the AANA was successful in obtaining the above clarification, the TEFRA conditions of payment for anesthesiologists have been inappropriately interpreted by many as quality of care standards for the practice of anesthesia instead of reimbursement criteria for anesthesiologists. The regulations have served to create disruptions in the overall delivery and flow of services in the operating room setting, causing needless and costly delays to the government and ultimately to consumers. In some cases, anesthesiologists have used the medical direction conditions of payment in negotiations with hospitals as justification to adopt the anesthesia care team model of practice. Assertions that the medical direction conditions are standards of care and assure a better level of quality than the care provided by a solo CRNA practitioner have been successfully used by anesthesiologists to support the anesthesia care team model, but such assertions are not supported by valid scientific research.

By 1996, AANA believed changes in healthcare and healthcare reimbursement favoring less restrictive conditions would allow flexibility in allocation of anesthesia personnel and more expedient service to consumers. In addition, studies began to support the opposite of the anesthesiologists' promotion that medical direction of CRNAs provided a higher quality of care. For example, the 1992 Center for Health Economics Research (CHER) report to the Physician Payment Review Commission (PPRC) recommended the following: "Refinements to the TEFRA provisions should be considered in view of the reductions in payments to the anesthesia care team. In particular, opportunities for increasing the flexibility of role functions should be reviewed. Considerations should also be given to the appropriateness of promulgating specific practice standards within a payment policy." The CHER report went on to say, "With the implication of a capped payment, the Health Care Financing Administration should consider whether to review the TEFRA requirements to see if modifications of the TEFRA rules would permit greater efficiencies without decreasing the quality of care (PPRC Report to Congress, 1993)."

In 1993, the PPRC Report to Congress on "Payments for the Anesthesia Care Team" noted: "The use of the anesthesia care team seems to be determined by individual preferences for that practice arrangement. There appear to be no demonstrated quality of care differences between the care provided by the solo anesthesiologist, solo CRNA, and the team (PPRC, 1993)."

In a study of medical direction conducted at a Los Angeles county hospital, findings concluded, "Anesthesiologists and nurse anesthetists in this study agreed in their perceptions that more than 70 percent of these cases did not need medical direction." The report further noted, "Even though this study was from one practice setting, it suggests that excessive medical direction may be contributing to the higher costs of anesthesia care teams. Revision of medical direction guidelines (TEFRA), focusing on patient and operative factors, is recommended to preserve the anesthesia care team as a practice option, while making it more cost effective (Fassett & Calmes, 1995)." In another study of medical direction, the findings were as follows: "Significantly, the protocol groups appear to have no difference from the retrospective group in all outcome criteria, meaning that medical direction can be reduced without a reduction in quality. This can result in a significant cost reduction when physician time is considered. It is possible to significantly reduce the costs of anesthesia care teams through reduction of unnecessary medical direction and revision of TEFRA guidelines. This study may have other applications in terms of provider job satisfaction and the ability to use physician resources most effectively (Stein, 1994)."

In 1997, based on studies such as the ones described above, the AANA initiated as part of its legislative agenda a congressional lobbying effort to revise the TEFRA conditions of payment for medical direction of CRNAs by anesthesiologists. In 1998, the AANA shifted its focus from legislative strategies for revision of TEFRA to revision through regulatory change. Healthcare reform, contrary to earlier predictions, brought an increase in surgical and anesthesia case numbers, and managed care companies put emphasis on increased operating room efficiency without a decline in quality of care. The TEFRA conditions, in many instances, hindered efficient utilization of operating rooms. Since the TEFRA conditions were not tied to quality of care, AANA, as did other healthcare organizations, used legislative and regulatory change as the avenue to advocate positively for the public, as well as for its members.

In a 1998 joint meeting that included the American Society of Anesthesiologists (ASA), AANA, and HCFA, proposals were advanced by both AANA and ASA for revisions to seven conditions of payment for physician medical direction. ASA and AANA reached consensus on a revised recommended set of medical direction requirements that are listed as proposed revisions in Table 18.1 (63 *F.R.*, June 5, 1998). However, it came to AANA's attention in a publication called *Anesthesia Answer Book—Action Alert* (1998) that ASA had second thoughts about the agreed-upon revisions. HCFA's response to the concerns posed by the ASA membership and several state anesthesiologist societies was to retain the current requirements established in 1983 (63 *F.R.*, November 2, 1998). HCFA decided that the medically directing physician must be present at induction and emergence for general anesthesia but only if applicable for other types of anesthesia, such as regional anesthesia (63 *F.R.*, November 2, 1998). HCFA plans to study the medical direction issue further, welcomes comments, and may propose changes in the future (63 *F.R.*, November 2, 1998).

Because the matter of fraud has been elevated to a level of serious concern (as it relates to the misapplication of the seven conditions), all providers should have a complete understanding of practice parameters allowable in a medically directed situation. The reader should be aware that an anesthesiologist who is concurrently directing the administration of anesthesia to not more than four surgical patients cannot ordinarily be involved in furnishing additional services to other patients. However, addressing an emergency of short duration in the immediate area, administering an epidural or caudal anesthetic to ease labor pain, or periodic rather than continuous monitoring of an obstetrical patient, does not substantially diminish the scope of control exercised by the physician in directing the administration of anesthesia to the surgical patients. It does not constitute a separate service for the purpose of determining whether medical direction criteria are met. Further, while directing concurrent anesthesia procedures, a physician may receive patients entering the operating suite for the next surgery, check or discharge patients in the recovery room, or handle scheduling matters without affecting fee schedule payment (*Medicare Carrier's Manual*, Part 3, Section 15018C).

It is important to note at the bottom of Table 18.1 the statement requiring the anesthesiologist to document that his/her medical direction involvement is a part of the final language that became effective January 1, 1999. Of particular importance in the compliance arena is HCFA's imposition of specific documentation requirements for the medically directing anesthesiologist. This documentation requirement by HCFA was at the recommendation of AANA (63 *F.R.*, November 2, 1998). The AANA asked that HCFA revise the medical documentation requirement mandating that the physician alone personally document the record. AANA's rationale for the request was that the CRNA should not have to document the physician's participation since the CRNA may not agree concerning the extent of the physician's participation in the case (63 *F.R.*, November 2, 1998).

AANA continues to monitor the

impact that the TEFRA rules for physician reimbursement for medical direction of CRNAs have on operating room efficiency, patient care, and CRNA practice. Making changes in these conditions for payment has been difficult for the AANA because these are conditions that do not impact CRNA reimbursement for anesthesia services. It is difficult for a healthcare provider organization to implement change regarding another provider's mechanism of payment; therefore, change in the TEFRA conditions for payment may come incrementally as more evidence supports the problematic impact they have on operating room efficiency and cost.

Since the inception of the medical direction guidelines, AANA has influenced changes in the TEFRA conditions for physician medical direction payment and reimbursement for CRNA services in the following ways:

- The adoption of a 1:4 medical direction ratio rather than a 1:2.
- A published statement by HCFA that the criteria for medical direction should not be considered quality-related standards, rather, payment criteria.
- Adoption of 1998 revisions that facilitate flexibility in practice.
- A published requirement that the physician document his/her personal and inclusive involvement in satisfying the conditions for medical direction payment.
- Adoption of a 50 percent split in payment by the anesthesiologist and CRNA for a case, as long as the ratio of medical direction does not exceed 1:4.
- Adoption of a 50 percent split in payment between the anesthesiologist and CRNA when the medical direction is 1:1.

SUPERVISION: MEDICARE CONDITIONS OF PARTICIPATION

The current Medicare regulations require physician supervision of CRNAs as a condition for hospitals, ASCs and CAHs to receive Medicare payment (Tables 18.2-18.4). These regulations do not require that a CRNA be supervised by an anesthesiologist.

During the 1990s, AANA pursued a revision of these Medicare conditions of participation that would remove the physician supervision requirement for CRNAs and instead defer to state statutory rules and regulations related to licensure. Currently, 31 states have no physician supervision or direction requirement concerning CRNAs in nurse practice acts, board of nursing rules/regulations, medical practice acts, board of medicine rules/regulations, or their generic equivalents. Clearly this is an indication that many states, as a matter of public policy, do not believe it is necessary to require physician supervision of CRNAs.

In December 1997, HCFA released for comment proposed revisions to the Medicare Conditions of Participation for Hospitals, ASCs and CAHs which would eliminate the requirement for physician supervision of CRNAs, deferring instead to state law (Tables 18.2-18.4). AANA supported these proposed revisions to the Medicare and Medicaid rule for facility reimbursement for the following reasons:

- The proposed rule brings HCFA into compliance with 42 U.S.C. section 1395 which prohibits "any Federal officer or employee to exercise any supervision or control over the practice of medicine or the manner in which medical services are provided, or over the selection, tenure, or compensation of any officer or employee of any institution, agency, or person providing health services; or to exercise any

Table 18.2: HHS/CMS (formerly HCFA) Medicare and Medicaid Programs: Hospital Conditions of Participation

CURRENT LANGUAGE	PROPOSED LANGUAGE
Medicare and Medicaid Guide ***Subpart D – Optional Hospital Services*** ***42CFR §482.52*** Condition of Participation: Anesthesia services.	***Sections 42CFR Parts 416, 482, 485 & 489*** ***42CFR §482.45*** Condition of Participation: Surgical and anesthesia services.
If the hospital furnishes anesthesia services, they must be provided in a well organized manner under the direction of a qualified doctor of medicine or osteopathy. The service is responsible for all anesthesia administered in the hospital.	If the hospital provides surgical or anesthesia services, they are provided through the use of qualified staff. The patient receives appropriate pre- and post-procedure evaluations, and all care is accurately documented.
(a) Standard: Organization and Staffing. *The organization of anesthesia services must be appropriate to the scope of the services offered. Anesthesia must be administered by only* (1) A qualified anesthesiologist; (2) A doctor of medicine or osteopathy (other than an anesthesiologist); (3) A dentist, oral surgeon, or podiatrist who is qualified to administer anesthesia under State law; (4) A certified registered nurse anesthetist (CRNA) as defined in §410.69(b) of this chapter who is under the supervision of the operating practitioner or of an anesthesiologist who is immediately available if needed; or (5) An anesthesiologist's assistant, as defined in §410.69(b) of this chapter, who is under the supervision of an anesthesiologist who is immediately available if needed.	(a) Standard: Staffing. (1) Surgical procedures are performed only by practitioners with appropriate clinical privileges. (2) Anesthesia is administered only by a licensed practitioner permitted by the State to administer anesthetics.
(b) Standard: Delivery of services. *Anesthesia services must be consistent with needs and resources. Policies on anesthesia procedures must include the delineation of preanesthesia and postanesthesia responsibilities. The policies must ensure that the following are provided for each patient:* (1) A preanesthesia evaluation by an individual qualified to administer anesthesia under paragraph (a) of this section performed within 48 hours prior to surgery. (2) An intraoperative anesthesia record. (3) With respect to inpatients, a postanesthesia follow-up report by the individual who administers the anesthesia that is written within 48 hours after surgery. (4) With respect to outpatients, a postanesthesia evaluation for proper anesthesia recovery performed in accordance with policies and procedures approved by the medical staff.	(b) Standard: Evaluations. (1) A comprehensive assessment of the patient's condition is performed before surgery, except in emergency cases where a modified assessment is acceptable. (2) A preanesthesia evaluation by an individual qualified to administer anesthesia is performed prior to the administration of anesthesia. (3) A postanesthesia evaluation for proper anesthesia recovery is performed by an individual qualified to administer anesthesia. (c) Standard: Documentation of care. (1) The comprehensive or modified presurgical assessment described in paragraph (b)(1) of this section is entered in the patient record before surgery, except in emergency cases, where the assessment may be entered following surgery. (2) A properly executed informed consent form for the operation is entered in the patient's record by the hospital before

(continued)

Table 18.2: HHS/CMS (formerly HCFA) Medicare and Medicaid Programs: Hospital Conditions of Participation (continued)

Source: As adopted 51 *F.R.* 22010 (June 17, 1986; effective September 15, 1986) and amended at 57 *F.R.* 33878 (July 31, 1992; effective August 31, 1992).	surgery, except in emergency cases where the delay needed to obtain consent would place the health or safety of the patient in serious jeopardy. (3) The hospital maintains a complete, up-to-date operating room register. (4) The hospital writes or dictates an operative report describing complications, reactions, length of time, techniques, findings, and tissues removed or altered immediately following surgery and enters it in the patient's record promptly following surgery. (5) The hospital maintains an intraoperative anesthesia record and enters it in the patient's record promptly following surgery or any other procedures requiring anesthesia. (6) The hospital writes a report of the results of the postanesthesia evaluation described in paragraph (b)(3) of this section and enters it in the patient's record promptly following completion of the procedure for which anesthesia was required. Source: 62 *F.R.* 66730 (December 19, 1997, Proposed Rules).

supervision or control over the administration or operation of any such institution, agency, or person (AANA President Scot D. Foster, CRNA, PhD, FAAN, 1998)."

- "HCFA routinely defers to state policy regarding licensure and practice acts regarding healthcare practitioners. HCFA's deferral to state law on the issue of physician supervision comports with other portions of the proposed rule as it relates to other healthcare practitioners as well as to prior HCFA policy (Foster, 1998)."
- Executive Order No. 12612 (October 27, 1987) directs executive departments and federal agencies from limiting the policy discretion of the states to the extent possible, unless the federal statute "contains an express preemption provision or there is some other firm and palpable evidence compelling the conclusion that the Congress intended preemption of State Law, or when the exercise of State authority directly conflicts with the exercise of Federal authority under the Federal statute (Foster, 1998)."
- "Requiring supervision can increase surgeon concerns about liability. These concerns, no matter how unwarranted, sometimes serve to increase cost. There are instances in which hospitals or ASCs with limited financial resources nevertheless feel compelled, because of surgeon liability

Table 18.3: HHS/CMS (Formerly HCFA) Medicare and Medicaid Programs: Ambulatory Surgical Services Conditions of Participation

CURRENT LANGUAGE	PROPOSED LANGUAGE
Part 416 *Subpart C—Specific Conditions for Coverage* *42CFR 416.42* Conditions for coverage: Surgical services.	*Part 416* *Subpart C—Specific Conditions for Coverage* *42CFR 416.42* Conditions for coverage: Surgical services.
Surgical procedures must be performed in a safe manner by qualified physicians who have been granted clinical privileges by the governing body of the ASC in accordance with approved policies and procedures of the ASC.	
(a) Standard: Anesthetic risk and evaluation. A physician must examine the patient immediately before surgery to evaluate the risk of anesthesia and of the procedure to be performed. Before discharge from the ASC, each patient must be evaluated by a physician for proper anesthesia recovery.	
(b) Standard: Administration of anesthesia. Anesthetics must be administered by only (1) A qualified anesthesiologist or (2) A physician qualified to administer anesthesia, a certified registered nurse anesthetist, or an anesthesiologist's assistant as defined in § 410.68(b) of this chapter, or a supervised trainee in an approved educational program. In those cases in which a nonphysician administers the anesthesia, the anesthetist must be under the supervision of the operating physician, and in the case of an anesthesiologist's assistant, under the supervision of an anesthesiologist.	(b) Standard: Administration of anesthesia. Anesthesia is administered only by a licensed practitioner permitted by the State to administer anesthetics.
(c) Standard: Discharge. All patients are discharged in the company of a responsible adult, except those exempted by the attending physician.	
Source: As adopted, 47 *F.R.* 34082 (August 5, 1982; effective September 7, 1982), and at 57 *F.R.* 33878 (July 31, 1992; effective August 31, 1992).	Source: 62 *F.R.* 66730 (December 19, 1997).

concerns, to hire anesthesiologists to supervise CRNAs (Foster, 1998)."

- "The proposed rule will not mandate changes in personnel in hospitals or ASCs. There will be no dramatic change in the way anesthesiologists, other physicians, and nurse anesthetists work in hospitals or ASCs, simply by virtue of the deferral to state law on supervision. In addition, nothing in the HCFA proposed rule would prevent a state legislature from enacting a physician requirement if they chose to do so (Foster, 1998)."
- "Supervision is unnecessary, as evidenced by the numerous states that do not require supervision but still maintain high-quality anesthesia care (Foster, 1998)."
- "HCFA's proposed rule confirms earlier HCFA intentions in the 1994

draft regulation removing supervision for hospitals, the 1997 draft regulation removing supervision for ASCs, and the 1995 Medicare reform package as agreed to by the Senate Finance Committee (Foster, 1998)."

- "CRNAs have the education and training to practice without physician supervision (Foster, 1998)."
- "No significant differences in quality of care between anesthesia outcome providers has been documented or proven (Foster, 1998)."
- "The federal government explicitly recognizes the value of CRNAs. CRNAs are reimbursed under a number of programs and they are the predominant anesthesia personnel in the military (Foster, 1998)."
- "Federal law does not require that anesthesiologists supervise or 'medically direct' CRNAs. What federal law does require is that if anesthesiologists supervise CRNAs, and want to bill for that supervision, anesthesiologists must satisfy the seven criteria listed in section 405.552. This is a critical distinction, because it is important to bear in mind that the Medicare requirements for medical direction are payment criteria only, and do not mandate any particular practice arrangement (Foster, 1998)."
- "Nurse anesthetists were the nation's first anesthesia personnel, giving anesthetics for more than 100 years. Nurse anesthetists are clearly qualified as anesthesia providers, even without physician supervision (Foster, 1998)."

HCFA's proposal was opposed by the ASA, which called for a national study comparing anesthesia outcomes between the two provider groups. However, undertaking such a study, which would have cost taxpayers approximately $15 million, was considered and rejected by the Centers for Disease Control and Prevention (CDC) in 1990. At that time, the CDC concluded that poor anesthesia outcomes were so rare it would be a waste of government money to conduct an anesthesia-outcomes study (AANA Quality of Care in Anesthesia, 1998).

Throughout the comment period, while HCFA deliberated on its final revisions to the Medicare and Medicaid conditions for participation, the AANA vigorously lobbied HCFA in support of the proposed supervision rule. The association emphasized that thanks to advancements in pharmaceuticals, monitoring technology, and anesthesia provider education, anesthesia care today is safer than ever before, with approximately one death for every 240,000 anesthetics as compared with two deaths for every 10,000 anesthetics just 20 years ago.

It is important for the reader to understand the efforts that were put forth by AANA to advocate its position on the supervision issue. These include but are not limited to the following:

- AANA representatives met with many key government personnel to advocate the position of CRNAs on the issue of supervision, including HCFA analysts, the administrator of HCFA, members of Congress and their staffs, the secretary of HHS, members of the White House staff, staff of the Office of Management and Budget, and a host of others.
- As ASA's opposition to the proposed rule increased, together with the delay in HCFA announcing the final rule, AANA called upon Senator Kent Conrad (D–ND) and Congressman Jim Nussle (R-IA) to introduce legislation to require HCFA to implement the new regulations related to CRNA supervision in the hospital conditions for

Table 18.4: HHS/CMS (formerly HCFA) Medicare and Medicaid Programs: Critical Access Hospital Conditions of Participation

CURRENT LANGUAGE	PROPOSED LANGUAGE
Part 485 ***Subpart F—Conditions of Participation: Critical Access Hospitals (CAHs)*** ***42CFR §485.639*** Conditions of participation: Surgical services.	***Part 485*** ***Subpart F—Conditions of Participation: Critical Access Hospitals (CAHs)*** ***42CFR §485.639*** Conditions of participation.
Surgical procedures must be performed in a safe manner by qualified practitioners who have been granted clinical privileges by the governing body of the CAH in accordance with the designation requirements under paragraph (a) of this section.	
(a) Designation of qualified practitioners. The CAH designates the practitioners who are allowed to perform surgery for CAH patients, in accordance with its approved policies and procedures, and with State scope of practice laws. Surgery is performed only by— (1) A doctor of medicine or osteopathy, including an osteopathic practitioner recognized under section 1101(a)(7) of the Act; (2) A doctor of dental surgery or dental medicine; or (3) A doctor of podiatric medicine.	
(b) Anesthetic risk and evaluation. A qualified practitioner, as described in paragraph (a) of this section, must examine the patient immediately before surgery to evaluate the risk of anesthesia and of the procedure to be performed. Before discharge from the CAH, each patient must be evaluated for proper anesthesia recovery by a qualified practitioner as described in paragraph (a) of this section.	
(c) Administration of anesthesia. The CAH designates the person who is allowed to administer anesthesia to CAH patients in accordance with its approved policies and procedures and with State scope of practice laws. (1) Anesthetics must be administered only by (i) A qualified anesthesiologist; (ii) A doctor of medicine or osteopathy other than an anesthesiologist, including an osteopathic practitioner recognized under section 1101(a)(7) of the Act; (iii) A doctor of dental surgery or dental medicine; (iv) A doctor of podiatric medicine; (v) A certified registered nurse anesthetist, as defined in § 410.69 (b) of this chapter; (vi) An anesthesiologist's assistant as defined in § 410.69(b) of this chapter; or	(c) Administration of anesthesia. The CAH designates the person who is allowed to administer anesthesia to CAH patients in accordance with its approved policies and procedures and with State scope of practice laws. Anesthesia is administered only by a licensed practitioner permitted by the State to administer anesthetics.

(continued)

Table 18.4: HHS/CMS (formerly HCFA) Medicare and Medicaid Programs: Critical Access Hospital Conditions of Participation (continued)	
(vii) A supervised trainee in an approved educational program, as described in §§413.85 or 413.86 of this chapter. (2) In those cases in which a certified registered nurse anesthetist administers the anesthesia, the anesthetist must be under the supervision of the operating practitioner. An anesthesiologist's assistant who administers anesthesia must be under the supervision of an anesthesiologist.	
(d) Discharge. All patients are discharged in the company of a responsible adult, except those exempted by the practitioner who performed the surgical procedure. Source: 60 *F.R.* 45851 (Sept. 1, 1995), as amended at 62 *F.R.* 46037 (Aug 29, 1997).	Source: 62 *F.R.* 66763 (Dec. 19, 1997, Proposed Rules).

payment for participation in the Medicare program.

- AANA retained outside legislative consultants to assist in the promotion of its legislative initiatives.
- AANA retained public relations consultants who assisted in the following endeavors to increase the public's awareness of the vital role that CRNAs play in anesthesia delivery in this country: (a) advertising in many publications, including the Capitol Hill newspaper *Roll Call* and *USA Today*, (b) assisting with media training for AANA officers and staff who have appeared on radio programs and been interviewed by a variety of publications, and (c) developing radio advertisements for use in Washington, D.C. to garner support for AANA's position.
- AANA retained grassroots consultants to assist in gaining letters of support for the new regulation from key members of Congress.

The effects of these advocacy efforts yielded an extensive base of support from a broad healthcare sector and the public. Support for the proposed rule came from the American Hospital Association, National Rural Health Association, Federation of American Health Systems, St. Paul Fire and Marine Insurance Company, Kaiser Permenante Central Office, California and Oregon Kaiser System, and numerous rural hospitals across the country. The list of national and health professional associations, individual nurses and physicians, and members of the public at large that wrote letters to HCFA/CMS on this issue is exhaustive.

From the beginning, ASA used as one of its major arguments that a change in this rule would be detrimental to Medicare beneficiaries. In an effort to obtain the views of a sample population of senior citizens, AANA commissioned a survey of Medicare patients conducted in October 1999 by the independent research firm Wirthlin Worldwide, which revealed the following: (1) 88 percent of Medicare beneficiaries surveyed would be comfortable if their surgeon chose a nurse anesthetist to provide their anesthesia care; (2) 81 percent surveyed preferred a nurse anesthetist or had no preference between a nurse anesthetist or physician anesthesiologist when it came to their anesthesia care; and (3) 62 percent of those surveyed found it acceptable for the nurse anesthetist to not be supervised by their surgeon, but to work collaboratively with the surgeon who would be present throughout the surgery (AANA advocacy advertisement, 2000).

On March 9, 2000, after deliberating for more than two years, HCFA announced that removal of the federal requirement that nurse anesthetists must be supervised by physicians when administering anesthesia to Medicare patients would be forthcoming. The final rule was to be published in the *Federal Register* in June 2000. However, the rule was not published in June as anticipated. The rule remained on hold through the following months with periodic reports that it was in progress at the Office of Management and Budget. AANA continued to press the administration to publish the rule. Because Congress did not complete its budget and legislative work until late in the year, implementation of the rule remained vulnerable to legislative threats from the ASA which was pushing for a legislatively mandated study that, if enacted, would preempt implementing a final rule.

It was not until January 18, 2001, with the approval of the Clinton administration, that the rule was published in the *Federal Register* (66 *F.R.*, January 18, 2001)—it was scheduled to become effective March 19, 2001. The rule eliminated the federal physician supervision requirement for CRNAs as proposed in the December 19, 1997, rule. However, on March 19, 2001, the effective date was delayed 60 days by the new Bush administration for purposes of review. On May 18, the rule was further delayed for 180 days to explore alternatives for implementation (66 *F.R.*, May 18, 2001). On July 5, 2001, CMS (formerly HCFA) published a proposed rule (66 *F.R.*, July 5, 2001) which would maintain the existing supervision requirement, but allow a state's governor, in consultation with the state's boards of medicine and nursing, to request an opt-out or exemption from the physician supervision requirement, consistent with state law.

AANA submitted extensive comments to CMS concerning the July 5, 2001, proposed rule. The essence of the AANA position was that CMS should reinstate the January 18, 2001, rule, which removed the federal supervision requirement and deferred to the states on the regulation of CRNAs. AANA noted in its comments that it agreed with the initial approach reflected in the December 19, 1997, proposed rule and January 18, 2001, rule which articulated the need to focus on outcomes of care and work toward eliminating unnecessary procedural requirements. AANA further noted that it believed CMS had been moving in the right direction toward streamlining outdated requirements and embodying an approach that more accurately reflects clinical practice, while maintaining high quality of care.

"In the January 18, 2001 rule, HCFA agreed with the AANA regarding virtually every major issue that was raised. These arguments were stated succinctly by HCFA in the January 18, 2001 *Federal Register*, leaving the AANA, hospitals, and supporters of the rule in Congress to assume that the 180-degree turnaround was not due to policy issues but rather political considerations (AANA President Deborah A. Chambers, CRNA, MHSA, 2001)."

AANA also noted considerable support from external entities for HCFA's proposed rule of December 19, 1997, and the January 18, 2001, final rule:

"The AANA has worked diligently with several administrations to bring about the January 18 rule change—a change supported by the American Hospital Association, the Federation of American Hospitals, Premier, Inc., VHA, Inc., the National Rural Health Association, the Center for Patient Advocacy, the TREA Senior Citizens League, the American Nurses' Association, Mutual of Omaha, United Healthcare of Arizona, dozens of individuals, hospitals, and many others. Several state governors have also written HCFA/CMS to support the approach reflected in the January 18 rule.

"The primary opposition to the January 18 rule change came from organized medicine, though physicians at CMS did approve the adoption of the January 18 final rule. Opponents to implementation of the January 18 rule have tried to exploit the unfounded fear that CRNAs would be providing anesthesia care without physician involvement if the rule were implemented. That is not the case, as existing Medicare Conditions of Participation require that every Medicare patient be under the care of a physician (see 66 *FR* 4678) (Chambers, 2001)."

Ultimately, however, CMS published in the November 13, 2001, *Federal Register* its final rule concerning the federal Medicare and Medicaid physician supervision requirement for CRNAs (66 *F.R.* November 13, 2001). The November 13 rule amended the requirement in the Anesthesia Services Condition of Participation for Hospitals, the Surgical Services Condition of Coverage for Ambulatory Surgical Centers, and the Surgical Services Condition of Participation for Critical Access Hospitals. The November 13 rule, which is virtually identical to the July 5, 2001, proposed rule, took effect immediately upon publication.

The rule allows states to "opt-out" of or be "exempted" from (the terms are used synonymously) the federal supervision requirement. For a state to "opt-out" of the federal supervision requirement, the state's governor must send a letter of attestation to CMS. The letter must attest that: (1) The state's governor has consulted with the state's boards of medicine and nursing about issues related to access to and quality of anesthesia services in the state, (2) it is in the best interests of the state's citizens to opt-out of the current federal physician supervision requirement, and (3) the opt-out is consistent with state law. A governor's opt-out request takes effect immediately upon submission to CMS.

Additionally, the rule states that a governor can request at any time that a previously granted opt-out be withdrawn. Such a request would be effective upon submission to CMS.

Less than one month after the rule took effect, Iowa became the first state to opt out of the federal supervision requirement.

Finally, in its November 13 rule comments, CMS states that the Agency for Healthcare Research and Quality (AHRQ) will "conduct a study of anesthesia outcomes in those states that choose to opt-out of the CRNA supervision requirement compared to those states that have not."

The AANA supports AHRQ conducting a scientific study of anesthesia outcomes of CRNAs and anesthesiologists working alone, but feels strongly that CRNAs must be fairly represented in defining the design parameters and methodology of such a study. A scientifically valid study should be governed by the following principles:

- It should compare important anesthesia outcomes of patients receiving anesthesia from unsupervised CRNAs with those receiving anesthesia from anesthesiologists personally providing the service. Any scientifically valid anesthesia outcomes study of CRNA practices must include anesthesiologists practicing without CRNAs (as indicated in the CMS July 5 proposed rule). Otherwise, there will be no valid basis for comparison of CRNA and anesthesiologist outcomes.

- It should be designed by a team of qualified researchers representing all stakeholders including, at a minimum, CRNAs, anesthesiologists, HHS, AHRQ or other designated agency, with no single group having a majority.

Throughout the four years that the federal physician supervision issue engaged the healthcare community, many individuals and organizations worked for the removal of this requirement. AANA clearly recognized that the efforts of many different groups and individuals outside of the association who believed the initial proposed rule was the right thing to do for patients and the healthcare system were essential to HCFA's decision to remove the supervision requirement in the final rule published on January 18, 2001. To its colleagues in the nursing community who worked tirelessly in support of this effort, AANA said "thank you" for staying the course, noting that the association believes as they do that the removal of restrictive barriers to the legitimate practice of nursing serves the public's interest and is sound healthcare policy.

STANDARDS FOR HEALTH PLANS/PROVIDER NONDISCRIMINATION LANGUAGE

From the inception of managed care reform, the AANA adopted a proactive position in support of the following: (1) legislation ensuring that consumers have healthcare choice and accountability, and (2) health plans that include provider nondiscrimination language prohibiting health plans from arbitrarily excluding providers based solely on their licensure or certification. The rationale for this position was that discrimination in any form would limit access, choice, and marketplace competition for CRNAs. The key concepts that AANA strongly supports for all health plans are: (1) patients have the fundamental right to choose their healthcare providers; (2) patients have a right to information; (3) patients and their healthcare providers have a right to due process; and (4) healthcare providers should be protected from unjustified liability.

In 1994, AANA strengthened its position on nondiscrimination by healthcare plans through membership in a coalition of nonphysician providers, and since 1997 has served as chair of the coalition working for the adoption of the Patient Access to Responsible Care Act (PARCA) that reflects the key principles of managed care reform outlined above. The PARCA alliance's major work resulted in the Patient Access to Responsible Care Act of 1997, introduced by Congressman Charlie Norwood (R-GA). Although this bill was ultimately unsuccessful, in 1999 both the House and Senate passed a comprehensive managed care reform proposal. However, it was not until 2001 that Patients' Rights legislation moved to its next significant stages of evolution. In August 2001, Patients' Rights legislation was approved by the Republican-majority House of Representatives with President Bush's support; a more expansive bill passed the Democrat-controlled Senate (S. 1052), but President Bush indicated he would veto this legislation.

Both the Senate and House bills include key provisions backed by AANA and PARCA, including language insisting on provider nondiscrimination and point-of-service assurance. Both bills also ensure that during internal and external appeals processes, at least one qualified healthcare professional who delivers the service in question—whether it is a physician or a nonphysician provider—will be represented on the review panel. Previous versions had only physicians doing the reviews. Although both the House and Senate measures are largely similar, Republicans and Democrats appeared willing to go to the mat to secure victory for their own perspectives on whether to make managed care plans liable for their decisions. The issue remained unresolved as 2001 came to a close.

AANA maintains its leading role in efforts to move final passage of effective Patients' Rights legislation. The PARCA coalition continues its meetings at AANA's Washington office, working to ensure, among other principles, that provider nondiscrimination language is included in whatever managed care reform bill is ultimately enacted into law.

ANTITRUST

Over the years, CRNAs and their state associations have been vigilant in monitoring both state and federal regulation for situations that would jeopardize a CRNA's ability to compete in the marketplace. Most often these situations involve CRNAs being coerced into unfavorable work or salary arrangements, or employment arrangements that could substantially affect their ability to practice.

In his 1998 book, *Not What the Doctor Ordered: How to End the Medical Monopoly in Pursuit of Managed Care*, Jeffrey C. Bauer offered a compelling view of how some physicians attempt to control the healthcare market: "The CRNA story illustrates perfectly the benefits of competition from qualified non-physician practitioners and the harmful effects of doctors' anticompetitive efforts to control the market. In particular, it shows why persistent enforcement of antitrust law, something very different from health reform, is needed to protect consumers' welfare from doctors' monopoly when acceptable substitutes are available. Nursings' early leadership in anesthesia was perfectly logical because anesthetic services require the professional skills at which nurses excel: monitoring patients, making decisions, and taking actions (which commonly includes administering medications). Nevertheless, state medical societies began challenging nurse anesthetists' rights to practice since the time of the Flexner Report, promoting legislation that would prevent anyone other than a physician from administering anesthesia. Doctor's efforts to eliminate or control the competition included not-so-subtle efforts to discredit nurse anesthetists in the eyes of the public..."

More specifically, there are situations in which antitrust ramifications are readily apparent. The first involves independent CRNAs who may function as independent contractors. As such they compete directly with physician anesthesiologists. Consequently, weakening of antitrust laws and regulations would not serve CRNAs well when competing for market share. A second example could be cited by CRNAs in anesthesia care team practice, where under the guise of facility reorganization they are not offered a stable employment situation, salary, or benefits.

AANA's federal lobbying activities related to antitrust have focused on opposing any legislation that weakens antitrust laws or any changes to the Federal Trade Commission antitrust guidelines as they relate to physicians. AANA's efforts have also included opposing legislation that eliminates the protection that nonphysician providers have under the antitrust laws from anticompetitive treatment by anesthesiologists and health plans. A recent example of AANA's advocacy for maintaining strong federal antitrust enforcement and protection was exemplified in the AANA's opposition in 1999 to the Campbell (R-CA) antitrust bill, H.R. 1304. Basically, H.R. 1304 would have created a broad new antitrust exemption for physicians and healthcare providers to negotiate terms, fees, and conditions with health plans, without fear of antitrust sanction.

AANA has a long history of monitoring legislation and regulatory change in antitrust law that could negatively impact CRNA practice. For example, in 1993 AANA testified in opposition to President Clinton's Health Security Act provisions, which would have granted an antitrust exemption to providers to negotiate collectively with regional alliances over fee schedules to be paid under certain fee-for-service plans. Although CRNAs were included in the definition of providers in the Clinton bill, CRNAs have historically had less negotiating power than physicians and therefore would have been at risk from being excluded from the fee-negotiation process.

CRNAs have the ability to compete in the healthcare marketplace due to their cost effectiveness and the quality of care they deliver. They can, however, only continue to do this if they have a level playing field on which to compete. AANA believes the current antitrust laws are intended to preserve competition and promote consumer welfare. Expanding antitrust exemptions beyond what current law permits would only serve to undermine these objectives by eliminating competition, limiting consumer choice, and increasing costs to consumers.

NURSE ANESTHESIA EDUCATION FUNDING

A primary mission of the AANA is to support the education of students and CRNAs. The AANA has been very active over the last decade in securing from federal sources this necessary and vital support for educational programs. There are two primary sources from which this money is derived. The first is from the Nurse Education Act. This act was established under Title VIII of the Public Health Service Act. The program has provided funding for grant programs administered by the Division of Nursing under the Health Resources and Services Administration at HHS. Historically funding has gone to nurse anesthesia students, faculty, and new programs. This federal program has served the nurse anesthesia community well in the past, and its continuation remains a high priority for AANA. Since 1994, over 75 percent of CRNA students have received student traineeships.

Nurse anesthesia education was historically allocated a line item of funding. In 1998, as part of the reauthorization of Title VIII, Congress replaced it with language allocating nurse anesthetist education a minimum percentage of total Title VIII funding. The legislated set-aside of 4.38 percent of Title VIII funds for nurse anesthetist education, about $3 million in fiscal year 2001, expires at the end of fiscal year 2002. Funding provided in fiscal year 2001 totaled $1.9 million in grants to eight schools, plus $1 million in traineeship grants to 66 schools. Reauthorization of Title VIII is of crucial concern to nurse anesthesia education because of the importance of federal funding to expanding nurse anesthesia programs, especially during this time of acute shortage of anesthesia providers. Congress is expected to address this issue in 2002.

Debate over the Title VIII funding allocation has been characterized by sharp disagreements among nursing organizations over nursing funding, rather than upon the perspective that nursing education funding generally should increase because Washington provides about $46 to medical education for every $1 to nursing education.

The other primary source of funding for nurse anesthesia comes from the Medicare program. In order to ensure a stable and adequate supply of qualified health professionals to care for the nation's elderly population, especially those in rural and medically underserved urban areas, Medicare has historically paid hospitals for their share of the cost that they incur in connection with approved educational activities. Hospitals that operate approved nursing and allied health programs are eligible for reimbursement under the Medicare Nursing and Allied Health program.

However, with the movement of the majority of nurse anesthesia programs to university-owned programs, reimbursement of training costs has been seriously curtailed by changes made to the inpatient and outpatient PPS and the current nursing and allied health regulations that will only reimburse hospital-operated programs for the net costs of clinical training programs. The effect of these requirements is a 55 percent decrease in eight years in the number of nurse anesthesia programs receiving Medicare funding.

Additional curtailments in reimbursement for CRNAs involved in clinical supervision of students occurred with the enactment into law of Medicare direct reimbursement of nurse anesthetists. Prior to the provisions for direct reimbursement, the full services of CRNAs, including clinical supervision of students, were reimbursed on a reasonable cost basis. Since direct reimbursement was implemented, Medicare will only reimburse a teaching CRNA for the anesthesia service if the CRNA is supervising the student in a 1:1 ratio and is continually present with the student. No reimbursement is provided for either services if the CRNA is supervising students in a 1:2 ratio.

AANA is addressing these reimbursement/funding issues as part of its federal agenda. Clearly, the lack of payment provisions discourages healthcare facilities from becoming involved in nurse anesthesia educational programs if they cannot recover the costs of CRNA clinical instructors. AANA believes that Medicare education funds should be utilized to promote a cost-effective health workforce with an appropriate balance of physician, nursing and related healthcare professionals. Services provided by advanced practice nurses such as nurse practitioners, clinical nurse specialists, and CRNAs have the greatest potential for increasing accessible, affordable, quality healthcare services to Medicare beneficiaries. APNs cost much less to prepare, and overall are lower-cost providers in the marketplace than their physician colleagues. Secondly, AANA believes that the nursing component of the Medicare education funds should be made available to education programs as well as to institutions currently eligible for Part A reimbursement.

SUMMARY

There are many other legislative issues that AANA has lobbied successfully, including military incentive pay and direct assistance to state organizations involved in particular issues of reimbursement, recognition and practice rights. The primary mission of the AANA—to support member well-being through effective advocacy—has been quite successful. In fact, in 1999 the AANA Office of Federal Government Affairs was named by *Fortune* magazine as one of the most effective lobbying groups on Capitol Hill—a tribute to both AANA's professional personnel and to its members who value effective advocacy efforts on their behalf. Further, many other professional organizations look to the AANA's experience and expertise to formulate, organize and deploy their own legislative plans. Clearly, the AANA must continue to be highly visible and influential in both federal and state governments on matters of public policy pertinent to its members and the patients they serve.

Most important to appreciate is the notion that a legislative agenda is only as successful as those involved in its implementation. This advocacy effort, though managed through AANA's Washington, D.C., office at the direction of the AANA

Board of Directors, is possible only through the dedicated efforts of AANA's members. It is the members themselves who provide grassroots efforts, participate in local and national campaigns of elected members of Congress, provide congressional testimony, participate in public relations campaigns, write letters, make phone calls, organize communications systems, meet personally with leaders of business, industry and governmental bureaucracies, and provide funds to the CRNA Political Action Committee. We can never loose sight of the concept that an organization is only as strong as its members, and their grassroots involvement is absolutely essential to achieving success in the public policy arena.

The authors of this chapter have relied on selective source documents developed by AANA staff in the Park Ridge, Ill., and Washington, D.C., offices in the course of writing this chronology of federal legislative advocacy. We gratefully acknowledge the expert contributions and commitment of these professional staff members.

REFERENCES

American Association of Nurse Anesthetists. (1998). *Quality of Care in Anesthesia.* Park Ridge, IL.

American Association of Nurse Anesthetists. November 12, 2001, press release. Park Ridge, IL.

American Association of Nurse Anesthetists. (2000). Nine out of 10 Medicare patients are comfortable with nurse anesthesia care. Advocacy advertisment. Park Ridge, IL.

American Assocation of Nurse Anesthetists. (2001). AANA State Government Affairs Department summary of essential elements of the November 13, 2001, CMS final rule. Park Ridge, IL.

ASA disagrees with AANA, in part, on medical direction. (1998). *Anesthesia Answer Book—Action Alert*, 1-2.

Bauer, J. C. (1998). *Not What the Doctor Ordered: How to End the Medical Monopoly in Pursuit of Managed Care* (2nd ed.). New York, NY: McGraw-Hill.

Center for Health Economics Research. (1992). *Payment Options for the Anesthesia Care Team.* Submitted to the Physician Payment Review Commission. Washington, DC.

Chambers, D.A. (2001). Comments of the American Association of Nurse Anesthetists on the Proposed Rule; Medicare and Medicaid Programs; Hospital Conditions of Participation; Anesthesia Services; 66 *F.R.* 35395 (July 5, 2001); File Code HCFA-3070-P. American Association of Nurse Anesthetists. Park Ridge, IL.

Fassett, S. & Calmes, S.H. (1995). Perception by an anesthesia care team on the need for medical direction. *AANA Journal.* 63: 117-123.

Fortune Magazine. (1999). The power 25. Vol. 140, No.11. New york, NY.

Foster, S. D. (1998). Comments of the American Association of Nurse Anesthetists on the proposed rule regarding the Medicare and Medicaid programs; hospital conditions of participation; provider and supplier approval. American Association of Nurse Anesthetists. Park Ridge, IL.

Gunn, I.P. (1997). Nurse anesthesia. In J. J. Nagelhout & K. L. Zaglaniczny (Eds.), *Nurse Anesthesia.* Philadelphia, PA: W.R. Saunders Co.

Medicare Carrier's Manual, Part 3 (HCFA-Pub. 14-3). Section 15018C.

PPRC Report to Congress. (1993). *Chapter 11 Payments for the Anesthesia Care Team.* Washington, DC.

Stein, C.S. (1994). A patient-based approach to medical direction within the anesthesia care team. *AANA Journal.* 62: 359.

47 *F.R.* 34082 (August 5, 1982; effective September 7, 1982) and at 57 *F.R.* 33878 (July 31, 1992; effective August 31, 1992).

48 *F.R.* 8902 (March 2, 1983; effective October 1, 1983).

48 *F.R.* 8938 (March 2, 1983; effective October 1, 1983).

51 *F.R.* 22010 (June 17, 1986; effective September 15, 1986) and amended at 57 *F.R.* 33878 (July 31, 1992; effective August 31, 1992).

60 *F.R.* 45851, (September 1, 1995, as amended at 62 *F.R.* 46037, August 29, 1997)

63 *F.R.* 39818 (June 5, 1998; effective December 31, 1998).

63 *F.R.* 58912 (November 2, 1998; effective January 1, 1999).

66 *F.R.* 4674 (January 18, 2001; effective March 19, 2001).

66 *F.R.* 7702 (January 24, 2001; effective March 19, 2001).

66 *F.R.* 27598 (May 18, 2001; effective November 13, 2001).

66 *F.R.* 35395 (July 5, 2001—proposed rule).

66 *F.R.* 56762 (November 13, 2001—effective immediately).

STUDY QUESTIONS

1. Describe the functions of Medicare Part A and Part B. Distinguish between medically directed and nonmedically directed payment systems. "Supervision" is a term used in both Parts A and B, yet has different meanings in both parts. Describe and distinguish each.

2. What barriers exist that make revision of the seven conditions for reimbursement for physician medical direction difficult?

3. How has TEFRA been inappropriately interpreted? How has that affected the practice of CRNAs?

4. Describe some of the more important reasons AANA has given CMS to support the removal of physician supervision.

5. What is the significance of provider nondiscrimination language in healthcare plans?

6. List three reasons related to anesthesia practice why CRNAs should support strong federal antitrust legislation.

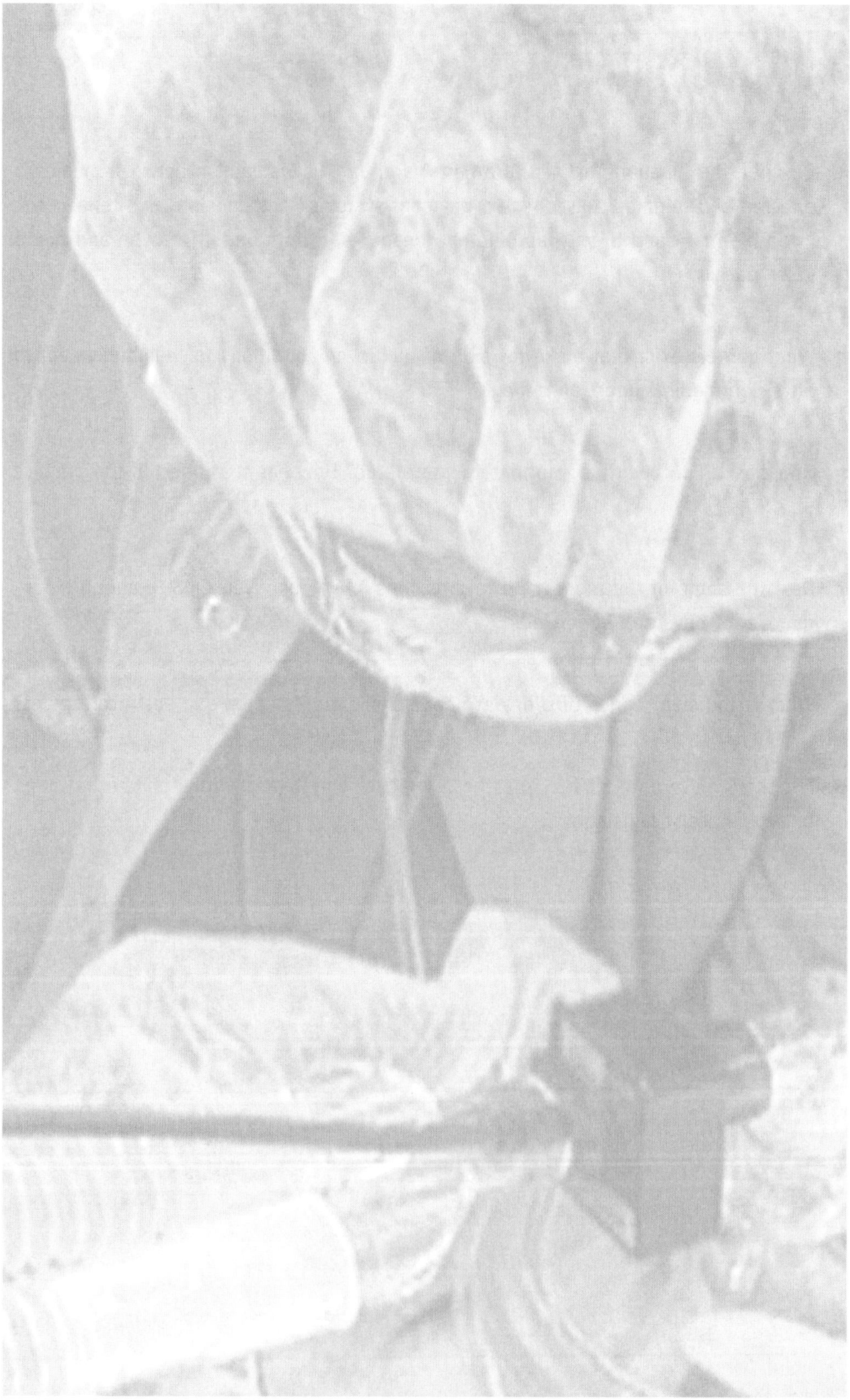

CHAPTER 19

THE INTERNATIONAL FEDERATION OF NURSE ANESTHETISTS

Ronald F. Caulk, CRNA, FAAN

Executive Director
International Federation of Nurse Anesthetists
Park Ridge, IL

Sandra M. Ouellette, CRNA, MEd, FAAN

Program Director, Anesthesia Program
Wake Forest University Baptist Medical/University of North Carolina at Greensboro
Winston-Salem, NC

KEY CONCEPTS

- The International Federation of Nurse Anesthetists (IFNA) is an international organization of nationally registered nurses with special education in nurse anesthesia.
- Standards as approved by IFNA are the ultimate mandate internationally for educational preparation and clinical and ethical behavior of the anesthetist.
- Nurses participate in the delivery of anesthesia services in 107 countries and participate in 70 percent to 80 percent of all anesthesia administered in the world.
- It is in the best interest of IFNA to align itself with established international organizations whose goals and programs are consistent with the aims of IFNA.
- IFNA is the second of only three international nursing specialties to be recognized by the International Council of Nurses.
- Future effectiveness of international professional organizations lies in their ability to provide international solutions to local problems.
- The IFNA Educational, Practice and Ethical Standards stand as international witness for the globalization of a profession in both preparation and practice.
- IFNA is the only international nursing organization to establish international standards.
- Each member country of IFNA exists in its own political and legal environment, and any assistance given must take those elements into consideration.

In 1978, two European nurse anesthetists, Jan Frandsen of Denmark and Hermi Löhnert of Switzerland, attended the Annual Meeting of the American Association of Nurse Anesthetists (AANA). Their interest in international cooperation among nurse anesthetists and AANA's agreement planted the seed for what would become the International Federation of Nurse Anesthetists (IFNA).

This chapter describes the historical development, philosophy, objectives, and functions of IFNA. Qualifications for membership, organizational structure, and educational and research activities are addressed. Future directions and the value of the federation to the profession conclude the chapter.

HISTORICAL DEVELOPMENT OF IFNA

It was not until 1978 that nurse anesthetists began to realize that they were a worldwide entity. Sparked by the interest of Löhnert and supported by the AANA Board of Directors, the idea of international cooperation began. From this concept, IFNA was born. IFNA, which represents 45,000 active practicing nurse anesthetists worldwide, is a growing organization whose members practice in both developed and developing countries.

The first International Symposium for Nurse Anesthetists, cosponsored by the AANA and the newly formed and then Schweizerische Fachvereinigung für Nichtärztliche Anästhesisten (Swiss Association), convened in Lucerne, Switzerland, in June 1985, and was attended by 250 nurse anesthetists from 11 countries. At a meeting of the official country representatives, the decision was made that another international symposium should be held in three years. The Symposium Organizing Committee (SOC) was formed to plan the next symposium, and the representatives requested that country organizations bid to host the symposium. The SOC was composed of a representative from Switzerland, the Netherlands, Denmark, Germany, and the United States and held its first meeting in Roskilde, Denmark, in February 1986. The offer of the Netherlands Association to host the Second International Symposium in Amsterdam was accepted for the 1988 2nd International Congress.

Three years later when the 2nd International Congress of Nurse Anesthetists convened in Amsterdam, the Netherlands, 511 nurse anesthetists from 16 countries attended. At the 1987 March meeting of the Congress Organizing Committee (COC) and country representatives, several European associates had already proposed the possibility of developing an international organization. It was decided that each representative would discuss the feasibility of an international organization with his or her board of directors. It was the suggestion of the AANA Board of Directors that Ronald Caulk, CRNA, FAAN, AANA representative to the COC, prepare a feasibility questionnaire to determine the objectives of such an organization. The questionnaire asked the nurse anesthesia leaders of each country organization to determine what they felt would be the goals, purpose, objectives, and composition of such an organization. The questionnaire was distributed to all official country representatives. The results were presented to the country representatives at the Amsterdam meeting. The responses to questionnaires indicated that the country representatives shared the same goals and objectives. The concept of forming an international organization was greeted with great enthusiasm at the Amsterdam meeting, and plans were made to continue to move ahead with the formation of an international organization. The name of the International Congress changed to "World Congress," and the committee changed to the "Congress Planning Committee (CPC)."

In September 1988, the first organizational meeting of the proposed international organization was held in Teufen, Switzerland. The meeting was chaired by Löhnert; Caulk was appointed secretary. The name of the organization and the philosophy were adopted. Caulk presented definitions of society, association, alliance, organization and federation. It was decided that membership would be by national organizations and that "federation" best described the intent of the proposed organization.

Federation was defined as the act of federating or uniting in a league; the formation of a political unity, with a central government by a number of separate states, each of which retains control of its own internal affairs; a league or confederation; a federated body formed by a number of states, societies, unions, etc., each retaining control of its own internal affairs.

It was the decision of the representatives that Switzerland be the site of the proposed federation. Subcommittees were formed to discuss structure and bylaws, membership, dues, functions, and objectives. Structure, bylaws, and dues and the official languages were planned. The dues were established at 0.50 Swiss francs per active member of each member organization, and these dues have not changed. The official language would be English with German and French being established as "working languages." Working languages have since been removed from the bylaws. Membership in IFNA presented the major obstacle, and subcommittees regarding categories of membership and conditions of membership were appointed to prepare recommendations for the March 1989 meeting in Oslo, Norway. Objectives and functions developed and agreed upon at this meeting are listed in Tables 19.1 and 19.2. It was agreed that a World Congress would be planned every three years (Caulk and Maree, 1990).

In March 1989, the CPC and representatives from various countries met to resolve the membership issue and the completed draft of the constitution (bylaws), which had been outlined by a committee of four. Since internationalism was new to the group, leaders had sought the advice and support of the International Council of Nurses (ICN) during the planning and development of the organization.

In May 1989, Sandra M. Maree, CRNA, AANA president, and Caulk, then the AANA representative to the CPC, attended the ICN 19th Quadrennial Congress in Seoul, Korea. The purpose of attending the meeting was to study the history of the organization and to attend the business session of the Council of National Representatives (CNR). It was believed that lessons learned from this nearly 100-year-old organization would undoubtedly be very beneficial in the formation of IFNA (Caulk and Maree, 1990). It was at this meeting of the ICN that a resolution was adopted by the CNR to recognize internationally organized nursing specialties.

In June 1989, country representatives met in Teufen, Switzerland, to finalize and adopt the proposed bylaws and review country applications for membership in IFNA. Eleven countries were admitted as charter members. The first meeting of the IFNA Board of Directors was held on June 10, 1989. Caulk served as acting chair for the formal acceptance of the proposed bylaws and the election of officers. The bylaws were adopted and officers elected. Lohnert was the first president. Other officers included Caulk, vice president; Hanna Birgisdottir, Iceland, secretary; and Svein Olaussen, Norway, treasurer. Committees were formed, and arrangements were made for incorporation in Switzerland. Switzerland was selected as the home of IFNA for several reasons: political neutrality, monetary stability, location, and the fact that it was also the home of ICN, the World Health Organization (WHO), the International Red Cross, and other international organizations.

Following the formation of the organization, the Board of Directors set out to address the objectives. During the first year, the IFNA Board of Directors requested the Education Committee to develop international educational standards for nurse anesthetists. The decision to develop the educational standards was intended to address the IFNA objectives based on the fact that the educational standards worldwide were very diverse. These standards were adopted in 1990. The following year, the Education Committee developed international standards of practice that were adopted by the IFNA Board of Directors in 1991. The code of ethics was adopted in 1992 (IFNA Education Committee, 1990, 1992a, 1992b). It was not until 1997 that IFNA leadership learned from the Center for Quality Assurance in International Education (CQAIE) that IFNA was the only international nursing organization to adopt such standards. At this organizational meeting it was agreed that Löhnert be recognized as the founder of IFNA based on his initial concept of an international symposium and his active participation in the founding of IFNA.

In November 1990, IFNA President

Table 19.1: Objectives of the International Federation of Nurse Anesthetists

- To promote cooperation between nurse anesthetists internationally
- To develop and promote educational standards in the field of nurse anesthesia
- To develop and promote standards of practice in the field of nurse anesthesia
- To promote opportunities for continuing education in anesthesia
- To assist nurse anesthetists' associations to improve the standards of nurse anesthesia and the competence of nurse anesthetists
- To promote the recognition of nurse anesthetists
- To establish and maintain effective cooperation between nurse anesthetists, anesthesiologists, and other members of the medical profession, as well as hospitals and agencies representing a community of interest in nurse anesthesia

Table 19.2: Functions of the International Federation of Nurse Anesthetists

- To promote continual high quality patient care
- To serve as the authoritative voice of nurse anesthetists and nurse anesthesia internationally
- To provide a means of communication among nurse anesthetists throughout the world
- To promote the independence of the nurse anesthetist as a professional specialist in nursing
- To advance the art and science of anesthesiology

Table 19.3: IFNA Member Countries and Year of Admission

*Austria (1985)	France (1985)	Jamaica (1997)	*Sweden (1985)
Benin (1994)	Gabon (1994)	Morocco (1997)	*Switzerland (1985)
Cambodia (1997)	*Germany (1985)	Netherlands (1995)	Taiwan (1999)
Croatia (1999)	Ghana (1993)	Nigeria (1993)	Uganda (1996)
Czech Republic (1996)	Great Britain (1995)	*Norway (1985)	*United States (1985)
Democratic Republic of the Congo (1992)	Hungary (1999)	Poland (1998)	
Denmark (1997)	*Iceland (1985)	*Slovenia (1985)	
*Finland (1985)	Italy (2001)	*South Korea (1985)	
	Ivory Coast (Côte d'Ivoire) (1994)	Spain (1992)	

*Charter countries.

Caulk and Vice President Löhnert visited ICN and WHO in Geneva, Switzerland. The purpose of the visit was to thank ICN for its assistance and support in the development of IFNA and to learn more about the process for ICN recognition of international nursing specialties. The purpose of the visit to WHO was to introduce IFNA to the offices of the Non-Governmental Organizations (NGOs) and nursing.

After the establishment of IFNA, 1,100 nurse anesthetists attended World Congress III in Oslo, Norway. By 1994, when the 4th World Congress convened in Paris, France, attendance had grown to more than 2,600 people representing 47 countries. The 5th World Congress in Vienna, Austria, in 1997 was attended by more than 1,700 people from 41 countries. The 6th World Congress was held in Chicago in August 2000. More than 4,000 nurse anesthetists attended.

Since IFNA was founded, membership has grown at a rapid pace. Table 19.3 lists the 31 countries that were members as of 2002. In 1995, the executive office of IFNA was established at the AANA headquarters in Park Ridge, Ill., with Caulk as the first executive director.

DEFINITION AND ROLE OF NURSES IN ANESTHESIA DELIVERY WORLDWIDE

IFNA is an international organization of nationally registered nurses with special education in nurse anesthesia. A nurse anesthetist is a person who has completed a program of basic nursing education and basic nurse anesthesia education and is qualified and authorized in his/her country to practice nurse anesthesia. Member countries of IFNA are dedicated to the precept that their individual members are committed to the advancement of educational standards and practices, which will advance the art and science of anesthesiology and thereby support and enhance quality patient care.

There has been and remains some confusion about nurse anesthesia worldwide. The role varies from country to country and continent to continent. Throughout mainland Europe, nurse anesthetists commonly practice in an "anesthesia care team" setting. This setting consists of physician anesthetists (or anesthesiologists) supervising the nurse anesthetists. The ratios for this supervision vary from 1:2 to 1:3 and are generally accepted as being cost effective in both the cost of education and the provision of anesthesia services. There is an agreement as to the respective roles, and the team works in harmony. The overall educational preparation of the nurse anesthetist is, on average, 18 months (Caulk, 1998).

In recent times there has been much discussion about the role of the anesthetic nurses that have been used in the past to assist the physician anesthetist. While they have been utilized in several areas of the world, more often they are found in the United Kingdom, Australia, New Zealand, Canada, and Hong Kong. Whether called a discussion or debate, current interest involves the role today and in the future of the anesthetic nurse. It is the understanding of IFNA that the role of the anesthetic nurse was originally to assist the physician anesthetist and that the educational preparation of the anesthetic nurse was approximately 22 weeks. It is the belief of IFNA that if nurses are utilized for the preoperative and postoperative preparation of the patient and if they perform venous and arterial cannulation, induction and emergence of anesthesia, intubation, and extubation, and if they are left alone for any reason, they should be appropriately educated. In addition to a defined scope of practice and appropriate educational background, there should be recognition for practice as well as oversight in the recognition of the educational process and credentialing. IFNA is not concerned about whether these countries utilize nurse anesthetists. If nurses are being utilized in such a manner, however, IFNA is concerned that their scope of practice is defined and the educational process is sufficient to support anesthesia practice and patient safety.

In the United States, nurse anesthetists practice in all 50 states, Puerto Rico, and the District of Columbia. While it is a common belief that all nurse anesthetists in the United States are independent practitioners and in competition with physician anesthesiologists, current practice does not support this perception. Seventy-five percent of all nurse anesthetists in the United States practice in the anesthesia care team model. The majority of the independent practitioners provide anesthesia services in rural areas where there are no physician anesthesiologists.

In the United States, nurse anesthetists are registered nurses with a baccalaureate degree who have successfully completed a nurse anesthesia educational program at the master's degree level. Nurse anesthesia educational programs are accredited by the Council on Accreditation of Nurse Anesthesia Educational Programs. This council is recognized by the U.S. Department Office of Education as the official accrediting agency. Following graduation, the nurse anesthetist must successfully complete a national examination administered by the Council on Certification of Nurse Anesthetists before utilizing the credential Certified Registered Nurse Anesthetist (CRNA). Nurse anesthetists then remain certified by a recertification process every two years. The Council on Recertification of Nurse Anesthetists oversees this process. Nurse anesthetists provide more than 65 percent of the anesthetics administered in the United States and are the sole anesthesia providers in approximately two-thirds of all rural hospitals.

Nurse anesthetists and other non-physician anesthetists in less developed countries or countries in transition play a major role in the provision of anesthesia services. Many of these countries have very few physician anesthesia providers, and some have none. The majority of physician providers are located in the universities and teaching hospitals as educators and team leaders. Outside of the teaching setting, nurse anesthetists provide 90 percent to 100 percent of the anesthesia services. Due to the practice setting and the situations in which they practice, there is concern about the educational preparation and continuing education opportunities for these individuals. IFNA is also concerned about the ratios of anesthesia providers in these countries. While Scandinavian countries enjoy ratios of approximately 1:3,000 of anesthesia providers to populace and the United States and central Europe have approximately 1:7,000, some countries in Africa and Southeast Asia have ratios of 1:200,000 to 1:300,000+.

QUALIFICATIONS FOR MEMBERSHIP IN IFNA

Being a federation, IFNA membership is by country. It is the belief that it takes a strong country organization to effectively address issues involving nurse anesthesia practice. While many nurse anesthetists are organized within their countries, some have organized in order to apply for membership in the IFNA.

Within a country, one national nurse anesthetist association or federation of nurse anesthetists may become a member of IFNA. Where neither of these exists, a separate nurse anesthetist section or chapter of a national association composed of other health workers may become a member. Member country organizations are controlled by nurse anesthetists, speak for nurse anesthetists on nurse anesthesiology matters, and are the most representative of nurse anesthetists in the country, according to the IFNA definition of nurse anesthetist.

Each national nurse anesthetist association has the right to define its own membership at the national level. Where there is more than one small group of nurse anesthetists within a region, nurse anesthetists may form a regional organization for representation within IFNA.

Duties of the member country associations include communication with the executive director of IFNA of names and addresses of officers, number of members, and bylaws of the country organization. Representatives of member associations are responsible for seeing that dues are paid. They also report to the CNR once a year, respond to requests for information from the board, and make recommendations to the CNR regarding amendments to the bylaws, policies, or position statements of the IFNA.

Nonnurse anesthesia provider organizations may apply for associate membership in IFNA. These members may participate at meetings of the CNR as observers with the right to speak but no voting privileges. Dues for associate membership are one half the regular membership dues. At this point in time, no non-nurse anesthesia provider organizations have applied for associate membership.

IFNA ORGANIZATIONAL STRUCTURE: BYLAWS, COMMITTEES, MEETINGS

IFNA business is governed by bylaws, which were approved initially in 1989. Several revisions to the bylaws have occurred since adoption. A summary of the current bylaws is found in Table 19.4. A complete copy of this document can be obtained from IFNA headquarters.

Committees are the backbone of IFNA. It is through committee activity that projects are developed, planning is accomplished, and research is promoted. Committee members are selected by the IFNA president with the approval of the CNR.

The IFNA CPC is responsible for the IFNA World Congress. The country selected to host the World Congress appoints a National Organizing Committee (NOC). The CPC plans, organizes, implements, and evaluates the World Congress in collaboration with the NOC. Members also maintain communication with the IFNA executive director, officers, and executive committee, and ensure continuity of IFNA traditions in relation to the scientific program and ambiance of the World Congress.

An IFNA World Congress is a professional highlight for nurse anesthetists internationally. Objectives of the World Congress are to: (1) provide a forum whereby major trends and issues of interest to the international community of nurse anesthetists are discussed by peers and experts; (2) share and disseminate new knowledge and professional experiences as related to topics of interest of nurse anesthetists; (3) provide an opportunity for nurse anesthetists occupying similar positions in different countries to gather to discuss matters of mutual interest; and (4) strengthen collaboration between nurse anesthetists internationally to improve standards for nurse anesthesia education, continuing education, and practice at a high scientific level (IFNA, 1997).

EDUCATIONAL ACTIVITIES OF IFNA

A major focus of IFNA has been improving anesthesia education and safety throughout the world. In keeping with that focus, education, practice, and ethical standards were adopted between 1990 and 1992. A standard represents what the prudent nurse anesthetist in similar circumstances must exercise. Standards as approved by IFNA are the ultimate mandate internationally for educational preparation and clinical and ethical behavior of the anesthetist.

The preamble to the IFNA Educational Standards for Preparing Nurse Anesthetists is given in Table 19.5. The standards were revised in 1996 and 1999. The preamble to the IFNA Standards of Practice appears in Table 19.6. These standards were revised in 1996. The preamble to the IFNA Code of Ethics appears in Table 19.7; that document was adopted in May 1992. Complete copies of these documents can be obtained from the IFNA headquarters.

In addition to standards, the Education Committee also prepared monitoring guidelines. In contrast with standards, guidelines are not mandated. They are suggested or advised. Patient Monitoring Guidelines as revised in 1998 are found in Table 19.8 (Aker and Rupp, 1994).

During the 1991 World Congress, a first attempt was made to ascertain whether nurse anesthesia teachers would be interested in establishing a forum at the World Congress that related to their interests. The initial forum consisted of 45 representatives from the following 13 countries: Tunisia, France, Poland, Sweden, Norway, Switzerland, Korea, Finland, Austria, Slovenia, the Netherlands, Denmark, and the United States. While it did not provide for simultaneous interpretation, the participants were eager to continue with the concept. The first IFNA Teacher's Session was held at the 4th World Congress. It was so successful that this session was expanded and is now a permanent part of the World Congress.

IFNA headquarters continues to receive many requests for information on starting new programs. In response to this need, the IFNA Education Committee prepared a document titled "Guidelines for Starting a New Program and Sample Curriculum." It was prepared in 1996 and revised in 1998. Members of the Education Committee from France, Norway, Ghana, and the United States are available for consultation to countries wanting to start a program. IFNA's goal is to provide compe-

Table 19.4: IFNA Bylaws*		
Article I	Name and description	The name is the International Federation of Nurse Anesthetists (IFNA). It is a federation of national nurse anesthetist associations that have been formally admitted for membership and that have complied with the dues for membership. IFNA is organized and functions unrestricted by consideration of nationality, race, creed, color, politics, sex, or social status.
Article II	Philosophy	IFNA is an international organization of nationally registered nurses with special education in nurse anesthesia. The members of this professional organization are dedicated to the precept that its members are committed to the advancement of educational standards and practices, which will advance the art and science of anesthesiology and thereby support and enhance quality patient care.
Article III	Purpose	The purpose of IFNA is to promote assistance in the development of strong national nurse anesthesia associations.
Article IV	Objectives	Adopted as illustrated in Table 19.1.
Article V	Functions	Adopted as illustrated in Table 19.2.
Article VI	IFNA languages	The official language of IFNA is English.
Article VII	Definition of nurse anesthetist	A nurse anesthetist is a person who has completed a program of basic nursing education and basic nurse anesthesia education and is qualified and authorized in his/her country to practice nurse anesthesia.

*This table represents a summary of the complete document, which is available from IFNA headquarters.

tent, safe anesthesia care to patients requiring such services. Only those nurses who have completed a program of instruction in nurse anesthesia or who are supervised nurse students within such educational programs should be allowed to provide or participate in the provision of anesthesia services.

IFNA'S RESEARCH IN ACTION

In response to a challenge in 1990 by Dr. Miriam Hirschfeld, chief nurse scientist, WHO, IFNA set out to document the existence, role, education, and recognition of nurse anesthetists worldwide. Maura S. McAuliffe, CRNA, PhD, was appointed the IFNA official nurse anesthesia researcher to embark upon an ongoing international study, "Nurse Anesthesia Worldwide: Practice, Education and Regulation," in collaboration with WHO.

Using the WHO address list of its member countries and the ICN address list of its member organizations, the study was started. The first two phases of the study were completed in 1994, with the third and final phase concluded in 2000. The results of the first two phases of this study were astonishing, even to IFNA. The results indicated that nurses were participating in the delivery of anesthesia services in 107 countries. It was even more surprising to learn that nurses were participating in 70 percent to 80 percent of all anesthesia administered in the world. In many of the less developed countries, results indicated that nurses are providing 90 percent to 100 percent of all anesthesia services. This valuable study was funded by the AANA Council on Recertification (USA) and IFNA (Caulk, 1998). The results of the first two phases of the study were presented at the 4th World Congress in 1994; results of the final phase of the study were presented at the 6th World Congress in 2000. Of concern to IFNA was the fact that many ministries of health and nursing leaders were unaware of who was providing anesthesia services within their respective countries. Of even greater concern was the fact that many of these providers have no formal education, are not officially recognized, and are pleading for continuing education opportunities.

LIAISON WITH OTHER INTERNATIONAL ORGANIZATIONS

It is clear today that it is in the best interests of IFNA to align itself with established international organizations whose goals are consistent with and whose programs dovetail with the stated aims of IFNA. To a degree, IFNA's eventual success depends on its ability to become associated with the international organizations and programs it supports. This vision led IFNA leaders to approach organizations with the widest possible constituencies for mutual support and affiliation (Caulk, 1992).

The European Economic Community

One of IFNA's objectives in having an early priority for defining standards of practice and education was to provide member countries with a document they could use to help upgrade education or practice. Specifically, defined standards could be used in planning for the anticipated formation of the European Economic Community in 1992 that is now known as the European Union (EU). The official committee in charge of developing rules for nursing within the EU is the Advisory Committee for Training in Nursing (ACTN), with members appointed by governments of the EU. Each country appoints three representatives, one health authority, one nurse practitioner, and one nurse educator to ACTN. In 1977, general care nursing education was defined by a specific sectarian directive and adopted by the Council of Ministers. Nursing specialties

Table 19.5: IFNA Educational Standards for Preparing Nurse Anesthetists

Preamble

Nurse anesthetists are prepared and utilized in many countries throughout the world to provide, or assist in the provision of quality [*] anesthesia services to patients. The following position on Educational Standards for Preparing Nurse Anesthetists [*] is written to accommodate the major variance in the scope of nurse anesthesia practice [*] within these countries as they relate to national organizational membership in the International Federation of Nurse Anesthetists (IFNA). Rather than writing minimal and optimal standards, the Education Committee of the IFNA has chosen to build such flexibility within a single set of standards. It is believed that such standards will have the capability to foster a responsible basis for preparing nurse anesthetists competent to provide anesthesia services, which adheres to qualitative standards and assures patient safety, comfort, and well-being while providing flexibility that allows for the identification of new goals and facilitates their achievement as scopes of practice grow and change in the years to come. (Note: Words, or groups of words, followed by [*] indicate that their definition is included in the glossary.)

Definition of a Nurse Anesthetist

A nurse anesthetist provides, or participates in the provision of, advanced specialized nursing and anesthesia services to patients requiring anesthesia, respiratory care, cardiopulmonary resuscitation, and/or other emergency, life-sustaining services wherever required. Advanced specialized nursing and anesthesia services incorporate the biological and behavioral sciences into practice as they relate to patients and their families.

Table 19.6: IFNA Standards of Practice

Preamble

The International Federation of Nurse Anesthetists is an international organization of registered nurses with special education in nurse anesthesia. A nurse anesthetist is a person who has completed a program of basic nursing education and basic nurse anesthesia education and is qualified and authorized in his/her country to practice anesthesia. The member countries of this professional organization are dedicated to the precept that their members are committed to the advancement of educational and practice standards, which will advance the art and science of nurse anesthesiology and thereby support and enhance quality patient care.

A characteristic of any profession is its responsibility to the public for developing standards, whereby the quality of practice rendered by its members can be judged. Establishing standards is essential in upgrading practice, and they are developed and subscribed to by all members based upon the profession's philosophy, theory, science, principle, and research. Standards provide a means to evaluate the practice and provide the practitioner with a level of expectation and a framework within which to operate.

Purpose of Standards

While nurse anesthetists' services are utilized in many countries throughout the world, anesthesia practice may vary from one country to another or from one geographic location to another within a country because of requirements or limitations imposed by local law or institutional characteristics. Additionally, the practice of the nurse anesthetist is governed by policies, rules, and regulations as established by the healthcare institution in which the anesthesia care is being provided. The standards are descriptive, providing a basis for evaluation of the practice and reflecting the rights of those receiving anesthesia care.

Table 19.7: IFNA Code of Ethics

Preamble

The fundamental responsibility of the nurse anesthetist is to provide or participate in the provision of advanced specialized nursing and anesthesia services to patients requiring anesthesia, respiratory care, cardiopulmonary resuscitation, and/or other emergency, life-sustaining services wherever required. Advanced specialized nursing and anesthesia services incorporate the behavioral and biological sciences into practice as they relate to patients and their families. Inherent in anesthesia nursing practice is respect for life, dignity, and rights of man. It is unrestricted by considerations of nationality, race, creed, age, sex, politics, or social status.

The purpose of a code of ethics is to acknowledge a profession's acceptance of the responsibility and trust conferred upon it by society and to recognize the international obligations inherent in that trust. The International Federation of Nurse Anesthetists Code of Ethics is devised from the premise that as healthcare professionals, nurse anesthetists must strive, both on an individual and collective basis, to pursue the highest possible ethical standards.

were not and currently are not addressed. Any new country members of the EU must agree to this directive. The EU Directorate XV, in charge of the inner market and free movement of professions, employs a permanent secretary for ACTN to whom IFNA submitted the IFNA Standards of Practice. The permanent secretary responded that "the Commission services consider that such initiatives contribute to facilitate the recognition of professional qualifications with the Community Directives called the 'General System' (Directive 89/48/CEE and 92/51/CEE) which concern the recognition of specialised nurses certifications." The professional self-regulation at the European level could be useful for competency authorities in the course of applying for recognition under the above directives in so far as if a professional has received an education in accordance with standards defined by the profession, that could signify that he/she has reached a certain level of professional competency. IFNA maintains close contact with the permanent secretary of ACTN.

In 1971, the Standing Committee for Nursing was formed, following the ICN meeting in Dublin, with Marie-Paul Florin (France) serving as the first president. The first formal meeting of the committee was held in Brussels, and the organization was the official liaison with the Europeoan Community Commission. The committee is composed of nursing leaders from EU national nurses associations that are members of ICN. The committee works collaboratively with ACTN and makes recommendations but does not have any authority. It is anticipated that in the future the Standing Committee of Nursing will have more influence. IFNA does work collaboratively with the committee, however.

The Council of Europe is the official committee of all European countries including the EU, except for Russia. This council has in the past developed recommendations for the European level and developed the guidelines concerning nursing specialties that IFNA used as reference in establishing the IFNA Educational Standards. Currently the council follows the decisions of the EU.

Another organization in which IFNA participates is the European Network of Nursing Organizations. This organization is composed of members from EU and non-EU countries and addresses nursing and nursing specialty issues. It is a branch of the Standing Committee for Nursing.

The IFNA president and other European nurse anesthetists have taken an

Table 19.8: IFNA Patient Monitoring Guidelines

Anesthesia safety is the goal of anesthesia delivery worldwide. Parameters that enhance safety include professional knowledge, vigilance, constant monitoring, and changes in the anesthetic plan based upon patient responses to the anesthetic.

Included in the International Federation of Nurse Anesthetists Standards of Practice is a standard (IV) that addresses monitoring. It states, "the nurse anesthetist will monitor psychological and physiological responses, interpret and utilize data obtained from the use of invasive and noninvasive monitoring modalities, and take corrective action to maintain or stabilize the patient's condition, and provide resuscitative care." The nurse anesthetist will monitor, record, and report the patient's physiological and psychological signs and provide resuscitative care that includes fluid therapy, maintenance of airway, and provision of assisted or controlled ventilation.

Patient monitoring guidelines are intended to assist the nurse anesthetist in providing consistent, safe anesthesia care. While these guidelines are intended to apply to patients undergoing general, regional, or monitored anesthesia care, they do not apply to epidural analgesia or labor or pain management. These guidelines may be exceeded in any or all respects at any time at the discretion of the anesthetist. In extenuating circumstances, the nurse anesthetist must use clinical judgment in prioritizing and implementing these guidelines. If there is reason to omit a monitored parameter, the reason for the omission should be documented on the record.

Ventilation:

Purpose: To assess adequate ventilation of the patient.

Guideline: Ventilatory adequacy shall be assessed by palpation or observation of the reservoir breathing bag, chest movement, and auscultation of breath sounds. Ventilation should be continuously assessed by the use of a precordial or esophageal stethoscope. Correct placement of an endotracheal tube must be verified by auscultation and chest excursion. When available, spirometry, ventilatory pressure monitors, and end-tidal CO_2 monitoring should be used. When a patient is ventilated by mechanical ventilator, the integrity of the breathing circuit must be monitored by a device that is capable of detecting disconnection.

Oxygenation:

Purpose: To assess adequate oxygenation of the patient.

Guideline: Adequacy of oxygenation shall be monitored by observation of skin color, color of the blood in the surgical field, and arterial blood gas analysis as indicated. The use of pulse oximetry is encouraged on all patients. During general anesthesia, the oxygen concentration delivered by the anesthesia machine shall be continuously monitored with an oxygen analyzer with a low oxygen concentration limit alarm. An oxygen supply failure alarm system shall be used to warn of low oxygen pressure in the anesthesia machine.

Circulation:

Purpose: To assess adequacy of the patient's cardiovascular system.

Guideline: Circulation shall be assessed by at least one of the following measures: digital palpation of pulse, auscultation of heart sounds, continuous intra-arterial pressure monitoring, or pulse oximetry. Skin color and capillary refill should be monitored. Blood pressure and heart rate shall be determined and recorded at least every 5 minutes. An electrocardiogram (EKG) continuously displayed from induction through emergence is highly encouraged.

Body Temperature:

Purpose: To assess changes in body temperature.

Guideline: During every anesthetic, there shall be readily available a means to measure body temperature. When changes in temperature are anticipated, the temperature shall be measured.

(continued)

Table 19.8: IFNA Patient Monitoring Guidelines (continued)

Neuromuscular Function:

Purpose:	To assess neuromuscular function.
Guideline:	When neuromuscular blocking drugs are used, neuromuscular function shall be assessed by respiratory strength, hand grip, sustained head lift, and negative inspiratory force. Assessment of neuromuscular function by a nerve stimulator is strongly recommended.

Anesthesia Equipment:

Anesthesia equipment should be selected to ensure appropriate delivery of available anesthetics and maintenance of physiological parameters adequate for organ preservation. Equipment should be checked thoroughly each day, and an abbreviated check of all equipment shall be completed before each anesthetic.

Nurse Anesthetist:

Continuous clinical observation and vigilance are the cornerstone for anesthesia safety. The nurse anesthetist shall be in constant attendance of the patient until care has been accepted by another qualified individual.

active role in the discussion of nursing specialties and continue to monitor and participate in activities regarding nursing specialties in the EU. Establishing the definition of a nursing specialty is difficult in that what is recognized as a nursing specialty in one country is not recognized as a nursing specialty in another. The post-basic nursing education for the specialties also varies from country to country. Within Europe, nursing and nurse-specialty organizations influence the decision-making process for the profession, but all regulations are determined by the EU ministries of health.

A common passport is planned for EU members, permitting free travel for its citizens and free trade for member countries across their borders. Further, the plan also permits professionals from one country to move to and practice in any of the member countries. To what extent this can be achieved is questionable, but if European nurse anesthetists are to have any part in shaping their futures as they relate to the EU, some standards upon which these countries could agree are needed. IFNA affords an appropriate forum for nurse anesthetists from various countries to cooperate and collaborate in these efforts.

While IFNA is frequently asked for assistance with career placement in other countries, it is not a role or function of IFNA. Membership in IFNA does not imply that reciprocity is available. Outside of the EU, there are many requirements such as working visas, licensure as a nurse, recognition of nurse anesthesia education, and language proficiency examination before a nurse anesthetist can work in a foreign country. There are exceptions, but generally, information regarding employment abroad can be obtained from the respective ministry of health.

International Council of Nurses (ICN)

Nurses' involvement in an early women's movement, organized at the national and international level, helped to coalesce nursing organizations in the United States and to form the ICN.

A group of nurses had attended the 1899 meeting of the International Council of Women in London and decided that a need existed for an analogous international organization of nurses; a committee of these nurses met in July

1900, adopted a constitution, and elected officers, thereby forming ICN. At the time of formation, membership consisted of individual nurses from various countries. The first meeting of ICN was held in Buffalo, N.Y., in 1901.

Because only one representative national group could join the U.S. National Council of Women—which was affiliated with the International Council of Women—the American Federation of Nurses (AFN) was formed in 1900. The AFN linked two nursing organizations: the Nurses' Associated Alumnae—a loose association of graduates of various nursing schools—and the American Society of Superintendents of Training Schools.

By 1904, it was decided that ICN should be a federation of national organizations representing nurses in each country, rather than a membership consisting of individual nurses. Accordingly, the AFN was invited, along with the German Nurses Association and the national Council of Nurses of England, to become charter members of ICN. The American Nurses' Association (ANA) was formed in 1911 as the representative organization of the Nurses' Associated Alumnae of the United States. After the AFN disbanded in 1913, the ANA became the official U.S. representative to ICN.

ICN has grown significantly over the years—it currently has a membership of 120 countries—and conducts an international congress for nurses quadrennially. It was to ICN that the planning committee of IFNA turned for assistance in its formation. While ICN has been made up principally of national organizations representing nurses in general, it has devised a mechanism for the recognition and affiliation of international specialty nursing organizations.

The ICN Professional Services Committee that defined qualifications for specialty organizational affiliation includes the requirement that such organizations have membership from two organizations representing 50 percent of the seven global areas adopted by ICN (i.e., representation from four of these global areas; IFNA had representation only from three). The problem that existed was the fact that the ICN North American voting area consisted of two countries, Canada and the United States. With Canada not having nurse anesthetists, it was impossible for IFNA to meet ICN requirements.

In 1995, ICN restructured the voting regions, including the reorganization of the European organizations and the addition of Mexico and the Caribbean basin to the North American voting area. In 1996, Mexico became a member of IFNA, and in 1997 the Jamaican Association of Nurse Anesthetists became an IFNA member. With the addition of these two organizations to IFNA, the ICN requirement of organizational representation from four of the global areas was met. In 1996, IFNA was officially recognized by ICN. IFNA was the second of only three international nursing specialties to be recognized by ICN. IFNA continues to enjoy this relationship on a formal basis and attends CNR meetings as observers.

World Health Organization (WHO)

IFNA has made contact with nurse anesthetists in a number of countries. The breadth of usage of nurse anesthetists includes both developed and developing countries. Because IFNA aims to foster and promote quality nurse anesthesia education and practice wherever nurses provide these services, it would be an important step to gain recognition or affiliation with WHO.

Persons involved in assisting developing countries to achieve adequate health delivery systems have questioned using nurses rather than physicians for anesthesia services. Two reasons apply: First, physicians from these countries trained elsewhere in anesthesia often do not return to their native countries to practice; even if trained in their own countries, they often emigrate elsewhere to practice. Nurses appear less prone to emigrate.

The second reason is that the precarious economic status of many developing countries suggests that nurses would be the more cost-effective anesthesia provider and would, as is evident in all IFNA member countries, practice throughout the country, wherever need exists.

In general, it appears to be WHO's primary aim to promote a strong primary care and disease prevention program in developing countries as a means to gain the most benefit for money spent. Although not often considered a primary care modality, anesthesia cuts across the various types of healthcare. Obstetrics, for example, is regarded as a primary care component, despite its involving high-risk patients and tertiary care; thus, access to selected anesthesia services in this healthcare area is essential to minimize both maternal and neonatal morbidity and mortality.

Further, anesthesia may be required to assist in preventing or correcting infection, pathology, traumatic injury, or congenital defects that, while not necessarily life-threatening initially, may over time cause disability and dependency and threaten life. Blindness, cleft lip or palate, conditions leading to deafness, and fractures with bone displacement exemplify such conditions.

It was at the first meeting with WHO, in November 1990, when Caulk and Löhnert obtained an appointment with Dr. Hirschfeld, chief nurse scientist, WHO, that the question of establishing a relationship or liaison with WHO was discussed. Dr. Hirschfeld, somewhat unfamiliar with nurse anesthetists and their practice, requested that additional information be furnished to her on the number of nurse anesthetists worldwide, the countries in which they are used, and the roles they fulfill. Unfortunately, other than the 11 member organizations, such information was virtually unknown to IFNA. IFNA had only unsubstantiated reports that nurses were involved in the provision of anesthesia services elsewhere.

Occasion for another meeting with Dr. Hirschfeld arose when she came to be the keynote speaker at the International Nursing Research Conference in October 1991. Dr. McAuliffe, then a doctoral student at the College of Nursing, University of Texas-Austin, and Caulk were present. At a subsequent meeting with Dr. Hirschfeld during the conference, it was discussed and proposed that a worldwide study of nurse anesthetists be conducted. Dr. Hirschfeld agreed that WHO would collaborate in the study. Funding was obtained, and the study is now complete. While IFNA is not yet recognized as an NGO, it does maintain an informal relationship with WHO.

Center for Quality Assurance in International Education (CQAIE)

The CQAIE is a consortium of higher education associations and quality assurance and competency bodies located at the National Center for Higher Education in Washington, D.C. The center is dedicated to monitoring quality issues in the globalization of U.S. higher education and provides assistance in the development and improvement of quality assurance systems throughout the globe. In 1996, the center became the secretariat of a new global organization of business, government, education, and the professions dedicated to issues of quality and access in education, and training that crosses national borders: the Global Alliance for Transnational Education (GATE) (Peace Lenn, 1997).

Dr. Marjorie Peace Lenn, executive

director of CQAIE, presented the keynote address at the IFNA 5th World Congress in April 1997. Dr. Lenn outlined for the group action steps for establishing a profession nationally or regionally. She also stressed that the dynamics of globalization leave no profession time to dwell in myopia without rendering the profession irrelevant in a changing world. According to her, future effectiveness of international professional organizations lies in their ability to provide international solutions to local problems or to be effective across borders as well as within borders. IFNA concurs with this statement and continues to work with this organization. It is through CQAIE that IFNA leaders have become aware of international trade agreements such as the North American Free Trade Agreement and the World Trade Organization with respect to trade in services affecting professional mobility. Many international organizations participate in CQAIE activities that include international accreditation and certification. While IFNA has not developed accreditation and certification internationally, it is an issue that will most probably be addressed in the future. IFNA has been an organizational member of CQAIE since 1997 and has both presented and participated at CQAIE and GATE meetings.

World Federation of Societies of Anaesthesiologists

A featured speaker at the 5th World Congress of IFNA in Austria was Dr. Anneke Meursing, Honorary Secretary, World Federation of Societies of Anaesthesiologists (WFSA). As a follow-up to this congress, IFNA representatives were asked to meet with the Executive Committee of WFSA.

On June 30, 1998, the president, executive director, and two members of the Education Committee (Sandra M. Ouellette, CRNA, MEd, FAAN, United States, and Jeanne Capron, France) of IFNA met with members of the Executive Committee of WFSA in Braunfels, Germany. The purpose of the meeting was to explore the possibility of forming a liaison with WSFA. Dr. Meursing suggested that two members of the IFNA Education Committee attend the meeting since many of the organizations' mutual interests involve education and continuing education in less-developed countries. The meeting focused on education and continuing education primarily in the less-developed countries and what the two organizations could do jointly to assist with these issues. Although it was emphasized by physician leaders that WFSA is a physician-based organization and views anesthesiology as a physician-based specialty, the existence and contributions of both nurses and clinical officers in various parts of the world was acknowledged. Overall, the meeting was cordial and productive. It provided IFNA with an opportunity to establish a working relationship with WFSA.

In May 1999, Ouellette, serving as IFNA Education Committee chair, joined Dr. Meursing in Blantyre, Malawi. The purpose of the trip was to participate in the 6th Anaesthesia Refresher Course Seminar and inauguration of the Association of Anaesthetists of Malawi.

International Hospital Federation

In 1998, IFNA Executive Director Caulk, and Glen Ramsborg, CRNA, PhD, met with the then International Hospital Federation (IHF) director general, Dr. Errol Pickering, to discuss the role of IHF and its relationship with other international organizations. IFNA was encouraged to become an organizational member of IHF and to participate in IHF activities. In 1998, IFNA became an organizational member of IHF and was encouraged to submit articles on nurse anesthesia for the IHF journal. Caulk prepared a paper, "The IFNA, an Introduction," which was published in *World Hospitals and Health Services* (Vol. 34, No. 2, 1998), the official journal of IHF. This journal has a worldwide circulation. While the predominate membership of IHF is hospital administrators, IHF addresses all issues in healthcare.

The International Society for Quality in Health Care

The International Society for Quality in Health Care (ISQua) is an independent, global organization with the following objectives: (1) promotion of quality improvement on a continual basis in healthcare internationally in both the public and private sectors; (2) development and maintenance of internationally agreed upon terminology of quality improvement; (3) organization of meetings on a regional and global basis; (4) provision of an internationally agreed method of accreditation for courses in quality improvement and related matters; (5) promotion of research in quality improvement in healthcare; and (6) maintenance of relationships with other relevant international and regional organizations.

ISQua membership includes many international professional organizations, national and regional accrediting bodies, and individuals participating in quality assurance. The Joint Commission on Accreditation of Healthcare Organizations has formed an international arm called the Joint Commission on International Accreditation. In July 1999, Caulk attended the "World Symposium on Improving Health Care Through Accreditation" in Barcelona, Spain. This symposium was cosponsored by the Fundacion Avedis Donabedium, a Spanish accreditation body, and by Underwriters Laboratories, and endorsed by the EU-sponsored External Peer Review Techniques Group and ISQua. This was the first such meeting attended by a leader of IFNA. International standards for hospital accreditation were proposed at this meeting. Of concern to IFNA is the fact that such standards address not only the standards for anesthesia departments, but also the credentials of "qualified anesthesia providers" within the department. The initiation of international standards met with mixed reviews, especially for the developing and less-developed countries where the cost for the accreditation of one hospital could well be the entire annual healthcare budget. When discussing ISQua activities, IFNA was advised that organizational membership in ISQua provided the only method for representation and addressing issues affecting anesthesia services. While some IFNA members have individual membership, it is only through organizational membership that the profession has an international voice. IFNA became an organizational member of ISQua in 1999.

GLOBALIZATION OF THE PROFESSIONS

Dr. Peace Lenn presented the keynote address at IFNA's 5th World Congress of Nurse Anesthetists in 1997. Her topic was "Nurse Anesthesia and the Globalization of the Professions" (Peace Lenn, 1997).

In this address, Dr. Peace Lenn stated there is an eagerness at the World Congress to accentuate differences in national practice rather than celebrate similarities in international practice. She believes that since IFNA has adopted international standards, it is well on its way to globalization of the nurse anesthesia profession. At the heart of professional practice is a core of common standards that, if adopted across borders and regions, defines the profession of nurse anesthesia in ways that not only protect

Table 19.9: Action Steps for Establishing a Global Profession

- Act as an international witness for the need for professional standards in nurse anesthesia.
- Interact effectively with appropriate regional and international organizations.
- Act as liaison to other globalizing professions.
- Consider development of an IFNA quality assurance process for nurse anesthesia educational and professional development programs.
- Monitor and record its own progress through research, publication, and international forums.

regulation and mode of practice, but also provide the world's people the best in anesthesia care.

IFNA's Educational, Practice, and Ethical Standards stand as international witness for the globalization of a profession in both preparation and practice. The global marketplace and new technology are contributing to the rapid globalization of higher education. Issues of quality, purpose, and responsibility abound in the new borderless educational arena, posing new challenges to the regulatory communities of accreditation, certification, and licensure, the three pillars of quality and competency assurance among the professions of the world.

Table 19.9 lists action steps for IFNA in establishing a global profession. IFNA remains committed not only to globalization of the nurse anesthesia profession, but also to national and regional development of the profession. With IFNA being the only international nursing organization to establish international standards, it will continue to work toward daily application of the standards in anesthetic care worldwide.

IFNA: ACCOMPLISHMENTS, NEEDS, FUTURE

Although IFNA has only been in existence since 1989, it has already accomplished many goals. Recognized strengths include adopted standards and increased networking among other international organizations interested in healthcare.

As with any new organization, IFNA has some weaknesses that it must strive to overcome. Lack of financial support is one of its major problems. Each member organization is assessed approximately 40 cents (0.50 Swiss francs) per year per active member. Many member countries are the size of some of the smaller states within the United States, and the number of nurse anesthetists in these countries is small. Many member countries have been financing their own representatives to the IFNA meetings, with money from the IFNA budget going only to those that cannot undertake any sponsorship.

There is a need to identify sources of revenue for the organization and the IFNA Education and Research Foundation whereby donations can be accepted and used for some of IFNA's planned activities and research. It would also be helpful if IFNA could sponsor scholarships or find other means by which nurse anesthetists could be financially assisted to obtain additional education so as to better prepare them as educators and leaders within their countries.

IFNA is not without potential for some internal political issues arising. National pride runs strong within each member country. While IFNA encourages global thinking, protection of one's own turf occasionally arises. Intent and desire to work together as equals are evident, but member nurse anesthesia organizations differ in size, in age, and in the development the specialty has attained. The principal fiscal support for the organization must come from the larger and longer-established organizations. This has the potential to leave the perception that one or two larger groups may attempt to dominate the group. Despite an organizational structure that can lend support to each member country, each must be sensitive to others' needs and offer support or assistance only when requested. Each country exists in its own political and legal environment, and any assistance given must take those elements into consideration.

SUMMARY

This discussion has centered on the first decade of IFNA activities. The extent to which IFNA will be successful in the future depends upon member countries' support for the goals of IFNA and IFNA's ability to align itself with the organizations and programs it supports. The speed of transportation and communication has made us all world citizens. It is only through IFNA that we have the best opportunity to fulfill our professional obligations to our world community. We believe the future is bright for both IFNA and the people we serve.

As we move forward in the 21st century, it is evident that IFNA has a need for more international research. While the recent IFNA international study provided much needed information (see abstract, Table 19.10) and worldwide publication for nurse anesthesia (McAuliffe, 1996), it is apparent that nurse anesthetists will need to be included as contributors to future healthcare and healthcare planning (Henry and McAuliffe, 1999).

Table 19.10: Nurse Anesthesia Worldwide: Practice, Education, and Regulation

The World Health Assembly, in 1977, determined that all member governments should have as their primary goal to achieve by the year 2000, a level of health that would allow their citizens to enjoy an economically and socially productive life. The main strategy for "Health for All by the Year 2000" is the development of a health system infrastructure, starting with primary healthcare, for the delivery of countrywide services that reach the whole population. Primary care includes maternal and child services and the identification and appropriate treatment of common acute diseases and injuries. The skills and resources required to provide these aspects of primary healthcare often involve relatively simple, yet life-saving or disability prevention procedures, such as is used in the management of acute labor and delivery complications of the mother and fetus, or the simple reduction of a displaced fracture of a leg or arm. These services, however, cannot be provided humanely without anesthesia.

In many countries, anesthesia is provided by nurses—a little known fact. This international study of nurse anesthesia was conducted to provide information with respect to the quantity and quality of anesthesia care delivered by nurses in countries in all regions as designated by the World Health Organization. This study provides information that can serve as a basis for future planning of anesthesia manpower resources and education.

STUDY METHODS AND FINDINGS: In phase I of the study, surveys were translated into five languages and mailed to ministries of health (164 countries); national nursing organizations (154 countries); and leaders in nursing administration (76 countries). The surveys asked if, in their countries, nurses gave or assisted in the giving of anesthesia, and requested respondents to provide names and addresses of nurse anesthetists who could participate in Phase II of the study. PHASE I RESULTS: Respondents from 107 countries (59% of all WHO member states) reported that nurses give anesthesia in their countries; 9 countries reported that nurses assist in the giving of anesthesia. In 18 countries the evidence was inconclusive, although it is highly likely that nurses in many of these countries give anesthesia. Respondents from 112 countries provided names and addresses of 624 nurse anesthetists.

In Phase II of the study, surveys containing items addressing anesthesia practice (80 items), education (16 items), and regulation (17 items) were translated into four languages and mailed to each of the 624 nurse anesthetists in Phase I of the study. PHASE II RESULTS: Respondents (n=299) from 92 countries validated the findings from Phase I. The Phase II subjects reported that nurse anesthetists provide as much as 77% of the anesthesia in urban areas and 75% of anesthetics in rural areas of their respective countries. The respondents reported that in the hospitals where they work, nurse anesthetists provide 85% of all anesthetics for cesarean sections; administer drugs to induce anesthesia (77%); perform tracheal intubation (74%); administer spinal anesthesia (57%); epidural anesthesia (44%); manage anesthetized patients intraoperatively (79%); perform tracheal extubation (77%); and manage patients in the immediate postoperative period (54%). Fifty-seven percent of the respondents reported they were required to have a physician anesthetist supervise their work (most were from the European region), 43% of the sample reported having no such requirement. All respondents had a formal course of study in anesthesia; however, many had to travel to other countries to receive their education. Fifty percent reported that continuing education was not available. Respondents (74%) reported that hospital policies as well as governmental regulations (60%) guide their practice of nurse anesthesia.

Improved access to continuing education and supportive legislation were most frequently cited as changes that would improve the anesthesia practice of nurses. An additional finding was that although nurse anesthetists currently provide much, and in some countries virtually all the anesthesia, their contribution to healthcare often goes unrecognized by their governments. If "Health for All" is to be achieved by any nation, fiscally responsible healthcare systems that maximally utilize the services of qualified classes of healthcare providers must be instituted. National healthcare policymakers should be made aware that nurse anesthetists currently provide much of the anesthesia care worldwide, and the most cost-effective and efficient anesthesia care includes the utilization of nurse anesthetists. To maximally utilize these healthcare providers, nurse anesthesia educational programs should be expanded, and supportive legislation should be initiated.

Maura S. McAuliffe, CRNA, PhD

Beverly Henry, RN, PhD, FAAN

REFERENCES

International Federation of Nurse Anesthetists brochure.

Caulk, R. & Maree, S.M. (1990). The international federation of nurse anesthetists. *AANA Journal*. 58(3), 158-164.

IFNA Education Committee. (1990). International educational standards for the preparation of nurse anesthetists.

IFNA Education Committee. (1992a). International standards of practice for nurse anesthetists.

IFNA Education Committee. (1992b). Code of ethics.

Caulk, R.F. (1998). The International Federation of Nurse Anesthetists (IFNA), an introduction. *World Hospitals and Health Services*. 34(2), 11-14.

International Federation of Nurse Anesthetists. (1999). Bylaws.

International Federation of Nurse Anesthetists. (1997). Congress planning committee policy and procedure manual. 1-46.

Aker, J.G. & Rupp, R.M. (1994). Standards of Care in Anesthesia Practice. In Foster, S.D. & Jordan, L.M. (Eds.), *Professional Aspects of Nurse Anesthesia Practice* (pp. 89-112). Philedelphia, PA: F.A. Davis Co.

IFNA Education Committee. (1998). Monitoring guidelines.

Caulk, R.F. (1992). The International Federation of Nurse Anesthetists (IFNA). *CRNA Forum*. 8(2), 3-19.

Peace Lenn, M. (1997). Nurse anesthesia and the globalization of the profession. *AANA Journal*. 65(5), 444-449.

McAuliffe, M. (1996). Countries where anesthesia is administered by nurses. *AANA Journal*. 64 (5), 469-479.

Henry, B. & McAuliffe, M. (1999). Practice and education of nurse anesthetists. *Bulletin of the World Health Organization, The International Journal of Public Health*. 77 (3), 267-270.

STUDY QUESTIONS

1. The work of IFNA in the last decade is a good example of collaboration with other healthcare organizations that have a world-wide influence. Why is this collaboration necessary or desirable?

2. What are the primary objectives of IFNA? How do they relate to those of AANA?

3. What is a federation and why is it a workable organizational framework for IFNA?

4. Contact several international organzations of nurse anesthetists who are members of IFNA and explore the ways in which their scope of practice compares to your own. How do they plan on further developing practice standards in their country?

PRACTICE CHALLENGES

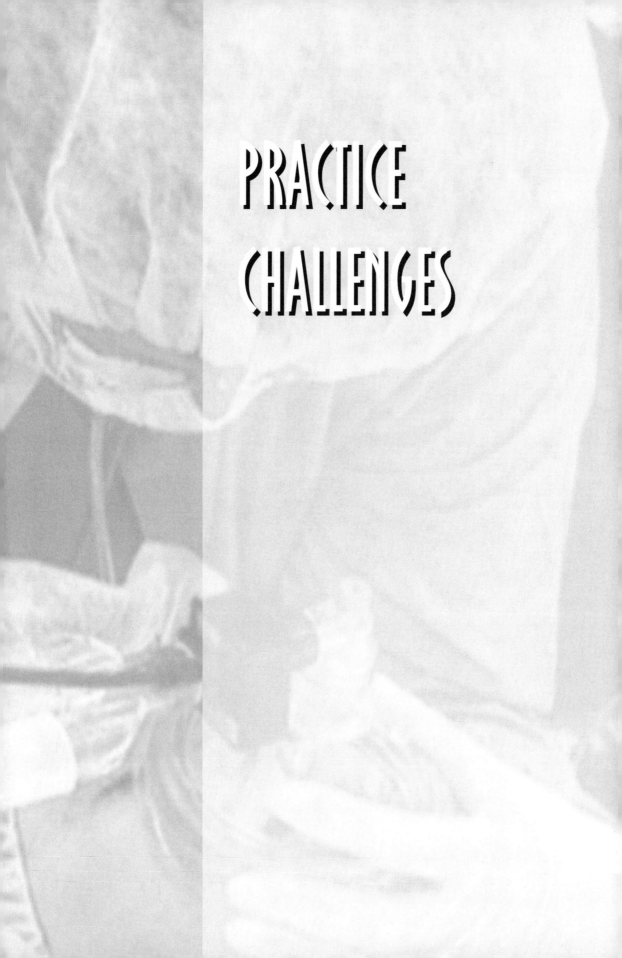

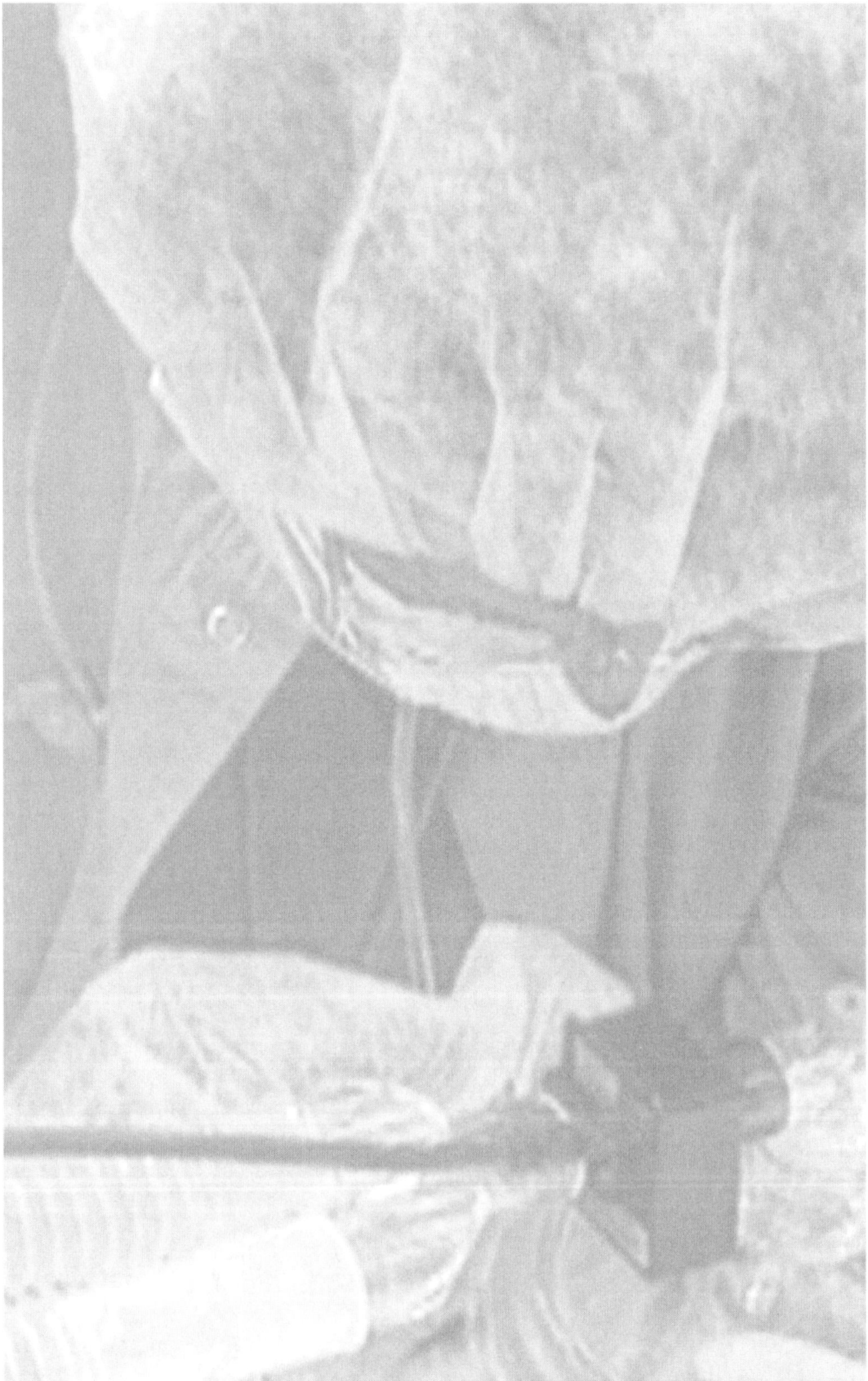

CHAPTER 20

ETHICAL DECISION MAKING IN ANESTHESIA

Marcia Bosek, DNSc, RN

Associate Professor,
Adult Health Nursing
Rush University College of Nursing
Chicago, IL

KEY CONCEPTS

- Ethical situations require Certified Registered Nurse Anesthetists (CRNAs) to consider professional and personal values, think about what is the right thing to do, identify options, and act upon the selected "right" option.
- In Western societies, autonomy is the most important goal during ethical decision making.
- Nonmaleficence, or do-no-harm, is a fundamental goal guiding a CRNA's actions.
- Beneficence requires that an action be implemented that will bring about good for the patient.
- Justice is concerned with equity or fairness in the distribution of scarce healthcare resources.
- Advocating for the welfare of patients is a responsibility CRNAs must uphold.
- Advance directives should never be consulted when the patient is competent and able to make healthcare decisions.

Nurse anesthetists face many problems and make many choices during their daily clinical practice. While all problems are not ethical problems and all choices are not moral choices, ethical problems do occur that require nurse anesthetists to consider their professional and personal values, think about what is the right thing to do, identify options, and act upon the selected "right" option. This chapter is concerned with issues of healthcare ethics and the role of the Certified Registered Nurse Anesthetist (CRNA) in promoting a humane, caring resolution to these difficult ethical quandaries.

The case study exemplars presented in this chapter are real ethical situations that CRNAs described during a recent research study, funded by the American Association of Nurse Anesthetists (AANA) Foundation, investigating how CRNAs resolve clinical ethical situations. Since every clinical situation is unique and no single, definitive, universal treatment protocol exists, the reader is cautioned not to get sidetracked by critiquing the specific clinical details, such as which drug was used. Rather, the reader should use the cases to promote thinking specifically as well as broadly about the ethical issues, values, and duties.

The terms ethics and morals are derived from Latin and Greek words meaning custom. Within each society, customs are developed. While a custom may be sanctioned by one society, the custom may not be evaluated as being right by other cultures or societies, for example, slavery, cannibalism, or polygamy. Every CRNA possesses a set of moral customs that have been influenced by family, neighborhood, religious community, and educational background. Just as each individual has a set of moral customs, every clinical practice setting also has a unique set of moral customs. Thus, the potential exists for ethical situations to occur when various customs and their associated beliefs conflict.

THE CRNA'S ADVANCED PRACTICE ROLE DURING ETHICAL ISSUES

While every nurse (as well as every healthcare professional) has an obligation to be an active participant in the resolution of clinical ethical situations, CRNAs by virtue of their advanced practice role have additional responsibilities. Bosek and Carpenter (as cited in Bosek & Savage, 1997) proposed that advanced practice nurses need to develop additional skills in:

- Fostering decision-making skills in patients and their significant others, as well as in other healthcare professionals.
- Inviting divergent opinions and interpersonal discussions.
- Resolving commonly occurring ethical issues in their area of clinical specialty.
- Engaging in prospective planning regarding recurrent ethical issues in their clinical specialty.

ETHICAL DECISION MAKING

Ethical Decision-Making Models

An assortment of ethical decision-making resources are available to help CRNAs resolve clinical ethical problems. First, a variety of ethical decision-making models exist (Francoeur, 1983; Jonsen, Siegler, and Winslade, 1998; Thompson and Thompson, 1985). Each model proposes a unique emphasis for guiding decision making, such as rights (Curtin, 1982). However, the majority of ethical decision-making models agree that the decision maker should: (1) identify the ethical dilemma, (2) identify and consider the pros and cons associated with each available option, (3) implement the selected option, and (4) evaluate the outcome and decision-making process (Bosek and Savage, 1999). These four steps are similar to the nursing process with the exception of identifying a goal.

Ethical Principles

Beauchamp and Childress (1994) advocate the use of four key principles to guide ethical decision making. These four principles can serve as the goals for ethical decision making and could be prioritized as follows: autonomy, nonmaleficence, beneficence and justice. In Western societies, autonomy (self-determination that is free from coercion) is the most important goal to be honored during ethical decision making. Nonmaleficence can be accomplished by implementing a specific action or by not performing a harmful act. While nonmaleficence or do no harm is a fundamental goal guiding a healthcare practitioner's actions, nonmaleficence may not be the patient's primary goal. For example, a fashion model made the autonomous decision to die (typically perceived as the ultimate of harms) rather than to undergo disfiguring surgery for appendicitis.

Beneficence builds on the concept of nonmaleficence. The principle of beneficence requires that a positive action be implemented that will bring about good or benefit the patient. Thus, a CRNA is promoting beneficence when an anesthetic with antiemetic effects is used during induction. Finally, justice is concerned with equity or fairness in the distribution of scarce resources (Beauchamp and Childress, 1994). Many justice questions are societal questions (such as right to healthcare). While social justice questions are extremely important and impact individual ethical decision making, healthcare professionals should resist the temptation to resolve these social questions at the individual patient's bedside. Social justice issues cannot be resolved in a case-by-case manner; rather, these questions require the CRNA, through individual as well as professional organizational and political involvement, to engage in community dialogues that can result in societal consensus and subsequent policy formation.

Evaluating Decision Making

Evaluation is an ongoing process that begins as soon as an option has been selected. The selected option is first evaluated for its potential to promote the identified values and ethical principles and then again after the ethical situation has been resolved to validate that the anticipated goals were achieved. During the evaluation phase, CNRAs should resist the temptation to claim "this action just felt right or things feel good now, so it must have been the right thing to do." Doing the ethically appropriate thing does not mean that one's emotions will also feel good or positive. Often implementing the ethically right option is an emotionally trying event. In addition, various participants in the ethical situation may evaluate outcomes differently due to differences in goals, values, and ethical commitments. Thus, at the end of any ethical situation, the outcomes should be evaluated from the identified decision maker's perspective and could include the following questions: "Were the identified goals achieved?" "Were the values and ethical priorities of the decision maker supported?" "Were any new ethical issues or questions raised as a result of implementing the chosen option?"

Decision-Making Resources

A variety of other ethical decision-making resources exist to facilitate the CRNA's ethical decision making. Institutional resources include policies and procedures, mission statements, and identified ethics mechanisms (either an ethics committee or an ethics consultant). Professional resources can be found through professional association codes and position statements (Bosek, 1993). For example, a CRNA should know the American Nurses' Association (ANA) Code for Nurses (1976, 1985), the AANA Code of Ethics (1992), and the ANA Position Statement on Nurses' Participation in Capital Punishment (1988). Finally, a wide variety of ethical information can be found in the published or Internet media (see Key References at the end of this chapter).

Casuistry

Nursing is a science and an applied art. Similarly, healthcare ethics is both theoretical and an applied science. The issue becomes how the CRNA can best apply theoretical ethics content to clinical practice problems. Rather than using a principled or moral ruled approach to ethics, this chapter will follow a casuistry ethics perspective. Proponents of casuistry ethics suggest that ethical reflection cannot be purely theoretical; rather, ethical reflection must consider the person's story and the contextual environment in which the scenario occurred. "What differentiates the new casuistry from applied ethics, then, is not the mere recognition that principles must eventually be applied, but rather a particular account of logic and derivation of the principles that we deploy in moral discourse (Arras, 1998)."

SCENARIO 1

Do-not-resuscitate (DNR) orders are a custom that Western society has promoted. In 1990, the Patient Self-Determination Act legislated the patient's right to refuse treatment as well as the right to make an advance directive, such as a living will or durable power of attorney for healthcare (DPOA) (Omnibus Reconciliation Act, 1990). Since the advent of cardiopulmonary resuscitation (CPR), many acute care and long-term healthcare agencies have developed the custom of initiating CPR for all patients experiencing a respiratory and/or cardiac arrest unless otherwise stipulated by a physician's DNR order. However, the custom of writing DNR orders and/or a patient's refusal of life-sustaining treatment can create an ethical situation for a CRNA, whose personal and professional customs may be different. For example:

> Mr. Smith became ill while on vacation in another state. After being ill for five days, the patient sought medical care. He was diagnosed with a necrotic bowel and scheduled for immediate surgery. When assessed by the CRNA, the patient stated, "I have a living will and a durable power of attorney for healthcare on file at my doctor's office back home. If I'm bad, you let me go." The CRNA's immediate thought was "Nobody dies in my operating room if I can help it!"

The major ethical conflict in this scenario is the patient's autonomous refusal of life-sustaining treatment versus the CRNA's commitment to nonmaleficence (do no harm). Maintaining Mr. Smith's autonomy while doing no harm would be key goals for the decision-making process.

AUTONOMY

The principle of autonomy, or patient self-determination, is a basic social value. An autonomous action is an act of intention that is free from coercion by others.

> "Clients have the moral right to determine what will be done with their own person; to be given accurate information, and all the information necessary for

> making informed judgments; to be assisted with weighing the benefits and burdens of options in their treatment; to accept, refuse, or terminate treatment without coercion; and to be given necessary emotional support." (ANA, 1976, 1985)

Patients may communicate their values and autonomous decisions about life-sustaining treatment through the creation of a written advance directive.

ADVANCE DIRECTIVES

Over the last three decades, medical technology has undergone explosive growth, especially in regard to life-sustaining technology, such as CPR, ventilators, feeding tubes, and renal dialysis. Inherent in these technological advancements are new problems associated with the ethical principle of respecting patient autonomy related to quality of life as well as the right to life versus the right to die. Thus, people are being encouraged to complete an advance directive.

An advance directive allows the person to communicate values and beliefs about healthcare decisions and life-sustaining treatment in the event that the person should become unable to participate in future healthcare decisions. An advance directive should never be consulted while the person is competent and able to make healthcare decisions. Two types of written advance directives exist: living wills and DPOA.

Living Wills

A living will, also called a directive to physicians, was first published in 1974 by the Euthanasia Educational Council, which later became the Concern for Dying and the Society for the Right to Die. While originally not designed as a legal document, living wills have gained legal standing in a majority of states in the United States. A living will is an instructional advance directive that typically directs the physician:

> "If at any time I should have an incurable and irreversible injury, disease, or illness judged to be a terminal condition by my attending physician who has personally examined me, and has determined that my death is imminent except for death-delaying procedures, I direct that such procedures which would only prolong the dying process be withheld or withdrawn, and that I be permitted to die naturally with only the administration of medication, sustenance, or the performance of any medical procedure deemed necessary by my attending physician to provide me with comfort care." (Illinois Living Will Act, 1992)

A living will is a useful document for guiding healthcare decisions regarding withdrawal of treatment for incompetent persons with terminal illnesses, such as cancer, who do not have a significant other to serve as a surrogate decision-maker. However, the living will has several limitations. First, the living will contains many ambiguous words or phrases that can be difficult to interpret. For example, at what point would the person be perceived to be imminently dying—when the person has six months, six weeks, six days, or six hours left to live? Second, the living will does not assist decision making for incompetent persons who are not terminally ill or imminently dying, but rather are in a persistent vegetative state or are incompetent due to illness such as Alzheimer's disease or head trauma. Third, the living will is not designed to facilitate decisions related to the initiation of healthcare interventions; it is designed to direct the removal of death-delaying procedures.

DURABLE POWER OF ATTORNEY FOR HEALTHCARE (DPOA)

A DPOA is a more powerful advance directive and addresses many of the limitations inherent in the living will. The first DPOA was adopted in California in 1984. The DPOA allows the person not only to refuse death-delaying procedures, but also to identify a surrogate decision maker and to specify which values and beliefs should be used to guide future healthcare decisions. In contrast with the living will, the DPOA is not limited to when a person is imminently dying of a terminal illness. Therefore, the DPOA may be used to guide healthcare decisions for any incompetent person regardless of the cause of the incompetence or prognosis.

While the federal Patient Self-Determination Act of 1990 requires that all patients have the right to complete an advance directive, advance-directive legislation remains at a state level and, thus, varies from state to state (Omnibus Reconciliation Act, 1990). Therefore, the possibility exists that Mr. Smith's living will and DPOA may not be legally binding in the state in which he is currently hospitalized. It would therefore be in Mr. Smith's best interest to complete (while he is still competent) a new DPOA form for the state in which he is hospitalized. Nevertheless, while Mr. Smith remains competent and able to participate in healthcare decision making, his DPOA and living will are not in effect and should not be used to guide decision making.

NONMALEFICENCE

Nonmaleficence is the concern for doing no harm or evil and is considered to be a foundational principle guiding actions by healthcare professionals. In the Hippocratic oath, physicians pledge, "I will apply dietetic measures for the benefit of the sick according to my ability and judgment; I will keep them from harm and injustice (Temkin and Temkin, 1967)." Harm is a broad term that includes not just physical or psychological injury, but also threats to the individual's life goals.

Actions that inflict harm always require moral justification. Surgery and anesthesia can cause actual and potential harm to the patient but are morally justified by the premise of bringing about good for the patient by correcting an injury or illness. In other words, the potential for good (or beneficence) is perceived to outweigh the actual or potential harms associated with surgery and anesthesia. This tension between doing good and preventing harm is a key to understanding the CRNA's immediate response to Mr. Smith's request to "let me go."

The CRNA's role during surgery is to maintain the patient's physical condition. The possibility exists for a patient receiving anesthesia to experience a life-threatening event related to hypotension, hypoxia, or a cardiac arrhythmia (Sommer, 1999). Thus, during a surgical intervention, the CRNA may be unable to discriminate when a life-threatening event is precipitated by an anesthetic agent or is the result of the patient's underlying illness. Based on the principle of nonmaleficence, many CRNAs believe that all actions must be taken to correct any life-threatening event occurring in the operating room.

DO-NOT-RESUSCITATE ORDERS

The DNR order has become well accepted and widely used in Western hospitals (Tomlison and Brody, 1988). A DNR order is a medical order, made by a physician and recorded in the patient's chart, to withhold resuscitation in case of cardiac or respiratory arrest. Cardiopulmonary resuscitation after a cardiac and/or respiratory arrest has been one of the most dramatic innovations of medicine in the last 50 years (Kouwenhoven and Jude, 1960). CPR has both positive and negative potentials. The potential good, the sustaining of life, is obvious, but the potential harms include anoxic encephalopathy, permanent ventilator dependence, or severe functional disability (Abramson, et al, 1985). This negative side to CPR has brought experts in medicine, bioethics, and medical law together. Special orders, no CPR, no code, or, most commonly, DNR, have been established to ensure that CPR is not performed inappropriately (Franklin, 1990). Many experts contend that a DNR order is fully compatible with aggressive care and should not imply that other life-sustaining treatment be withheld or withdrawn (The Hastings Center, 1987). However, the presence of a DNR order creates ethical quandaries for anesthesia providers. While a DNR order prohibits the initiation of CPR, a DNR can also prohibit the use of intubation, mechanical ventilators, vasoactive drugs, and defibrillation (Franklin, 1985), which are interventions anesthesia providers may need to implement to provide safe and effective anesthesia.

Options

Prior to identifying options, the CRNA should clarify Mr. Smith's comments and related values. Is Mr. Smith refusing all medical intervention or selected therapies? What does Mr. Smith mean by "If I'm bad let me go"? Does "bad" refer to dying, a specific quality of life level, or seriousness of the injury? Does Mr. Smith understand the technology (intubation, ventilator support, intravenous therapy, and anesthetic agents) that will be required to successfully correct his necrotic bowel? In addition, the institution's DNR policy should be reviewed. After Mr. Smith's values and beliefs are validated, several options exist for resolving this ethical situation:

- A DNR order may be written for the perioperative period (which may result in the CRNA refusing to provide anesthesia).
- No surgery.
- Surgery with a postoperative DNR order.
- Contacting his primary care provider for more information and/or assistance in determining short-term and long-term treatment goals for Mr. Smith.

SCENARIO 2

CRNAs may also find themselves involved in ethical conflicts with other members of the healthcare team.

> Late one evening, a 20-year-old woman fell while roller blading and fractured her ankle. The surgeon has spent six hours trying to fix the fracture, putting screws in and taking them out numerous times. The operating room walls are "papered" with 14 x-rays, and it is now early in the morning. The surgeon has contaminated the surgical field several times. The patient has been transferred to general anesthesia from a spinal. The CRNA is now concerned that the woman is at risk for serious complications, including the possibility of losing her foot, if this surgeon continues to operate.

The ethical problem in this scenario involves the CRNA's obligation to advocate for the patient. Initially, the obligation to act as a patient advocate seems obvious; however, this CRNA is experiencing an ethical dilemma due to conflict between personal and professional values. Specifically, the CRNA is torn between the professional obligation to promote a "good" outcome for the patient and the desire to avoid any personal harm to the CRNA's working relationship with the surgeon and within the institution. In this scenario, the CRNA's primary decision-making goal should be to promote a beneficent outcome for the patient with a secondary goal of doing no harm (nonmaleficence) to the CRNA's job security as well as the various healthcare professional relationships and reputations involved in this scenario.

BENEFICENCE

The principle of beneficence requires first that harm be avoided (the principle of nonmaleficence) and second that a benefit or good be created. Thus, beneficence is action-oriented and requires positive steps. The CRNA in the scenario was correctly acting to avoid harm by following the standards of practice for anesthesia as demonstrated by converting the patient to general anesthesia. However, the second component of the principle of beneficence requires the CRNA to purposefully act to cause good to occur. Good for this patient includes regaining full range of motion of her ankle. Since the CRNA cannot perform the surgical intervention, the CRNA will need to identify other ways to promote good for this patient, such as advocacy.

ADVOCACY

Both the AANA (1992) Code of Ethics and the ANA Code for Nurses (1976, 1985) stipulate that nurses must act to safeguard patients from the incompetent practice of any healthcare provider. One way that a CRNA can safeguard the patient is by fulfilling the role of advocate. In fact, the AANA Code of Ethics claims that advocating for the welfare of patients is a responsibility CRNAs must uphold. To be an advocate means to "plead the cause of another; an intercessor; defender (Funk & Wagnalls, 1996)." This definition presumes that the advocate holds the belief that patients have rights that must be supported and that the patient's rights do in fact come before other priorities and obligations (Bandman and Bandman, 1995).

Therefore to act as an advocate, the CRNA must first know the patient's goals or cause. The ability to know and/or validate the patient's goals or cause is complicated in this case by the fact that the patient is under general anesthesia and, thus, unable to participate in decisions about her surgical treatment. Therefore, the CRNA's knowledge of the patient's goals is limited to preoperative assessment data and assumptions that may be universalized to all surgical patients, such as "patients, who consent to a surgical procedure, want their physical problem corrected to the fullest extent possible." Based on this assumption, the CRNA would be ethically justified to act on the belief that this particular patient also has a commitment to regaining optimal function of her ankle.

Second, the CRNA must identify to whom the intercession must be directed. In this scenario, the CRNA needs to intercede to the surgeon by verbally promoting the patient's cause. When promoting the patient's cause, the CRNA may need to create a distance between the patient and the source of harm. For example in this scenario, the CRNA could suggest that the surgeon needs a break and/or needs to seek consultation or assistance from an orthopedic surgeon. However, creating a distance between the patient and the perceived source of harm can be difficult during the perioperative phase since creating distance may result in the need to suspend the surgical procedure, which can be of equal or greater threat to the patient's safety and recovery.

When intercession is insufficient to ensure the patient's rights are protected, the CRNA advocate will need to assume the defender advocacy role. The defender role builds on the CRNA's legitimate role and positional power as a member of the healthcare team (Bandman and Bandman, 1995). The defender role may require the CRNA to work through the institutional hierarchy to gain political support for the patient's rights, as well as to identify supplemental resources that can be accessed to promote the patient's rights and to facilitate a beneficent outcome. For example, the CRNA could notify the surgeon's supervisor or the chief of orthopedic surgery about the patient's current status and the perceived need for immediate assistance. The ability to successfully implement the defender role is contingent upon the CRNA's professional reputation and clinical skills and judgment. In other words, to successfully fulfill the defender advocate role, the CRNA must be able to capitalize on an established clinical expertise and dedication to patient safety and rights. Thus, prerequisites to being an advocate are recognized clinical expertise and an existing dedication to patient rights and beneficent care.

IMPAIRED PRACTITIONERS

Unfortunately, the need for advocacy often occurs because a healthcare professional is incompetent or impaired. Carpenter (1994) identified that healthcare professionals can be impaired from chemicals (drugs and alcohol); professional burnout or environment factors, such as fatigue from working extended hours or short staffing patterns; or knowledge deficits related to working outside of one's specialty area.

In this scenario, the surgeon may be experiencing a variety of environmental impairments, such as fatigue from a protracted surgery that is extending into the night and possibly limited knowledge and experience regarding ankle orthopedics. CRNAs have an ethical obligation to work within their agencies and professional organization to enact policies and procedures that proactively address the antecedents of environmental impairment, as well as the stresses that result in the abuse of chemicals or professional burnout. In addition, CRNAs should be cognizant of institutional and state licensure policies for reporting healthcare professionals with chemical impairments. Finally, in the event that a CRNA experiences a chemical impairment, support is available through the AANA's Peer Assistance Advisors.

VALUE CONFLICTS

Each CRNA holds a variety of professional as well as personal values. Curtin (1982b) defined values as "those assertions or statements that individuals make, either through their behavior, words, or actions, that define what they think is important and for which they are willing to suffer and even die—or perhaps to continue living." Personal values are developed throughout one's life, and are shaped by parents, family members, friends, teachers and school groups, and community and religious groups, in addition to both good and bad personal experiences (Steele and Harmon, 1983).

Professional values build upon an individual's personal values. CRNAs develop their professional values throughout their professional career. However, it is unclear whether professional educational programs can really create an ethical practitioner with strong professional values if the person has a limited and/or superficial personal value system.

The CRNA in this scenario seems to be experiencing a conflict between professional and personal values. The CRNA appears to value professional skills and a commitment to helping patients, and to potentially value advocacy. However, a commitment to acting on these professional values is potentially or actually threatening key values. This CRNA may be thinking, "If I act on my professional values, I may be threatening my reputation as a team player. This surgeon is a powerful person in this institution. I'm not certain that I'm willing to risk my job and, thus, my family's financial security over this incident."

Before deciding how to act, the CRNA needs to undergo a process of values clarification. The CRNA seems to have already freely chosen a variety of values from existing alternatives. However, merely "choosing a value" is insufficient; the CRNA must also willingly share the values with others and consistently use the values to guide actions. Ideally, values clarification occurs within a group prior to the need to act on the value. However, this CRNA does not have the luxury of trying out the professional values first in a safe, nonthreatening environment since the CRNA is being forced to simultaneously share and act on these professional values. Thus, the process of clarifying one's values will create risks in addition to promoting self-actualization (Steele and Harmon, 1983).

Options

Before problem solving begins, the CRNA should first clarify the professional and personal values influencing the CRNA's perception of the situation and willingness to intervene. In addition, the CRNA needs to have clearly identified and prioritized the ethical issues involved in this situation. How the agency customarily deals with issues of professional disagreement should also be considered. Ideally, this time of clarification and prioritizing should bring the CRNA to the realization that a professional nurse anesthetist's primary professional obligation is to protect the patient from harm and to promote good whenever possible. This obligation is supported by professional as well as personal values regarding the value of human life and promoting autonomy by maintaining function and independence.

Thus, the CRNA has several options available, including:

- Address concerns directly to the surgeon about the actual and potential outcomes or harms and ask the surgeon to request assistance or consultation.
- Ask the circulating nurse for assistance and/or ideas for dealing with the situation.
- Notify the surgeon that the CRNA is calling in the orthopedic surgeon for consultation or assistance.
- Contact the on-call orthopedic surgeon for consultation or assistance without first notifying the surgeon.
- Notify the medical director of anesthesia on call of the CRNA's need to be removed from this case.
- Seek consultation from the medical director of anesthesia regarding how to proceed.
- Say nothing and allow the surgery to continue.

SCENARIO 3

One of the hardest ethical situations a CRNA may face is the situation where the CRNA's professional standard of practice and the CRNA's professional and personal values are challenged by another professional.

> I was moonlighting at a surgical center. This center did therapeutic abortions. The first day, I used propofol and alfentanil for anesthesia with haloperidol for postoperative nausea. The second day, the owner of the center, who also is a CRNA, told me I couldn't use propofol because the

drug was too expensive. In addition, the owner didn't want me to change the circuits on the anesthesia machine between patients because the circuits were too expensive. I felt like I was being asked to compromise care to these women because of the financial cost.

CONSCIENTIOUS REFUSAL

"Conscientious ... is not a special moral or psychological faculty. Rather, it is a form of self-reflection on and judgment about whether one's acts are obligatory or prohibited, right or wrong, good or bad. It is an internal sanction calling attention to the actual or potential loss of a sense of integrity and wholeness of the self (Beauchamp and Childress, 1994)."

Conflicts of conscience occur when a person is directed (often by someone with positional authority and power) to act against the person's standard of conduct, thus threatening the person's sense of integrity and self-worth. In the preceding scenario, this CRNA is not experiencing any conflicts of conscience related to participating in abortions that might be the case for other CRNAs. Rather, the CRNA is experiencing a conflict of conscience when the owner directs that the CRNA's standard of care is not obligatory and in fact is creating a financial harm to the surgical center, which would ultimately affect patient care by escalating surgical costs.

When a conflict of conscience occurs, the CRNA must determine how to respond to the recognition that a conflict of conscience has occurred. Ultimately, the CRNA will have to decide whether to ignore the conflict of conscience (or in other words learn to live with the dissonance) or to express opposition to the direction causing the conflict.

During a conflict of conscience, CRNAs must be able to clearly describe the basis for refusing to comply. First, the CRNA may realize "I can't do that, because I could not live with myself if I were to do it (Brushwood, 1993)." This type of refusal is referred to as conscientious refusal since it illustrates an insult to the individual's personal conscience. However, before making such a claim, the CRNA must be knowledgeable of how the state defines conscientious objection. For example, the Illinois Right of Conscience Act (1977) defines conscience as "a sincerely held set of moral convictions arising from a belief in and relation to God, or which, though not so derived, obtains from a place in the life of its possessor parallel to that filled by God among adherents to religious faiths." Therefore, if the CRNA was employed in Illinois, the CRNA could not claim to have a conscientious objection since religious values were not involved in the conflict of conscience. Thus, the CRNA is not acting to avert personal harm to self.

Rather, the CRNA is expressing a beneficent refusal. When claiming a beneficent refusal, the CRNA is attempting to avoid harm to the patient. Thus, the CRNA's objection to the owner's direction is based on professional knowledge and commitment to promoting the patient's welfare. An act of beneficent refusal may receive legal support from employment laws protecting the employee's right to decline to carry out acts required by an employer if such acts are inconsistent with current policies and professional codes (Brushwood, 1993).

It is imperative that the CRNA use language accurately and be able to verbalize specific rationale for objecting. For example, a CRNA expressing a conscientious objection to participating in the abortion would explain, "I believe that a fetus is a living being and I am commanded by God not to kill. Therefore, my conscience will not allow me to participate." In contrast, the CRNA in the preceding case would be expressing an objection based on beneficence when stating, "I cannot comply with your directive to reuse the anesthesia circuits because the circuits would be contaminated and subsequent patients will be put at risk."

JUSTICE

The CRNA could respond to the owner's request by stating, "It would not be fair to not change the circuits between patients." A similar claim could be made related to not providing propofol. But what does the CRNA mean by "fair"? If the use of fair by the CRNA means "harmful," then this would be another example of objection based on beneficence. However, if fair refers to justice and how scarce resources (money, time, and supplies) are distributed, then the CRNA would be basing the response on the principle of distributive justice.

Distributive justice is concerned with how scarce resources are used and distributed. The decision of how scarce resources should be distributed can be answered in a variety of ways. First, one would need to decide if the scarce resources should be distributed to each person equally or based on the person's need, merit, potential for or actual contribution(s) to society, or, finally, based on free market price (Beauchamp and Childress, 1994).

Second, the principle of justice requires that equals should be treated equally. Therefore, the CRNA would need to determine if every woman treated at the surgical center was in fact equal to every other patient in terms of the need to be protected from infection and/or nausea. Assuming that every woman undergoing an elective abortion is generally in normal health, then the CRNA would be justified to determine that each woman needs equal protection from nosocomial infections. In addition, the CRNA would be hard pressed to explain how the first patient of the day differs from the second patient of the day, thus, deserving of a new circuit when the remaining patients do not.

Finally, comparing the owner's perceived need for financial gain to the patient's need to be protected from infection seems ludicrous at best. First, the owner and the patients are not equals and, thus, should not be compared. Second, the needs being compared are not equal. Based on the principles of nonmaleficence and altruism, the patient's right to be free of harm should have precedent over any need the owner may have.

Options

- Follow the owner's direction.
- Follow normal protocol for changing circuits.
- Provide care in a manner that does not require circuits to be used.
- Refuse to provide general anesthesia care.
- Perform assessments only.
- Perform local anesthesia.
- Refuse to work at this surgical center.

OTHER ETHICAL ISSUES EXPERIENCED BY CRNAS

Many other ethical issues have been identified in the anesthesia literature that CRNAs should become knowledgeable about. In particular, CRNAs are becoming more involved in clinical research investigations. When engaged in research activities, the CRNA's ethical commitment to promote nonmaleficence toward the study's subjects must be nonnegotiable. While each research study will have obtained Institutional Review

Board approval prior to beginning, the CRNA must remain vigilant in recognizing the potential for conflict of interests which may threaten the subjects' rights and safety at any point during the research project.

The CRNA may become knowledgeable about ethical issues by learning about the various ethical positions and nuances, professional codes and standards, and by engaging in personal and professional values clarification regarding these frequently occurring ethical issues in the perioperative setting. CRNAs may want to organize professional continuing education programs, "brown bag" discussions, journal club readings, and/or inservices as forums to encourage lifelong learning in addition to professional dialogue and debate on these frequently occurring ethical topics.

Frequently occurring ethical issues that CRNAs have or may encounter include:

- Animal research requiring anesthesia (Riopelle, 1992).
- Potential conflict of interests when industry provides economic support of anesthesia research (Peterson, 1994).
- Obtaining informed consent when the patient is a minor, emancipated, or mentally incompetent.
- Parental consent issues due to religious preferences, abuse, neglect, or inability to obtain care in emergency situations.
- Aggressiveness of care and/or resuscitation in the delivery room (Truog and Rockoff, 1992).
- Conflicts between the mother and fetus (Miller, 1991).
- Using cost to determine choice of anesthetic (Wetchler, 1992).
- Refusal of blood products by Jehovah's Witness patients (Benson, 1989).
- The use of genetic testing for malignant hyperthermia and atypical pseudocholinesterase preoperatively (Lysaught and Schwinn, 1991).
- Euthanasia and assisted suicide (Jonsen, 1993; Truog and Berde, 1993).
- Conflict of conscience when the CRNA's personal values do not match the patient's.
- Challenges to the anesthesia provider's professional decision making due to the responsibility of sharing care with the surgeon (Benson, 1989; Fine, 1992).
- Providing lethal injections for capital punishment cases (Aprile, 1995).
- Participating in abortion.
- Competition for employment contracts (Simpson and Foster, 1992).

SUMMARY

CRNAs experience a variety of ethical situations in the perioperative setting. While a variety of decision-making models and resources are available to assist the CRNA in resolving these ethical situations, the CRNA will need to consider each ethical situation as a unique situation involving specific values, customs, policies, and nuances. Thus, there is no one right answer that the CRNA can memorize for resolving clinical ethical situations. Rather, the CRNA will need to develop expertise in assessing and discussing values and beliefs, identifying options, and communicating the ethical justifications for each option.

REFERENCES

Abramson, N.S., Safar, P., Detr, K.M., Kelsey, S.F., Monroe, J., Reinmuth, O., & Snyder, J.V. (1985). Neurologic recovery after cardiac arrest: Effect of duration of ischemia. Brain Resuscitation Clinical Trial I Study Group. *Critical Care Medicine.* 13(11), 930-93-1.

American Association of Nurse Anesthetists. (1992). *AANA Code of Ethics.* Park Ridge, IL: Author.

American Nurses' Association. (1976, 1985). *Code for Nurses with Interpretive Statements.* Kansas City, MO: Author.

American Nurses' Association. (1988). *Position Statement on Nurses' Participation in Capital Punishment.* Kansas City, MO: Author.

Aprile, A.E. (1995). Ethical issues involving medical personnel and the administration of lethal injection in capital punishment. *CRNA—The Clinical Forum for Nurse Anesthetists.* 7(3), 116-117.

Arras, J.D. (1998). Getting down to cases: The revival of casuistry in bioethics. In J.F. Monagle & D.C. Thomasma (Eds.), *Health Care Ethics: Critical Issues for the 21st Century* (pp. 541-553). Gaithersburg, MD: Aspen Publishers, Inc.

Bandman, E.L., & Bandman, B. (1995). *Nursing Ethics: Through the Life Span* (3rd ed.). Norwalk, CT: Appleton & Lange.

Beauchamp, T.L., & Childress, J.F. (1994). *Principles of Biomedical Ethics* (4th ed.). New York, NY: Oxford University Press.

Benson, K.T. (1989). The Jehovah's Witness patient: Considerations for the anesthesiologist. *Anesthesia & Analgesia.* 69, 647-656.

Bosek, M.S.D. (1993). A comparison of ethical resources. *MEDSURG Nursing.* 2(4), 332-334.

Bosek, M.S.D., & Savage, T.A. (1997). Teachable moments: Integrating ethics into clinical education. *Dean's Notes.* 18(5), 1-4.

Bosek, M.S.D., & Savage, T.A. (1999). Ethics. In D.D. Ignatavicius, M.L. Workman, & M.A. Mishler (Eds.), *Medical-Surgical Nursing Across the Health Care Continuum* (3rd ed., pp. 75-91). Philadelphia, PA: W.B. Saunders Company.

Brushwood, D. B. (1993). Conscientious objection and abortifacient drugs. *Clinical Therapeutics.* 15(1), 204-212.

Carpenter, M. (1994). The impaired nurse. *MEDSURG Nursing.* 3(2), 139-141.

Curtin, L. (1982a). No rush to judgment. In Curtin, L. & Flaherty, M.J. (Eds.), *Nursing Ethics: Theories and Pragmatics* (pp. 57-63). Bowie, MD: Robert J. Brady Co.

Curtin, L. (1982b). What are human rights? In Curtin, L. & Flaherty, M.J. (Eds.), *Nursing Ethics: Theories and Pragmatics* (pp. 1-16). Bowie, MD: Robert J. Brady Co.

Fine, P.G. (1992). Anesthesiology and the discipline of medical ethics: Challenges and opportunities. *Anesthesia & Analgesia.* 74, 327-328.

Francouer, R. T. (1983). *Biomedical ethics: A guide to decision making.* New York, NY: John Wiley & Sons.

Franklin, C. (1985). Do not resuscitate policies. *Acute Care.* 11(3-4), 208-211.

Franklin, C. (1990). When and how to write do-not-resuscitate orders. *Journal of Critical Illness.* 5, 938-952.

Funk & Wagnalls New International Dictionary of the English Language (comprehensive ed.). Chicago, IL: World Publishers Inc.

Illinois Right of Conscience Act. (1977). 745ILCS 70/1, et seq.

Illinois Living Will Act. (1992). 755ILCS 35/1, et seq.

Jonsen, A.R. (1993). To help the dying die: A new duty for anesthesiologists? *Anesthesiology.* 78, 225-228.

Jonsen, A.R., Siegler, M., & Winslade, W.J. (1998). *Clinical Ethics* (4th ed.). New York, NY: McGraw-Hill.

Kouwenhoven, W.B., Jude, J.R. & Knickerbocker, G.G. (1984). Closed-chest cardiac massage. *JAMA.* 251(23), 3133-6.

Lysaught, M.T., & Schwinn, D. (1991). Promises and pitfalls: Ethical dimensions of genetic engineering and anesthesiology. *Seminars in Anesthesia.* 10(3), 141-156.

Miller, F.H. (1991). Maternal-fetal ethical dilemmas: A guideline for physicians. *Seminars in Anesthesia.* 10(3), 157-162.

Omnibus Reconciliation Act (1990). Title IV. Section 4206, *Congressional Record.* October 26, 1990.

Peterson, C.J. (1994). Industry support of research and conflict of interest. *Anesthesiology.* 81(1), 270.

Riopelle, J.M. (1992). The ethics of using animal models to study treatment of phantom pain. *Anesthesiology.* 76, 1069.

Simpson, J.S., & Foster, S.D. (1992). Legal and ethical aspects of nurse anesthesia practice. In W.R. Waugaman, S.D. Foster, & B.M. Rigor (Eds.), *Principles and Practice of Nurse Anesthesia* (2nd ed.). Norwalk, CT: Appleton & Lange.

Sommer, B. (1999). Patient health and safety. In W.R. Waugaman, S.D. Foster, & B.M. Rigor (Eds.), *Principles and Practice of Nurse Anesthesia* (3rd ed., pp. 81-92). Stamford, CT: Appleton & Lange.

Steele, S.M., & Harmon, V.M. (1983). *Values Clarification in Nursing* (2nd ed.). Norwalk, CT: Appleton-Century-Crofts.

Temkin, O., & Temkin, C.L. (Eds.). (1967). *Ancient Medicine: Selected Papers of Ladwig Edelstein.* Baltimore, MD: Johns Hopkins Press.

The Hastings Center (1987). *Guidelines on the Termination of Dying.* Briarcliff Manor, NY: Author.

Thompson, J.E., & Thompson, H.O. (1985). *Bioethical Decision-Making for Nurses.* Norwalk, CT: Appleton-Century-Crofts.

Tomlinson, T., & Brody, H. (1988). Ethics and communication in do-not-resuscitate orders. *N Engl J of Med.* 318(1), 43-46.

Truog, R.D., & Berde, C.B. (1993). Pain, euthanasia, and anesthesiologists. *Anesthesiology.* 78(2), 353-360.

Truog, R.D., & Rockoff, M.A. (1992). DNR in the OR: Further questions. *Journal of Anesthesia.* 4, 177-180.

Wetchler, B.V. (1992). Economic impact of anesthesia decision making: They pay the money, we make the choice. *Journal of Clinical Anesthesia.* 4(suppl 1), 20S-24S.

KEY REFERENCES

McGraw, K.S. (1998). Should do-not-resuscitate orders be suspended during surgical procedures? *AORN*. 67(4), *794-799*.

President's Commission for the Study of Ethical Problems in Medicine and Biomedical and Behavioral Research. (1983). Deciding to forgo life-sustaining treatment decisions. Washington, DC: Author.

Reich, W.T. (Ed). (1995). *The Encyclopedia of Bioethics* (Rev. ed.). New York, NY: MacMillan Publishing Co.

Walters, L. (1977 to date). *Bibliography of Bioethics* (Vols. 1-24). Washington, DC: Georgetown University.

STUDY QUESTIONS

You are scheduled to provide anesthesia during an emergent abdominal vascular surgery that often requires a minimum of four units of packed red blood cells. The patient is a 35-year-old mother of three children under the age of 12 and is a professing Jehovah's Witness. The patient stated that she does not want to receive a blood transfusion (donor or via cell saver) under any circumstances.

1. What questions would you need to ask the patient to verify her refusal of blood transfusions during surgery?

2. What questions would you ask or actions would you take to verify that her refusal of a blood transfusion was a deep fundamental value for this patient and not just an attempt to "please the elders of the church"?

3. What professional and personal values are influencing how you view this case?

4. What is your agency's policy about refusal of blood by persons with expressed religious convictions?

5. Does the fact that this woman is the sole support for three minor children influence how you view this case?

6. What is your state's legal position about refusal of blood by persons with expressed religious convictions?

7. If the CRNA's goal is to "do no harm," should the CRNA be concerned about potential spiritual harm as well as potential physical harm associated with administering blood products to a patient professing religious objections?

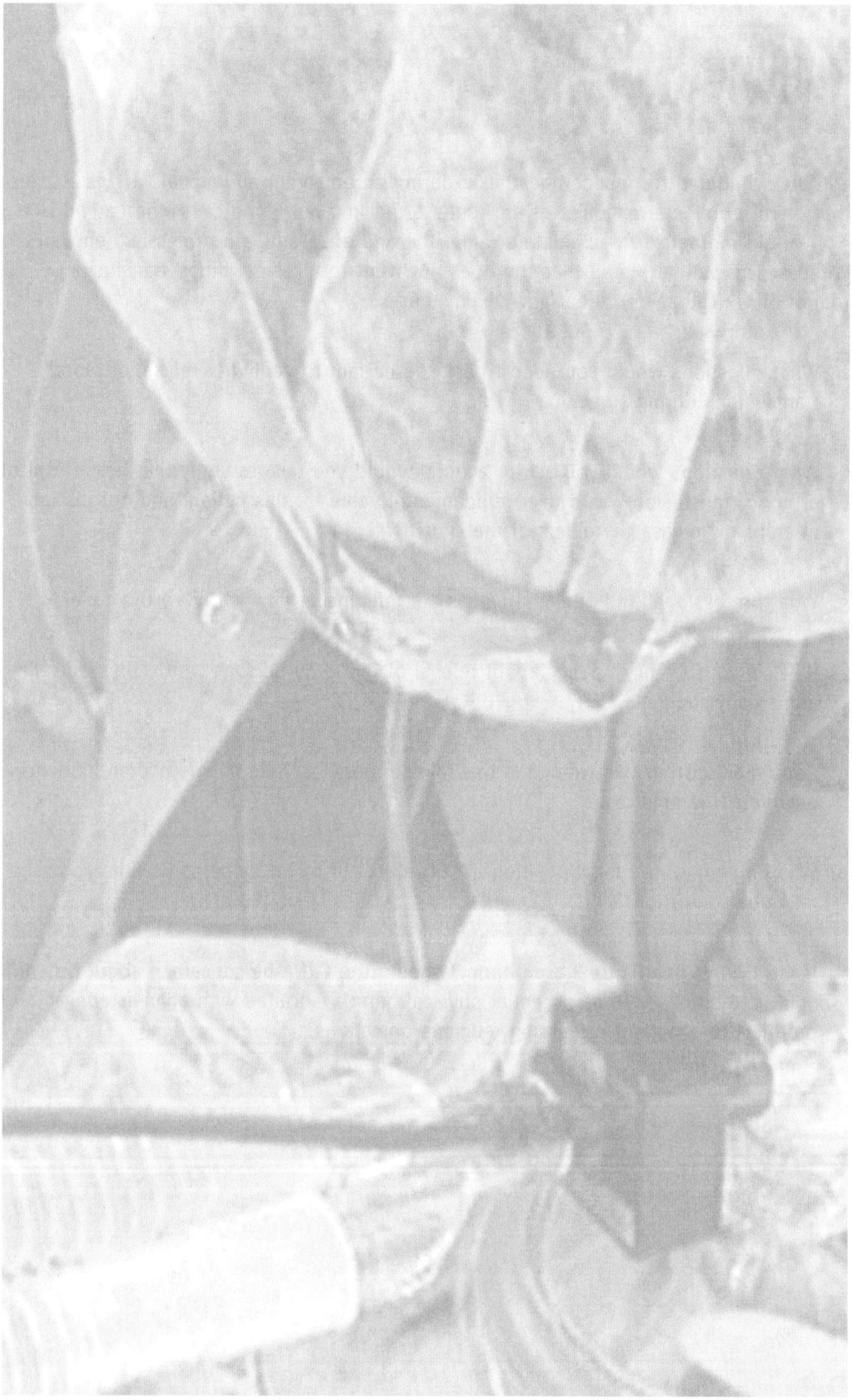

CHAPTER 21

PEER ASSISTANCE – PART 1

Diana Quinlan, CRNA, MA

Chair, AANA Peer Assistance Advisors Committee
Jacksonville, FL

KEY CONCEPTS

- The incidence of substance abuse in anesthesia personnel is alarming and Certified Registered Nurse Anesthetists (CRNAs) are an at-risk population from stress and access to drugs. Studies confirm a high fatality rate in anesthesia abusers.

- There are four major theoretical models of addiction. The models to be explored are: genetic/biological, disease, psychological, and familial.

- Risks and compounding factors make anesthetists more vulnerable to addiction than other healthcare personnel due to what Farley and Talbott identified as five specific "anesthesiology trigger mechanisms" for addiction.

- The symptoms and behaviors associated with dependence follow typical patterns or characteristics related to the specific substances being abused.

- Diversion behavior includes increased time in or near the narcotic supply, or unusual choices and amounts of drug sign-outs.

- Anesthesia departments have a responsibility to prevent or reduce harmful behavior, address addiction should it occur, and have department policies that include narcotic accountability and drug-testing procedures.

- A quality assurance process should be in place that includes audits of anesthesia records/narcotic sheets; department documentation should include observations of behavior, performance evaluations, and due process.

- Insurance provisions should be adequate to provide reasonable coverage that reflects the risk of addiction in anesthesia providers.

Almost 40 years ago an article appeared in the *Journal of the American Association of Nurse Anesthetists* (AANA) that suggested addiction was an occupational hazard within the anesthesia community (Lundy and McQuillen, 1962). As time progressed, the American Medical Association (AMA) and others concluded that addiction is a disease that is progressive and often fatal if left untreated. Although the disease concept is now widely accepted, the moral stigma remains when the addict is a doctor or nurse. Increasing demands within the field of anesthesiology; newer, more potent drugs; and erratic practice constraints contribute to an increasing problem of addiction among anesthesia providers.

It is a sad commentary on a profession whose goal it is to restore health and prolong life that those involved in the healthcare system are often the last to receive assistance. Any other disease afflicting one in 10 individuals of a select society would be deemed an epidemic, or a disaster of great proportion. Only through support, education, and research can we begin to comprehend the scope of this disease and its impact on the professional.

HISTORY

Chemical dependency (CD) has existed for centuries, perhaps even since the beginning of man. Knowledge of man's attempt to pharmacologically manipulate his perception of the world dates back to ancient history. Wine, henbane, mandragora, opium, cocaine, and countless other mood-altering substances offered comfort and escape to ancient man, as have other addicting substances to every major civilization through recorded history.

In early America, abuse of medicinal substances was commonplace. Dr. Crawford Long and his 1840s contemporaries frequently held ether-sniffing parties in Philadelphia. Other physicians of the 19th and early 20th century had a similar history of abuse. Many used themselves as subjects in an attempt to discover the therapeutic potential of test substances. The renowned British discoverer of chloroform, James Simpson, and the famous American surgeon, Halstead, are among the more notable physicians who became addicted during their attempts to gain firsthand knowledge about the properties of anesthetic agents (Talbott and Wright, 1987). Sigmund Freud used cocaine extensively and even recommended it for the treatment of morphine and alcohol dependence (Health Communications, 1983).

Medical professionals were not the only ones to naively succumb to addiction. The Civil War converted thousands of soldiers into morphine addicts. Early patent medicines contained opium or morphine salts that made any recipient prone to addiction. Coca-Cola, as it was dispensed at soda fountains at the turn of the century, contained addicting amounts of cocaine. It was eventually reformulated under federal law.

Historically, attempts have been made to address the issue of addiction among healthcare providers. Early in the 20th century, a report by Abraham Flexner prompted state medical associations and legislatures to regulate medical practice and to pass laws that required physicians to be free of "vice, moral turpitude, and the intemperate use of alcohol and drugs (Flexner, 1910)."

By 1920, England passed the Dangerous Drugs Control Act that sought to register addicts. That attempt revealed that nearly 25 percent of those listed were doctors, dentists, nurses, or veterinary surgeons (Stimson, Oppenheimer, and Stimson, 1984).

Despite this early knowledge of the addictive behavior of certain healthcare professionals, it is rare to find literature concerning addiction among nurses before 1975. The AANA Program Committee in 1962 asked the executive director, a nurse anesthetist, and a prominent anesthesiologist to provide a paper on the professional hazards of narcotics to anesthetists. Although their search of the literature was exhaustive and yielded many revelations that still hold true, one major exception of that time was the belief that addiction was caused by an underlying emotional disturbance (Lundy and McQuillen, 1962).

A more contemporary "disease concept" of predisposition to addiction being biogenetically transmitted has been proposed. Numerous reports have confirmed that less than 5 percent of impaired health professionals have psychiatric problems that contributed to their disease (Talbott, 1983).

Sullivan, et al (1988) mention multiple studies that suggest dual impairment; psychopathology and addiction may coexist in some cases. The depressant effects of alcohol, for example, may manifest in anxiety and depression. Other emotional, social, and family problems may manifest as addiction progresses, masking the primary disease. For this reason, it is essential to diagnose and treat CD before other psychological problems, as treatment will likely be ineffective for other disorders if the individual is still actively using drugs.

Bissell and Jones (1981) estimated in 1978 that there were more than 40,000 alcoholic nurses in the United States. Beck and Buckley (1983) stated in their *Newsweek* exposé that nearly 4 percent of doctors and nurses were narcotic dependent.

Despite well-intentioned attempts to determine estimates, there are few reliable data relative to the incidence of alcoholism and drug addiction within the nursing profession. One reason for this lack of information was inherent in the nature of the disorder. Since self-delusion and denial are primary characteristics of addiction, most nurses are not aware of their own plight (Bissell and Jones, 1981). Additionally, coworkers forge what Talbott (1983) names a "conspiracy of silence." Even when a colleague was a suspected abuser, peers perpetuated the "conspiracy" by covering up the abusing nurses' poor work performance. A fear that confrontation attempts would result in loss of licensure and, thus, livelihood for their colleague was weighed heavily by those who would have liked to help (Green, 1984).

One index of the increasing number of chemically dependent nurses has been the rise in addiction-related disciplinary actions taken by state boards of nursing. In a survey reported in 1981, 35 of 37 participating boards commented that drug addiction was significant and increasing (Mereness, 1981). During the same period, the National Council of State Boards of Nursing (NCSBN) determined that for a one-year period, 67 percent of 971 actions against licensees were for chemical dependency (Green, 1984). A written survey of member boards of the NCSBN in 1992 looked specifically at discipline of advanced practice nurses (NCSBN, 1993). Certified Registered Nurse Anesthetists (CRNAs) accounted for 75 percent of the drug-related complaints reported. However, other categories of nurse practitioners accounted for the higher percentage of complaints for scope of practice, prescriptive authority, and other practice-related complaints. Interestingly, this study did not state what percentage of the nurse practitioner population was nurse anesthetists. The authors commented that CD is a problem for all nurses, but CRNAs appear to be at greater risk due to the nature of their work and their access to substances (NCSBN, 1993).

Older statistics are likely to be misleading since most hospitals, wary of bad publicity, were reluctant to report abuse. Most hospitals fired the offending nurses, leaving them untreated and free to seek employment elsewhere. Since the initiation of the National Practitioner Data Bank (NPDB), most credentialing bodies, currently mandated to report chemically dependent physicians, are similarly reporting nurses to their licensing body (NPDB, 1986; Quinlan and Bodenhorn, 1990).

IMPAIRMENT

The term impairment is often used to describe declining performance or decreasing health as a result of certain factors or conditions. The effects of these factors may cause deterioration in personal and professional lives. Impairments in practice may be caused by psychiatric conditions such as depression or personality disorder, by advancing age or changing physical limitations, or by CD on drugs or alcohol.

As the healthcare community makes progress in advocacy for its own, the term impairment has been refined to apply only to impaired practice, not impaired individuals. This is reflected in name changes of advocacy groups from impaired nurse committees to wellness committees, health professionals programs, or resource networks.

This chapter will focus on the factors that are related to dependency on drugs or alcohol. But it is important to keep in mind that dual disorders (mental health and substance abuse) often coexist. Chemical dependence is a chronic, relapsing disease that affects individuals in all walks of life. Although some claim it occurs no more frequently in the healthcare professional than in the general public (American Society of Anesthesiologists, 1998), it does occur much more frequently among anesthesia providers than other health professionals (Angres, Talbott, and Bettinardi-Angres, 1998).

Those who still harbor beliefs that drug abuse is purely a moral or ethical issue do not accept the disease concept of addiction. This moral model of thought is in direct conflict with the medical model of thought defined eloquently by Maxwell (Maxwell, 2000). The medical model of thought has a belief system based on empirical clinical findings with a constant interplay of information, diagnoses, and treatment plans. In contrast, the moral model of thought has beliefs based on faith, and empirical information will not alter these beliefs.

The AMA and the American Psychiatric Association (APA) recognize CD as a diagnosable, treatable disease. This concept based on the medical model of thought believes for addiction to develop, there must be a drug that is readily available and an urge to use that drug. This urge or craving is part of the neurochemical makeup of any individual and has its foundation in the central nervous system neuroreceptors. It is CRNA and anesthesiologists' access as anesthesia providers to highly potent and very pure drugs that keeps them high-risk. This, coupled with a genetic or behavioral urge to use those drugs, may make anesthesia providers inherently susceptible to the disease of addiction.

The disease is progressive, with rapidity of onset dependent upon the abused substance or "drug of choice." While addiction to alcohol may take decades to become apparent, addiction to potent opioids may become apparent within weeks. Unless the disease is recognized and treated appropriately, it will result in social, psychological, and physical harm to the abuser and may be fatal (ASA, 1998).

A cascade of behavioral changes occurs when an individual begins to use substances. This order of deterioration reveals problems to family long before coworkers and makes early detection difficult. Sadly, addiction may not be discovered in the workplace until its later stages, or until death. Many nurse anesthetists have been discovered dead in the hospital setting to the shock and surprise of their unknowing coworkers. It is because of this natural progression of deterioration that family members, as well as colleagues, need to be educated about chemical dependence.

INCIDENCE

Statistics regarding the incidence of substance abuse among healthcare providers typically range from 3 percent to 6 percent, about the same as the general public, to as high as "30 times higher than the general public (Garb, 1965)."

Until 1998, confirmative data specific to nurse anesthetists was nonexistent. However, a survey by Bell et al (1999) identified a 9.8 percent incidence of anesthesia drug misuse among the CRNA population studied. The survey was a random sampling of a demographically representative group of AANA members certified as actively practicing and representing almost 10 percent of the national CRNA population. A list of 50 anesthesia-specific pharmaceuticals, including inhalation agents, narcotics, sedatives, induction drugs, and other adjunctive drugs used primarily in anesthesia, was the key component of the survey. The list included all scheduled drugs plus those not often kept under lock. The drugs were not over-the-counter, prescribed for their personal use, or for a purpose other than as an adjunct for anesthesia. The participants were asked which drugs on the list they had misused by self-administering. This study alone verified the perception by many that the incidence of misuse is high, that availability is a major factor in use, and that access needs to be more closely examined by anesthesia department and pharmacy managers.

Past studies have clearly shown that potent opioids, fentanyl and sufentanil, were the drugs most frequently used by anesthesia providers, comprising about 70 percent of substance abuse cases. Alcohol and cocaine accounted for about 10 percent, while the remaining 20 percent was divided nearly evenly among drugs such as benzodiazepines, inhalation agents, sodium thiopental, lidocaine, and propofol. As seen in Figure 21.1, Bell et al found the trend was away from opioids and toward drugs of less accountability.

Prior surveys conducted within anesthesia communities were mostly anecdotal or relied on information from the heads of departments to report the number of suspected or confirmed abusers. Gravenstein conducted a survey of 15 southeastern academic anesthesia departments for the period 1974 through 1979 (Gravenstein, Kory, and Marks, 1983). The survey asked department chairs to recall information on the incidence of and the outcome from drug abuse by their personnel. It also asked all anesthesia personnel and a control group of medical students to respond to certain statements to assess attitudes toward drugs. The results of the chairs' reports indicated a 1 percent to 2 percent abuse rate (abuse significant enough to come to the chair's attention). Of that group of 44 identified abusers, 7 died of their disease, a high mortality rate for any disease.

A study of all U.S. anesthesia training programs by Ward and Saidman (1981) found that 30 of 235 confirmed anesthesia personnel who abused drugs died of their disease. Three were not suspected abusers until their deaths. This retrospective survey included the 10-year period ending in

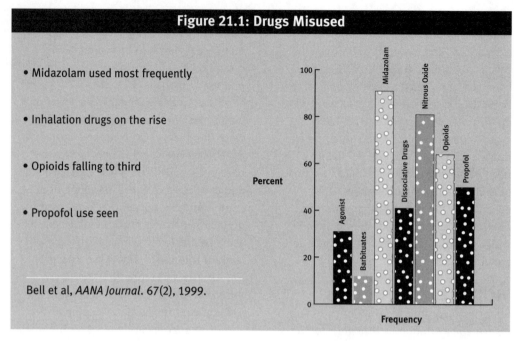

Figure 21.1: Drugs Misused

- Midazolam used most frequently
- Inhalation drugs on the rise
- Opioids falling to third
- Propofol use seen

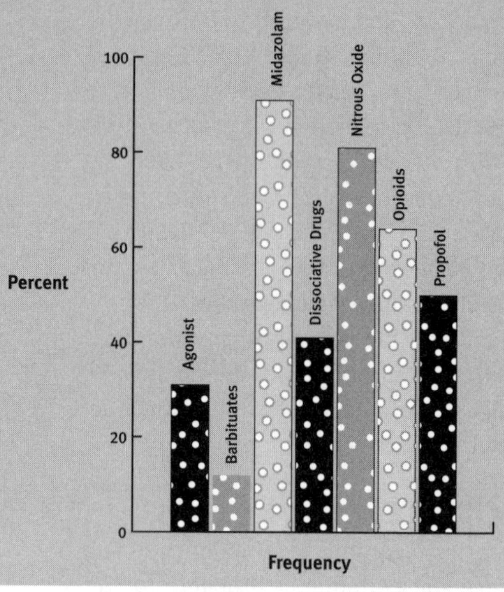

Bell et al, *AANA Journal*. 67(2), 1999.

1980. The Ward study questionnaires were distributed to 289 resident and nurse anesthetist training programs with an 85.5 percent response rate. Of the 247 respondents, 168 (68 percent) indicated at least one incident of suspected abuse; of those suspected respondents, approximately 80 percent were confirmed. Initial suspicion of abuse was raised by a staff anesthesiologist in 47 percent and by a staff CRNA in 31 percent of cases. The three most prevalent indicators that prompted suspicion were behavioral changes, inappropriate drug requests, and mood swings. Suspected abusers were more likely to be residents and student nurse anesthetists. While the Ward and Saidman study queried training programs, the study by Bell et al sampled anesthesia providers directly. What is alarming about the 9.6 percent drug misuse rate found by Bell et al is that it is probably an underestimate. Researchers agree that those addicted to substances are hesitant to admit to this unless confronted.

A 1983 analysis of the Medical Association of Georgia's Impaired Physicians Program (MAG-IPP) reported alcoholism and drug addiction at 10 percent to 14 percent with anesthesiologists included in the highest rate by medical specialty (Farley and Talbott, 1983). Of the first 507 chemically dependent physicians treated in this program, 9.6 percent were anesthesiologists. A follow-up review of MAG-IPP data revealed that anesthesiologists were still overrepresented as a physician specialty in the program. Of the more than 1,200 physicians seen, 11.9 percent were anesthesiologists, yet they represent only 3.9 percent of all U.S. physicians. Anesthesia residents were grossly overrepresented in this same program. Over a third of the physician population at the treatment program consisted of anesthesia residents, yet they represent only 4.6 percent of the U.S. physician population (Gallegos et al, 1988).

Talbott studied the group of anesthesiologists (including residents) in his treatment program and contrasted them with the remaining physician population. Table 21.1 demonstrates distinct differences in the two groups that help develop a profile

Table 21.1: Impaired Anesthesiologists Compared with Other Physicians

Impaired Anesthesiologists	Other Physicians in Treatment
• 3-7 times prevalence	• 1-2 times prevalence
• 69 percent intravenous drug users	• Oral route
• Fentanyl, morphine	• Alcohol, demerol, amphetamines
• 50 percent under 35 years	• 19 percent under 35 years
• 20 percent single	• 10 percent single
• 28 percent residents or fellows	• 8 percent residents
• Higher unemployment, retirement, suicide (2 times) rates	

of the anesthesia abuser. Another comparative method to develop a profile of today's abuser is to contrast characteristics of abusers from two different generations. Table 21.2 compares the addicted doctor of the 1970s to the 1990s, showing the evident changes.

Of the anesthesia providers initially mentioned in the 1983 MAG-IPP, 49 were anesthesiologists and 21 were nurse anesthetists. It has often been stated that the rise in the rate of narcotic addiction among nurses clearly parallels that among medical doctors (Bissell and Haberman, 1984). Garb (1965) suggested that the equivalent of three medical school and 10 nursing school graduating classes were lost to narcotic addiction each year. A review of five states' impaired physician programs in the early 1980s revealed 79 percent to 87 percent of cases were for substance abuse as opposed to physical or psychological impairments. There was a similar correlation for nurses when comparing the reasons for disciplinary action by state boards of nursing, with over 95 percent of actions being drug related (NCSBN, 1997).

There is no consensus regarding the incidence of CD among healthcare providers. Some authors quote an addiction rate 30 to 100 times that of the general population, but this inflated statistic has been traced back to a study done in Germany in the 1940s (Jefferson and Ensor, 1982). David Smith, MD, former director of the Haight-Ashbury Clinic of San Francisco, believes the prescription drug dependence is two to three times higher among healthcare professionals than among those in other occupations (Naegle, 1988).

Others believe that estimates of lifetime occupational prevalence are only slightly higher than those for the general population. One significant difference is that the history of alcoholism in professionals also includes multiple drugs, presumably a result of increased drug availability (Talbott and Wright, 1987).

Gender Considerations

Another interesting factor in the incidence of substance abuse comes from an ASA survey that showed while women represent 25 percent of anesthesia residents, only 10 percent of addicted residents are women. A study from Texas examining the profile of the disciplined nurse recognized that although this group is composed predominately of females, men are represented three times more often than in the general nursing population (Green, 1996).

Table 21.2: Profile of User

1970s	1990s
• Alcohol, pills	• Injectables
• One drug	• Multidrug use
• Average age, 54 years	• Average age 35 years
• Years of abuse	• Days or months of abuse
• Weaker drugs	• Higher potency drugs

The activity on the AANA peer assistance hotline also confirms an overrepresentation of male CRNAs. Although men account for more than 40 percent of the CRNA population, they represent about 80 percent of the callers with addiction. This gender difference merits further investigation, although some speculate that men are simply more likely to experiment than women. Some of this speculation arises from theories that personality traits are implicated in who may become an addict.

THEORY

Several theoretical models have been utilized to help us understand addictive behavior (Swain and Stasiak, 1990). These models fall into four major categories: biogenetic, disease (medical model), psychological, and familial.

Genetic/Biological Model

The biogenetic model is defined as a physiologic predisposition caused by multiple factors that influence metabolism of substances. This genetic link is supported by several studies of the general population. One survey of chemically dependent nurse anesthetists found that 71 percent reported a relative, usually a father, who was also chemically dependent (Norris, Pierson, and Waugaman, 1988).

Studies of twins adopted during infancy but raised apart have demonstrated that children born of alcoholic parents are four times more likely to become alcoholics regardless of the environment in which they are raised (Swain and Stasiak, 1990). The incidence of substance abuse is similarly much greater in children of addicts. Racial differences may also account for other biogenetic causes. One such example is acetaldehyde, a breakdown product of alcohol, which is poorly metabolized by Asians and Native Americans (Arnold, 1989).

A brain difference has been discovered in children of alcoholics by a team of researchers at Johns Hopkins University (Wand, 1998). These offspring have an altered brain chemistry that may predispose them to become alcoholics. A difference in natural opioid activity in the brain may make them more vulnerable to alcoholism for two reasons. It alters the brain's reward/craving pathway, and it also changes the brain's response to stress. Stress is involved in many types of drug-seeking behavior. This research was conducted on nonalcoholic young adults with a strong family history of chronic drinking. It also offered another connection between brain chemistry and predisposition to alcoholism. Cortisol, a stress hormone, when elevated is thought to increase growth of the brain's reward system, making it easier for the brain to be stimulated by drugs of abuse. The resultant effect is that a drink would produce a larger reward to this overdeveloped system, thus amplifying the reward. So children of alcoholics have a flawed response to stress, plus a heightened reward to drugs in the brain.

Disease Model

Chemical dependency is now widely accepted as a primary disease. Studies have linked neurotransmitter deficiencies to a variety of addicting substances and even deviant behavior. One such study conducted on rapists in one southern prison system found the same neurotransmitter substance deficient in the entire group. Many are thus concluding that, like Parkinson's disease, a biochemical deficiency in the brain may be a real culprit in chemical addiction.

Psychological Model

The psychological theory views addiction as a function of personality disorders or traits. One example is the correlation between excitement-seeking tendencies and addictive behavior seen in certain healthcare workers (McDonough, 1990). Studies have drawn a parallel between these personalities and vocational choices, such as working in the emergency department, intensive care unit, or anesthesia. Other traits common to substance abuse include extraversion, impulsivity, and nonconformity (Forgays, 1986). Substance abuse is often seen concurrently with other psychological manifestations (Mullan et al, 1986). Mullan et al found that 32 percent of alcoholics were also neurotic. Abuse may mask or precipitate an underlying, pre-existing disorder.

Familial Model

The social pathology of family dynamics may have a strong impact on addictive tendencies. Family illness or dysfunction may be prevalent for generations and have long-lasting effects on primary family members. Issues such as codependency, sexual addiction, incest, and child abuse have detrimental effects on the entire family unit. They may elicit latent responses decades after the incident or offending behavior is discontinued.

Of all the theoretical models postulated, the disease model is now the most widely accepted rationale for CD among healthcare professionals. When linked with certain genetic predispositions or familial dysfunctions, the risk of becoming addicted escalates dramatically.

SYMPTOMS AND BEHAVIORS

Addiction is confirmed by the symptoms of specific drugs (or alcohol) based on selected criteria for diagnosis according to *Diagnostic and Statistical Manual of Mental Disorders, Edition 4 (DSM-IV)*, the reference used by those in the mental health community (APA, 1994).

According to the *DSM-IV,* substance dependence is manifested by three or more of the following, within a 12-month period:

- Tolerance (increased amount, or diminished effect with same dose).
- Withdrawal, or substance use to avoid withdrawal.
- Larger amounts over a longer period than anticipated.
- Unsuccessful effort to cut down use.
- Time spent in activities to obtain, use, or recover from the substance.
- Social, occupational, or recreational activities diminish.
- Use continues despite persistent physical or psychological problems.

This dependence pattern can be observed for a variety of substances, including opioids.

Opioid intoxication coincides with recent use, euphoria followed by apathy, dysphoria, or impaired occupational

Table 21.3: Behaviors Associated with Chemical Dependency

- Isolates and withdraws from peers
- Increasing or unexplained tardiness or absenteeism
- Unwilling or unable to communicate feelings
- Mood lability with frequent, unexplained anger; overreacts to criticism
- Frequent illness or physical complaints
- Dishonesty, often over trivial or unimportant matters
- Increasing difficulty with peers, supervisors, and authority
- Frequent home crises: family illness and situational problems
- Gradual and subtle deterioration of routine work performance
- Inappropriate dress and hygiene
- Disappears and disappoints patients and peers during work
- Evidence of alcohol or drug use, odor of alcohol or strong mouthwash
- Tremors, "Monday morning shakes"
- Waits until alone to open narcotics cabinet
- Wears long sleeves all the time
- Consistently signs out more narcotics than peers
- Forgetful, unpredictable
- Frequent bathroom breaks
- Makes preoperative rounds or visits at unusual hours
- Shows up during time off and around departmental drug supply
- Intoxicated at social functions
- Inappropriate choice or amount of drug
- Use of infrequently used drugs
- Using narcoleptic drugs on simple cases

functioning during or shortly after use. Also seen may be pupillary constriction (or dilation with severe overdose), drowsiness, slurred speech, and impaired memory. These symptoms may not be typical of those seen in someone abusing fentanyl. Anecdotal accounts abound of astronomical doses taken intravenously by an abuser who remains totally coherent, highly functional, and without any of the aforementioned signs. The drugs available to the anesthetist are so pure and the abuser so skilled in administration that few report any effects other than escalating need or tolerance. An occasional overdose occurs, but this is generally with the abuser who tries a drug such as sufentanil for the first time, or with an addict who relapses and uses the same amount after months of abstinence.

Opioid withdrawal is characterized by three or more of the following signs that on the surface look like a bad case of the flu. The symptoms include dysphoria, nausea and vomiting, muscle aches, lacrimation or rhinorrhea, pupillary dilation, piloerection or sweating, diarrhea, yawning, fever, or insomnia.

Alcohol intoxication symptoms,

Table 21.4: Johnson's Four-Stage Model of Progression

1. Learning the mood swing
   - Recreational or medicinal
   - Experience is pleasant
   - Relaxing, no side effects
   - Aware of substance's positive effects
2. Seeking the mood swing
   - Using to repeat effect
   - May occasionally overdo it
   - *Many* remain at this stage
3. Harmful dependency
   - Begin to lose control
   - Experience is no longer fun
   - Adverse effects, costly
   - Unacceptable behavior
4. Using to feel normal
   - Total loss of control
   - Use to avoid withdrawal, pain
   - Consumed with compulsion

which most people have seen socially, include the following:

- Inappropriate sexual or aggressive behavior
- Mood lability
- Impaired judgment
- Impaired social or occupational functioning
- Slurred speech
- Incoordination
- Unsteady gait
- Nystagmus
- Impaired attention or memory
- Stupor or coma

Alcohol withdrawal is seen with cessation of (or reduction in) use that has been heavy and prolonged. Two (or more) of the following changes develop within several hours to days after cessation or reduction:

- Autonomic hyperactivity (sweating, tachycardia)
- Increased hand tremor
- Insomnia
- Nausea or vomiting
- Transient visual, tactile, or auditory hallucinations or illusions
- Psychomotor agitation
- Anxiety
- Grand mal seizures

Since symptoms are mostly physical manifestations, they are easily recognized. Anesthetists are experts at constantly interpreting changes in physical signs and conditions. Behaviors are more difficult to attribute to substance use. Table 21.3 lists typical behaviors associated with CD (Health Communications, 1983; Hyde, 1990).

Suspicion of chemical dependency should not be presumed by a single sign or symptom, but rather by increasing changes in behavior. Because the career is so sacred to the healthcare professional, evidence of the disease on the job usually indicates a late stage. Johnson describes a four-stage model of progression to addiction: learning the mood swing, seeking the mood swing, harmful dependency, using to feel normal. This last stage is where total loss of control ensues with compulsive use to avoid the pain of withdrawal. Table 21.4 details all the stages in Johnson's model of progression.

Tolerance

Opiate addiction may progress rapidly in the anesthesia setting. Generally, fentanyl abuse will lead to addiction within a few months, where the anesthetist may

Figure 21.2: Rendition of Arnold's Time Versus Drug Continuum

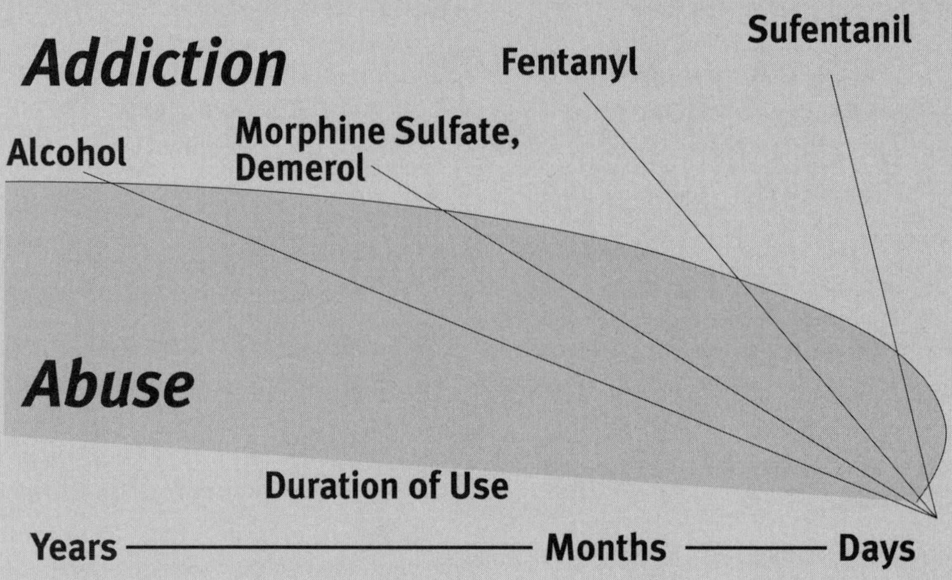

Arnold (1990)

attain a habit of 50 to 100 mL per day. With sufentanil, the onset of addiction is within weeks, and daily use may reach as high as 10-20 mL. These doses easily exceed what a nonabuser could tolerate, and yet this amount is often necessary "just to feel normal." Tolerance to fentanyl and sufentanil develops much more rapidly than to morphine, meperidine, or alcohol. Figure 21.2 represents the time/drug continuum developed by Arnold (1990).

Many addicts report that they are never able to attain the same sensation or "high" as the initial time they used. They will progressively escalate the dose and frequency to achieve the same feeling, but never reach that point. Eventually the addict will use to avoid the pain of withdrawal associated with abstaining from the drug (ASA, 1998).

RISK FACTORS

Multiple risk factors for addictive behavior have been identified for the anesthesia provider. Farley and Talbott (1983) commented on certain similarities among anesthesiologists and nurse anesthetists treated in the MAG-IPP that they labeled "anesthesiology trigger mechanisms." Table 21.5 lists triggers specific to anesthesia providers.

More specific stress-related risk factors include life and death decision making, long working hours, and altered sleep patterns associated with call. Depression may also manifest itself in the professional due to fatigue, stress, the death of patient, and the juggling of family and social life with a demanding career (ASA, 1989).

Risk Factors for Anesthesia Students

Similar risk factors exist for the nurse anesthesia student, the most predominant being stress. Students have high expectations of their own performance in both the classroom and the clinical arena. Perception of poor performance, be it accurate or not, may put them at risk because of decreased self-esteem

Table 21.5: Trigger Mechanisms for Anesthesia Providers	
• Ease of drug availability • Prior experimentation with mood altering drugs (common among younger generation of anesthesia providers) • Job-related stress in highly specialized vocation	• Respect not equivalent to responsibility • Intimate knowledge of the powers of drugs; instant relief of stress, pain, fatigue are offered almost mechanically to their patients, making its use an almost "chemical way of life"

(Kless, 1989). Other factors for students may be related to increasing financial problems, decreasing time for self and family, lack of coping skills, and depression from being overwhelmed by the associated demands.

While a student in nurse anesthesia, Ross conducted a study to examine the reported incidence of substance abuse among nurse anesthesia students that covered the period of January 1991-December 1996 (Ross, 1997). With an 80 percent response rate from a total survey of 87 program directors, 20 percent of programs reported at least one incident of abuse. Geographical location may also be a factor. Programs located in an area with a population of less than 50,000 were least likely to have an incident.

Other Risk Factors

Attitudes about alcohol, being so highly acceptable in our society and almost mandatory in certain social situations, contribute further pressure. Another factor continues to be the lack of education in the health professions regarding substance abuse. Clark (1988), and Clark and Stone (1999), suggest that such education be offered to all health personnel and integrated into new staff orientation.

DENIAL

There are many misconceptions about the disease of CD, by both addicts and their coworkers. As a profession at risk, it is alarming that colleagues know so little about an occupational hazard that will likely affect them at some time in their career, either directly or indirectly (Quinlan, 1985). A study conducted for the Alabama Association of Nurse Anesthetists revealed negative bias on the part of nurse anesthetists who had worked with impaired anesthetists, as well as poor performance on a knowledge test about the disease. The anesthetists who were most knowledgeable were recent graduates and those falling within the 30-39 year age group.

Over 60 percent of those responding to the survey had some exposure to a chemically dependent individual, and over 70 percent of those listed "coworker" as their relationship to that individual. When respondents were asked if they would be able to recognize CD in themselves, almost 80 percent answered in the affirmative; yet less than 8 percent had any confidence in their ability to recognize dependency in a colleague. These responses support the frequently cited characteristic of the disease—denial—and further emphasize the fact that CRNAs may not know how to handle the problem of CD alone.

Denial is the most difficult obstacle to overcome for both chemically addicted healthcare workers and their colleagues. The worker often performs adequately while impaired; many anecdotal accounts attest that there are those who actually excel at their tasks while under the influence of drugs. Even when job performance deteriorates, most managers and colleagues are quick to accept excuses like stress, fatigue, and use of cold remedies. Employers sustain the denial even at termination by offering rationales that have nothing to do with addictive behavior. One such account tells of an employer who, upon finding a nurse on the floor of the bathroom with a narcotic syringe in her thigh, dismissed her on the grounds that she was late reporting back from lunch (Sullivan, Bissell, and Williams, 1988).

Despite the fact that alcoholism is designated a primary disease by the AMA, the healthcare industry and the public continue to view alcohol and drug use as a personal choice, manageable by willpower. Nurses are expected to maintain composure in the face of disaster. When able to do this despite other questionable behaviors, the problem of abuse is often ignored.

Healthcare professionals are trained to perceive medication and its applications as beneficial. Therefore, many colleagues fail to question a worker's drug use, and instead, assume the coworker is knowledgeable about its effects and addictive potentials. Professionals are trained observers of physical symptoms. By the time features of substance abuse are evident, coworkers have generally supported the impaired colleague's dependency through denial and enabling.

An often forgotten contributor to the denial of addiction is the family. One of the reasons healthcare professionals are so highly esteemed by our society is the personal sacrifice made by many of them. Coupled with enormous responsibilities, long hours, and a deep commitment to patient care, one wonders why anyone would pursue such a vocation. The family unit understands this sense of commitment from the inside. The family is therefore apt to accept changes in personal behavior as job-related without questioning.

Overwhelming denial of the disease also hinders identification by coworker and family. This problem may actually be compounded by our professional role as caregivers or by a family member who encourages the continuation of a bad behavior by letting it go unchallenged.

ENABLING

Enabling is often considered empowering or encouraging. However, in CD, enabling only shields the addict from consequences and is an obstacle to ultimate help. Coworkers and managers often enable impaired colleagues to continue bad behavior and poor performance. By making excuses, ignoring problems, covering up mistakes, and accepting incomplete work, coworkers and managers become enablers (Krames, 1989). The message sent to the chemically dependent health professional is that the behavior is acceptable and performance need not change. Table 21.6 offers typical feelings or actions by others that are enabling.

To be a part of the solution, coworkers need to stop enabling and talk clearly about the behaviors seen at work. They need to acknowledge that a problem may exist for the colleague and put the colleague on notice that they will no longer be responsible for the colleague's share of the workload. In a study of chemically dependent nurse anesthetists, Norris et al (1988) found that 75 percent believed their colleagues knew they were actively abusing substances while administering anesthesia and did nothing.

In many ways, the profession itself perpetuates the addictive process by rewarding behaviors such as competitiveness, self-sacrifice, and perseverance at all costs. Furthermore, the profession is reluctant to seek outside help, often called the "white coat" syndrome for fear that ensuing punitive action or bad press will impact every associate. Thus, the

Table 21.6: Feelings or Actions of Colleagues that Enable the Chemically Dependent	
• Accepting chemically dependent (CD) person's responsibilities and duties	• Believing the CD person can control use and behavior
• Avoiding, withdrawing from situation	• Accepting CD person's rationalizations, excuses, promises
• Believing they can fix CD behavior	• Reasoning with or enduring behavior of the CD person
• Moralizing, judging, blaming the CD person for own bad feelings	• Confronting with generalities, opinions, judgments
• Denying condition, minimizing severity of problem	• Expressing vague, general demands for change that provoke denial
• Protecting the CD person from consequences of using by lying; protecting the CD person's image	• Failing to follow through on ultimatums

Table 21.7: Stages of Enabling
• Anxiety, increasing tension, denial
• Preoccupation, assuming responsibility
• Coping mechanisms, dysfunctional behavior
• Crisis, suicide, overdose

conspiracy of silence is perpetuated, and enabling worsens the situation. There are escalating stages of enabling as shown in Table 21.7.

The manager may further enable by accepting commonly held beliefs such as "offering treatment will damage the anesthetist's career," "any abusing nurse should be fired," "it's only a personal problem," or "if they ignore it, it will all work out." The manager may also fear liability. The major problem with these beliefs is that they are a real threat to life—a CRNA whose employment is terminated will likely lose the very benefits needed for treatment, plus the incentive to participate in treatment. It may also encourage coworkers to remain silent or cover up if they find that termination is the only alternative to managing addictive behavior. Another approach is to just ignore the situation, but this also worsens the problem. Often the situation escalates, thereby reinforcing denial and avoidance of the real issue. Treating the situation as if it were only a personal problem increases risk for everyone—the department, patients, and the CRNA. It ultimately erodes staff morale and leaves the disciplinary process and job standards unclear.

DEPARTMENTAL RESPONSIBILITY

It is imperative that managers and employers comprehend the many aspects of maintaining a work environment that is structured. They should have adequate record keeping and accountability (narcotic accounting, quality assurance [QA] process, employee evaluations), and be prepared for the potential of a substance abuser within the anesthesia department (Quinlan, 1995). Others to include in the development of this responsibility are the hospital or group administrators. Policy manuals should contain procedures for managing addicted healthcare workers. The goals of all these educational efforts and policies are to ensure (1) timely identification of the addict, (2) intervention to facilitate rapid assessment, (3) adequate leave of absence for treatment, and (4) aftercare for successful reentry into the workplace. This life-saving sequence can lead to an excellent prognosis and retention of a valued professional. Planning will also significantly decrease the turmoil that often falls upon an unprepared department.

Policy Development

Perhaps the policy that frightens most practitioners deals with drug testing. Whether or not a department has a recovering anesthetist on its staff, it should have a well-described policy regarding drug testing. There is much debate nationally about this issue in job settings where there is potential for public harm. The transportation industry set the standard long ago with airline pilots, railroad engineers, bus drivers, and others.

Public trust of the healthcare profession has eroded in the last decade partly because of decreased services, increased costs, and gate keeping by health maintenance organizations. Occasionally one will see an editorial where the writer is shocked that doctors and nurses are *not* tested, especially given their accessibility to highly addicting drugs. So it may be that, whether or not testing contributes to improved patient services, the public perception of healthcare may be improved if we agree to abide by some of the same standards currently required of other professionals.

The American Nurses' Association opposed random (without cause) drug tests for healthcare workers in a 1997 position statement titled "Drug Testing for Health Care Workers." It gives qualified consent to testing where there is reason to believe drugs or alcohol are affecting the work of the employee and proper restrictions are applied. The position statement can be viewed on the Internet at www.aana.com/peer.

The AANA Peer Assistance Advisors Committee (PAAC) developed a sample chemical dependency policy for departments of anesthesia that includes useful criteria on drug testing. This policy is proactive in that it is useful to establish such criteria as a precaution to drug abuse. When a recovering anesthetist returns to the workplace, more rigid criteria will also apply. These will generally be found in the specific return-to-work contract, a sample of which is available at www.aana.com/peer. Section II of the sample policy is excerpted below:

A Sample Policy/Procedure for Departments of Anesthesia on Chemical Dependency (developed by the AANA PAAC, March 1999)

II. Drug Testing

Anesthesia providers shall be required to submit to drug testing as a condition of employment. Failure or refusal to cooperate with any aspect of this policy including, but not limited to, refusal to sign forms consenting to drug testing or the refusal to submit to urine or blood sampling for testing to determine use of, or impairment by, a controlled substance or intoxicant will result in disciplinary action up to and including discharge and the reporting of use to the appropriate authorities.

Applicants and employees will be required to sign an acknowledgment form and consent to this policy. An employee may be required to undergo a blood test or urinalysis under any of the following circumstances:

A. When there is reason to believe in the opinion of this facility that an employee is under the influence of intoxicants, nonprescribed narcotics, hallucinogens, marijuana, or other nonprescribed controlled substances.

B. After the occurrence of a reported work-related injury/illness, or accident while on the facility property or during work hours.

C. During any physical examination provided by the facility.

D. When employees have been on leave of absence, or have not worked within the 12 weeks proceeding their return date.

Testing Procedure

Drug testing will be conducted utilizing the following measures:

A. Employees will be required to sign the facility's consent forms.

B. Employees will be required to sign the chain of custody forms provided by the testing laboratory.

C. Employees should disclose any medication, whether prescribed or over-the-counter, as well as any dietary intake that could alter a drug screen.

D. The facility will use a laboratory for testing which meets the current scientific and technical guidelines for drug testing programs.

E. A second test will be used on any positive screen.

F. All positive drug tests will be verified by a medical review officer. If it is determined there is a legitimate medical explanation for the positive result, the medical review officer shall report the test results as negative.

Confidentiality

Testing and test results will be handled confidentially with disclosure of results provided only to those individuals with a need to know. Upon request, employees will be provided a copy of test results.

Prescription Drugs

Employees and applicants who have been taking legally prescribed drugs or over-the-counter medications should disclose this use prior to testing. A confidential consent form requesting information concerning this drug usage will be provided each employee or applicant prior to testing.

(A copy of the entire policy may be obtained on the AANA peer assistance Web site at www.aana.com/peer.)

Many common substances interfere with drug test results. Several popular over-the-counter (OTC) cold remedies interfere with immunoassay and mimic opiates. Dextromethorphan will give a false-positive PCP result. Several bronchial medications mimic barbiturates and amphetamines, some for weeks following use. Commonly used OTC medications for menstrual cramps mimic opiates on assay. Benadryl will appear as methadone on certain drug tests. Even medication and conditions related to diabetes and vaginal yeast infections can alter the analysis of a drug test (NCSBN, 1997).

It is therefore vitally important that one inquire about all dietary and medicinal intake within a two-week period of testing and follow up any positive screen with a more reliable assay method utilizing gas chromatography–mass spectrometry on the original specimen. When testing for drugs that could have been diverted from the workplace, it is important to do a split specimen. This is a technique that reserves, by freezing, half of the original specimen for follow-up analysis at a future date.

For this reason alone it is imperative that a proper "chain of custody" is observed when collecting, handling, and shipping any specimen for analysis. If one cannot document each person who handled the specimen from the moment the container was offered for specimen collection until the final reporting of the results, then the test will not be recognized in legal settings. The reporting of assays where a chain of custody has been interrupted may constitute liability for the employer, testing laboratory, and any other handlers.

Narcotic Accountability

A written, consistent process of narcotic accountability is essential for the efficient use and documentation of narcotic dispensing, recording, and wasting (Quinlan, 1994). It should be written and followed uniformly by all departmental members and meet the guidelines of regulatory agencies such as the Drug Enforcement Agency and hospital protocol. In 1985, Adler et al described a narcotics control program in use in anesthesia training. This model supposes that narcotics and other drugs of potential abuse pose an occupational risk to physicians and nurses. They advocate a system that limits access and encourages strict accounting.

Narcotics should *not* be exchanged between department members, not even narcotics signed out for the same patient between primary and relieving anesthetists. This also applies to patients taken to the postanesthesia care unit (PACU) where transfer of care is made to another nurse. This time of transfer is fraught with opportunities for poor record keeping. Many CRNAs have been disciplined for poor accountability at this juncture. It is wiser to have the PACU nurse sign out fresh narcotics for use in the recovery area than to compromise the accounting of the anesthetist's record. Additionally, it is not prudent for PACU nurses to accept, let alone administer, a drug they have not drawn up themselves. All unused portions of drugs should be accounted for.

Departments should evaluate the efficacy of their narcotic accountability system and pay particular attention to poor institutional habits and complacency. Some old habits are hard to break, such as keeping the keys in a "secret" drawer for easier access by the staff. There are no secrets in an operating room (OR), and everyone from the chief surgeon to housekeeping will know where the keys are kept. The only adequate method is for someone to keep them in their possession and to have a log of everyone (name and time) who takes possession of the keys.

All scheduled drugs should be kept under double lock and signed for only by authorized individuals according to regulatory guidelines. All unused portions of drugs should be returned to a centralized, mail slot type of locked compartment that can be opened only by the pharmacy or departmental narcotics control officer, or the unused portions may be returned to a staffed pharmacy. The use of a satellite pharmacy within the OR has met with great success, as have automated dispensing systems like the Pyxis (Pyxis Corporation, San Diego, CA). Syringes returned to these locations should be randomly assayed for content.

Assays can be conducted on a random basis by a chemical analysis of the syringe for drug and concentration or more frequently and inexpensively by the use of a handheld refractometer. The refractometer is calibrated differently for each type of drug used in anesthesia and merely looks at how that drug refracts light. It is an exceptional device that can distinguish between drug types and also can pick up dilutional effect. Either pharmacy personnel or a designated member of the anesthesia department can utilize this refracting technique to screen every returned specimen. The process takes a very small droplet and requires about 20 seconds to accomplish its task. In the absence of a centralized accountability system as described, all narcotic wastage should follow facility guidelines with documented double witnessing of wastage. However, the ideal method remains a policy of "no wasting," and a preserved potential for assay.

Random assays may raise suspicion of department members and should be followed by observations of behavior and audits of anesthesia and PACU records of persons suspected of diverting drugs. These audits should be conducted periodically and when suspicion warrants. They also make an excellent QA project for a department.

Quality Assurance

The assaying of drugs for waste and review of records makes an excellent ongoing QA process for any anesthesia department. This is also an excellent opportunity to look at customary habits that may have evolved in a facility and to set a standard for accountability that is consistent, regardless of time of day and level of provider. Sequestering excess drugs for late night call or duty in remote areas such as obstetrics or radiology signals a problem in the system. The same process, or at least the same level of accountability, should apply everywhere the department provides service, no matter the hour. Opportunity is created where there are holes in the system. This availability coupled with the strain of the hour and isolated location may create the situation where the anesthetist uses for the first time.

Valuable QA should also include written periodic evaluations of department members and random audits of written records. Questionable outcomes that point toward drug use should remain confidential and undiscoverable until such time that intervention or discipline may be required. The review should include anesthesia records, PACU notes, and narcotic inventory and usage. Unusual trends, violations, or errors should be documented and investigated within the department. When sufficient evidence exists that inappropriate narcotic usage has occurred, a specific investigation should begin with a more in-depth review of specific records.

Insurance Provisions

Because anesthesia providers are at increased risk of becoming addicted, departments should make available as part of their benefits package both healthcare and disability insurance policies with provisions for CD and mental health treatment (Quinlan, 1995). Quality treatment is expensive and, for the anesthetist, can be a lengthy process. Few are prepared to meet day-to-day expenses for a year with no income and then pay for an extensive costly treatment on top of that. Unless a CRNA has sufficient savings to live for two years without a salary, the CRNA needs to rely on alternative methods of income.

Addicts new to treatment may find themselves jobless, in a restricted environment for months, and financially strained. Adequate disability insurance can ease the strain, provide for the family, and make the recovery process much less painful. Worse yet, a higher percentage of addicted CRNAs are men and the primary wage earners of their families. As previously mentioned, while men represent more than 40 percent of CRNAs, they account for approximately 80 percent of the peer assistance hotline callers. Men are more inclined to succumb to the emotional and financial devastation of being discovered. Some die at their own hand rather than face potential professional humiliation and the disappointment of family. They may feel obligated to care for their family in a final exit that leaves their family more financially secure as beneficiaries.

A department with adequate insurance provisions can offer hope to the addict and peace of mind for those at risk. For those in recovery seeking to reenter the workplace, the only insurance available will be with a group policy. The waiting period to apply for individual disability or malpractice insurance is generally five years of uninterrupted recovery.

Employees also need to be informed of their right to continue their health insurance plan for up to six months after an employer stops providing this benefit. Employees may continue to pay the employer portion of their insurance premium and keep their entire policy in force. This is important not only for possible addiction treatment, but also for a family health policy, especially if they are the only family member able to access coverage.

This continuation of coverage is assured workers through the Consolidated Omnibus Budget Reconciliation Act of 1985 (COBRA). It requires employers with group health plans to offer continued coverage to employees and their dependents. This coverage may be restricted if it is not triggered by a qualifying event (termination, leave of absence). Misconduct or reduction in hours are not qualifiers, but most employers will grant a leave for substance dependency if drug diversion on the job has not triggered criminal charges. Coverage is continued for at least 18 months from the date of the event and if the employee is declared disabled, coverage may be extended to 29 months. This benefit also includes beneficiaries, such as spouse or dependent. Drug and alcohol treatment is considered medical care that must be offered as part of coverage.

Another important consideration that impacts time away from work but is not a direct insurance provision is the Family Medical Leave Act (FMLA) of 1993. This federal law grants a leave of absence for child care or for serious health problems of employees, their children, spouse, or parents. It applies only to workplaces with 15 or more employees, but does allow up to 12 weeks of unpaid leave. A serious health problem is defined as "an illness, injury, impairment, or physical or mental condition that involves continuing treatment by a healthcare provider." Substance abuse is included if it rises to the level of an illness or impairment that requires continuing treatment, such as a rehabilitation program. Alcohol or drug abuse that results in the employee periodically missing time from work (one to two days at a time) would not qualify.

A medical certification can be required before the employee is granted a family medical leave or before returning to work. An employee under some circumstances may request intermittent leave (taking off blocks of time, i.e., attending family therapy week for a spouse in treatment) or may request the reduction of the normal weekly or daily work schedule to accommodate this illness. At the end of the leave period, the employee must be restored to the same job, site, and level of benefits as before leave began. Or if the job is unavailable, the employee should be placed in an equivalent position with equal pay and benefits. During leave, the employee is *not* entitled to accrual of seniority or benefits. Employers must, however, continue health insurance coverage on the same terms.

It may be an unreasonable expectation on the part of the anesthetist to expect an employer to hold a position for the amount of time it may require to get appropriate treatment and establish a recovery program for long-standing narcotic addiction, as this may take six to 12 months. However, an alcoholic, someone treated for a mood or compulsive disorder, or someone who has been misusing substances but is not addicted, may be able to return to work within the allotted 12-week leave period.

Documentation

Documentation of work performance and behavior of a suspected colleague is essential to objective evaluation of the situation, as well as crucial to an effective resolution or intervention. It must be written, clear, and concise, and must include specific dates, times, and the names of other witnesses. Appropriate documentation should commence upon suspicion of misuse of departmental pharmaceuticals or signs of drug or alcohol abuse. Note changes in behavior such as appearance, demeanor, attendance, and being in the department when off duty. Hearsay must never be recorded, only observable behavior or the results of poor or questionable performance (anesthesia records, narcotic inventory). The department head or supervisor should keep documentation in nondiscoverable files. These are private personnel files that are protected from mandatory disclosure. The information may be made a part of the employee's record should disciplinary action be warranted.

When the documented evidence warrants, the manager should seek appropriate assistance to confront the individual, or the manager may refer the suspected abuser to trained intervention professionals. Major hospitals and universities often have access to employee assistance programs (EAPs). Other facilities may have an established network with regional peer assistance programs or other specialized facilities. CRNAs should consider addiction an occupational hazard and lobby for the availability of resources to deal effectively with this increasing problem.

CONFRONTATION OR INTERVENTION

When there is sufficient documented evidence of impaired practice, or when evidence exists that the employee is diverting controlled substances from the department, a confrontation should be planned. An intervention consultant should be sought who is knowledgeable about the ethical and legal issues of the locality, the facility dynamics, and the roles of the coworkers who will be essential to the intervention process (Crosby and Offer, 1988). Employees should be offered the option to voluntarily self-report to an alternative-to-discipline program for professionals with impaired practice (if such a program or legislation exists within the state of practice).

A meeting or intervention should be planned to confront the employee with documented questionable behavior. The planning and conduct of this confrontation includes:

- Sufficient documented evidence.
- The presence of the principal observers of the questionable behavior.
- A trained individual capable of conducting an intervention.
- Potential immediate placement of the employee in a facility for assessment and possible treatment or any occasion when an acute crisis warrants (e.g., inebriated on duty).

An extended leave of absence should be granted to an employee for chemical dependency treatment that leaves intact all applicable insurance plans and benefits. The individual should be advised if and/or how to make payment for the continuance of such benefits (i.e., COBRA). If employees refuse to comply with a request that they be evaluated for CD, they should be informed that the informa-

Table 21.8: Persistent Behavioral and Performance Problems

• Absenteeism – unauthorized, excessive, patterned	• Escalating error or incident rate
• Loss of time on duty – increased breaks, missing from post	• Job "shrinkage" – mistakes, missed deadlines
• Confusion, lack of concentration, distant	• Deteriorating relationships with others
• Spasmodic work pattern	• Proximity to source off and on duty

tion collected will be submitted to the appropriate regulatory agency for further investigation and probable discipline. It is this option to avoid reporting to the regulatory authorities that is most influential in the addict's decision to cooperate. Initially it is seen as a measure to preserve license and career. Ultimately it is recognized as the turning point in a downward spiral.

Managerial Role in Identification

Managers play a crucial role in the identification and intervention of a chemically dependent employee (Quinlan, 1994, 1995). However, they should only supervise, assess, and document performance. Diagnosis must be left to those trained in intervention and treatment. The critical factor is recognition of persistent behavioral and performance problems. Characteristics often typical of those who raise suspicion are found in Table 21.8.

The manager will most likely be the individual who coordinates the efforts leading to an intervention. This will include gathering supporting documentation from coworkers; researching options, financial resources, and treatment opportunities; contacting a professional interventionist; and possibly participating in the actual intervention. The manager also needs to be prepared for the possibility that the intervention may fail and know how to report the suspected addict to the appropriate authorities. Table 21.9 details the steps required in the intervention process and what may transpire with a failed intervention.

Managers and administrators concerned about liability from an angry employee after an intervention should not be overly fearful. Courts have not upheld defamation suits when the intervention was done in good faith, confidentially, with reliable documentation, and without malice.

DEPARTMENT GUIDELINES

Managers who seek to develop their own guidelines for chemical dependency by sampling a broad spectrum of resource organizations will find a helpful list at the end of chapter 22. The ASA published guidelines specifically for departments of anesthesiology (1998), and the AANA PAAC published a booklet about chemical dependency in CRNAs offering very specific direction to managers (2000). Both resources clearly advise each department to have a well-established policy that defines dependence as a medical disease that, if left untreated, is incompatible with safe clinical performance. They further suggest that it is the duty of all members of the department to share their concerns about substance abuse.

The anesthesia manager, chair of the department or a designee is encouraged to act as a confidential resource to be informed on how to judge whether someone is addicted and to act judiciously to place any member of the staff on medical

Table 21.9: Steps Toward Intervention

1. Documentation
   - Gather data to support observations
   - Note inappropriate behavior
   - Illogical charting or drug selection
   - Inaccurate narcotic records
   - Witnesses to the above
   - Specific factual accounts
   - Variability of outcomes (patients in pain)
2. Research all options
   - Explore all policies (institutional, departmental, insurance)
   - Assess disciplinary options
   - Determine leverage
   - Select intervention team
3. Identify financial resources
   - Review employee benefits
   - Leave time (FMLA)
   - Medical insurance (COBRA)
   - Disability coverage
   - Facility support (EAP, referral center)
   - Family situation, loans
4. Identify treatment programs
   - Gather information on available sites
   - Check with state nurses association, or state peer assistance program
   - Alternative discipline programs
   - State health department (mental health)
   - Council on alcoholism or drug dependency (local, state, or regional)
5. Meet with the team
   - Review key points (documentation)
   - Develop a plan of action
   - Assign key roles
   - Make contingency plans
   - Choose time and place
   - Review facts about chemical dependency (treatable, chronic, progressive disease; denial; enabling; long-term recovery)
6. Conduct intervention
   - The *goal* is getting the nurse to accept help
   - Present documentation
   - Ask nurse to sign agreement for evaluation, release of information
   - Escort nurse to treatment, do *not* send off alone; report to licensing authority if nurse fails to agree
7. Debriefing and closure
   - Allow participants to decompress and ventilate feelings
   - Obtain counseling after the event
   - Brief on confidentiality
   - Follow up with treatment facility

(continued)

Table 21.9: Steps Toward Intervention (continued)
Failed intervention occurs when: • Plan falls apart, team turns confrontational • Nurse refuses evaluation: report to licensing authority and allow it to conduct investigation with your documentation • Treatment facility not available

leave whose conduct is suspect. The guidelines further advocate that all staff members retain medical insurance coverage that includes CD treatment.

To further assist the anesthesia department, the AANA PAAC has developed a CD policy for departments of anesthesia. This comprehensive model, which will assist managers in developing their own unique policy by selecting applicable segments, can be viewed at www.aana.com/peer.

Having a recovering member within the department should also encourage employers to make certain they have written policies governing fitness for duty, health benefit coverage for drug dependency, and effective evaluation mechanisms for overall performance. These adjustments in policies and procedures should make a department stronger and better prepared to respond to the occupational hazard of chemical dependency.

For members of departments of anesthesia to fully comprehend the addiction sequence, the treatment process, recovery, reentry to the workplace, and relapse must be addressed. This component of the complete addiction cycle is discussed in chapter 22.

References

Adler, G.R., et al. (1985). Narcotics control in anesthesia training. *JAMA.* 21;3133-3136.

American Association of Nurse Anesthetists. (2000). *Chemical Dependency and the Certified Registered Nurse Anesthetist* (brochure). AANA PAAC. Park Ridge, IL.

American Psychiatric Association. (1994). *The Diagnostic and Statistical Manual of Mental Disorders (DSM-IV)* (4th ed.). Washington, DC.

American Society of Anesthesiologists. (1998). *Chemical Dependence in Anesthesiologists: What You Need to Know When You Need to Know It* (brochure). Park Ridge, IL.

American Society of Anesthesiologists. (1992). Retrospective survey of substance abuse in anesthesia training programs. *ASA Newsletter.* April, 10.

American Society of Anesthesiologists. (1989). The impaired physician in anesthesiology: An overview. *ASA Newsletter.* 53(9), 4-5.

Angres, D.H., Talbott G.D., & Bettinardi-Angres, K. (1998). *Healing the Healer: The Addicted Physician.* Madison, CT: Psychosocial Press.

Arnold, W.P. (1995). Substance abuse survey in anesthesiology training programs: Brief summary. *ASA Newsletter.* 59(10), 12-13, 18.

Arnold, W.P. (1991). Legal aspects of chemical dependence. *ASA Newsletter.* 55(2).

Arnold, W.P. (1990). Environmental safety including chemical dependency. In Miller, R.D. (Ed.), *Anesthesia* (3rd ed). New York, NY: Churchill Livingstone, Inc.

Arnold, W.P. (1989). Disease or not disease, that is the question. *ASA Newsletter.* 53(8), 7-8.

Beck, M. & Buckley, J. (1983). Nurses with bad habits. *Newsweek.* August 22:54.

Bell, D.M., McDonough, J.P., Ellison, J.S. & Fitzhugh, E.C. (1999). Controlled drug misuse by Certified Registered Nurse Anesthetists. *AANA Journal.* 67(2), 133-140.

Bissell, L. & Jones, R. (1981). The alcoholic nurse. *Nursing Outlook.* 29, 96-101.

Bissell, L. & Haberman, P.W. (1984). *Alcoholism In the Professions.* New York, NY: Oxford University Press.

Clark, G.D. & Stone, J.A. (1999). The assessment of substance abuse curriculum in schools of nurse anesthesia. *Journal of Addictions Nursing.* 11(3).

Clark, M.D. (1988). Preventing drug dependency: Part 1, recognizing risk factors. *J Nurs Adm.* 18, 12-15.

Crosby, L.R. & Offer, P.L. (1988). Intervention with chemically dependent nurses: A paradigm for professional retention. *QRB.* April, 111-115.

Farley, W.J. & Talbott, G.D. (1983). Anesthesiology and addiction (editorial). *Anesth Analg.* 62, 465-66.

Flexner, A. (1910). Medical education in the United States and Canada: A report to the Carnegie Foundation for the advancement of teaching. Carnegie Foundation, New York.

Forgays, D.G. (1986). Personality characteristics and self-abusive behavior. *NIDA Monograph Series.* 45-58.

Gallegos, K.V., Browne, C.H., Veit, F.W. & Talbott, G.D. (1988). Addiction in anesthesiologists: Drug access and patterns of substance abuse. *QRB.* April 116-122.

Garb, S. (1965). Narcotic addiction in nurses and doctors. *Nursing Outlook.* 13, 30-34.

Gravenstein, J.S., Kory, W.P. & Marks, R.G. (1983). Drug abuse by anesthesia personnel. *Anesth Analg.* 62, 467-72.

Green, A. (1996). Texas Creates a profile of the disciplined professional nurse. *Issues.* 17(2).

Green, P.L. (1984). The impaired nurse: Chemical dependency. *Focus on Critical Care.* 11(2), 42-46.

Health Communications, Inc. (1983). *Do you know the facts about drugs?* Deerfield Beach, FL.

Hyde, G.L. (1990). Management of the impaired person in the OR. *Plastic Surgical Nursing.* 10 (2), 77-79.

Jefferson, L.V. & Ensor, B.E. (1982). Help for the helper: Confronting a chemically impaired colleague. *AJN.* 4, 574-577.

Krames Communications (1989). *Chemical Dependency: Reaching Out To the Impaired Caregiver.* Daly City, CA.

Kless, J.R. (1989). Use of a student support group to reduce student stress in a nurse anesthesia program. *AANA Journal.* 57, 75-77.

Lundy, J.S. & McQuillen, F.A. (1962). Narcotics and the anesthetist: Professional hazards. *AANA Journal.* 30(3), 147-178.

Maxwell, S. (2000). Concepts of addiction. National Nurses Society on Addictions Conference, Chicago.

McDonough, J.P. (1990). Personality, addiction, and anesthesia. *AANA Journal.* 58, 193-200.

Mereness, D. (1981). Protect your patients from nurse addicts. *Nursing Life.* 1(1), 71-73.

Mullan, M., et al. (1986). The relationship between alcohol and neurosis. *British Journal of Psychiatry.* 48, 435-441.

Naegle, M. (1988). Drug and alcohol abuse in nursing, an occupational hazard? *Nursing Life.* 8(1), 42-54.

National Council of State Boards of Nursing, Inc. (1997). *Chemical Dependency Handbook for Boards of Nursing.* 33-36, 54-56.

National Council of State Boards of Nursing, Inc. (1993). Advanced nursing practice discipline survey results. *Issues.* 14(2), 1,4.

National Practitioner Data Bank. (1986). US Government Printing Office, C.F.R. Title 45, Volume 1, Parts 1-199, Sec. 60.1, p. 130.

Norris, J., Pierson, F. & Waugaman, W. (1988). Critical factors associated with substance abuse and chemical dependency in nurse anesthetists. *Journal of Alcohol and Drug Education.* Winter, 6-11.

Quinlan, D.S. (1995). The impaired anesthesia provider: The manager's role. *AANA Journal.* 63(6), 485-491.

Quinlan, D.S. (1994). Chemical dependency. In Foster, S.D. & Jordan, L.M. (Eds.), *Professional Aspects of Nurse Anesthesia Practice.* Philadelphia, PA: F.A. Davis Publishing.

Quinlan, D.S., & Bodenhorn, K.A. (1990). Update: The National Practitioner Data Bank. *Specialty Nursing Forum.* 2(1).

Quinlan, D.S. (1985). A study of the opinions of Alabama certified registered nurse anesthetists regarding selected factors related to chemical dependency (unpublished thesis). University of Alabama at Birmingham.

Ross, T.K. (1997). The reported incidents of substance abuse among student registered nurse anesthetists in the United States from 1991 through 1996 (abstract). *AANA Journal.* 65(5), 503-504.

Stimson, G.V., Oppenheimer, B.A. & Stimson, C.A. (1984). Drug abuse in the medical profession. *Br J Addiction.* 79, 395-402.

Sullivan, E.J., Bissell, L. & Williams, E. (1988). *Chemical Dependency in Nursing: The Deadly Diversion.* Menlo Park, CA: Addison-Wesley Publishing Company.

Swain, E.A. & Stasiak, D.B. (1990). Chemical dependency and the student nurse anesthetist: A strategy for caring. *CRNA: The Clinical Forum for Nurse Anesthetists.* 1(2), 50-53.

Talbott, G.D. & Wright, C. (1987). Chemical dependency in health care professionals. *Occupational Medicine: State of the Art Reviews.* 2(3), 581-591.

Talbott, G.D. (1983). Mirror image therapy. Address at the annual meeting of the American Association of Nurse Anesthetists. New Orleans, LA.

Wand, G.S. (1999). Brain difference discovered in children of alcoholics (findings published in Annals of General Psychiatry, December 1998). Substance Abuse Letter, Parrish, M.R. (Ed.). PaceCom Publications. March 17, (5)18.

Ward, C.F. & Saidman, L.J. (1981). Controlled substance abuse: A survey of training programs 1970-1980. *Anesthesiology.* 55(3), A345-A346.

STUDY QUESTIONS

1. How would you explain the increased incidence of substance abuse in the healthcare community over the general population? What differences exist in the types of substance abuse and their addictive patterns? Are anesthesia providers more prone to abuse of certain substances? If so, what do current trends indicate they may be?

2. Your father was an alcoholic before he died at 60; you experimented with marijuana, and then a little cocaine when in college. You like to hang out with your coworkers after a long day in the OR. People offer to drive you home but you know you are just fine. Your wife thinks you might have a drinking problem. As an anesthetist and a child of an alcoholic, statistically what are your chances of being a substance abuser in the course of your career?

3. You recognize some suspicious symptoms and behaviors of potential drug abuse, but the abuser is your best friend and your coworker. How do you work through the enabling and denial?

4. As a coworker, you are pretty sure that one of your colleagues is using. What steps do you take now?

5. How would your activities as a manager differ from that of the coworker mentioned in question 4? What specific steps should the manager take to preserve order in the department and still be an advocate for the CRNA?

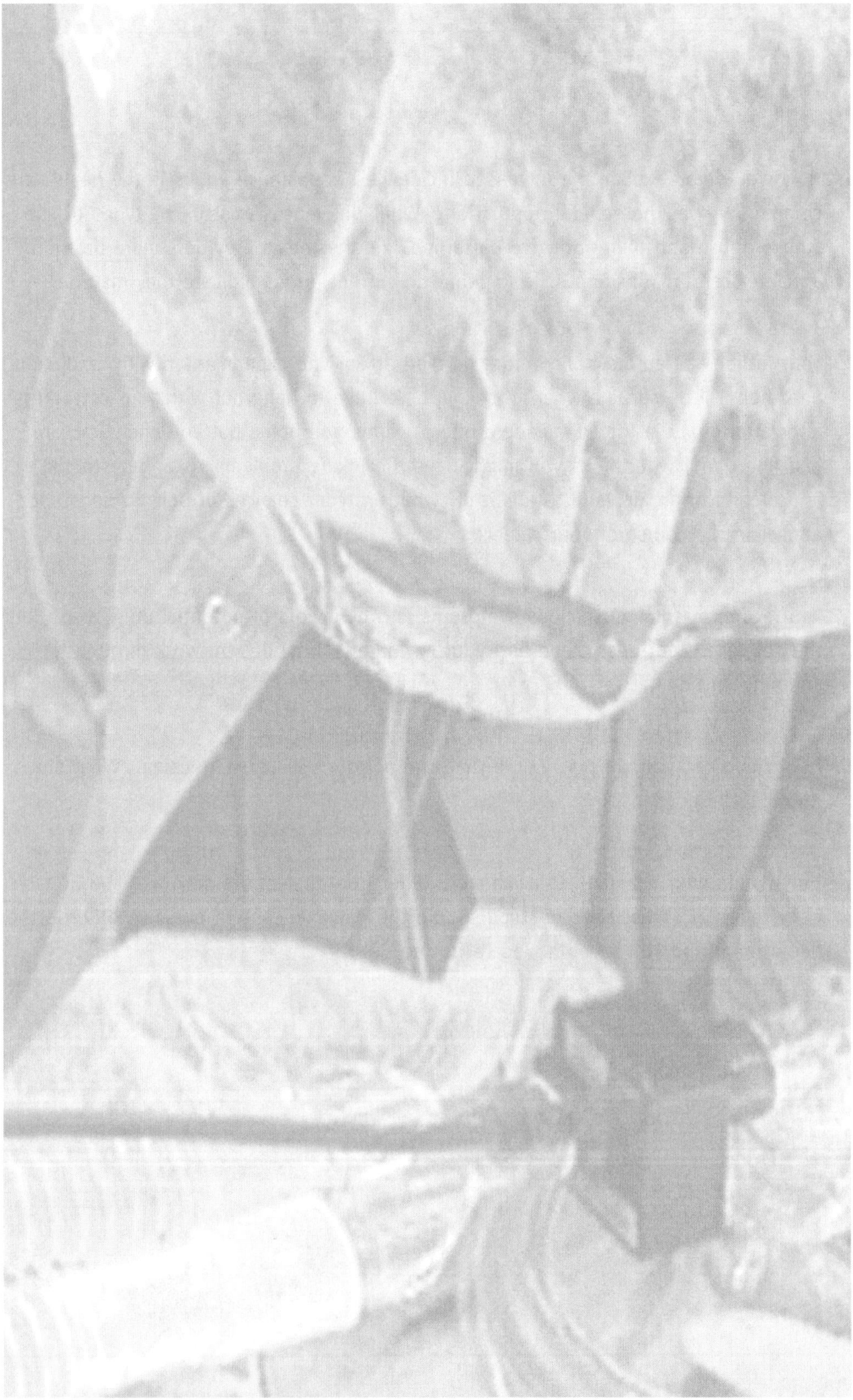

CHAPTER 22

PEER ASSISTANCE – PART 2

Diana Quinlan, CRNA, MA

Chair, AANA Peer Assistance Advisors Committee
Jacksonville, FL

KEY CONCEPTS

- Intervention and/or disciplinary action need to be anticipated and planned.
- All personnel should know the disciplinary options in their state, especially whether they have access to alternative programs in lieu of board of nursing action.
- The treatment process should include a model based on abstinence and the 12 steps, provide detoxification services and residential programs that are very important to the anesthetist addict, and be designed specifically to meet the needs of nurses/doctors in treatment.
- Reentry into the workplace is possible after a good treatment program but must include an aftercare contract, supervision, appropriate work hours, random drug screening, and frequent evaluations.
- Ethical and legal aspects need to be considered regarding the returning Certified Registered Nurse Anesthetist which must balance the employee's rights and the duty to protect the patient.
- Prevention strategies make the entire identification, treatment and reentry process manageable.
- The American Association of Nurse Anesthetists offers many resources in peer assistance, including a network of state peer advisors, a national support group, and a Web site of informational tools.
- Local resources and departmental in-services can provide necessary support information while institutions should have an overall employee wellness philosophy that encourges advocacy and prompt intervention.

The preceding chapter lays the foundation for this chapter by reviewing the history and incidence of chemical dependence in nurse anesthesia professionals. It cites theories, symptoms, and risk factors for addiction among the helping professions and discusses its relationship with the workplace by looking at departmental responsibilities, including intervention and guidelines for managers. This companion chapter will take the reader to the next logical step by discussing treatment options and disciplinary processes and their alternatives. Issues related to recovery, reentry, and relapse are addressed, as are pain management, prevention strategies, and peer assistance efforts.

TREATMENT

Chemical dependency is a treatable disease. Those who have it, and their families, should be entitled to the same care as those who have any other disease. Treatment should be found in the mainstream of the American healthcare system with a full range of services. Treatment of an addictive disease is different from any other disease because denial, guilt, and shame inhibit the individual from asking for help. Furthermore, the disease cannot be eradicated with antibiotics or surgery, there are few laboratory tests that can predict the progress of treatment, and success in treatment requires the complete commitment of the patient (Angres, Talbott, and Bettinardi-Angres, 1998).

Programs

The predominant format for facilities in the treatment of chemical dependence is abstinence-oriented and introduces a 12-step program. Inpatient or residential treatment programs offer the best options for the healthcare provider. However, personal financial constraints, as well as constraints imposed by the increasing use of health maintenance organizations and other insurance restrictions, now make this a rarity. The alternative when residential treatment is not feasible is the use of intensive outpatient (IOP) therapy. With this eventuality in mind, it is important to stress to managers and anesthetists the importance of being adequately insured with both health and disability policies to avoid financial catastrophe. Table 22.1 lists specific elements essential to a modern inpatient program.

This residential treatment approach is holistic in nature as it attempts to address the physical, emotional, and spiritual needs and wounds of the addict. Anesthesia providers seem better served in programs that are geared specifically to health professionals. These innovative treatment programs use other recovering healthcare professionals in the process. Mirror image therapy, a concept pioneered by Talbott (1983), helps the newest arrivals to treatment see the progress made by other addicts with the same professional background. Goals become tangible when seen through the eyes of a professional colleague who has had a similar experience.

Whether someone can access a residential program or must rely on IOP, there are essential characteristics of either that should be indicative of a good program for the professional with impaired practice. It is vital to screen treatment programs, preferably before the need arises. If a crisis occurs, there will be a plan of action and confidence in the type of care preselected. Table 22.2 lists the essential components to look for when screening treatment programs.

Process

The treatment process is generally divided into four major components of care: detoxification, evalution, therapy and dis-

Table 22.1: Elements of Modern Inpatient Programs
• Detoxification from alcohol and drugs
• Monitored abstinence from mood-altering agents
• Treatment of current medical ailments
• Positive health habits in diet, exercise, sleep
• Participation in supervised group and community therapy
• Diagnostic evaluation and self-revelation
• Evaluation and intervention with the family
• Mediation with the employer and authorities
• Introduction of Alcoholics Anonymous or Narcotics Anonymous
• Short-term limited objective counseling
• Instruction in short-term recovery skills
• Discharge planning and continued aftercare
Source: Talbott Recovery System, Atlanta, GA. 1987. Used with permission.

Table 22.2: Screening Treatment Programs
• Consider chemical dependency a primary disease
• Multidisciplinary team—medical, psychological, and neurobehavioral components with nurses, therapists, social workers, and physicians
• Alcoholics Anonymous (AA) or 12-step model
• Focus is physical, mental, emotional, and spiritual needs of nurse
• Staff experienced, well-credentialed
• Significant census of other healthcare practitioners
• Family therapy component
• Provides comprehensive evaluation and then individualized treatment plan
• Accredited by the Joint Commission on Accreditation of Healthcare Organizations
• Aftercare plan individualized prior to discharge
• Follow up and consultation with employer
• Introduction to AA, Narcotics Anonymous, healthcare professional support group
• Long-term follow-up (2-5 years)
• Availability *after* discharge
• Flexible payment plan

charge planning. Not everyone requires detoxification from drugs or alcohol, so many enter treatment at the evaluation stage. If the assessment indicates treatment would be advantageous, the addict is encouraged to stay and begin the therapeutic portion of the process. The last part of the treatment is discharge planning. This service can be invaluable in helping addicts communicate effectively with their employers and licensing bodies, and in planning reentry to practice. Table 22.3 shows the four-pronged process for treatment.

Selection

Of all the criteria to consider in selecting a quality treatment program for the anesthetist, one of the best indicators is the patient census. Sending nurses or doctors to treatment where they are the sole health professional client may not be in their best interest. Having an anesthetist in an environment where group therapy is the cornerstone of treatment is important, but an anesthetist who is the lone health professional becomes the resident "expert" in the group, rather than the patient. The healer reverts back to trying to heal others and does not get the help needed. The caretaking that got the nurse into trouble initially may resurface and the situation may become nontherapeutic.

Cost

The cost of residential treatment currently ranges from $15,000 to $30,000. It usually includes one 28-day inpatient course and two years of follow-up (aftercare). Most major health plans are accepted by treatment facilities, but declining reimbursement has hit the mental health community very hard. If health insurance pays this expense, it is considered a one-time coverage. Treatment for relapse, lost wages, and drug screening tests are generally not compensated by any health insurance plan.

Because treatment is so costly, yet vital to survival, it is imperative that managers and employers permit a leave of absence during this time frame. In most cases, this assures continued health insurance coverage. Employers who react by terminating the employment of the professional create a situation in which the addict may perceive the only options as suicide or fleeing to another job, thus perpetuating the problem.

Disability coverage is often difficult to obtain, or maintain, after treatment. Malpractice insurance was long unaffected by the diagnosis of addiction because there was no public record of patient injury directly resulting from an impaired anesthesia provider (Polk, 1991). Recent changes now restrict a provider from obtaining an individual liability policy for a minimum of five years of uninterrupted recovery. However, one may still access coverage by joining a group with an existing policy. The restrictions are less prohibitive with a group, and the situation is more ideal for the returning professional, since supervision, not isolated practice, is recommended.

Ultra-Rapid Opiate Detoxification

Although current, mainstream treatment approaches do not support ultra-rapid opiate detoxification (UROD), it is a trend with promise if claims of its success hold true as research continues. During UROD, patients are managed under a general anesthetic and given opiate antagonists to flush the opiate from the body and block its effect on the brain. It is designed to treat addictions to opioids such as heroin, acetaminophen-oxycodone (Percocet), codeine, methadone, and fentanyl.

Gooberman, a New Jersey internist and member of the American Society of Addiction Medicine (ASAM), provided this treatment to approximately 300 patients in one year as a four-hour outpa-

Table 22.3: Screening Treatment Programs

TREATMENT: DETOXIFICATION

- Opiates may require 3-5 days; purer, larger doses; high dependence
- Medically supervised withdrawal
- May require hospital and nursing care for seizures, tremors, nausea and vomiting, diarrhea, respiratory failure, anxiety
- Ultra-rapid opioid detoxification may be option
- Multi-phased evaluation begins
- Suicidal precautions, isolate

TREATMENT: EVALUATION

- Medical history and physical
- Addiction history
- Psychiatric and family assessment
- Team conference to develop care plan
- Review detoxification outcome, history and physical, intervention report, evaluation teams, nurse's notes

TREATMENT: THERAPY

- Group, individual, and 12-step
- Overcoming denial
- CD education about disease concept
- Learn nonchemical coping
- Abstinence-based recovery model
- Continued medical care
- Recreation, art, music therapies
- Introduction to self-help groups
- Family therapy

TREATMENT: DISCHARGE PLAN (A SIGNED CONTRACT)

- Type of follow-up care
- Peer assistance program (monitor)
- Local therapist, medical doctor
- Limitations on practice
- Alternative disciplinary program or state board of nursing
- Meetings (support groups)
- Random drug screens
- Re-evaluation before reentry

tient process. The treatment allows the patient to undergo physical withdrawal while under anesthesia, and the patient wakes up drug free, bypassing the agony that an addict would normally experience (Drug Benefit Trends, 1999).

Loimer, in Austria, introduced UROD in 1988. He wrote that heroin and other opiates produce a "high" by chemically linking with receptors in the brain associated with pleasure from food, sex, and sometimes exercise. In a patient undergoing UROD, opiate antagonists displace the opiates by attaching themselves to the receptors. The opiates are flushed out of the body in the detoxification process. If the patient continues taking an antagonist drug such as naltrexone (ReVia) after detoxification, the antagonist blocks opiates and a high is not achieved (Loimer, 1988).

While Gooberman agrees that UROD is not a cure, he believes that the naltrexone therapy the patients are asked to maintain for six months to a year increases their chances of staying "clean and sober." He encourages patients to use a support system of family, religion, or a 12-step program with the naltrexone.

Another provider of rapid detoxification, the Center for Investigation and Treatment of Addictions (CITA), uses a similar method. The CITA program has treated thousands of addicts in Italy, Spain, Mexico, Germany, and Israel and is currently offered in the United States in various locations. The CITA treatment includes a 24-hour hospital stay and a six-month aftercare program.

Other programs are offered in an outpatient setting with general anesthesia and at less cost but do not include the follow-up therapy so vital to the addiction recovery process. Detoxification alone is insufficient for continued recovery. It needs to be utilized in conjunction with strong aftercare. The issues that cause an individual to become chemically addicted continue to be issues until ameliorated with proper counseling and therapy.

Addicts say that UROD's quick and less painful detoxification gives many the courage to quit. The National Institute on Drug Abuse (NIDA) does not endorse rapid detoxification treatment, but has not taken an official position. NIDA researchers say the method is "without ethical, medical, scientific, or financial justification as a clinical treatment at the present time." Other critics call UROD expensive and unproved because the volume in this country to date is insufficient to provide an adequate sample for study, and there has been little peer-reviewed scientific publication in this area.

NIDA admits that opiate detoxification has "no known mortality risks in uncomplicated cases," but that the risk of serious adverse events, including death, with anesthesia is about one in 15,000. The article also points to the risk of aspiration and choking during UROD. However, CITA and other centers' patients are intubated and ventilated when treated, so there is a protected airway. The risk of anesthesia is small compared with the risks associated with continued heroin use, since heroin addicts have a 20 percent mortality rate if left untreated (Hellinghausen, 1996).

While both CITA and Gooberman support rapid detoxification therapy, they disagree on the best practice. CITA is opposed to anesthesia use in a nonhospital setting and relies on weekly individual and group therapy to enhance outcomes. CITA claims 70 percent of overseas patients were "clean" a year after detoxification (Drug Benefit Trends, 1999).

According to NIDA, studies have indicated "a small but significant incidence of cardiovascular complications including cardiac arrest and pulmonary edema" with the use of naloxone, one of the opiate antagonists used to accelerate the detoxification process. However, David Glatts, a CRNA at the Gooberman clinic, restricts patients with a history of cardiac problems or asthma from the procedure and applies the same precautions for anesthesia as any standard outpatient setting (Drug Benefit Trends, 1999).

UROD supporters admit it is not a cure but rather another weapon in a limited arsenal. They argue that the high rate of return to drugs for graduates of inpatient detoxification and rehabilitation programs indicates that addiction is a disease state and, therefore, like any other disease, the emphasis of care should be on the most efficient and humane treatment.

NIDA reserves its hopes for UROD as a treatment of last resort. If it is subsequently proven safe and effective with rigorous scientific investigations, NIDA contends UROD may have some use in the treatment of extremely high-risk individuals who are dependent upon opiates and who would otherwise turn down more conventional detoxification procedures.

As the nation's healthcare system focuses on the least expensive way to provide only the most necessary care, a comparatively inexpensive method to treat addiction will appeal to healthcare cost-cutters (Hellinghausen, 1996). NIDA estimates the daily rate for inpatient detoxification programs in the United States at $285 a day. Even though UROD allows acute withdrawal from drugs within hours under general anesthesia, rather than days, at present "it is estimated that the cost of UROD is about two to three times the cost of more traditional inpatient methadone detoxification procedures of 10 to 13 days in duration," said the NIDA article. It also emphasized that medication without psychosocial support has little impact on opiate addiction and long-term relapse prevention (Drug Benefit Trends, 1999).

Methadone Maintenance

A National Institutes of Health panel convening on the effective treatment of opiate addiction decided that methadone maintenance therapy has clear medical and economic benefits for both the individual and society (Drug Benefit Trends, 1999). The panel called for insurance coverage, improved training for physicians, and a reduction in unnecessary federal and state regulations. This endorsement for methadone maintenance has not been met eagerly by all in the treatment community. Many believe that giving another addicting substance to treat addiction only compounds the problem. Much controversy remains regarding the safest, most cost-efficient method of detoxification and maintenance of recovery.

Rational Recovery

An alternative method of treatment was founded by Trimpey in 1986 and is touted as an aggressive "self-recovery" program (Trimpey, 1996). The basic premise of this "addictive voice recognition treatment" is that one can come to recognize one's own inner voice, override it's influence, and remain abstinent. Trimpey contends that this simple thinking skill permits anyone to recover immediately and completely from addiction. Rational recovery (RR) does not see addiction as a disease, but rather as a failure of the addict to take control by recognizing the recurring thoughts that feed the inappropriate or addictive behavior.

It is important to note that ASAM and most leading treatment facilities do not recognize RR as an effective option. RR does not believe that denial is a symptom of the disease of addiction or even that addiction is a disease. Instead, proponents of RR advocate that an addict deny using ("never incriminate yourself"); refuse to participate in Alcoholics Anonymous (AA), even as an option to jail for driving under the influence; and assert constitutional rights (hire an attorney and fight for First Amendment rights—freedom of religion) rather than submit to an imposed treatment program. This confrontational approach is in opposition to current advocacy program philosophy and places most addicts in a position of conflict with licensing boards that work with alternative programs (Trimpey, 1996).

DISCIPLINE

Disciplinary actions taken by state nursing licensure boards involving the use of drugs or alcohol range from 67 percent to as high as 90 percent (Fowler, 1986). These actions are highest for the advanced practice nurse, with the CRNA being the nursing specialist with the highest percentage of disciplinary action related to substance abuse.

State boards of nursing have varying philosophies regarding their role as it relates to the impaired nurse. Despite a resolution by the American Nurses' Association (ANA) which advocates offering treatment antecedent to disciplinary action, many boards of nursing continue to take a punitive approach to addiction. A 1986 study conducted of these boards confirmed that the majority, believing their primary obligation was to the public, took a very caustic posture toward the addicted nurse. Few states then had any interest in developing programs for nurses with impaired practice and believed they had little latitude for alternatives to discipline (Markarian and Quinlan, 1986).

Many boards of nursing that offer only discipline clearly do not understand the disease concept of addiction. If they did, they would afford nurses the same quality of care and consideration they expect nurses to provide their patients with a disease. Instead, there remains a pervasive prejudice against addicted nurses who are instead treated as if their addiction is a moral or ethical dilemma rather than an illness. Keep in mind that the American Medical Association (AMA) and other leading medical authorities clearly categorize chemical dependency as a treatable disease. Since making this pronouncement, the AMA instituted a movement that led to the establishment of an alternative approach for physicians in *every* state. Each state medical board supports a process that enables the physician to voluntarily seek assistance and safely reenter practice under contract.

Nursing and medicine began this process of offering alternatives at the same time, in the early 1980s. The medical community achieved total state participation over 10 years ago, nursing is still debating the issue. Nurses face a disciplinary process that may include criminal prosecution, incarceration, and revocation of license. Sadly, this is often accompanied by lack of treatment and even death or suicide.

Legislative Models

The National Nurses Society on Addictions (1985) published a legislative model for the establishment of diversion programs. This model supports the intent of the ANA resolution in that it provides an avenue for treatment before disciplinary action. States that have enacted such legislation report success in retaining, treating, and returning nurses to the workforce.

In 1990, the ANA published a monograph titled *Suggested State Legislation: Nursing Disciplinary Diversion Act* that included a rehabilitation model with an immunity provision that is helpful in negotiating reentry agreements (ANA, 1990). The term "diversion" was an unfortunate choice, since it is often confused with the diversion of controlled substances from the workplace, rather than diverting the nurse into a nonpunitive program. The term "diversion program" was replaced with terms like "alternative programs" or "nondisciplinary."

The National Council of State Boards of Nursing (NCSBN) published a handbook to be used as a model resource for its member state boards of nursing (NCSBN, 1997). Its introduction gives a glimpse of the discrepancies in states' disciplinary approaches. The handbook clearly states that the resource contains materials that support the "alternative program approach," while others support the "discipline philosophy." Because member state boards of the NCSBN are voluntary, the NCSBN has no authority to mandate that states take a singular approach to chemical dependency.

Alternative Approaches to Traditional Discipline

New models for approaching chemical dependency in nurses were introduced during the 1970s and 1980s that combined aspects of both the traditional discipline process and the preventive peer assistance approach. As knowledge increased about the disease of addiction and alternative approaches provided services with improved outcomes, more states moved toward the alternative model (ANA, 1990).

Nonpunitive disciplinary options vary from established peer assistance committees that advocate for the impaired nurse to the state board of nursing issuing a charge letter that offers the nurse an opportunity to negotiate a settlement prior to a full evidentiary hearing. In the second case, the license is suspended or revoked but with a stay of action that places the individual on probation. As long as the nurse complies with the terms of probation (treatment and aftercare), the stay protects the license. Nurses may actually return to work with the stay in place under close monitoring. This is another example of a nonpunitive approach that serves both the public and the professional (Dorsey and Scheer, 1987).

ALTERNATIVE PROGRAMS

Alternative programs are recognized by the appropriate state regulatory board, such as a board of nursing, and offer a voluntary, nonpublic opportunity for healthcare professionals whose practice is potentially impaired. This is done with close monitoring by program staff in lieu of formal disciplinary action on the professional license. Where these programs function, legislative authority has generally been granted by the state and approved by the board of nursing to conduct such activity. The nonpublic aspect of this approach maintains monitoring and licensure activity in closed files that are usually purged after five years of successful recovery. Public disciplinary approaches publish in the board of nursing newsletter the name of the nurse, the nurse's town of residence, and action on license indicating substance abuse.

Recently the public has questioned the fairness of nondisclosure, especially in states operating under the "sunshine law." If the process for investigation and action by the legislatively approved alternative program is well established, consistent, and well documented internally, and outcomes are tracked objectively, there should be less cause for alarm by the public. An interim report on a study conducted by Yocom and Haack (1996) that compared the two regulatory approaches—traditional discipline versus alternative—revealed that the retention rate after reentry for the alternative model was almost twice that of the disciplinary approach (68 percent versus 37 percent). This presumably is attributed to the quality of aftercare during monitoring.

By 2000, 60 percent of states offered formal legislation or alternative programs that permitted treatment without an adverse judgment upon the license. At present, even the states with some advocacy offer a variety of models for alternatives to disciplinary proceedings. Each may have a different legal or professional provision since the state maintains the authority to decide which model best serves the public. Therefore, a consensus within nursing does not exist. That translates to differences in discipline, treatment, monitoring, and reentry for the addicted nurse based solely on geography.

There currently is a movement of national advocacy groups, including the AANA Peer Assistance Advisors Committee (PAAC), to urge nursing to take a consensus approach to impaired practice. Many state boards are hesitant to offer an alternative to discipline, citing duty to patient safety. These organizations fail to see that the alternative approach actually provides better patient safety because it identifies chemically dependent (CD) nurses sooner and removes them from practice within hours to days. The traditional discipline method often requires six to 18 months of documentation, investigation, and hearings before the nurse is removed from practice. Within the same time frame, a CD nurse can often be identified, treated, and reentered to safe practice under a rigid monitoring program.

The saying, "Nursing is an army that shoots its wounded," has been used many times by those exasperated with the lack of progress within nursing. While it is

Table 22.4: Aftercare Contract
• Group or individual therapy (nurse support or caduceus groups)
• 12-step meetings (AA, Narcotics Anonymous)
• Total abstinence from *all* mood-altering substances, including alcohol
• Continued medical care by a contract physician with addiction education
• *No* medication without prescription from contract physician (over-the-counter medication included)
• Random drug screens (including "drug of choice")

hoped that advocacy groups can turn this tide, it ultimately will take the concerted effort of countless nurses to petition their own state boards or state legislators to create and fund alternative programs. It will also take the cooperation of colleagues to urge appropriate policies and guidelines within their workplaces that provide advocacy and support.

It is hoped that positive results with alternative programs will lead all boards of nursing to eventually take an uniformed approach to chemical dependency among nurses. To date it has been a tedious process, and this slow response by the nursing profession has contributed to the continued and often permanent loss of skilled nurses to a treatable disease.

It would be wise for CRNAs to know the provisions for disciplinary action related to impaired practice within the states in which they hold licensure. Information on disciplinary action is provided to other states so that multiple licensures will be affected by the action on one license. A CRNA who has the misfortune to become addicted in a state with no alternative discipline, despite being licensed in other states with less punitive approaches, will be disciplined by the state in which the activity occurs. Therefore, it would benefit the nurse to work toward an ideal model that affords the disciplinary alternatives, access to evaluation and treatment, monitoring contracts, and reentry assistance. With at least one in 10 CRNAs statistically at risk, every anesthetist in this country will be involved in some manner with a colleague needing this service. How it is handled impacts the entire department as well as the addict. One can best be prepared by supporting legislation that provides the best alternative program for the practice area and by creating or revising departmental chemical dependency policies.

CONTEMPLATING REENTRY

For CRNAs who have successfully completed treatment and are in active recovery from drug addiction, reentry into the workplace may be contemplated. The time away from the job will be dependent upon multiple factors, including the drug of choice, the disciplinary process, the quality and efficacy of treatment, and adequacy of aftercare, among others. After treatment, but prior to reentry, the health professional should be adapting to the new life with the aid of an "aftercare contract" (AANA, 2000). These contracts are generally developed while in initial treatment and continued as a follow-up therapeutic plan. They act as a bridge of continued care when the anesthetist returns to the workplace. Table 22.4 lists the salient features in a model aftercare contract.

Specific considerations for reentry to practice must include elapsed time, legal constraints, licensure, credentials, clinical and cognitive skills, emotional readiness, job availability, insurability, and willingness. The addicted nurse must really consider, "Do I really want to return?"

Talbott devised a rating system to determine if anesthesiologists are fit to return to practice (Angres, Talbot and Bettinardi-Angres, 1998). Category I indicates they can return as soon as they are judged to have accepted their disease, demonstrated a balance in recovery of bonding with AA and Narcotics Anonymous (NA), have healthy family support, have no presence of psychiatric disease, and are fully committed to a recovery contract. Category II suggests they are not prepared to reenter and should be reassessed after two years of well demonstrated recovery. These individuals experienced some relapse, remain dysfunctional but show improvement, are not yet bonded with AA or NA, still have a healthy attraction to anesthesia practice, remain in some denial with occasional mood swings but are demonstrating that their recovery skills are improving. Basically, they just need more time removed from the stressor of anesthesia practice and continued remediation.

Category III advises that no return to practice be pursued. This practitioner had prolonged intravenous drug use, previous failed treatments, and relapses, and has a component of severe psychiatric disease or personality disorder, severe family dysfunction, and poor recovery skills. It is difficult for the untrained to easily differentiate these categories because so much of an employer's assessment would be based on the addict's own interpretation of his or her own progress. For this reason it is imperative that employers obtain appropriate evaluation documents from the treating facility as well as from the program monitoring the practitioner in recovery. Negative drug screens alone are not sufficient determinants of one's compliance in recovery or readiness for reentry.

Some departments of anesthesia have had success with early reentry (less than six months after treatment) by using naltrexone as an adjunctive drug. Naltrexone therapy is indicated for opioid addiction and was also approved for alcoholism treatment in 1995 (Hudson, 1998). It is a useful pharmacological adjunct in the prevention of relapse, as it blocks opiate receptor sites and negates the desired effect should the recipient use a substance. If the person uses, detection in a positive drug screen would indicate a need for reevaluation and possibly return to treatment.

Simulator Assessment

Another innovative approach to reentry includes the use of an anesthesia simulator for both the self-assessment of readiness and the updating of clinical skills (Quinlan, 1998). Since there are a myriad of triggers for relapse in the surgical environment (sights, sounds, smells, tactile sensations), this situation can be invaluable to determine relapse potential. The recovering CRNA spends blocks of time in a fully simulated surgical environment, surrounded by all these triggers and managing clinical anesthesia scenarios.

The simulator is a life-sized "patient" mannequin fully integrated to a computerized system that will allow the operator to intubate orally or nasally, cannulate veins or arteries, auscultate heart and lungs, check pupillary changes, defibrillate, and even catheterize. It has a drug recognition system that interprets the actual administered dosage, producing an appropriate physiologic response on the monitors in concert with the inspired gases.

These devices are ideal for educational institutions to use as teaching tools and one can see the obvious advantage to utilizing this for someone contemplating reentry. This process would sharpen clinical skills and help the anesthetist regain confidence while in a controlled, fully observed environment. Although the simulation will be stress producing, none of the anxiety will be associated with patient safety. Rather, the stress can be used constructively to evaluate the recovering individual's reaction to old triggers.

The entire scenario is recorded on video and can be reviewed with the anesthetist for further education, as well as insight into the emotional aspect of the experience. Any process that would allow the impaired provider opportunity for regaining clinical skills in a protected environment has definite benefits. Ideally these opportunities for clinical simulation can begin during aftercare as individual progress dictates. For some this may affirm early in their recovery that a return to the workplace is possible; for others it may indicate that a change in profession might be appropriate. This information would be valuable to those situated in states where punitive licensing boards have mandatory terms that restrict reentry up to five years. Anesthetists may discover potential problems before committing to a job, before placing a patient in their care, or before embarrassing themselves to prove something they are not equipped to handle at this time. For some it may be the ultimate test in which they determine that the triggers bring back too much, and they have time to reconsider whether they truly want to reenter that stressful environment.

Refresher Courses

While the simulator experience has great potential, there is also a need for an educational component to bring the reentering anesthetist up to date with newer agents and adjunctive therapies. Several nurse anesthesia programs are entertaining the idea of refresher tracks for this purpose. It will benefit not only the recovering nurse, but also anyone who has experienced an extensive lapse in clinical time (i.e., child rearing, research, education, or administrative work). Additionally, the PAAC is seeking ways to offer Web-based instruction for continuing education credit specific to addiction to satisfy an increasing number of boards of nursing stipulating this on their monitoring contracts. There is currently one AANA-approved refresher course that provides instructional materials over the Internet. It requires that the recovering nurse find his or her own site for the clinical component of the course. This requires an intact nursing license.

Employment Considerations

Whether a recovering anesthetist has the benefit of naltrexone therapy or simulator retraining, there are other assessments that focus on the prospective job setting (Quinlan, 1995). The potential to participate in group insurance policies, have set limitations on the accessibility of the departmental drug supply, and be given adequate supervision initially with work schedules that do not permit isolation, are key elements. Written contracts with specific consequences or instructions regarding drug screening, timely evaluations, adequate departmental policies for narcotic accountability, and specified consequences for relapse are all issues to discuss up front. These considerations are summarized in Table 22.5.

Coworkers

Barriers to reentry can include institutional prejudice, lack of coworker support, and some practice restrictions (Hughes, Smith, and Howard, 1998). Prior to reentry, addressing the concerns of coworkers is essential. Management personnel should honestly explain the need for any special considerations (supervision, key control, drug screens), conduct an in-service on chemical dependency, and tighten all pertinent policies and accountability procedures. Every effort should be made

Table 22.5: Employment Considerations
• Liability insurance availability
• Position limitations (supervision, no call or shifts, no access to keys to drug storage cabinets)
• Signed written contract (with specified limitations, testing protocol, policies)
• Random drug screens (on demand, toxicology specific, chain of custody, CRNA pays for own screens)
• Departmental policies in place
• Performance evaluations at one, three, and six months, then every six months
• Continuing aftercare plan from treatment program
• Specified consequences for relapse

to make the coworker feel comfortable with the situation. Most CRNAs in recovery find it easier to work in an environment in which they can share their recovery rather than hide it. This level of openness leads to greater collegial support and understanding. It also reduces potential enabling if the situation is well understood by all colleagues. Perpetuating "the secret" in the workplace only puts additional stress on all parties.

REENTRY

The American Society of Anesthesiologists (ASA) has addressed the issue of whether successful reentry is possible in the field of anesthesiology. Citing a 60 percent to 80 percent recovery rate for physicians, and having no specific data for anesthesiologists, many wondered if returning to the work environment is in the addict's or the patient's best interest. A survey of residency program directors by Menk revealed a success rate of only 34 percent for anesthesiology residents who were narcotic addicts compared with 70 percent for nonnarcotic addictions (Polk, 1991). The lasting effects of this survey do a disservice to the anesthesia community, as Menk did not ascertain critical comparative information, such as the type of treatment, length of time out of the workplace, and aftercare contracts. It is not uncommon to hear reports of residents returning to training within weeks of treatment and without the benefits of a strongly structured recovery program. A later study by Paris and Canavan (1999) demonstrated that anesthesiologists have no statistically different relapse rate than other physicians; however, they do have a higher opiate abuse rate (78 percent versus 42 percent).

Neal Gray, MD, a certified addictionologist and an anesthesiologist at the University of Texas at San Antonio, credits strong institutional policies and rigid aftercare contracts for the successful return to work by all anesthesiologists he has treated. The follow-up care includes the usual regimen of abstinence from mood-altering substances, regular AA or NA meetings, and random drug screens. It also includes naltrexone therapy for opiate abusers and a strict sample-collection protocol. Additionally, recovering anesthesiologists must pay for their own drug screens (Polk, 1991).

Confidentiality

An important legal issue is the right of the nurse as opposed to patient or public responsibility (Quinlan, 1994). Confidentiality of information and records concerning substance abuse is addressed by the Department of Health and Human

Services (HHS) under Part 2 of Section 42 of the Code of Federal Regulations (CFR) (Arnold, 1991; HHS, 1987).

When the facility employing the recovering healthcare provider (patient) is a recipient of federal funds, information obtained during that patient's management may be disclosed only with written consent of the patient. The regulation permits "communication of information within a program" during management of the patient's care and between a program and a "qualified service organization." The latter would include impairment committees or state diversion programs. The intervention process could also be interpreted as patient management and, therefore, disclosure of this information, except to a treatment program, could be illegal.

Disclosures

It is wise to secure a written consent from the recovering addict before disclosing anything related to the person's substance abuse. A letter of recommendation, for example, should be composed only after up-to-date permission has been obtained. This consent must include "the name of the person making the disclosure, the recipient of the information, the name of the patient, the need for disclosure, the extent of information to be disclosed and a statement that permission may be revoked at a later date" (Arnold, 1991).

It must also include a declaration indicating that its confidentiality is protected by the aforementioned federal regulation and that further disclosure without the written approval of the addict is prohibited.

Institutional Liability

Institutions have a responsibility to their employees (or credentialed staff) to develop policy, provide education, be consistent with discipline, and provide adequate preventive measures regarding chemical dependency. Schools and universities have additional responsibilities, especially if they receive any federal funding. Table 22.6 outlines the five key areas of this responsibility.

Federal Protections for the Handicapped

Regulations found in Title 45 of CFR Part 84 concern the rights of handicapped individuals (Quinlan, 1994). Under those regulations, "handicap" applies to "any person who has a physical or mental impairment which substantially limits one or more major life activities" including work or employment. "Mental impairment" is defined as "any mental or psychological disorder" and includes both alcoholism and drug addiction.

The regulations state that any individual who "can perform the essential functions of the job in question" is considered by law to be "qualified handicapped." Furthermore, the regulations state: "No other qualified handicapped individual shall solely by reason of his handicap be excluded from the participation in, be denied the benefits of, or be subjected to discrimination under any program receiving federal assistance." This is broadly interpreted to include hospitals reimbursed under Part A of Medicare (Arnold, 1991; DHEW, 1977).

This law then raises the question as to whether a recovering addict may be a "qualified handicapped." That judgment must be made individually based on the facts surrounding the abuse, the job to be performed, and the risks involved for the employer (HHS, 1987).

The history of substance abuse makes the issue difficult. A case could be made that the recovering provider is not trustworthy. Some older studies claim that recovering anesthesiologists who have been addicted to opiates are more likely to relapse than are those who have

Table 22.6: Institutional Responsibility

1. Policies and Procedures
    - Philosophy of employee well-being
    - Recognition of CD as a disease that *can* effect job performance
    - Fitness for duty policy
    - Supportive intervention and treatment
    - Protocols for drug screening
    - Supervision for reentry
2. Education
    - In-service training on CD for *all* employees
    - Managers trained to identify and intervene with chemical dependent employee
    - Consultation services for manager
3. Consistent Discipline
    - *All* suspected employees offered same disciplinary process
    - Awareness that enabling behaviors are reinforced with inconsistent approaches
    - Consistent policy implementation so others will not be fearful to report
4. Provisions
    - Adequate healthcare coverage
    - Disability coverage offered (especially for anesthesia providers)
    - Routine performance evaluations
    - Employee assistance program
    - Protocol to follow to seek services
5. Universities and Schools
    - Student assistance programs
    - Referral of students to treatment
    - Educational course on CD
    - Train instructors and faculty to identify CD, intervene, and find treatment options

been addicted to alcohol or nonopiates, including cocaine (Arnold, 1991). Nevertheless, 45 CFR Part 84 prohibits discrimination based solely on a history of substance abuse. Therefore, legal recourse is available if employment is refused.

Americans with Disabilities Act

The Americans with Disabilities Act (ADA) was passed in 1990 and provided broad legislation with significant implications for regulatory agencies, such as boards of nursing. The ADA has taken shape during the last 12 years as case law and review articles interpret the law. Congress designed the legislation to protect disabled persons from discrimination in employment among other things. The ADA defines disability as "...with respect to an individual, a physical, or mental impairment that substantially limits one or more of the major life activities of such individual; a record of such an impairment; or being regarded as having such an impairment." Mental impairment is broadly defined and includes "... any mental or psychological disorder such as mental retardation, organic brain syndrome, emotional or mental illness, and specific learning disabilities...."

Within the ADA, chemical dependency *is* classified as a disability as long as the individual is in active *recovery*. Therefore the ADA requires "reasonable accommodation for *recovering* chemically dependent employees." This does not mean that an employer has an obligation to hire the recovering individual. But given equal qualifications, the addiction history should not be a restriction to employment (NCSBN, 1997).

Title II regulations require that boards of nursing not arbitrarily discriminate against qualified individuals with disabilities. The U.S. Supreme Court held in *Southeastern Community College v. Davis* (1979), under section 504 of the Rehabilitation Act, that an "otherwise qualified person is one who meets *all* requirements in spite of his handicap, not except for his handicap." Licensure differs from employment in that demonstrating the ability to perform a full range of duties was found essential, and courts have tended to defer to the judgment of licensing boards.

The ADA does *not* prohibit discrimination against persons who are currently using illicit drugs or who demonstrate continued use of a drug. The illicit use, possession, or distribution of drugs is considered unlawful under the Controlled Substances Act; it does exclude those taken under the supervision of a licensed healthcare professional, and it also excludes alcohol. The regulations do make provisions for individuals who are in active recovery or participating in a supervised rehabilitation program. This provision is the basis of state legislation that supports the concept of nursing peer assistance programs, offering an alternative to the traditional disciplinary approach.

A blanket position that a chemically dependent nurse can never practice again would not survive a challenge under ADA. Boards of nursing may need to focus less on the status of being chemically dependent and more on the effects on nursing practice. Needed is a tailored case-by-case approach with clear rationales for licensure decisions that explain how their determinations protect the public.

Title III prohibits discrimination on the basis of disability by private entities operating as places of public service; this would obviously apply to almost all patient care facilities in this country. If an individual can perform, with or without accommodation by the employer, the essential functions of the position, he or she is considered qualified for the job. Reasonable accommodation would include job restructuring, part-time or modified work schedules, or reassignment to another position. Pre-employment inquiries must be limited to questions covering the ability of the individual to perform the job. Employers may not inquire about an individual's disability or require medical examination until after a conditional job offer has been made. An offer can be conditioned on the results of such examination only if all applicants are required to have such an examination or drug screen. The information must be treated as confidential and filed separately from other personnel data (Arnold, 1991).

If the potential employer "can demonstrate that the accommodation would impose an undue hardship on the operation of its program," then the employer is in compliance when refusing to hire (DHEW, 1977). Recent case law further defines the ADA, and chisels away at the protection initially offered to those with addiction. A decision by the federal Equal Employment Opportunity Commission (EEOC) in March 1996 ruled that federal agencies are not required to offer an employee a "firm choice" between treatment for alcoholism or discharge, but may terminate the person's employment even when the deficiency in question is addiction-related. In response to this case (*Johnson v. Babbitt*) and many similar ones, the ASAM recommended that this type of employee be offered opportunity for rehabilitation, and that the ADA should be amended by Congress to remove discriminatory language regarding alcoholism and drug dependency (ASAM, 1996).

National Practitioner Data Bank

The federal government is taking an active role in addressing the issue of substance abuse as it relates to public safety. One legislative act established a national clearinghouse for the reporting of adverse actions against licensees or credentialed professionals. Formally opened in 1991, the National Practitioner Data Bank (NPDB) collects and releases information related to the professional competence and conduct of physicians, dentists and, in some cases, other healthcare practitioners (Quinlan and Bodenhorn, 1990). This information is intended to direct discrete inquiry into specific areas of a practitioner's licensure, professional society memberships, medical malpractice payment history, and record of clinical privileges (NPDB, 1986).

The information is intended to augment, not replace, traditional forms of credential review. The flow of information is two-way. Credentialing bodies are mandated to report chemically dependent physicians and dentists and may voluntarily report nurses. Those entities granting licensure or clinical privileges similarly query the bank for adverse actions on any practitioner applying for privileges. It is highly recommended that practitioners periodically query the NPDB itself to ascertain whether their name has been submitted erroneously. The self-query can be accomplished by requesting the appropriate application over the Internet (www.npdb-hipdb.org/docs/QA.htm#Self Query); a valid credit card is accepted for the fee, which is currently $10.

This self-query by law cannot be sent to a third party, like a board of nursing, preferred provider organization, or insurance company; its remains a confidential request between the inquirer and the NPDB. There is a mechanism for disputing either the factual accuracy of the information in the report or whether the report was submitted in accordance with NPDB's requirements. These requirements include whether the reporting entity was eligible to report to the NPDB. This discourages libelous characterizations by allowing entries only from authorized agencies, credentialing bodies, and insurance providers with firsthand information. A guidebook to the NPDB printed in May 1996 and with recent chapter revisions is offered on the Web site.

Healthcare Integrity and Protection Data Bank

Congress recognizes that healthcare fraud burdens the nation with enormous financial costs and threatens healthcare quality and patient safety. Even with the NPDB, it was thought that there was not a comprehensive source of adverse action information on healthcare providers, suppliers, and practitioners. Congress recognized this void and in 1996 the Health Insurance Portability and Accountability Act was enacted as Public Law 104-19, Section 221(a). This act directed the secretary of HHS to create the Healthcare Integrity and Protection Data Bank (HIPDB) to help combat fraud and abuse in the healthcare delivery system. The goal is to provide a resource to help health plan or federal and state programs determine if the providers they seek to employ are ethical and professionally competent.

Since 1999, federal and state government agencies and health plans are required to report to the HIPDB all final adverse actions taken against a healthcare provider, supplier, or practitioner since August 21, 1996. The types of adverse actions that must be reported to the HIPDB include:

- Healthcare-related civil judgments against healthcare practitioners, providers, and suppliers.
- Healthcare-related criminal convictions against healthcare practitioners, providers, and suppliers.
- Adverse actions taken by federal or state agencies responsible for licensing and certification of healthcare practitioners, providers, or suppliers.
- Exclusions of healthcare practitioners, providers, and suppliers from participation in federal or state healthcare programs.
- Any other adjudicated actions or decisions as established by regulation.

The HIPDB is a central repository of information for use by federal and state agencies, licensing boards, law enforcement agencies, and health plans when conducting thorough investigations of healthcare providers, suppliers, or practitioners. Eligible users can obtain information on healthcare-related adverse actions taken against any licensed or certified healthcare professional, such as a physician, dentist, nurse, or physical therapist, by submitting a query to the HIPDB. This information is intended to augment, not replace, traditional forms of review and investigation, and it is intended to be an important supplement in a careful review of a provider's, supplier's, or practitioner's past actions (HRSA, 1999). Information from both the NPDB and the HIPDB is available on their joint Web site (www.npdb-hipdb.org).

Wrongful Determination

Ward addressed the issue of liability for a well-meaning colleague who attempts to intervene and then finds the coworker is not suffering from chemical dependency (Polk, 1991). It is unlikely that suspicion of substance abuse would rise to the level of intervention without irrefutable evidence such as behavioral changes, work performance, and narcotic count discrepancies. Unless a secondary diagnosis, such as a personality disorder, complicates assessment or judgment of the accuser, it is highly unlikely that a defamation case would be supported. If the colleague's and the patient's safety are the paramount reasons for pursuing action, and the intervention has been conducted in a confidential manner, the accused, in Ward's judgment, would probably not risk publicizing the case by bringing suit. "In either event, liability is much more likely to be due to *not* taking action when a colleague and his patients are in jeopardy because of the disease."

Coworker Legal and Ethical Responsibilities

Coworkers have certain legal responsibilities in identifying and reporting a CD CRNA. Many state boards of nursing have mandatory reporting laws that may hold a colleague responsible for harm to patients if the colleague fails to report a coworker suspected of impairment. Documentation of performance and behavior of a suspected colleague is essential to objective evaluation of the situation, as well as crucial to an effective resolution or intervention. Collegial responsibility also includes documenting behavior, participating in the plan to get a nurse to evaluation and/or treatment, lobbying for alternative programs, supporting education and research, and insisting the department update its policies and procedures.

Major hospitals and universities often offer employee assistance programs. Other facilities may have established networks with regional peer assistance programs or other specialized services. CRNAs should consider addiction an occupational hazard and lobby for the availability of resources to effectively address this increasing problem.

Reentry into the Workplace

Reentry into anesthesia after a period of absence creates a stressful time of readjustment. A person who has been in treatment for an addictive disease will need the same period of adjustment as a person who has been away from clinical anesthesia for any other reason. Recovering persons should be encouraged not to rush back to work, but to allow time to develop a new abstinence-based lifestyle and new coping mechanisms. People who are in recovery from substance abuse may enter the profession more aware of their feelings, who they are, and what their goals are, and be better equipped to seek support from peers than prior to seeking treatment.

CRNAs reentering a department of anesthesia fear rejection by their peers. They are ready and willing to work to regain the trust and respect from their peers, but they need to be met halfway in this effort. Recovering anesthetists are aware of their disease of chemical dependency—a disease requiring their attention—and strategies for a lifetime to prevent relapse. The "internal critic" is well developed in the professional. Thus, recovering professionals make dedicated and grateful employees who will be dependable and willing to work hard and will expend great effort in keeping their personal and professional lives in balance.

Informing Colleagues

Before a recovering nurse reenters an anesthesia department, the department manager should assess the feelings and concerns of the staff working directly with that individual about chemical dependency, the recovery process, the recovering CRNA's needs, and the support needed from the staff for a successful reentry. The manager will need to monitor the reentry and keep in close contact with the recovering employee. Evaluations should be performed periodically as stipulated in the return-to-work contract. Sensitivity and support from the staff are essential to help the recovering anesthetist adjust to new employment.

Educating the staff about alcoholism and drug addiction can facilitate reentry to practice. Initial reentry should be as free of stress and temptation as possible. Therefore, it is highly desirable that the anesthetist be assigned initially to only day-shift duty without night call. Rotating shifts or overtime are best avoided early in the recovery as well. Because this may add a burden on other department members, it would be therapeutic to have a session that allowed colleagues an opportunity to express their feelings and concerns.

The employing institution has a legal obligation to the public. Historically, most institutions do not want to accept the potential legal liability by employing a recovering professional. However, trends are changing slowly. More institutions are establishing peer assistance programs to help and support the recovering substance abuser during recovery. Aftercare contracts and new laboratory screening techniques have given the institution the tools necessary to assure the public and protect itself. New medications such as naltrexone and disulfiram (Antabuse) are also available to complement the recovery process.

Aftercare

Returning to the workforce after appropriate treatment is challenging for both the recovering anesthetist and the employer. To make reentry smooth for both parties, a written contract is recommended that clearly states the expectations of both (Robbins, 1987; Sullivan, 1988). The contract is necessary for the employer and the agency overseeing the recovery process, e.g., treatment facility, state diversion program, or impaired nurses committee. Table 22.4 lists the essential components of an aftercare contract to demonstrate the range of expectations present in early recovery.

Before reentry into the workplace, a return-to-work contract should be established between the employer and recovering anesthetist (AANA, 2000). Each contract should be geared toward the particular individual involved according to his or her particular situation. Also, state board of nursing rules and guidelines should be taken into consideration when designing a reentry contract. A reentry contract, though similar to the aftercare contract, may be more restrictive than the state's monitoring requirements, but must not be more lenient. Privileges for the CRNA to resume administration of scheduled drugs such as narcotics should be made by the individual responsible for supervising the CRNA's progress in the workplace, in conjunction with the addictionologist and/or primary physician. Rigid drug accountability policies must be in place as part of this expanded scope of practice. Legal counsel should draft the actual reentry contract. A sample chemical dependency policy for departments of anesthesia, which fully details the types of conditions expected by all staff within the department regarding drug testing, narcotic accountability, and education, can be found on the AANA peer assistance Web site at www.aana.com/peer. Such a policy provides groundwork for consistency and avoids the pitfalls of multiple layers of accountability and mixed expectations. A model reentry contract is also found at www.aana.com/peer. It lists essential components of a good recovery plan for the prospective employee and clearly articulates what the department expects of the employee and the consequences for failure to comply.

Reentry Guidelines

Anesthesia providers with a history of chemical dependency may (re)enter the department if they can show sufficient evidence of successful completion of treatment and documentation of uninterrupted active recovery. Applicants or employees with a history of chemical dependency should provide evidence of successful completion of drug or alcohol rehabilitation and sustained active recovery and sobriety. They should possess a current nursing license and any required registration or certification, including active recertification as a CRNA, as determined by the AANA Council on Recertification of Nurse Anesthetists. Anesthetists can reenter practice under a provisional recertification with approval by the council. These individuals should have their history kept in confidence and their anonymity protected until such time that they choose to divulge their anonymity, and be treated with respect and afforded all opportunities granted to others with disabilities. Last, they should abide fully with all departmental policies and comply with the conditions set forth in a rigid written reentry contract.

An ASA survey of anesthesia training programs found that only about 50 percent of physicians with a history of fentanyl abuse returned to the specialty following treatment (Arnold, 1995). Of those who returned, the employment of nearly half was terminated either voluntarily or involuntarily. In that group, the apparent relapse rate was nearly 20 percent per year over a maximum period of 18 months. In contrast, for those who abused nonopioid drugs, the relapse rate was about 4 percent. The use of naltrexone as an adjunct was not mentioned. This must, however, be placed in context. The rate for relapse in the general population is approximately 70 percent with a recovery rate of 30 percent. When compared with the public, healthcare providers maintain a higher level of recovery in both quality and longevity.

Evaluation

In addition to the contract, there should also be mechanisms for ongoing evaluation of work performance. These assessments should be more frequent at first, weekly then tapered to monthly. Recovering anesthetists should also contribute to the process by providing written objectives for their own progress.

All reporting and assessments should remain confidential. However, department coworkers should know that the anesthetist is in recovery. This is beneficial for several reasons. It actually assists the anesthetist to remain compliant when supporting staff are knowledgeable about the disease. It also decreases enabling behaviors of well-meaning colleagues and explains the need for rigid supervision of narcotic administration. The self-disclosure also helps the addict deal with the new work situation with complete honesty. Keeping secrets is stressful and a trigger for relapse.

Naltrexone (ReVia)

Naltrexone is an agonist used to block the effects of opiates and most recently alcohol (Hudson, 1998). It can be an effective adjunct to a quicker reentry time since it places another level of confidence in the aftercare process. To begin therapy, the patient must be narcotic free for seven to 10 days. It is dispensed in tablet form for oral use. Because some addicts have been known to "cheek" their drug by slipping the pill inside their buccal mucosa rather than swallowing it, some advocate that the tablet be crushed and given in a small amount of liquid. The manufacturers recommend a simple syrup solution in this situation so that the drug is not altered by the pH of acidic juices. Dosing begins with a test dose of 25 mg, increased in increments up to 150 mg/day by the third day. One 50 mg tablet will block the euphoric effects of 25 mg of heroin. Liver enzymes should be followed up during the course of treatment, which may extend several years. The screening costs to check liver enzymes and the blood level or naltrexone, plus the cost of the treatment drug, make it somewhat expensive.

Side effects are minimal, with the exception of a 13 percent incidence of nausea. The remaining effects of insomnia, fatigue, dizziness, and/or vomiting average around 2 percent. The benefits include ease of administration (oral), rapid gastric absorption, and a good narcotic-negating effect should the patient use. Like any drug treatment, an addict may learn to use the drug of abuse in an amount sufficient to override the effects of naltrexone. Naltrexone does not block the effects of cocaine or benzodiazepines. Addicts who try to override the narcotic blockade by using while taking the drug often experience profound respiratory depression. Random screens and close supervision should be adequate to determine whether an individual is attempting to override the naltrexone block. Individuals receiving naltrexone should wear a Medic-Alert device.

The person's condition should be stabilized on naltrexone therapy at least one week prior to return to work. This therapy is initiated and maintained under medical direction and should not be terminated suddenly. A contract that is written with naltrexone as an adjunct should include a board hearing (attorney, chief anesthesiologist/CRNA), be a three- to five-year contract that begins upon reentry, and should include a staff in-service (operating room, postanesthesia care unit, others). Naltrexone administration should continue for two years and be discontinued only upon the agreement of an evaluating team.

The issue of whether to utilize naltrexone as part the recovery process requires considerations beyond the risks and benefits of the adjunctive therapy. CRNAs often relapse within two weeks, even after a year or more off from work, despite excellent intentions, a rigid contract, and being cleared for return to work. For the first six months to a year, naltrexone or disulfiram may be used as an adjunct to the return-to-work program. The certified addictionologist or primary physician in charge of the medical and psychological care of the recovering CRNA should determine the advisability of these two drugs, as well as other medications prescribed for the anesthetist.

Managers should always remember that naltrexone is only an adjunct to quality aftercare. It is also important to have a highly functional narcotic policy that requires returning unused narcotics to a central drop box, periodic audit of anesthesia and narcotic records, random drug screens, and frequent performance evaluations. The benefits of utilizing this technique can be great for both addicted CRNAs and their coworkers. The CRNA is able to return to work sooner and administer narcotics to patients with added confidence. The anxiety for the staff should be reduced with these checks in place. It is perhaps the best option for recovered opiate abusers who are able to reenter, and it can be individually tailored over time to fit the situation.

RELAPSE

Relapse is a recurrence of disease symptoms after a period of improvement. It is a progression of cognitive and behavioral patterns reactivating feelings like isolation, elevated stress, denial, and impaired judgment. It is important to distinguish a "slip" from a relapse. A nurse inadvertently taking over-the-counter cold medication containing some type of mood-altering substance may cause a "slip" that generates a positive drug screen. These kinds of singular events, though a lapse in judgment, may not indicate a return to addictive behavior and should be remedied with counseling and tighter screening. Relapse in anesthesia personnel appears to be higher with opiate addiction. Several studies have indicated it is highest in anesthesia residents, leading to a response by some medical societies to not advocate for a return to anesthesia practice for these residents (Polk, 1991). However, it may well be that the resident relapse rate is higher with opiate addiction because appropriate advocacy, support, and accountability are not in place for reentry and the resident is often rushed back into training within days to weeks of leaving.

Relapse rates are very difficult to determine and useless if not considered on a case-by-case basis. Length and quality of treatment, time away from work before reentry, rigid aftercare contracts, narcotic accountability policies, and reentry contracts are just some of the considerations to compare when determining why relapse occurred in a specific person. Statistics without qualifiers do a great injustice.

A retrospective study of recovering anesthesiology residents who reentered service under monitoring found that relapse rates remained fairly constant during the entire 10-year study period. The annual relapse rate was 14.4 percent overall and 18.9 percent among opioid abusers (Arnold, 1995).

Thomas Hornbein, MD, of the University of Washington, developed a policy in which resident and staff anesthesiologists were granted one chance to reenter practice after treatment but were not allowed to return if they had one relapse (Polk, 1991). The Medical Society of New Jersey will "not advocate for anesthesia residents in recovery to return to their programs and will give practicing anesthesiologists only one chance at reentry to the specialty" (Polk, 1991).

Some people are likely to experience relapse just because they reside in a geographic location that lacks advocacy. Others experience relapse because their employers expect them to return to work full time with call and full access to narcotics less than a month after treatment. Still others experience relapse because their entire treatment plan consisted of only one week of therapy and an hour per week with a counselor.

The Intervention Project for Nurses (IPN), Florida's alternative program for nurses, has been in existence for more than 10 years (Hughes, Smith, and Howard, 1998). The project has assisted over 6,000 nurses, includes 70 nurse support groups and trained facilitators throughout the state, and has approximately 800 nurses in these groups at a time. In the program, the relapse rate is less than 5 percent and well documented. It succeeds because it is consistent in its restrictions, allows reasonable time away from the job, and provides excellent follow-up and rigid contracts for all nurses, including CRNAs. In determining relapse rates, it would be inaccurate then to average this state's rate of 5 percent with states without any advocacy or those with only tentative support and lack of structure.

Anecdotal information gathered by the AANA PAAC indicates that CRNAs can reenter the workplace safely and enjoy long-term recovery. A study conducted by Seibert and Demenes (1996) while members of the AANA PAAC clearly indicates this is most successful when the CRNA has received quality in-patient treatment and long-term follow-up.

The continuation of an aftercare contract is also an essential feature of long-term recovery. There appears to be a trend toward relapse in those with long-term sobriety or recovery of five to 10 years or more. Many of these individuals acknowledge a gradual slip once the formal contract period is over, all practice restrictions are lifted, *and* the rigors of anesthesia practice escalate. Addicts must work on their recovery daily, especially those who return to active practice. It would be wise to consider a lifelong plan for recovery as long as the anesthetist is actively practicing anesthesia. This would include continued attendance at support groups such as AA, plus random urine drug screens on a quarterly basis. This will keep the CRNA grounded in the recovery plan and provide some measure of long-term accountability.

Others are also beginning to see this trend toward relapse after long-term recovery. The IPN in Florida initiated a three-year relapse prevention program as part of its aftercare contract with licensees. It includes one continuing education (CE) credit per month, offered at the nurse support group meeting, as part of a 36-CE credit curriculum. This curriculum is specific to relapse prevention techniques using the Gorski method. Participants gain the skills needed to identify relapse triggers, learn coping techniques, and earn valuable CE credit at the same time.

PAIN MANAGEMENT CONSIDERATIONS

Management of chronic as well as acute pain for the substance abuser is fraught with controversy. Regardless of whether the pain is acute or chronic, the goal of treatment should be the alleviation of pain. There are tools within the armamentarium to consider before utilizing narcotics. These should be explored thoroughly with a pain management specialist. Addicts have experienced relapse because their medical provider was not well versed in either the options to managing pain or the delicate nature of selecting adjuncts with addiction in mind.

Therapeutic agents such as heat, cold, transcutaneous electrical nerve stimulation, massage, psychotherapy, hypnosis, relaxation techniques, regional anesthetic blocks, and medications may play a role. Again, the written contract is a vital part of the treatment plan. The optimal contract will have provisions for pain management that suggest limitations on healthcare provisions. When chronic pain is an issue, there should be only *one* prescriber, *one* pharmacy, and specific delineation of times to take medications (e.g., 8-4-10, rather than TID). In this way, medication can be dispensed and accounted for in a manner that is least likely to be abused.

In establishing a chronic pain management regimen, the treating provider needs to ascertain that the addict is properly detoxified from addictive substances and stabilized on appropriate alternative medications if possible. The addict should increase recovery activities by increasing counseling or therapy, adding more 12-step meetings, obtaining drug-specific screens, and making more frequent office visits. Attempts should be made to use nonmedical therapies. These efforts should all be documented and agreed upon within the confines of a written contract.

The monitoring program managing the addict's aftercare contract will need to update the contract by including the name of the pain management specialist, a list of approved medications, and a drug-screening protocol that takes into account the new drugs or therapies. It would be counterproductive to have a positive drug screen and disciplinary action initiated for failure of the treating provider to communicate these special needs in writing. There should be a scrupulous accounting of all medications dispensed on follow-up visits, accounting for any missing pills or prescriptions. And deviation from the established plan should constitute a breech of contract and grounds for referral for either evaluation in a treatment program or disciplinary action.

For the nurse in a methadone maintenance program, a baseline dosage needs to be established. In the presence of pain, dosing with the addict's usual amount will not adequately treat pain. In this situation, the addict may need to exceed the daily baseline dose. Methadone maintenance has been used primarily in this country for heroin addiction. There is much controversy regarding the use of methadone for treatment of other opioid addictions, as many believe it is merely trading one addictive substance for another, much like morphine and cocaine addiction were initially treated with heroin.

Without the combination of long-term aftercare that includes drug-screen monitoring, 12-step meetings, and group therapy, *no* adjunct to care appears to be the "magic bullet." Perhaps the best cited advantage to methadone therapy has been in the abuser of intravenous street drugs. Many of these abusers have a high criminal likelihood attached to their drug-seeking behavior. Proponents of methadone maintenance cite its longer duration of action, less frequent need for dosing, and witnessed administration as rationales for better control of the street-drug abuser.

Opponents to this therapy argue that *any* mood-altering substance, despite its substitution benefits, is still an addictive substance that only perpetuates the problem.

Treating acute pain is more complicated since practitioners unfamiliar with the addict's recovery limitations may treat the addict on an emergency basis. Reports abound of nurses being dismissed from monitoring programs because they were treated in an emergency room after an injury with medications that caused relapse. Being traumatized and in pain is a difficult situation for anyone. It is understandable that one might not be thinking clearly in these situations. Hopefully, as pharmacological alternatives become increasingly available and healthcare practitioners begin to understand the ramifications of addiction, these circumstances will decline.

ASAM reminds us that chronic pain and addiction act to exacerbate or reinforce each other (1996). They are two distinct disease processes that closely mimic one another. The essential factors in the management plan are to not *undertreat* the pain, to acknowledge the addiction, and to recognize relapse risks and triggers.

If the pain will be related to surgery, the plan should begin prior to the surgical event. Prepare in advance, have a clear understanding of what the addict was using, the level of tolerance, and prior drugs of choice. Many addicts, afraid of relapse, will put themselves in harm's way by either avoiding any postoperative pain medication or by accepting only local or regional anesthetics. Inadequate surgical anesthesia or pain relief may also be endured because addicts think they do not deserve any better. Care providers need to be observant about the signals the addict gives and, above all, treat addicts just like any other patient but with the knowledge that more drug may be needed than one would traditionally use.

One way to manage postsurgical pain is with regular, scheduled dosing rather than an as-needed schedule or patient-controlled analgesic method. Addicts should not be put back into the role of self-administration. If they have to ask for pain medication, they fear it will be perceived as drug-seeking behavior.

If the recovering nurse or person with pain is to be seen on an outpatient basis, it is important to evaluate the baseline dosage and to send the person home with as little drug as possible. If daily dispensing can be achieved with a pain clinic or other facility, this would be ideal. A week's supply should be the maximum amount sent home; never send an addict home with a month's supply of any potent drug.

Some addicts have devious drug-seeking aberrant behavior that may trigger relapse. Some of the hallmarks include needing more drug than expected and requesting specific drugs by name. A real tip-off is when the person knows more about the substance than the prescribing physician, or the person is utilizing several sources, either prescriber or pharmacy, and escalating doses without approval. Frequent refills, unapproved use of medications, resisting change in the treatment plan, and deteriorating function can also be signs of relapsing triggers.

PREVENTION

Talbott and Wright, pioneers in the treatment of health professional addiction, believe chemical dependency should be "managed like cancer, with careful attention to host and environmental factors, screening programs, investigation of alternative methods of induction and maintenance of remission, prompt detection and treatment of recurrence, and long-term follow up" (Talbott & Wright, 1987).

While the medical community quickly moved to institute an advocacy-based program for physicians in every state in the mid-1980s, nursing still lags behind. Perhaps the hope of uniting the nursing community in a similar manner rests with the networks and coalitions that are finally emerging. The National Organization of Alternative Programs was founded in 1999 with a mission of public safety, rehabilitation, and monitoring. This group is currently composed primarily of alternative programs for nurses, but its bylaws and intent are to include all types of alternative programs serving the cadre of healthcare professionals.

Other networking activities are currently underway, with the AANA PAAC taking a leadership role. A variety of nursing specialty groups rely on the expertise and information made available through this AANA effort by accessing the peer assistance Web site, the resource directory of state peer activities, informational packets, hotline, and committee members.

AANA Peer Assistance

The changing climate in nursing regarding addiction, prompted by formal resolutions from both the ANA and the National League for Nursing, led to the AANA establishing in 1983 an Ad Hoc Committee on Chemical Dependency (Quinlan, 1996). The resolutions of both organizations can be found at www.aana.com/peer. The visionary activities of this initial AANA committee included the development of one of the first position statements on substance abuse of any national nursing organization. This position statement was updated with the AANA Board of Directors' approval in 1998 and is available at www.aana.com/peer. This statement recognized addiction as a disease and its risk to the anesthesia profession. The initial position statement also established the PAAC and outlined its function.

Another outcome of the original ad hoc committee was the organization of a superb educational seminar on impaired practice. Many of the attendees became the nucleus of the peer assistance network for AANA. During this meeting, it was suggested that recovering CRNAs begin a national support group and suggested the name Anesthetists in Recovery (AIR). Other activities evolved from this nucleus group: a series of well-being newsletters and the introduction of *CRNA Well-Being: Helping Ourselves*, a peer assistance manual. This manual was revised several years later and eventually broken down into component packets specific to the needs of the users (managers, students, recovering anesthetists). Much is owed to this original ad hoc committee that boldly articulated the need and laid the groundwork for increasing activities and resources from the AANA.

Peer Assistance Advisors Committee

The AANA recognized that anesthesia providers, because of their exposure and the nature of their work, appear to be at high risk for substance abuse. In order to address these concerns within the profession, the AANA established the PAAC in 1986, building on the work of the original Ad Hoc Committee on Chemical Dependency. These peer assistance advisors serve as a resource and support for nurse anesthesia practitioners and students.

The functions of the AANA PAAC include assessing the impact of the disease of addiction on nurse anesthesia practice and educating nurse anesthetists, students, employers, and the public about addiction. They are also charged with investigating the availability and effectiveness of treatment modalities, plus advocating for research into the education, prevention, intervention, treatment, and recovery of addiction. They also assist individuals or organizations in the formulation of guidelines regarding intervention, treatment, aftercare, and reentry into the workplace.

The PAAC generally consists of three or four CRNAs and/or one nurse anesthesia student, appointed annually by the incoming president of AANA as an ad hoc committee. The members have diverse backgrounds as managers, clinicians, educators, and administrators with expertise in addictive disorders and are often reappointed to the committee to provide continuity to a service that is highly confidential and sensitive in nature.

Now in its second decade, much progress by the PAAC is evident. Legislation or alternative programs offering treatment without adverse action on nursing licenses are now available in 30 states (all 50 states offer such service to physicians). Each state nurse anesthetist association appoints a state peer advisor and committee, many offering much needed continuity by serving many consecutive years. A list of these advisors, state nursing boards, and any affiliated state chemical dependency program is updated continually by the PAAC and is available from the AANA Peer Assistance Advisors Web site under "Resource Directory."

This networking directory was expanded in 1999 to include national and international advocacy groups when it was discovered that many agencies outside AANA were utilizing this directory as a key networking resource. The directory also lists contact information by state regarding chemical dependency programs and boards of nursing. There is also an indication as to the type of programs available, e.g., alternative, disciplinary, peer assistance, or resource only.

The network of state peer advisors is maintained to provide a more personal local resource within each state as an informed contact regarding resources and provisions of their own state's nurse practice act as it relates to impaired practice. They are informed about whether the current methods used by their state board of nursing are alternative or disciplinary. There are instructional materials for state peer advisors, as well as for educators and managers.

The original committee established the concept of peer advisors or resource CRNAs from each state that would serve as a network of information and support. They were also encouraged to establish peer advisory committees within each state association to work on the local level by encouraging legislation for alternatives to discipline, assisting CRNAs to obtain treatment, and providing education about impairment. These advisors are volunteers who devote some of their time to assisting colleagues with issues that impair practice. Many of these dedicated peer advisors have been functioning as their state's resource for 10-15 years, since the inception of AANA peer assistance activities. Responsibilities and suggested functions of these advisors can be found at www.aana.com/peer.

The PAAC has maintained a peer assistance hotline since the middle of the 1990s. Assistance may be sought by calling this confidential and informational hotline, available nationwide for CRNA members, at (800) 654-5167, or help may be found by contacting a peer assistance advisor. An updated listing of all available resources is found on the Web site (www.aana.com/peer). The phone number appears in every issue of the *AANA NewsBulletin* and is posted on the AANA Web site. Many find the information recorded on the automated message sufficient to connect them with necessary resources. Still others choose the option of calling one of the PAAC members listed for more personal assistance. The nature of these calls has evolved over the years. Initially the majority of callers were seeking assistance in confirming suspicions about impaired colleagues. Current hotline callers are fairly well informed about substance abuse symptoms and are generally seeking clarification on matters of licensure, certification and credentialing, or resources for treatment. With the advent of the Web site in 1999, many hotline calls are now "Hot Email" queries.

One of the many educational activities of the committee has been to provide models to nurse anesthesia schools for the development of a drug and alcohol program that meets the requirement of federal mandates. A survey conducted by a PAAC member in 1996 demonstrated that all nurse anesthesia educational programs were in compliance with the law mandating the inclusion of policies and guidelines regarding substance abuse by students or faculty within programs that receive any federal funding, including reimbursement through Medicare for clinical sites. A model of the "Required Components of a Drug and Alcohol Program Within Schools Receiving Federal Funding" may be of further assistance to schools that would like to review their program for compliance (www.aana.com/peer).

The PAAC-member survey of nurse anesthesia programs confirmed that all offered some content on chemical dependency, ranging from one to 10 hours total (Clark, 1996; Clark & Stone, 1999). While school directors should feel some sense of relief that all nurse anesthesia educational programs are currently offering curricula on chemical dependency and abiding by federal guidelines, this is not always the case in departments of anesthesia. Unless managers see that similar offerings are available through a departmental in-service or at state association educational seminars, they cannot be assured that all CRNAs receive the message. A listing of resource organizations and educational aids useful in developing a departmental educational program can be found at www.aana.com/peer.

The PAAC will assist department managers in meeting their needs regarding in-service programming. To this end, a lending library has been established by the PAAC at AANA to provide resources such as books, videos and audiocassettes to facilitate instruction. The committee is also available through the hotline and via email to any CRNA or student anesthetist who desires information on treatment options, needs support in recovery, or simply needs questions answered. Committee members also provide seminars at state meetings, schools, and anesthesia departments.

The AANA PAAC continually works to create resources to educate members about chemical dependency. Recent additions include a Web site (www.aana.com/peer) that includes the previously mentioned model policies and guidelines, a suggested reading list for faculty and students, links to other resource sites, and key articles written by the committee on peer assistance, including management issues and anesthetists in recovery. Another resource is a brochure on "Chemical Dependency among Certified Registered Nurse Anesthetists," written by the committee and available for distribution through the AANA office (AANA, 2000).

Anesthetists in Recovery (AIR)

AIR is a national support organization of CRNAs recovering from chemical dependency (Ratliff, 1996). It is an organization involved with both education and networking for reasons of peer assistance. An attempt is made at every AANA Annual Meeting to provide an AIR meeting on site. AIR meetings are also encouraged for every state nurse anesthesia association meeting. Contact information for AIR is maintained on the AANA PAAC

Web site (www.aana.com/peer).

Members of AIR agree with the definition set forth by the AMA, that chemical dependency is a primary psychosocial and biogenetic disease. The symptoms of the disease are cunning and baffling, as is the disease itself. Although AIR knows there is no cure for this disease, it affirms that there can be lifelong remission contingent on prompt detection, intervention, treatment, and a closely followed aftercare program involving 12-step groups, peer support groups and, of most importance, carefully timed and placed reentry into the anesthesia profession.

It is the belief of AIR's recovering anesthetists that reentry must be structured and that tools such as back-to-work contracts should be utilized. There are recovering anesthetists working all over the country today. They are disciplined professionals who are grateful to be in recovery. Recovering CRNAs reentering the profession can be role models. Much is to be learned and shared by this group of anesthesia providers.

Support for the family is also vital to the anesthetist's continued recovery. Partners of Anesthetists in Recovery was founded in 2000 as a voluntary support group in conjunction with the PAAC.

SUMMARY

Addiction *is* an occupational hazard in anesthesia, as McQuillen and Lundy (1962) understood when they described it as a professional hazard almost four decades ago. Chemical dependency *is* a treatable disease. Those who suffer from it, and their families, should be entitled to the same care and support as those who suffer from any other disease.

As newer, highly addicting synthetic drugs become part of the armamentarium of the anesthetist, and the demands on the profession increase, it becomes vital that studies be conducted that continue to identify risk factors, causality, and treatment. Much of this should come from the anesthesia profession in conjunction with the treatment community. Since all nurse anesthesia programs have moved to a master's framework, opportunity for graduate research has increased. Hopefully, programs will partner with the AANA PAAC and other advocacy groups to advance the knowledge about this high-risk disease and to further develop avenues for treatment, recovery, and retention.

Education about chemical dependency in the professions should begin in nursing school, continue in nurse anesthesia curricula, and be mandated as part of CE for the CRNA. Many states now require mandatory biannual courses on hepatitis and Acquired Immune Deficiency Syndrome because they believe the healthcare worker bears a significant risk. Anesthesia providers, who have at least a 10 percent risk of becoming dependent from workplace drugs, should be offered mandatory courses in addiction with the same purposes of informing them about their occupational risk.

Recovery is *a life-long process* and a new pattern for living that is *abstinence-based.* Having a recovering member within the department should encourage employers to make certain that they have written policies governing fitness for duty, health benefit coverage for drug dependency, and effective evaluation mechanisms for overall performance. These adjustments in policies and procedures will make a department stronger and better prepared to respond to the occupational hazard of chemical dependency.

Each state board of nursing has the ability to discipline differently. There is no continuity in "punishment or advocacy" in this country when it comes to nursing. With the incidence of addiction being highest among CRNAs than in any other practice specialty, CRNAs should work for equity in treatment and disciplinary options before the need arises. This is a great dilemma the AANA PAAC is working aggressively to change through networking, policy development, educational offerings, and the Web site. It *is* time for nursing to speak with one united voice and bring about a consensus on impaired nursing practice, just as the medical community did over a decade ago. The future of peer assistance and advocacy is looking brighter. However, there is still much that needs to be changed. In this new millennium, one can hope that nursing will stop being the "army that shoots its wounded" and become the profession that cares for its own.

GLOSSARY

Many terms are utilized to explain addiction and its related processes. Each expert in the field of addictionology may have his or her own vocabulary that best describes that expert's experience in the field.

Abstinence – Commitment to nonuse of alcohol and other drugs as part of the process of recovery.

Addiction – A chronic, progressive disease characterized by compulsion to use and loss of control.

Aftercare – The period of time following formal outpatient or inpatient treatment during which performance, conduct, and compliance with an established plan of recovery from abuse or addiction are closely monitored.

Alcoholics Anonymous (AA) and 12-Step Programs – Self-help groups or fellowships that provide support and promote sobriety and recovery.

Alternative Program – A voluntary, nonpublic disclosure opportunity for chemically dependent nurses who meet specific criteria to have their recovery closely monitored by program staff in lieu of disciplinary action.

Assay – The analysis of a substance to determine its composition.

Chemical Dependency – A state in which an individual experiences compulsion to take a drug, either continuously or episodically, in order to experience its psychic effects or to avoid withdrawal.

Cage Test - A questionnaire that asks four basic questions regarding alcohol consumption. A score of two or more positive responses requires further evaluation.

Have you ever felt that you had to cut down on your drinking?

Have people annoyed you by criticizing your drinking?

Have you ever felt bad or guilty about your drinking?

Have you ever had a drink first thing in the morning to steady your nerves, or to get rid of a hangover?

Codependence – The pattern of enabling behavior and denial by those living with an addict.

Conspiracy of Silence - A phenomenon of the family, friends, or coworkers becoming involved in a manner that enables the addict to maintain the appearance of normalcy. They will conceal the problem by shifting responsibility to themselves and providing rationalizations for the addicted individual's poor behavior. (Term coined by G.D. Talbott).

Cross Addiction – The use of multiple drugs (polypharmacy) to achieve drug effect.

Detoxification – Structured treatment to overcome the withdrawal symptoms of physical dependence to become drug free.

Disciplinary Process – Procedures and activities involved in the investigative review, prosecution, and case resolution of a licensee by a regulatory board.

Drug of Abuse – Chemicals taken to produce a rapid rise of brain levels of the substance to produce a "high" rather than relief from an illness. Taken in a self-medicating style to produce euphoria or ameliorate an uncomfortable feeling (emotional or physical).

DSM IV- The *Diagnostic and Statistical Manual of Mental Disorders* of the American Psychiatric Association, Edition 4, 1994. This manual defines diagnostic criteria for psychoactive substance abuse and dependence.

Enabling - The actions, or inactions, of an individual that encourage the chemically dependent person to continue substance abusing behavior.

Gas Chromatography–Mass Spectrometer (GC-MS) – Laboratory instruments up to 1,000 times more sensitive than thin-layer chromatography that specifically identify extremely small quantities of drugs through the analysis of body fluids.

Intervention – A preplanned meeting often structured and conducted by a trained professional that is designed to confront the addict with documentation and observations of the questionable behavior. The goal of the intervention is to get the addict to admit to the behavior and agree to an assessment at an approved treatment facility.

Monitoring – The use of drug screens and input from workplace supervisors, support group monitors, and/or treatment providers to track the drug-free progress of the nurse in an attempt to ensure patient safety and competency in practice.

Physical dependence occurs when a user cannot stop taking the drug without experiencing withdrawal. Symptoms include tremors, vomiting, delirium, cramps, convulsions, or even death, and vary according to the specific drug, the amount used, and length of time abused.

Psychological dependence may be characterized as an intense craving, compulsion to use, and preoccupation with the taking of drugs. It is more difficult to treat than physical dependence since the underlying behavior must be treated.

Recovery - A lifelong process of abstaining from the drugs or triggers that brought about substance abusing behavior. For health professionals, this begins the moment they admit they are chemically dependent and continues through the process of compliance with a program designed to maintain a drug-free life.

Reentry - The return to the workplace after appropriate treatment. As part of the recovery process, conditions of reentry are often outlined and agreed upon by the chemically dependent person in an aftercare contract. Such conditions usually include continued abstinence, submission to random drug testing, evaluations of work performance, and attendance at 12-step meetings.

Relapse - Failure to maintain a drug-free status during the recovery process. A break in abstinence that often begins with distancing from participation in group meetings, results in the reemergence of denial, and leads to the resumption of addictive behavior and substance abuse.

Return-to-Work Contract (Reentry Contract) – An agreement between the recovering nurse and employer that specifies the terms and conditions for the nurse to resume or continue practice.

Slip – A brief return to drug use while in recovery. It may consist of a single use or may last for several days. The addict's response is critical: Unless the addict immediately acknowledges the event and returns to aggressively participating in the therapeutic process, the addict should be reevaluated and possibly reenter treatment.

Sobriety – The state of abstinence from mood-altering substances.

Substance Abuse – The consumption of "mood-altering agents in dosages sufficient to result in physical, situational, or emotional harm." When such behavior continues over time, a biological, physical, and behavioral process of addiction will occur in about three out of five individuals, and chemical dependence will develop.

Thin Layer Chromatography (TLC) – Laboratory procedure used to detect a very high and recent dose of drug (potentially toxic levels). Useful in the emergency department but not sensitive enough for routine screening of drugs in the workplace or as part of a monitoring program.

Tolerance - Indicated by the user requiring larger amounts of a substance to achieve a given level of effect.

Treatment - A formal program that seeks to rehabilitate the chemically dependent individual by helping the person to acknowledge the disease, return to a healthier physical and emotional state, and develop lifelong coping skills that will help maintain a drug-free existence.

REFERENCES

American Association of Nurse Anesthetists. (2000). *Chemical Dependency and the Certified Registered Nurse Anesthetist* (brochure). AANA PAAC. Park Ridge, IL.

American Nurses' Association. (1990). *Suggested State Legislation: Nursing Disciplinary Diversion Act.* Kansas City, MO: Author.

American Society of Addiction Medicine. (1996). Public policy, fair treatment of persons whose job performance is impaired by alcoholism. ASAM Web site.

Angres, D.H., Talbott, G.D. & Bettinardi-Angres, K. (1998). *Healing the Healer: The Addicted Physician.* Madison, CT: Psychosocial Press.

Arnold, W.P. (1995). Substance abuse survey in anesthesiology training programs: Brief summary. *ASA Newsletter.* 59 (10), 12-13, 18.

Arnold, W.P. (1991). Legal aspects of chemical dependence. *ASA Newsletter.* 55 (2).

Clark, G.D. & Stone, J.A. (1999). The assessment of substance abuse curriculum in schools of nurse anesthesia. *Journal of Addictions Nursing.* 11(3).

Clark, G.D. (1996). The assessment of substance abuse curriculum in schools of nurse anesthesia. Poster abstract. Substance Abuse. 17 (2), 123.

Department of Health, Education and Welfare. (1977). 45 CFR Part 84: Nondiscrimination on the basis of handicap. *Federal Register.* May 4, 22676-22702.

Department of Health and Human Services. (1987). 42 CFR Part 2: Confidentiality of alcohol and drug abuse patient records. *Federal Register.* June 9, 21796-21814.

Dorsey, D.M. & Scheer, R. (1987). Licensing boards and impaired professionals. *Maryland Med J.* 36 (3), 238-40.

Drug Benefit Trends (1999). Medscape.com/2207.rhtm. 11(1):5-6

Fowler, M.D. (1986). Doctoring or nursing under the influence. *Heart & Lung.* 15, 205-207.

Health Resources and Services Administration (1999). Healthcare Integrity and Protection Data Bank. *Issues.* 20 (4).

Hellinghausen, M.A. (1996). Rapid opiate detox therapy expands options for addicts. *Nursing & Allied Healthweek.* Sunnyvale, CA.

Hudson, S. (1998). Reentry using naltrexone: One anesthesia department's experience. *AANA Journal.* 66 (4), 360-364.

Hughes, T.L., Smith, L. & Howard, M.J. (1998). Florida's Intervention Project for Nurses: A description of recovering nurses' reentry to practice. *Journal of Addictions Nursing.* 10 (2), 63-69.

Lundy, J.S. & McQuillen, F.A. (1962). Narcotics and the anesthetist: Professional hazards. *AANA Journal.* 30 (3), 147-178.

Markarian, C.J. & Quinlan D.S. (1986). A study of disciplinary attitudes of state boards of nursing. Unpublished research.

National Council of State Boards of Nursing, Inc. (1997). *Chemical Dependency Handbook for Boards of Nursing.* 33-36, 54-56.

National Nurses Society on Addictions. (1985). *Statement on model diversion legislation for chemically impaired nurses.* Evanston, IL: Author.

National Practitioner Data Bank (1986). U.S. Government Printing Office, C.F.R. Title 45, Volume 1, Parts 1-199, Sec. 60.1, p. 130.

Paris, R.T. & Canavan, D.I. (1999). Physician substance abuse impairment: Anesthesiologists vs. other specialties. *Journal of Addictive Diseases.* 18 (2).

Polk, S.L. (1991). Substance abuse in anesthesia: Patient safety among issues. *Anesthesia Patient Safety Foundation Newsletter.* 6 (1), 1-3.

Quinlan, D.S. (1998). Retrain to retain. *Treatment Today.* (10) 1, 48-49.

Quinlan, D.S. (1996). Peer assistance: A historical perspective. *AANA NewsBulletin.* 50 (1), 14-15.

Quinlan, D.S. (1995). The impaired anesthesia provider: The manager's role. *AANA Journal.* 63 (6), 485-491.

Quinlan, D.S. (1994). Chemical dependency. In Foster, S.D. & Jordan, L.M. (Eds.), *Professional Aspects of Nurse Anesthesia Practice.* Philadelphia, PA: F.A. Davis Publishing.

Quinlan, D.S. & Bodenhorn, K.A. (1990). Update: The National Practitioner Data Bank. *Specialty Nursing Forum.* 2 (1).

Ratliff, C. (1996). Chemical dependency in the profession. *AANA NewsBulletin.* 50 (1), 16-17.

Robbins, C.E. (1987). A monitored treatment program for impaired health care professionals. *J Nurs Adm.* 17 (2), 7-21.

Sibert, R. & Demenes, M. (1996). Criteria for successful re-entry as a CRNA provider post-addiction treatment [abstract]. *AANA Journal.* 64 (5), 454.

Sullivan, E.J., Bissell, L. & Williams, E. (1988), *Chemical Dependency in Nursing: The Deadly Diversion.* Menlo Park, CA: Addison-Wesley Publishing Company.

Talbott, G.D. & Wright, C. (1987), Chemical dependency in health care professionals. *Occupational Medicine: State of the Art Reviews.* 2 (3), 581-591.

Talbott, G.D. (1983). Mirror image therapy. Address at the annual meeting of the American Association of Nurse Anesthetists, New Orleans, LA.

Trimpey, J. (1996). *Rational Recovery: The New Cure for Substance Addiction.* New York, NY: Pocket Books.

Yocom, C. & Haack, M. (1996). *Interim Report: A Comparison of Two Regulatory Approaches to the Management of the Chemically Dependent Nurse.* Chicago, IL: NCSBN.

STUDY QUESTIONS

1. You are the supervisor of your anesthesia department. Assess the current guidelines for narcotic accountability and determine how they could be improved to minimize the potential for abuse of narcotics.

2. Distinguish the difference between a recovering employee having a "slip" versus a "relapse." What considerations need to be made by you, the supervisor, and the monitoring program in determining which it is and what to do next?

3. A nurse anesthesia student during the first year of clinical rotation in your department develops an acknowledged addiction to fentanyl. How would you intervene or advise the student? What do you believe the school should do, and who should make decisions regarding what to do next? Should the clinical site or the school determine this student's fate?

4. A recovering CRNA removed from practice for one year after abusing midazolam (Versed) and propofol is returning to your department. As manager, what will you do to prepare the department? What guidelines or practice stipulations do you need to develop or consider? How do you legally and ethically prepare the CRNA's colleagues and the facility?

5. You are a new solo CRNA practitioner in a rural hospital. The operating room, postanesthesia care unit, and anesthesia department share a common narcotic inventory. The keys are sequestered in a drawer under the narcotic cabinet. You officially waste drugs by grabbing any nurse you find to witness and countersign your drug sheet. The last CRNA was fired, despite his protests of innocence, when the count came up short. No employees were screened for drugs. Now the Joint Commission on Accreditation of Healthcare Organizations is planing to conduct their next inspection in three months. As the "head" of the department, what are your concerns about this accountability policy? Design a quality assurance process that will improve this situation and dazzle the inspectors when they arrive.

6. What peer assistance activities, research, and efforts have been made over the past 15 years by the AANA on behalf of its members? How does this compare with other nursing organizations, and how do you utilize this progress in your own practice setting?

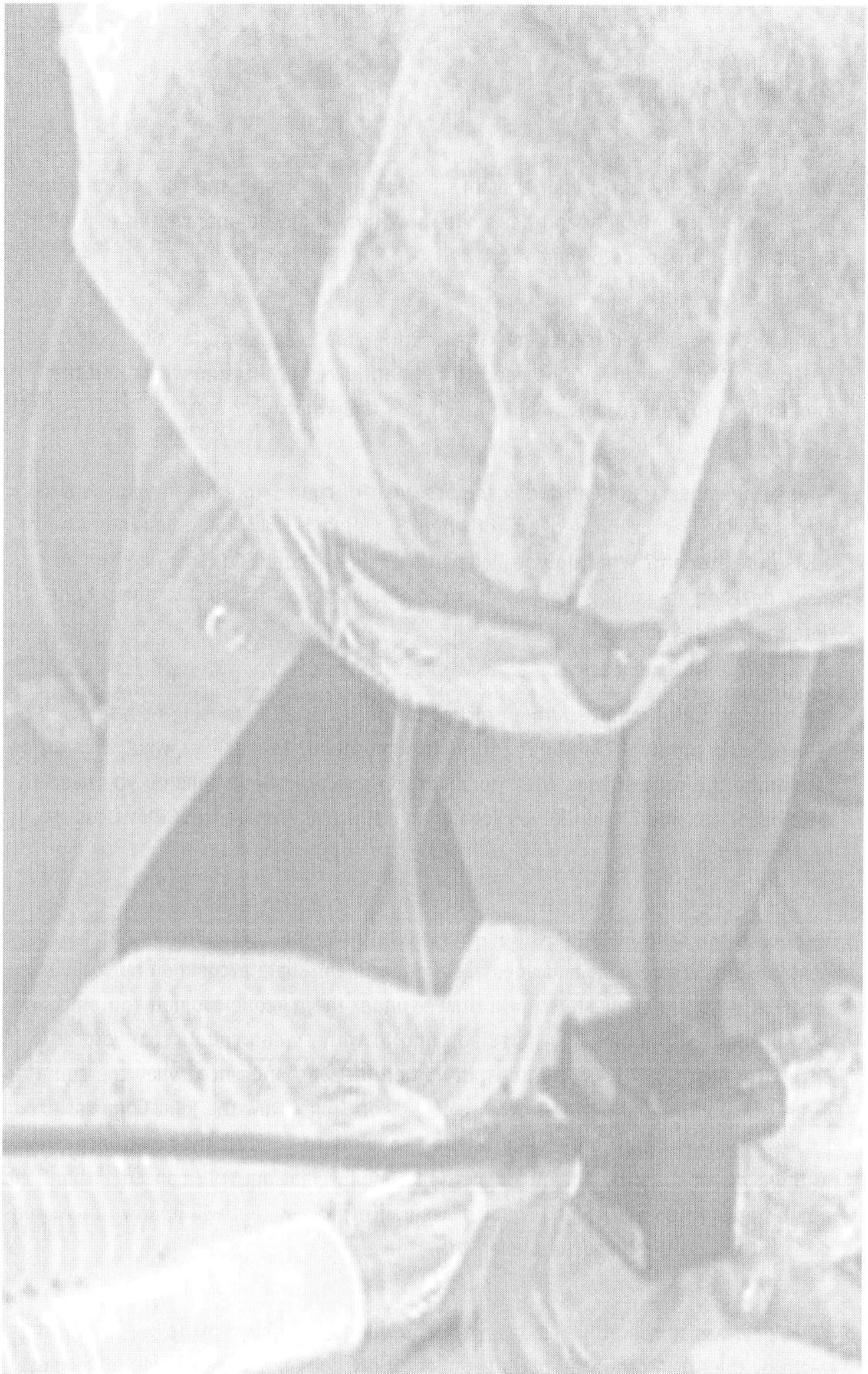

CHAPTER 23

INFORMATICS IN CLINICAL PRACTICE

Kathleen Charters, PhD, RN

Assistant Professor
University of Maryland School of Nursing
Department of Administration, Health Policy and Informatics
Columbia, MD

CAPT Cynthia S. Cappello, CRNA, MAE (USN)

Acting Chair and Program Director
Department of Nurse Anesthesia
Uniformed Services University of the Health Sciences
Bethesda, MD

KEY CONCEPTS

- Health informatics include the various approaches that have been used in medicine, nursing and clinical areas
- Computer-based patient records offer many opportunities to improve patient care and enhance patient care data.
- Standards that facilitate information retrieval include understanding principles of nomenclature and minimum data sets.
- Key terms related to decision support include data warehousing, data mining, data visualization, protocols, and expert systems.
- Technological advancements such as voice recognition, portable/wireless healthcare computers, telemedicine and the Internet have changed the way data is collected and reviewed.
- Concerns related to security and confidentiality of electronic healthcare information are now regulated through legislation such as the Health Insurance Portability and Accountability Act.
- Advances in health informatics and related technology offer many opportunities to enhance integrated health systems.

Healthcare professionals using sophisticated information technologies turn data into information and information into knowledge (Graves and Corcoran, 1989). This use of information technology is transforming healthcare. Economic forces and professional development drive the transformation. Managed care as a cost-control mechanism requires high-level access to massive amounts of low-level data, with intense analysis of that data to yield relevant information. Provider management to achieve optimal clinical care has the same requirement. According to the Healthcare Information and Management Systems Society (HIMSS, 1996a) and van Bemmel and Musem (1997), informatics is the field applying information technology and information management to business practices.

The cornerstone of healthcare information is patient data. Progress since the 1970s toward a computer-based patient record (also known as an electronic or computerized patient or medical or health record) is slow but steady (Ball, Peterson, and Douglas, 1999). Standards for common nomenclature and minimum data sets provide the necessary infrastructure for communication of healthcare data (Dick, Steen, and Detmer, 1997). Once patient data are available, the question of how to best support analysis leads to clinical decision support systems (Berner, 1998).

Healthcare data collection and review is changed by the use of information technology. One example is the use of voice recognition as a way to enter data without having to type or use mark-sense forms (Gardner-Bonneau, 1999). A second example, telemedicine, applies telecommunication and computing technology to the discipline of medicine. Portable or wireless technology is another example of changing data-collection patterns. It is possible to connect a patient with geographically distant providers in a real-time visual image with sound and simultaneously share data electronically (Coiera, 1997). The Internet has dramatically expanded access to information about healthcare for both patients and providers. For example, patients have the option of joining online help groups. Providers may electronically network and gain quick and easy access to the latest technical and professional information (Keinholz, 1997; Nicoll, 1998; Kiley, 1999; Mascara, 1999).

The use of information technology in healthcare also raises concerns (Commission, 1997). There are technical and professional challenges in maintaining security and confidentiality (Hagland, 1998; Frawley, Goldman, and Hudson, 1999). The security and privacy implications of the Health Insurance Portability and Accountability Act (HIPAA) are significant for both patients and providers (Hellerstein, 1999). As a consequence of this act, the Centers for Medicare & Medicaid Services assigns a national provider identifier to every medical doctor, nurse practitioner, and physician assistant. Medical groups, agencies, claims payment organizations, and employers are also assigned unique identifiers (Buppert, 1999). The use of electronic information raises legal issues. For example, there are legal ramifications when providers use the Internet to share health information via Web sites, communicate with patients using email, or transmit data or images for consultations (Schanz, 1999).

The greatest challenge is the need to integrate healthcare services. In the past, stand-alone systems used by specific healthcare professions and applied to specific areas of practice provided adequate support. However, the new generation of smaller affiliated facilities and the emergence of outpatient clinics, imaging centers, physician networks, home healthcare agencies, and nursing homes requires strategically rethinking and reengineering healthcare information systems. The need for community health information networks is growing. Accreditation requires improving interdisciplinary communication. Economic survival requires increased effectiveness and productivity. Government mandates require standards-based transmission of healthcare data and information. Integration of information across disciplines and between areas of healthcare delivery is essential. Anesthesia information system support fits within this paradigm. Information technology is central to healthcare organizations achieving their business goals (Kissinger and Borchardt, 1995).

INFORMATICS DEFINED

The field of informatics in the business of healthcare evolved from focusing on the discipline of the caregiver to focusing on the recipient of care. Health profession-specific informatics focuses on the discipline of the caregiver (Ball, Hannah, Newbold, and Douglas, 1995; Degoulet and Feischi, 1996; Friedman and Wyatt, 1997; Hebda, Czar, and Mascara, 1998). The first term used to describe the application of informatics to healthcare was medical informatics. Hannah, Ball, and Edwards (1999) define medical informatics as "those collected informational technologies which concern themselves with the patient care decision-making process performed by healthcare practitioners." As the field developed there was a shift to focusing on the recipient of care. The broad umbrella under which healthcare professions use information technology in combination with information management to focus on the recipient of care is health informatics (Hannah, Ball, and Edwards, 1999; Hebda, Czar, and Mascara, 1998).

Nursing informatics support the information handling work of all nursing specialties in all sites and settings of care, at both the basic and the advanced practice level (ANA, 1994, 1995; Saba and McCormick, 1995; Saba, Pocklington, and Miller, 1998). According to the American Nurses' Association (1994), "Nursing informatics is the specialty that integrates nursing science, computer science, and information science in identifying, collecting, processing, and managing data and information to support nursing practice, administration, education, research, and the expansion of nursing knowledge."

Informatics nurses develop and evaluate applications, tools, processes, and structures that assist nurses with the management of data in taking care of patients or in supporting the practice of nursing. They collaborate with other healthcare and informatics professionals to adapt or customize information technologies to the requirements of nurses (ANA, 1994, 1995; HIMSS, 1997). Informatics nurses study the flow of nursing information and use information technologies to facilitate that flow.

Clinical informatics covers healthcare providers using information systems to collect patient and client data. Information technologies support provider identification of desired outcomes for patient and clients, development of plans for achieving identified outcomes, implementation of plans, and measurement and evaluation of outcomes (ANA, 1995). Clinical systems support clinical protocols, the creation of individualized clinical pathways, and benchmarking for outcome measurement (Degoulet and Feischi, 1996). This support facilitates identification of best clinical practices and continual improvement of heathcare delivery (HIMSS, 1996a).

Information systems support decision making for all functions of providers, including clinical practice, administration, research, and education. Administration includes finance, budgeting, billing, and inventory control (Johns, 1997; Shapiro, 1999). Management engineering supports the healthcare delivery system through facilitating total quality management, analysis of operations and productivity, planning and management of facilities, and forecasting and cost-benefit analysis (HIMSS, 1996b).

COMPUTER-BASED PATIENT RECORD

In the late 1960s, visionary leaders saw the potential for using computers in healthcare information handling and developed prototype information systems (Weed, 1969). Since the early 1970s, when healthcare information systems were first used commercially (as billing systems), providers recognized the potential for improving patient records. In the 1980s, the Institute of Medicine of the National Academy of Sciences formed the multidisciplinary Committee on Improving the Patient Record. This committee (Ball and Collen, 1992) conducted an 18-month study to:

- Examine the current state of medical record systems.
- Identify impediments to the development and use of improved record systems.
- Identify ways to overcome impediments to improved medical records.
- Develop a research agenda to advance medical record systems.
- Recommend policies or other strategies to achieve these improvements.

The committee's conclusions and recommendations are described in *The Computer-Based Patient Record: An Essential Technology for Health Care* (Dick and Steen, 1991). By the 1990s, healthcare professionals widely recognized an imperative for replacing paper-based medical records with computer-based patient records (Ball and Collen, 1992). Government, professional organizations, and private industry are working to meet that goal (Ball, Peterson, and Douglas, 1999). An update is given in the revised edition of *The Computer-Based Patient Record: An Essential Technology for Health Care* (Dick, Steen, and Detmer, 1997).

Advocates for computer-based patient records include patients, clinicians, healthcare administrators, record administrators, healthcare researchers, and third-party payers. Patients are mobile and seek healthcare from a variety of providers; they need transportable records. Clinicians need readily transferable patient records and online decision-making support. Administrators need databases that support analysis of healthcare delivery. Record administrators need access to primary patient records and standards for the minimum core data set that makes up a patient record. Healthcare researchers need patient record data to support sample identification, quality of care evaluation, identification of patterns or variations in services, utilization studies, and outcome analysis. Third-party payers need faster, lower-cost electronic claims reimbursement processes (Ball and Collen, 1992).

Computer-based patient records and information systems are an essential technology in the management of healthcare quality and cost. The computer-based patient record, linked to knowledge bases and communication gateways, provides possibilities for systematic delivery of high-quality, cost-effective care. The vision includes a comprehensive lifetime view of legible, uniform patient data; collecting data only once then looking at that data in many different ways; decision support and knowledge-based aids; and increased communication. The computer-based patient record provides tools to improve quality, tools to support patient teaching, and the ability to manage care delivery and duration. The result is improved care through informed healthcare choices based on increased access to the complete and accurate patient record, studies of effectiveness and appropriateness of care, and real-time monitoring of care (Ball and Collen, 1992; Dick, Steen, and Detmer, 1997).

STANDARDS FACILITATING INFORMATION RETRIEVAL

Providers and researchers desire information relevant to particular practice and research questions. This information is distributed among many different electronic sources, including the computer-based patient record, scientific literature databases, factual databanks, knowledge-based expert systems, and directories of individuals and institutions. There are significant barriers separating potential users from healthcare information in electronic format. According to Lindberg and Humphreys (1992):

> The barriers include the variety of ways the same concepts are expressed in the different information sources and by the users themselves, the difficulty of identifying all the available sources and selecting those most appropriate to particular questions, and the range of access paths and conditions that must be negotiated to retrieve information from multiple sources.

Overcoming these barriers and developing interfaces between the various information sources requires healthcare information systems to support certain features. Key elements in the patient record must be standard and have explicit designation. Indices to the patient record and displays of patient record data must include full terms in addition to codes, acronyms, or abbreviated words.

Selected elements of patient records must have controlled vocabularies (Degoulet and Feischi, 1996). By combining existing controlled vocabularies, many of the concepts in patient records are already captured in a standard nomenclature, and ongoing work is developing other standards. Consider the nursing diagnosis standards developed by the North American Nursing Diagnosis Association and the nursing intervention and outcome classifications developed by University of Iowa researchers (McCloskey and Bulecheck, 1996; Johnson and Mass, 1997; McCloskey and Maas, 1998). Vocabulary control begins with identified minimum data sets (e.g., the Nursing Minimum Data Set as described by Werley and Lang [1988] or the Uniform Hospital Discharge Data Set) and will expand as more comprehensive data sets are developed (e.g., the Nursing Management Minimum Data Set described by Huber and Delany, 1998).

Since vocabularies and classifications may undergo substantial changes from edition to edition, detailed documentation of the various vocabularies used must be maintained. Locally developed classifications and vocabularies should be minimized. Development is difficult and time consuming, so the preferred course of action is to extend an existing system rather than create a new one. Lindberg and Humphreys (1992) promote reliance on controlled vocabularies in automated patient record systems to enhance the likelihood that these systems can be effectively linked to other information sources via the Unified Medical Language System.

DECISION SUPPORT

Providers combine clinical data within the context of health status to create information about an individual. Information from many individuals is then combined to create knowledge about a population. Knowledge is applied to decision making, as in considering the odds of a certain diagnosis given the clinical data, health status, and epidemiological prevalence. Since decision making is a process, information technology support for decision making falls along a continuum from basic (gathering data into one location to facilitate review) to intermediate (providing protocols with feedback on choices) to advanced (decision analysis and expert systems) (Berg, 1997; Warner, Sorenson, and Bouhaddou, 1997; Berner, 1998).

At the basic level of decision support, information technology provides the means of combining data then transforming data into information through data warehouses, data mining, and data visualization techniques. When electronic data from multiple sources have known meaning (as in a controlled vocabulary supporting a minimum data set), those data can be combined as required for analysis. There are two main ways this is done. One way is to build interfaces between the multiple sources. Another way is to combine the data from each source in one comprehensive database, a data warehouse. Users extract subsets of data from the data warehouse for analysis.

The following is an example of interfaces between multiple information systems. Information about a patient exists in a patient data management system, in a laboratory system, and in a radiology system. One way to get the data from three different information systems together in one place for clinical review is to build an interface between each individual system. If there is a need to see the data from each separate information system in each separate system, the interfaces will have to be bidirectional, and six interfaces are built. If only one information system is chosen as the place where all data are reviewed, the interface is from the two other sources into the one comprehensive information system. An interface is built to transfer data from the laboratory system to the patient data management system and from the radiology system to the patient data management system. Each time a change is made in any of the three information systems, the interface is adjusted to keep the data flowing as intended. Supporting the dynamic healthcare environment requires frequent changes to healthcare information systems. Therefore, maintaining interfaces between multiple information systems is costly and onerous.

Another way to approach the problem of gathering together data that reside in multiple-source systems is to create one comprehensive data warehouse. In this example, the patient data management system, laboratory system, and radiology system send their data to the warehouse. Data mining occurs when subsets of the data are extracted for analysis. Object-oriented technology is a promising means for combining data from different sources. In this example, the object is the patient, and the clinical, laboratory, and radiology data are attributes of the patient. The advantage of this approach is fewer interfaces to build and maintain, and an easier technique for adding on new sources of data.

Data visualization is looking at data in a way that facilitates understanding of the relationships between the data elements. Information technology allows data to be viewed in more than the two dimensions possible on paper. Virtual reality makes it possible to literally walk through a data set, viewing the data from any angle along the dimension of time. The ability to have multiple views of data is a critical step in moving from information to knowledge.

At an intermediate level of decision support, information technology provides protocols or care paths. Documentation of care is compared with the predetermined standards, and variances are automatically noted. The provider may override the recommendations, but annotation is expected. These tools serve as reminders of the expected course and do not supplant clinical decision making.

At a higher level of decision support, information technology provides online analytical processes and intelligent agents, supporting decision making and problem solving. Expert systems are rule based, probabilistic, or a hybrid combining knowledge-based reasoning with formal methods of decision analysis. Information technologies are best used to handle uncertainty that occurs when decision making is based on partial information. Expert systems may be used for consultation, critiquing, or simulation. Computer-aided decision analysis assists both providers and patients. Providers may benefit from diagnostic support. Patients may seek assistance in making difficult treatment decisions (Field, 1996; Coiera, 1997). One example is an intelligent decision support system consulted by an infertile couple making decisions about medical alternatives in light of their specific circumstances and preferences. Providers supply medical alternatives, physiological information, and pathological information for the knowledge base. Patients provide personal preferences and details of their individual circumstances. The intelligent decision support system works interactively to analyze the decision and produces a recommendation based on all information available (Holtzman, 1989).

Development of expert systems is generating opposing points of view. Advocates point out that the process of developing expert systems increases understanding of clinical practice and clinical judgment. Critics question the feasibility and desirability of making clinical practice more rational, uniform, and efficient. Expert systems are a tool, and any tool may be used for good or misused. Issues raised by decision support techniques need to be addressed: standardization, universality, localization, and the politics of technology (Degoulet and Feischi, 1996; Berg, 1997).

TECHNOLOGIES CHANGING DATA COLLECTION AND REVIEW

Information tools used for collecting and reviewing data are changing the way healthcare providers work. Gardner-Bonneau (1999) predicts automatic speech recognition will replace medical transcription in many medical specialties within the decade. The example of a voice recognition system for radiologists illustrates the human-factors work necessary to make a voice-recognition system useful (Gardner-Bonneau, 1999). When interactive voice-response systems are well designed, they are cost-effective time-savers.

The umbrella of telecommunication in the HIMSS includes nurse call systems, dispatch systems for code and trauma teams, network integration, application development, and telecommunication services for voice, data, and video technologies, voice processing, telephone and wireless communication systems, and telehealth systems (HIMSS, 1996c). The use of telecommunication in healthcare delivery is extensive and growing. One trend is increased use of wireless technology. For example, this technology supports traveling (for a finite distance) with a notebook computer communicating through radio frequency to a host system. This means a provider is not tied to a location by the length of a cable and does not lose network connectivity just to be mobile.

Another trend is the advance of telemedicine in supporting healthcare delivery when the participants are separated by distance (Field, 1996; Bashshur, Sanders, and Shannon, 1997). Driven by an increasingly mobile population and the geographic concentration of healthcare resources, demand is growing for remote access to care. Rural, military, and correctional systems populations are primary beneficiaries of telemedicine. The trend is increasing as specialties adapt this technology to their specific information needs, e.g., transmitting images and doing remote consulting. Established specialties include teledermatology, telegenetics, teleoncology, telepsychiatry, and teleradiology.

Use of the Internet is growing for both healthcare providers and patients. Providers use the Internet to network with colleagues, gain quick and easy access to the latest technical information, and review healthcare information. As a result, providers expand both their knowledge and capabilities. This is an opportunity to improve the quality of care through the large volume of healthcare information that providers can access (Kienholtz, 1997; Nicoll, 1998; Kiley, 1999; Mascara, 1999). Slack (1997) makes a strong case for information technology empowering patients to take a greater role in their own healthcare. The Internet brings patients together in online help groups and provides information for self-care and prevention of illness, which transfers more control to the patient.

CONCERNS

Requirements to protect privacy and confidentiality of health data include electronic health information. Health information increasingly flows through the national information infrastructure to deliver current, consistent, and accurate healthcare data at multiple sites to diverse users. Ironically, the information essential for integrated healthcare systems also creates potential for abuse and violations of security and confidentiality (Olson, Peters, and Stewart, 1998). Legal issues are raised as providers share health information via Web sites, communicate with patients by email, and transmit data or images for consultations (Schanz, 1999).

The government plays an active role regarding security issues. In 1998 the United States, at the urging of high-technology companies, loosened policies restricting export of encryption products despite concerns expressed by law enforcement and military intelligence agencies. Healthcare organizations use encryption to protect patient privacy. Public concerns over privacy and security spur legislative protection of privacy. The HIPAA legislates health information security provisions. Implementation of these provisions proactively forces organizations to be security conscious. Otherwise, they may suffer criminal sanctions as patients challenge organizations to prove patient information has not been used inappropriately. The issues have always been there, but HIPAA legislation provides an incentive to raise security and confidentiality awareness among all handlers of health information (Hagland, 1998).

Availability of health information in electronic format raises two major types of privacy and security concerns. There is increased potential for inappropriate release of information. Systemic concerns derive from open and widespread sharing of data among various parties. Health information flows from patient to provider, payer, analyst, employer, government agency, and beyond. Security encompasses both technological and organizational aspects. Technological solutions provide user authentication, access control, and encryption. The organization has a responsibility to provide training, monitoring, and enforcement (Commission, 1997). Citing the organizational requirement for establishing a security program, Johns (1997) discusses the components of security, audit, and control of health data. Moschella (1999) argues that, although there are legitimate risks that watchdog groups monitor, technology greatly increases individual privacy.

Use of the Internet carries with it additional privacy challenges driven by electronic commerce. Technology to allow trusted connections also allows collection of personal information. Internet privacy is multidimensional (Gogan, 1999). One form of privacy invasion is identity theft, another form is to gather information on children, and a third is to disclose patient record data to someone without a need to know or without informed consent of the patient. The debate is over the role the government should play versus the role the business community should play. Privacy advocates want the government to pass legislation regulating acceptable behavior regarding sensitive information whether or not it is on the Internet. Protection for patient record data requires informed consent of the patient before disclosure, law enforcement agency access only with a court order, and permission for patients to get treatment without having to agree to widespread dissemination of patient record information for peer review, research, or other purposes. Fair information practices should include the prohibition of using personal information gathered for one purpose for a second, incompatible purpose without consent of the individual (Zurier, 1998).

Commerce advocates argue the law of customer satisfaction drives self-regulation, so there is no need for government protection of consumer information. The Direct Marking Association advocates developing and posting privacy policies as a matter of conscious ethical business practices. The association supports regulation only in areas where there is potential for real harm to the consumer, such as protecting information exchanged between a healthcare provider and patient, fraud prevention, fraud protection against identity theft, and prevention of using a list to harm a child. Such laws are commensurate with the harm that comes from use of the data (Zurier, 1998).

INTEGRATED HEALTH SYSTEMS

As health informatics advances, the practice of using information technology to manage healthcare organizations and support the delivery of clinical care is extended to community and regional health networks. Information technology must meet demands for support of managed care networks, guidelines for case management, and community education and resource centers (Ball, Simberg, Albright, and Douglas, 1995). Meeting the demands and challenges of rapidly changing healthcare organizations requires reengineering information technology uses and information management systems. A dramatic shift from stand-alone hospitals to affiliated facilities requires a shift in information management strategies. The emergence of much needed standards affects information flow and organizational structure, providing an opportunity to construct an optimal information technology/information management organization. Information systems must create a more efficient and productive environment. To help healthcare organizations achieve their business goals, existing information systems must be assessed for readiness and ability to change (Kissinger and Borchardt, 1995).

INFORMATICS IN ANESTHESIA

In 1979 the introduction of an electronic anesthesia documentation system was attempted. This early attempt failed to gain widespread acceptance. Monitor manufacturers slowly developed anesthesia information management systems (Heinrichs, 1995).

In 1992, a computerized database supported tracking problems associated with anesthesia. The data were collected from a combination of handwritten records and other databases and transcribed into the anesthesia care database. Items tracked included preoperative status, anesthetic technique, drugs, physicians, surgical procedures, and events. The database provided reports of adverse outcomes following anesthesia, resident expertise profiles, and administrative data (Rose, Cohen, Wigglesworth, and Yee, 1992). This early experience was valuable in defining requirements for what data to collect, sources of data, and analysis of data.

By 1995, there were several anesthesia documentation systems available commercially. Weiss, Cotev, Drenger, and Katzenelson (1995) defined the ideal system for patient data management, then tested three anesthesia systems. The systems tested fell short of the ideal:

- Communicate with and capture data from monitors, anesthesia machines, and electronic equipment such as infusion pumps.
- Present relevant values and trends on a screen.
- Flag deviations from preselected limits of physiological and technical values.
- Provide algorithm-based decision support.
- Communicate with the hospital information system, transferring demographic data, laboratory and imaging results, and records created during preoperative consultations.

Heinrichs (1995) also found the existing anesthesia systems lacking, as they could not exchange data with other systems and there were a number of ergonomic problems.

In 1997, automated documentation systems were still underused by anesthesia. Gibby (1997) reviewed problems and possible solutions to establishing more user-friendly and effective anesthesia systems. Three studies identified the need for standardized definitions (Heinrichs, 1995; Weiss, Cotev, Drenger, and Katzenelson, 1995; Gibby, 1997). Gibby extended expectations to include reporting correlation of outcomes to care choices, based on capture of the clinical context and establishment of a standard postoperative evaluation. This brings the search for an anesthesia system back to the paradigm that information technology is central to healthcare organizations achieving their business goals.

The expected outcome of using an anesthesia system is an anesthetic record with relevant data collected automatically as well as entered manually by the provider. Ideally, the data are archived for later analysis. Advantages of an electronic anesthesia system include continuous high-quality documentation, comparability of data (assuming an anesthesia data bank), workload reduction for the provider, and availability of additional information. Concern that mental processing of data might not occur if data are automatically captured and recorded has not proven to be a problem. Therefore, the advantages outweigh the cost (Weiss, Cotev, Drenger, and Katzenelson, 1995). The benefit of anesthesia using an information system for documentation of care delivery, and using the data generated to improve care delivery, is congruent with the goals of the healthcare organization. The barriers to an anesthesia information system are the lack of standards and the lack of interfaces.

REFERENCES

American Nurses' Association (1994). *The Scope of Practice for Nursing Informatics* (NP-90). Washington, DC: American Nurses Publishing.

American Nurses' Association. (1995). *Standards of Practice for Nursing Informatics. (NP-100).* Washington, DC: American Nurses Publishing.

Ball, M.J. & Collen, M.F. (1992). *Aspects of the Computer-based Patient Record.* New York, NY: Springer-Verlag.

Ball, M.J. Hannah, K.J., Newbold, S.K. & Douglas, J.V. (Eds.). (1995). *Nursing Informatics: Where Caring and Technology Meet* (2nd ed.). New York, NY: Springer-Verlag.

Ball, M.J., Peterson, H. & Douglas, J. V. (1999). The computer-based patient record: A global view. *MD Computing.* 16 (5), 40-46.

Ball, M.J., Simberg, D.W., Albright, J. W. & Douglas, J. V. (Eds.). (1995). *Healthcare Information Management Systems: A Practical Guide* (2nd ed.). New York, NY: Springer-Verlag.

Bashshur, R.L., Sanders, J.H. & Shannon, G. W. (1997). *Telemedicine: Theory and Practice.* Springfield, IL: Charles C. Thomas.

Bemmel, J. van & Musen, M.A. (1997). *Handbook of Medical Informatics.* New York, NY: Springer-Verlag.

Berg, M. (1997). *Rationalizing Medical Work: Decision-support Techniques and Medical Practices (Inside Technology).* Cambridge, MA: MIT.

Berner, E.S. (Ed.). (1998). *Clinical Decision Support Systems: Theory and Practice (Health Informatics).* New York, NY: Springer-Verlag.

Buppert, C. (1999). PAs/NPs prepare for "enumeration," HCFA to impose national ID numbers. *Clinician News.* 1, 7, 8, 13.

Coiera, E. (1997). *Guide to Medical Informatics, the Internet, and Telemedicine.* Oxford, UK: Oxford University Press.

Commission on Physical Sciences, Mathematics, and Applications: Committee on Maintaining Privacy and Security in Health Care Applications of the National Information Infrastructure, National Research Council. (1997). *For the Record: Protecting Electronic Health Information.* Washington, DC: National Academy Press.

Degoulet, P. & Feischi, M. (1996). *Introduction to Clinical Informatics (Computers in Health Care).* New York, NY: Springer-Verlag.

Dick, R.S. & Steen, E.B. (Eds.). Committee on Improving the Patient Record, Institute of Medicine. (1991). *The Computer-based Patient Record: An Essential Technology for Health Care.* Washington, DC: National Academy Press.

Dick, R.S., Steen, E.B. & Detmer, D.E. (Eds.). Committee on Improving the Patient Record, Institute of Medicine. (1997). *The Computer-based Patient Record: An Essential Technology for Health Care* (Revised ed.). Washington, DC: National Academy Press.

Field, M.J. (1966). *Telemedicine: A Guide to Assessing Telecommunications in Health Care.* Washington, DC: National Academy Press.

Frawley, K.A., Goldman, J. & Hudson, Z. (1999). Countdown to privacy: Striving to strike a balance. *MD Computing.* 16(3), 36-39.

Friedman, C.P. & Wyatt, J.C. (1997). *Evaluation Methods in Medical Informatics.* New York, NY: Springer-Verlag.

Gardner-Bonneau, D. (1999). *Human Factors and Voice Recognition Interactive Systems (Kluwer International Series in Engineering and Computer Science).* Dordrecht, the Netherlands.

Gibby, G.L. (1997, April). Anesthesia information-management systems: Their role in risk-versus cost assessment and outcomes research. *Journal of Cardiothoracic and Vascular Anesthesia.* 11(2 Suppl 1), 2-5, discussion 24-25.

Gogan, J.L. (1999, February 8). Privacy vs. protection: Balancing privacy with free speech and e-commerce means protecting ourselves against impostors. *Information Week.* 184.

Graves, J.R. & Corcoran, S. (1989). The study of nursing informatics. *Image.* 21, 227-231.

Hagland, M. (1998, November). Six opinions on IT security. *Health Management Technology.* 16.

Hannah, K.J., Ball, M.J. & Edwards, M.J.A. (Eds.). (1999). *Introduction to Nursing Informatics* (2nd ed.). New York, NY: Springer-Verlag.

Healthcare Information and Management Systems Society. (1996a). *Guide to Effective Health Care Clinical Systems.* Healthcare Information and Management Systems Society. Chicago.

Healthcare Information and Management Systems Society. (1996b). *Guide to Effective Health Care Management Engineering.* Healthcare Information and Management Systems Society. Chicago.

Healthcare Information and Management Systems Society. (1996c). *Guide to Effective Health Care Telecommunications.* Healthcare Information and Management Systems Society. Chicago.

Healthcare Information and Management Systems Society. (1997). *Guide to Nursing Informatics.* Healthcare Information and Management Systems Society. Chicago.

Hebda, T., Czar, P. & Mascara, C. (1998). *Handbook of Informatics for Nurses & Health Care Professionals.* Menlo Park, CA: Addison-Wesley.

Heinrichs, W. (1995, February). Automated anaesthesia record systems, observations on future trends of development. *International Journal of Clinical Monitoring and Computing.* 12, 17-20.

Hellerstein, D. (1999). HIPAA's impact on healthcare. *Health Management Technology.* 20(3): 10-15.

Holtzman, S. (1989). *Intelligent decision systems.* Reading, MA: Addison-Wesley.

Huber, D. & Delaney, C. (1998). Nursing management data for nursing information systems. *Series on Nursing Administration.* 10, 15-29.

Johns, M.L. (1997). *Information Management for Health Professionals.* New York, NY: Delmar.

Johnson, M. & Maas, M. (Eds.). (1997). *Nursing Outcomes Classification(NOC): Iowa Outcomes Project.* St. Louis, MO: Mosby.

Keinholz, M. (1997). *Online Guide to Medical Research: Valuable Internet Resources for Medical Research, Practice and Advice.* Overland Park, KS: Ventana Communications.

Kiley, R. (1999). *Medical Information on the Internet: A Guide for Health Professionals.* Dallas, TX: Churchill Livingstone.

Kissinger, K., & Borchardt, S. (Eds.). (1995). *Information technology for integrated health systems: Positioning for the Future (Ernst & Young).* New York, NY: Wiley.

Lindberg, D.A.B. & Humphreys, B.L. (1992). The unified medical language system (UMLS) and computer-based patient records. In Ball, M.J. & Collen, M.F. (Eds.), *Aspects of the Computer-based Patient Record* (pp. 165-175). New York, NY: Springer-Verlag.

Mascara, C. (1999). *Internet Resource Guide for Nurses & Healthcare Professionals.* Menlo Park, CA: Addison-Wesley.

McCloskey, J.C. & Bulecheck, G.M. (Eds.). (1996). *Nursing Interventions Classification* (2nd ed.). St. Louis, MO: Mosby.

McCloskey, J.C. & Maas, M. (1998). Interdisciplinary Team: The nursing perspective is essential. *Nursing Outlook.* 46 (4), 157-163.

Moschella, D. (1999, March 1). Technology is increasing privacy, not threatening it. *Computerworld.* 33.

Nicoll, L.H. (1998). *Computers in Nursing's Guide to the Internet.* Philadelphia, PA: Lippincott, Williams & Wilkins.

Olson, L.A., Peters, S.G. & Stewart, J.B. (1998). Security and confidentiality in an electronic medical record. Available at: www.himss.org/publications/news.htm

Rose, D.K., Cohen, M.M., Wigglesworth, D.F. & Yee, D. A. (1992, September). Development of a computerized database for the study of anaesthesia care. *Canadian Journal of Anaesthesia.* 39, 716-723.

Saba, V.K. & McCormick, K.A. (1995). *Essentials of Computers for Nurses* (2nd ed.). New York, NY: McGraw-Hill.

Saba, V. K., Pocklington, D.B. & Miller, K.P. (Eds.). (1998). *Nursing and Computers: An Anthology.* 1987-1996. New York, NY: Springer-Verlag.

Schanz, S.J. (1999) *Using the Internet for Health Information: Legal Issues.* American Medical Association. Chicago.

Shapiro, J. (Ed.). (1999). *Guide to Effective Healthcare Information and Management Systems and the Role of the Chief Information Officer* (3rd ed.). Healthcare Information and Management Systems Society. Chicago.

Slack, W.V. (1997). *Cybermedicine: How Computing Empowers Doctors and Patients for Better Health Care.* San Francisco, CA: Jossey-Bass.

Warner, H.R., Sorenson, D.K. & Bouhaddou, O. (1997). *Knowledge Engineering in Health Informatics (Computers and Medicine).* New York, NY: Springer-Verlag.

Weed, L.L. (1969). *Medical Records, Medical Education, and Patient Care.* Chicago, IL: Year Book Medical Publishers.

Weiss, Y.G., Cotev, S., Drenger, B. & Katzenelson, R. (1995, October). Patient data management systems in anaesthesia: An emerging technology. 42, 914-921.

Werley, H.H. & Lang, N.M. (Eds.). (1988). *Identification of the Nursing Minimum Data Set.* New York, NY: Springer-Verlag.

Zurier, S. (1998, September 21). Privacy sound off: Regulation vs. self-regulation. *Internet Week.* 35.

KEY REFERENCES

Berner, E.S. (Ed.). (1998). *Clinical Decision Support Systems: Theory and Practice (Health Informatics).* New York, NY: Springer-Verlag.

Coiera, E. (1997). *Guide to Medical Informatics, the Internet, and Telemedicine.* Oxford, UK: Oxford University Press.

Commission on Physical Sciences, Mathematics, and Applications: Committee on Maintaining Privacy and Security in Health Care Applications of the National Information Infrastructure, National Research Council. (1997). *For the Record: Protecting Electronic Health Information.* Washington, DC: National Academy Press.

Degoulet, P. & Feischi, M. (1996). *Introduction to Clinical Informatics (Computers in Health Care).* New York, NY: Springer-Verlag.

Dick, R.S., Steen, E.B. & Detmer, D.E. (Eds.). Committee on Improving the Patient Record, Institute of Medicine. (1997). *The Computer-based Patient Record: An Essential Technology for Health Care* (Revised ed.). Washington, DC: National Academy Press.

Friedman, C.P. & Wyatt, J.C. (1997). *Evaluation Methods in Medical Informatics.* New York, NY: Springer-Verlag.

Gardner-Bonneau, D. (1999). *Human Factors and Voice Recognition Interactive Systems (Kluwer International Series in Engineering and Computer Science).* Dordrecht, the Netherlands.

Hagland, M. (1998, November). Six opinions on IT security. *Health Management Technology.* 16.

Hannah, K.J., Ball, M.J. & Edwards, M.J.A. (Eds.). (1999). *Introduction to Nursing Informatics* (2nd Ed.). New York, NY: Springer-Verlag.

Healthcare Information and Management Systems Society. (1996a). *Guide to Effective Health Care Clinical Systems.* Healthcare Information and Management Systems Society. Chicago.

Hebda, T., Czar, P. & Mascara, C. (1998). *Handbook of Informatics for Nurses & Health Care Professionals.* Menlo Park, CA: Addison-Wesley.

Kissinger, K. & Borchardt, S. (Eds.). (1995). *Information Technology for Integrated Health Systems: Positioning for the Future (Ernst & Young)*. New York, NY: Wiley.

Schanz, S. J. (1999) *Using the Internet for Health Information: Legal Issues*. American Medical Association. Chicago.

STUDY QUESTIONS

1. Compare and contrast healthcare informatics with medical, nursing, and clinical informatics.

2. List five advantages of a computer-based patient record.

3. Describe the role of nomenclature and minimum data sets in information retrieval.

4. List three possible approaches to decision support.

5. In what way are the following technologies changing healthcare data collection and review?
   - Voice recognition
   - Portable/wireless healthcare computing
   - Telemedicine
   - Internet

6. Describe three concerns about electronic healthcare data and the role of regulation in addressing those concerns.

7. What are the requirements for an anesthesia information system to fit in an integrated health system?

CHAPTER 24

IMPROVING QUALITY IN THE 21ST CENTURY

Denise Martin-Sheridan, CRNA, PhD

Professor of Anesthesiology
Associate Graduate Director
Nurse Anesthesiology Program
Albany Medical College
Albany, NY

Cathy A. Mastropietro, CRNA, PhD

Independent Contractor
Youngstown, OH

KEY CONCEPTS

- The process of improving quality in healthcare must be ongoing and have strategic components for review and assessment.
- In order to improve patient safety and error management in healthcare, the punitive nature of the culture and of the environment must be changed.
- Quality assessment should never be undertaken for its own sake, but should be linked to improving patient outcomes.
- The American Association of Nurse Anesthetists (AANA) has a long history of involvement in quality assessment and patient safety activities.
- Best practice protocols provide data-driven approaches to patient care and fiscal planning by analyzing and applying results of rigorous research to clinical decision making.
- Clinical pathways are logically sequenced prospective plans of care developed by all disciplines involved in the management of patients with specific diagnoses.
- Clinical pathways improve quality of care and reduce hospital expenditures by streamlining interventions, human product resources, and documentation.
- Evidence-based clinical pathways should be continuously reviewed and revised to reflect current theory and improved patient outcomes.

In order to remain competitive in the healthcare market place, hospitals need to provide quality services, be cost-effective, and ensure customer satisfaction. Escalating healthcare costs, the oversupply of hospital beds per capita, and reduction in reimbursement from payers have changed the playing field for hospitals trying to conduct business. Increasingly, federal initiatives to regulate the cost of healthcare have forced institutions to reevaluate their delivery systems. As a result, hospitals must change and respond to the initiatives by decreasing costs while improving quality and patient outcomes.

The incentives for change fostered the development of a movement where a variety of committees, boards, and departments were charged with the responsibility of monitoring quality in performance and identifying what strategies are required to ensure that the highest quality of care is provided at the lowest possible cost (Martin-Sheridan, 1999). The quality movement in the United States has its conceptual foundation in work by Demming whose organizational theory was employed in the business sector in problem-solving techniques and productivity development. An expert in quality methodology, Demming's techniques have been utilized to increase a company's market share and support continued growth in the face of competition for scarce resources (Zonsius and Murphy, 1995).

In the hospital sector, plans to ensure quality began to emerge when the American College of Surgeons (ACS) published the American College of Surgeons' Hospital Standardization Program in 1913 (Table 24.1) outlining requirements for professional staff, case reviews, audits, medical records, and support services. The elements of this program served as the basis for hospital accreditation developed in the 1950s by a newly formed organization that included the American Medical Association (AMA), the Canadian Medical Association, the American College of Physicians, and ACS. The new organization was called the Joint Commission on Accreditation of Hospitals, later known as the Joint Commission on Accreditation of Healthcare Organizations (JCAHO). Among other functions, the JCAHO establishes standards, or measures, of assuring quality in hospitals accredited by them. These standards for quality assurance (QA) may be viewed as the consensus of what constitutes adequate, acceptable, and excellent care. A QA program determines what level of care is being given and received and then takes whatever actions are required to maintain or improve that care (Lang and Marek, 1995). It is important for institutions to meet these established standards, not only from a quality perspective, but also from a reimbursement perspective. Hospitals and other healthcare institutions that seek Medicare reimbursement must meet certain predetermined conditions of participation established by the Social Security Amendments of 1965, Public Law 98-97. Meeting the JCAHO standards satisfies Medicare conditions of participation.

Following the establishment of standards of care came the review and regulation of practice through professional standards review organizations (PSROs) and professional review organizations (PROs) created in conjunction with Medicare and Medicaid legislation enacted in the 1960s. In 1982, as part of the Tax Equity and Fiscal Responsibility Act (TEFRA), the Peer Improvement Act created 54 PROs whose responsibility was to review the appropriateness and quality of care provided to Medicare beneficiaries. However, in a 1990 report on quality

Table 24.1: The Minimum Standard

1. That physicians and surgeons privileged to practice in the hospital be organized as a definite group or staff. Such organization has nothing to do with the question as to whether the hospital is "open" or "closed," nor need it affect the various existing types of staff organization. The word "staff" is here defined as the group of doctors who practice in the hospital inclusive of all groups such as the "regular staff," the "visiting staff," and the "associate staff."
2. That membership on the staff be restricted to physicians and surgeons who are (a) full graduates of medicine in good standing and legally licensed to practice in their respective states or provinces, (b) competent in their respective fields, and (c) worthy in character and matters of professional ethics; that in this latter connection the practice of the division of fees, under any guise whatever, be prohibited.
3. That the staff initiate and, with the approval of the governing board of the hospital, adopt rules, regulations and policies governing the professional work of the hospital; that these rules, regulations, and policies specifically provide:
   a. That staff meetings be held at least once each month. (In large hospitals the departments may choose to meet separately.)
   b. That the staff review and analyze at regular intervals their clinical experience in the various departments of the hospital, such as medicine, surgery, obstetrics, and the other specialties; the clinical records of patients, free and pay, to be the basis for such review and analysis.
4. That accurate and complete records be written for all patients and filed in an accessible manner in the hospital—a complete case record being one that includes identification data, complaint, personal and family history, history of present illness's physical examination, special examinations, such as consultations, clinical laboratory, x-ray and other examinations, provisional or working diagnosis, medical or surgical treatment, gross and microscopic pathologic findings, progress notes, final diagnosis, condition on discharge, follow-up, and, in case of death, autopsy findings.
5. That diagnostic and therapeutic facilities under competent supervision be available for the study, diagnosis, and treatment of patients, these to include, at least (a) a clinical laboratory providing chemical, bacteriologic, serologic, and pathologic services; and (b) an x-ray department providing radiographic and fluoroscopic services.

From the Minimum Standard of the American College of Surgeon's Hospital Standardization Program, 1913.

assurance commissioned by Congress, it was found that PSROs and PROs emphasized utilization of care rather than quality of care and failed to make a significant impact on the quality of care provided to patients (Dettmann, 1995).

Beginning in 1984, the primary methodology employed for QA can be described as a planned and systematic process to monitor and evaluate the quality and appropriateness of care. Many organizations adopted the JCAHO's 10-Step Model of Monitoring and Evaluation. This systems approach propagated by the JCAHO is basically a variation of the management concept of the closed loop. The purpose of the closed management loop and its incorporation into the 10-step model is to require within a management unit (such as a hospital department) a mechanism by which aspects of the management process can be documented.

Within the closed loop paradigm, all evaluative processes are linked together cyclically rather than being disjointed and disconnected. Consequently, when decisions or goals are made, tasks and activities necessary to implement them are assigned and implemented, resulting in conclusions being reached and recommendations being made. Results are then compared with the original decision and corrections are made if needed. The process is then repeated.

This process offered a solution to many of the causes of quality-related problems that the JCAHO frequently found during years of conducting accreditation surveys. When an institution studies quality problems, the underlying cause is usually due to a lack of effective communication and coordination between operational departments and subunits. The 10-step model was designed to ensure greater interaction among caregivers and ensure that every step of the process was complete and incorporated by components of the system. The tasks and activities of the 10-step model are:

1. Assign responsibility.
2. Delineate scope of services.
3. Identify important aspects of care.
4. Identify indicators.
5. Establish thresholds for evaluation.
6. Collect data.
7. Analyze data.
8. Take actions to improve services.
9. Assess the impact of actions taken.
10. Communicate the results to relevant components of the organization.

Indicators in step 4 and the thresholds in step 5 are key features that describe the system linkages found within the historical-implicit review process. Indictors are defined by the JCAHO as measurement tools used to monitor and evaluate the quality of important governance, management, clinical, and support functions. Common types or categories of indicators are the desirable indicator, outcome indicator, process indicator, rate-based indicator, sentinel event indicator, structural indicator, and undesirable indicator. Typical indicators employed in most hospitals are derived from an analysis of cases, including such indicators as patient death, medical complications, unexpected events, medical complications, complaints about services, and other failed outcomes.

A threshold, for the purposes of the model, is the level at which a trigger point is reached that signals the need for management to begin the process of evaluation and determine why the threshold was crossed. For instance, if an institution has set the acceptable nosocomial infection rate at 4 percent, and institutional data demonstrate that the rate has increased to 5 percent, a systematic process of focused evaluation of cause and remediation is triggered.

When the QA process first emerged, the emphasis was placed on retrospective review of patient records to monitor variances (problems) in care. This problem-oriented approach failed to comprehensively evaluate the hospital as a system, and instead focused on a static point in time. The objective of the process was to identify the variance, correct it, and remediate (often perceived as punishment) the responsible practitioner. While the QA movement made strides toward ensuring quality standards of care were met, it typically stopped at the person or group who were determined could have acted in a way that could have led to a different outcome (Leape et al., 1998).

This punitive approach to quality management made it difficult for the providers of care in healthcare institutions to buy into the process. Providers generally considered it a personal affront to their professionalism to have the conduct of their care scrutinized and questioned in a punitive manner. At the administrative level, it was perceived to be yet another responsibility in an increasingly more complex environment, constrained by rules that did little to significantly decrease the overall costs of doing business or improve the overall quality of care.

Contemporary quality assurance activities are generally derivatives of implicit strategies, the components of which include structure-process-outcome review. The nature of the review includes measurement and monitoring of achievement of certain structural criteria (e.g., is there evidence of written anesthesia department policies?), process criteria (e.g., is there evidence the department followed its policies?), and outcome criteria (e.g., is there evidence that appropriate interventions for change were made and evaluated?). Striving to continuously improve performance, effectiveness, and efficiency while promoting excellence, the healthcare industry adopted the approaches referred to as total quality management (TQM) and continuous quality improvement (CQI) (Martin-Sheridan, 1999).

Following the lead of managers in the business sector, healthcare managers began to emphasize quality improvement rather than quality assurance. The focus of quality improvement is to review or evaluate the organization as a system, as opposed to looking at a particular variance. Systems-oriented CQI methods require investment of institutional resources, which include time and personnel. A healthcare organization's goals and objectives for improving care are developed in a strategic plan that serves as the infrastructure for planning improvement initiatives. CQI methods accomplish improvements by measuring process and outcomes, assessing the reasons for current practices and the barriers to change, and intervening to improve current practices. Typically, QI methods assume that the individuals in an organization who are most involved in current practices, either as patients or potential patients or as members of the healthcare provider team, are the most able to understand and modify current practice.

QI often is carried out in small structured groups composed of individuals involved in current practice, with assistance from those who have experience with QI. The groups review data, develop QI interventions, and help implement as well as evaluate them. QI methodologies vary in their specifics, but include a focus on systems of care, ongoing change, interdisciplinary teams, measurement, analysis, and intervention. QI emphasizes improvement in outcomes by making a series of incremental or major improvements in the process of care, rather than emphasizing identification and removal of a few individual bad apples. Figure 24.1 is an example of a cause-and-effect diagram used to examine data in a QI process.

An essential piece of any CQI program that has as its objective to quantify and assess the quality of service provided to patients is evidence of its effectiveness. Identifying the link between a particular intervention and benefit is a measurement of outcome.

THE LINK BETWEEN OUTCOMES MEASUREMENT AND CONTINUAL QUALITY IMPROVEMENT

There is growing interest in patient outcomes and how they can be improved. An underlying reason for this interest is because there is growing evidence of variations in the outcomes of care, utilization of resources, and costs of care. Concerns

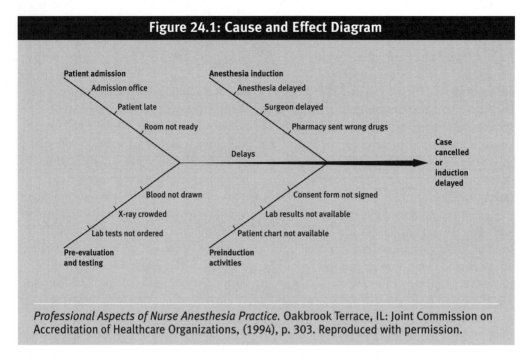

Figure 24.1: Cause and Effect Diagram

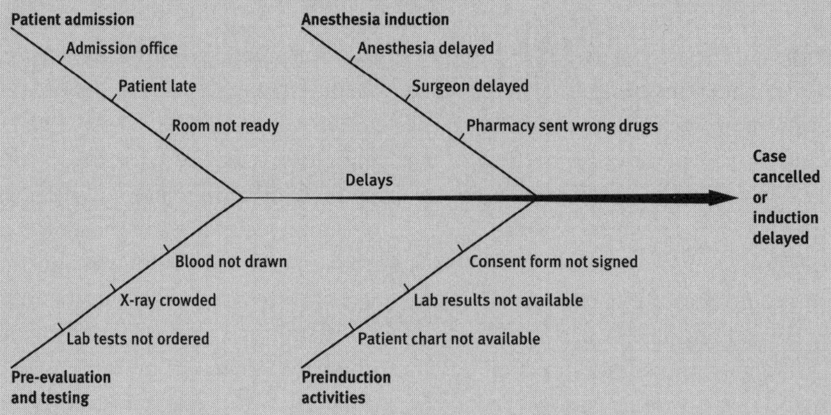

Professional Aspects of Nurse Anesthesia Practice. Oakbrook Terrace, IL: Joint Commission on Accreditation of Healthcare Organizations, (1994), p. 303. Reproduced with permission.

about undesirable variations have triggered increased funding for outcomes research, efforts to promote rational decision making and common practice by using practice guidelines, and activities to standardize utilization through external review and the need for care.

Outcomes can be described from several perspectives. As measurements, or variables, outcomes describe the result or effect of particular interventions. When a patient is the focus, the measurement may be the effect of a method of treatment. For the patient who undergoes an anesthetic, a desirable outcome might be defined as discharge from the facility within a predetermined period of time. Patient outcomes also can be expressed in physiologic terms (cardiac output, respiratory rate), in physical terms (ability to assume activities of daily living), in mental and psychological terms (cognitive and affective skills), in social terms (ability to interact with members of the family), and in other quality of life areas (level of pain, recollection under anesthesia) (Batalden, Nelson, and Roberts, 1994). Other examples of outcome measures include the incidence of morbidity and mortality, complication rates, patient satisfaction, length of stay, and overall cost (Bidwell-Cerone, Krainovich-Miller, Haber, Penney, and Carter, 1995).

While measurement of outcomes is important, measurement without plans for improvement would render the entire process only an academic exercise. In order to improve patient outcomes, a structured approach outlining what actions can be taken in the patient care process must be defined. For example, Davies et al. (1994) characterize an outcome assessment project in terms of a series of steps to be accomplished. Among the most important reasons for establishing the initiative in a healthcare setting is to evaluate the effectiveness of care and identify opportunities for improvement. Linking outcomes to the clinical process in order to enhance patients' quality of life should be the primary incentive.

Several methods or tools are used to link outcomes and improvement. Often in QI projects a flow chart is employed to provide a pictorial representation of the steps. A plan-do-check/study-act (PDCA) model has been described to help clarify the steps and identify inefficiencies. The model proceeds in the following manner:

- State aim.
- Identify measures of improvement.
- Describe and predict changes.
- Plan.
- Do pilot test.
- Check and study results.
- Act to improve.
- Reflect on learning.

The first step requires that the goal or purpose of the project is stated and the strategies by which any actual change can be measured are identified. After careful scrutiny and evaluation of possible changes, the most suitable and practical are adopted. Generally a small pilot testing period follows, during which qualitative and quantitative data are analyzed. The data are evaluated to determine the probable effects the changes will have on the system. Last, based on the experiences, some action is taken to implement the change, complete a system redesign, and continually evaluate the change in the improvement cycle (Batalden, Nelson, and Roberts, 1994). In Figure 24.2, the PDCA model is viewed as a continual cycle of improvement incorporated into daily work processes.

There are other tools utilized to link outcomes to practice that serve as markers in the QI process. Markers in this sense mean certain expectations, established by a profession for example, against which certain conduct of practice is evaluated and judged. The markers are established to avoid variations in patient care, utilization of resources, and costs of care, which may lead to undesirable outcomes. An example of these markers in healthcare includes practice standards.

Figure 24.2: Model for Improvement

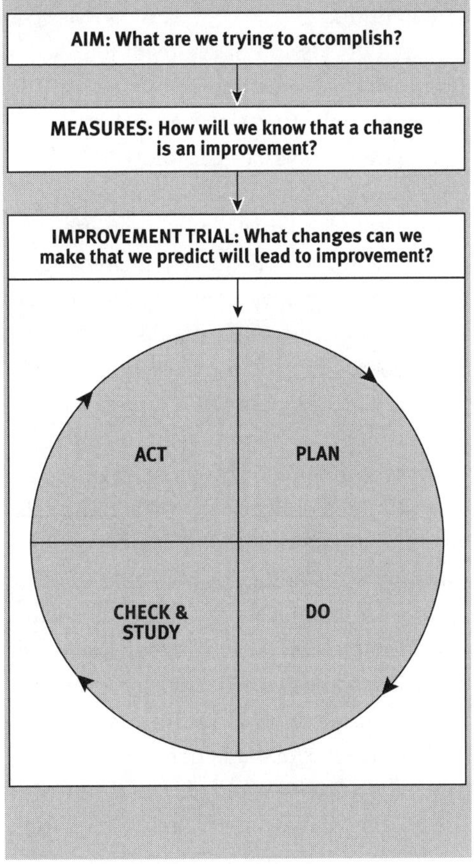
AIM: What are we trying to accomplish?
MEASURES: How will we know that a change is an improvement?
IMPROVEMENT TRIAL: What changes can we make that we predict will lead to improvement?
ACT
PLAN
CHECK & STUDY
DO

Standards

A standard is something established for use as a rule, or basis of comparison, for measuring or judging value or quality. In nurse anesthesia practice, for example, standards are used by general agreement to determine whether a certain level of care is provided. From the aspect of QI, standards may be viewed as expectations that drive the achievement of certain behaviors. In some situations, standards are used as yardsticks to measure results of care. They are established by a profession as a means of self-regulation to ensure quality in performance (Lang and Marek, 1995) and are perceived to be actions that any reasonable professional would take when faced with a similar set of conditions.

In a discussion of the legal foundations of nurse anesthesia practice (Blumenreich, 1999), the American Association of Nurse Anesthetists (AANA) legal counsel describes other sources of standards of care that affect Certified Registered Nurse Anesthetists (CRNAs). Licensing laws, which in many cases authorize certain regulatory bodies (e.g., boards of nursing) to issue rules and regulations, constitute a part of the standard of care. Criminal statutes that address standards of care also regulate a practitioner's obligations and actions relative to the patients in their care. As nurse anesthetists, standards applicable to all nurses are applicable to CRNAs as well.

Blumenreich goes on to say that other agencies, bodies, and boards, by virtue of their expertise in the healthcare field, also may establish standards of care. An example is the JCAHO, which has developed a list of clinical indicators (Table 24.2) which could be used to evaluate performance data. Additionally, the AANA Anesthesia Apparatus Checkout Recommendations are used as evidence of what parameters must be monitored when patients undergo an anesthetic.

The AANA has established standards for CRNA practice. These standards are published in the *Professional Practice Manual for the CRNA,* which describes the practice of the CRNA, delineates standards for nurse anesthesia practice, and offers guidelines for CRNAs and healthcare institutions that employ them (AANA, 1999). In 1999, the AANA Board of Directors adopted the Standards for Office Based Anesthesia Practice. Since CRNAs have been the predominant anesthesia practitioner in the physician's office, these standards reflect the experience CRNAs have providing quality anesthesia services in this setting. (See chapter 14, Table 14.1 to read the Standards for Office Based Anesthesia Practice.)

In addition to the standards established for practice, the Council on Accreditation of Nurse Anesthesia Educational Programs (COA) of the AANA uses the Standards for Accreditation of Nurse Anesthesia Educational Programs. These standards are utilized to evaluate graduate education programs in the specialty practice of nurse anesthesia in order to improve the quality of education, to educate competent nurse anesthetists who are prepared to meet the demands of the workforce, and to protect the consumer (COA, 1999).

Organizations also establish and publish guidelines. Although some would argue they fail to have the same weight as standards, guidelines nonetheless are utilized to evaluate whether certain tenents of practice are met. For example, the Centers for Disease Control and Prevention guidelines for universal pre-

Table 24.2: JCAHO Indicators for Anesthesia

Airway	General	Cardiovascular	Pulmonary
Failed intubation	Severe postoperative pain	Excessive blood loss	Aspiration
System disconnect	Postoperative nausea and vomiting	Hypotension	Pneumothorax
Esophageal intubation	Explicit recall	Hypertension	Pulmonary edema
Traumatic intubation		Cardiac arrest	

cautions (1995) define what body fluids should be considered infectious, and the method by which the fluids should be disposed. Failure to adhere to the "Universal Precaution" guidelines could violate the Occupational Safety and Health Act of 1970, which provides protection for healthcare workers from errors and work-related injury and illness. Reducing errors, and promoting safety of the patient and provider, is an essential component of systems to improve quality in healthcare.

PROMOTING PATIENT SAFETY AND REDUCING ERRORS IN HEALTHCARE: EFFECTING A CHANGE IN CULTURE

In 1996, President Clinton established the Advisory Committee on Consumer Protection and Quality in the Health Care Industry. The commission was charged with evaluating the changes occurring in the healthcare system and to make recommendations on how best to promote and assure consumer protection and healthcare quality. In 1998 the commission delivered its final report. Essentially, four categories of quality problems were documented. The following is from the final report addressing those categories.

Avoidable errors: Too many Americans are injured during the course of their treatment, and some die prematurely as a result. For example, a study of injuries to patients treated in hospitals in New York state found that 3.7 percent experienced adverse events, of which 13.6 percent led to death and 2.6 percent to permanent disability, and that about one fourth of these adverse events were due to negligence (Brennan et al, 1991). A national study found that from 1983 to 1993, deaths due to medication errors rose more than twofold, with 7,391 deaths attributed to medication errors in 1993 alone (Phillips, Christenfeld, and Glynn, 1998).

Underutilization of services: Millions of people do not receive necessary care and suffer needless complications that add to healthcare costs and reduce productivity. For example, a study of Medicare patients with myocardial infarction found that only 21 percent of eligible patients received beta blockers, and that the mortality rate among recipients was 43 percent less than that for nonrecipients (Soumerai et al, 1997). An estimated 18,000 people die each year of heart attacks because they did not receive interventions (Chassin, 1997).

Overuse of services: Millions of Americans receive healthcare services that are unnecessary, increase costs, and often endanger their health. For example, an analysis performed by seven healthcare plans estimated that one in six hysterectomies was inappropriate (Bernstein et al, 1993).

Variations in service: There is a continuing pattern of variation in healthcare practice, including regional variations and small-area variations (Wennberg and Cooper, 1998). This is a clear indicator that the practice of healthcare has not caught up with the science of healthcare to ensure evidence-based practice in the United States.

These categories will be the basis upon which quality improvement strategies are developed in the 21st century. Two of these categories, evidence-based practice and patient safety/reducing errors, are the focus of the last section of this chapter.

Evidence-Based Practice

Historical Perspective: Healthcare and the 1990s

The 1990s were a decade of great transition for healthcare providers, recipients, and payers. Sparked by the need for a more efficient healthcare delivery system, the movement of managed care and health maintenance organizations infiltrated the healthcare market and began to mold the future of healthcare. The proliferation of managed care was at its greatest during 1993-1996. During this period, the outcry to reduce hospital utilization and expenditures was deafening. Intense scrutiny of all aspects of healthcare began, and providers of healthcare were challenged to respond to priorities that mandated the delivery of comprehensive, rational, cost-efficient quality care.

The impact of these healthcare initiatives was dramatic. Consumers, administrators, and all varieties of healthcare providers found themselves under new dictates. Recipients of health services found themselves subservient to payers of healthcare; in many instances they lost the right to choose their primary physician or facility for services. Several years of established physician-patient interpersonal relationships were exchanged for selecting a physician from a list of unknowns. Often, recipients were given no option but to travel to unknown medical facilities for care under the guise of cost efficiency and effectiveness. Consumers were outraged.

Administrators also found themselves subservient to the drivers of healthcare. With cost containment the driving force behind managed care, product and human resources were streamlined, diagnostic procedures curtailed, and length of hospital stay reduced. Smaller hospitals, unable to withstand the penetration of managed care, merged with larger ones in order to survive. Competition among organizations grew intense. Increased accountability, performance documentation, and outcomes measurement weighed heavily in this competitive arena, as providers were held responsible for services rendered and results of treatment (Rosenstein, 1994). Healthcare providers were challenged to make clinical decisions with fewer diagnostic tools, provide the best treatment in a timely and less costly manner with reduced resources, and meet patient expectations for care.

Current State of Healthcare

The current climate in the healthcare community is the result of economic, political, and technological changes that occurred during the 1990s. Managers continue to define which changes in practice patterns focus on maximizing care while minimizing financial and human resources. At first thought, the two appear in discord. However, a paradigm shift has occurred in medical and nursing practice that embraces planned research utilization and collaborative work to effectively meet the developing changes in healthcare. Evidence-based practice and clinical pathways are emerging as quintessential strategies for clinical decision making for therapeutic interventions and as measurable benefits of total quality management.

Evidence-Based Practice Defined

Scientific reporting was born in the 1940s when clinicians began to value comparison of outcomes of treatment versus historical and concurrent control groups in evaluating interventions (Kennedy, 1998). Subsequently, the double-blind, randomized clinical trial emerged as the "gold standard" for evaluating the effects of therapy on morbidity and mortality and quality of life.

The proliferation of randomized clinical trials to assess therapeutic interventions was spawned by the Cardiac Arrhythmia Suppression Trial (CAST) conducted in 1989. In this well-publicized study, researchers relied on the historic hypothesis that lidocaine was an effective therapy for treating ventricular arrhythmias in postmyocardial infarction patients to evaluate newer local antiarrhythmic agents. Follow-up analysis revealed that the mortality rate was increased threefold in patients who received treatment versus the control group. The researchers erred clinically by failing to incorporate therapies such as beta blockers or angiotensin converting enzyme inhibitors that were scientifically supported to be the treatment of choice for ventricular arrhythmias in post-myocardial infarction patients (Cardiac Arrhythmia Suppression Trial Investigators, 1989). The CAST study intensely highlighted the value of outcomes-based clinical research. Concomitantly, the Agency for Health Care Policy and Research (AHCPR), created in 1989 to advance access to and quality of care, and the Food and Drug Administration demanded evidence-based outcomes data to establish guidelines for practice and determine efficacy and safety of interventions (Kennedy, 1998).

Evidence-based practice refers to clinical decision making that is influenced by aggressive, comprehensive analysis and use of current scientifically supported approaches to patient care. Less emphasis is placed on clinicians' personal experiences, knowledge of pathophysiological processes, and intuitive approaches to diagnosis and treatment. The primary underpinning of an evidence-based approach to decision making is examination of results of sound clinical research and patient outcomes. Critical strategies in providing quality patient care are determined following analysis of research results and methodological rigor of studies supporting specific management of select diagnoses or procedures. Synthesis of the studies results in a categorization of practice patterns that are rejected, modified, or incorporated into routine care of patients. Results of the analysis are compared with current institutional practices, and changes are made to improve delivery of care based on scientific data.

Guyatt, Cairns, Churchill et al (1992) assert that evidence-based practice requires precisely identifying a patient problem, conducting a comprehensive literature search, extracting relevant studies, determining validity by applying rules of scientific rigor, deducting the relevant clinical information, and applying best interventions to care of the patient. This "critical appraisal exercise" (Guyatt, Cairns, Churchill et al, 1992) can then be initiated to control variability in practice and address concerns about the effectiveness of management for specified diagnoses or procedures. Thus, empirically measured practices provide a data-driven approach to the care of the patient and fiscal planning.

Implementation of an Evidence-Based Practice Pattern

Implementing evidence-based practice begins with appointing an institutional multidisciplinary committee that includes representation from all professionals who contribute to the care of the patient. Open communication, intense collaboration, and familiarity with group process are the themes behind committee membership. Members should be selected based on clinical expertise and ability to influence decision making and effect change (Simpson, 1999). Each should be knowledgeable in critiquing research and recognizing scientific integrity.

The purpose of the committee is to develop a template for identifying best institutional practice patterns by evaluating the current theoretical basis for practice and implementing changes in present practices using literature synthesis, professional guidelines, and regulatory requirements in developing evidence-based practice protocols. The committee addresses the framework for evaluating current clinical practices and implementation of new protocols using a philosophy congruent with the overall philosophy of the institution to garnish conceptual support from administrative officials.

The process of defining evidence-based approaches to decision making for therapeutic interventions is initially arduous. A dedicated committee, focused on best patient care, will devote numerous hours and exhaust a multitude of resources developing protocols that are comprehensive, accurate, and resourceful. In addition to scientific literature, government regulatory agencies such as the JCAHO impose standards of care. Also, the AHCPR is continuously developing guidelines of care for specific diagnoses or procedures. For example, The Clinical Practice Guideline for Acute Pain Management: Operative or Medical Procedures and Trauma (AHCPR, 1992) directs current, effective, appropriate processes in the management of acute pain. It serves as the gold standard for anesthesia personnel in developing departmental policies and procedures for acute pain management.

In addition to the AANA standards for practice, many professional organizations have standards and guidelines that define minimal practices to be followed to promote patient safety. The various sources of practice guidelines can be accessed via the Internet through the United States National Library of Medicine MEDLINE Database, educational CD-ROM periodicals, or through the Web pages of professional organizations. Also, the AHCPR, in collaboration with the American Association of Health Plans and the AMA, developed the National Guideline Clearinghouse as a comprehensive database of clinical practice guidelines from professional organizations and other policy makers. Table 24.3 provides a sample of specialties with standards and guidelines and online resources that relate to anesthesia.

Once the committee examines relevant standards of care, the next step in information gathering is a retrospective analysis of a significant number of randomized clinical trials specific to the patient population of interest. A selective literature search is followed by examination of the relevancy of the report (i.e., design, methodology, interpretation of results, replication of findings). The retrospective report provides validation of current practice.

In contrast with retrospective analysis, another approach to establishing a strong knowledge base is research meta-analysis. Meta-analysis is performed as a prospective exercise to combine qualitative evidence from randomized trials to arrive at conclusive evidence that supports clinical interventions. Properly performed, meta-analysis leads to reliable evidence about the efficacy and safety of clinical interventions (Pogue and Yusuf, 1998). A well-designed meta-analysis uses a prospective protocol, describes key outcomes, controls data, evaluates sample size and statistical methods, and determines if results are conclusive (Pogue and Yusuf, 1998). Recently, proponents of meta-analysis have embraced collaborative groups (i.e., the Cochrane Collaboration) to write a prospective meta-analysis protocol. The group identifies trials to be included, defines key outcomes, and standardizes methodology subsequently optimizing statistical power. Meta-analysis provides less biased quantitative summary of existing evidence by allowing for statistical precision that may be lost in the single trial approach. Both approaches are useful in estimating a population effect, but do not prescribe individual treatment (Lau, Ioannidis, and Schmid, 1998).

Table 24.3: Online Resources for Standards and Guidelines Related to Anesthesia

Agency	Website
Agency for Health Care Policy and Research	www.ahcpr.gov
American Association of Nurse Anesthetists	www.aana.com
American College of Obstetricians and Gynecologists	www.acog.org
American Academy of Pediatrics	www.aap.org
American Nurses Association	www.ana.org
American Society of Anesthesiologists	www.asa.org
Association of Operating Room Nurses	www.asra.com
Best Practice Network	www.best4health.org
Cochrane Database of Systemic Reviews	www.cochrane.com
Joint Commission on Accreditation of Healthcare Organizations	www.jcaho.org
National Guideline Clearinghouse	www.guideline.gov
Society of Ambulatory Anesthesia	www.sambahq.org

Once consensus has been reached on best-supporting evidence in the literature, the processes should be measured against current institutional practices, services, and resources. Evaluation compares institutional practices against national standards and findings from deductive empirical research that emphasizes scientific method, measurement, and statistical principles.

Simpson (1999) suggests separating each institutional process into two categories: those performed out of habit without scientific support and those based on scientific evidence, measured against nationally recognized standards. Practices, procedures, or products that are not scientifically supported are eliminated from routine care. Costs for products, services, or procedures can then be compared and standards of practice developed that are theoretically and statistically supported and feasible within the institutional setting. Consequently, best care is harmoniously derived, scientifically driven, germane, and cost effective.

To be competitive in today's health market, healthcare resources must be used judiciously. Simpson (1999) describes differing philosophies for managing resources: cost containment and cost consciousness. She describes cost containment as an attempt to reduce expenses using preset budgets, while cost consciousness allocates financial and human resources after in-depth scrutiny of existing research including risks, benefits, and outcomes. Cost containment is dollar driven; cost consciousness is data driven relying on professional consensus to determine efficient, best practices. This concept is best accomplished by implementing clinical pathways.

Clinical Pathways

Clinical pathways focus on reaching predetermined outcomes, within a designated time frame, using specified resources. The concept of systemized project plans originated in skilled labor management to steer complex industrial projects, and it was not until the late 1980s that path-

Table 24.4: Key Concepts of Clinical Pathways

- Paths are developed by multidisciplinary teams.
- Paths integrate care for all disciplines.
- All disciplines are accountable for patient outcomes.
- Paths are not cookbooks but guides that can be modified to individual patient needs.
- Paths streamline care by stating outcomes on a timeline. They help eliminate duplication and bottlenecks that extend stays and waste resources.
- Paths may be a framework for documentation.
- Paths may be the basis for an outcomes-management and quality-improvement program in which variances are collected, analyzed, and used to revise the plan of care.
- Patients are involved. Patient satisfaction is monitored.

Reproduced with permission from *OR Manager.* (1994). Volume 10, 7.

ways were embraced for healthcare. Credit is given to nurse colleagues at the New England Medical Center for developing the first pathways for the healthcare industry (Zander, 1988). Case management plans (precursors to clinical pathways) were developed to coordinate care across all services that manage the patient with complex conditions. Designed for the patient with complicated needs, the plans are extensive documents of care.

In keeping with the changes in healthcare, the promoters of case management plans applied the concept of care plans to patients with predictable courses of treatment, response, and length of hospital stay. The format was tailored to offer the caregiver a snapshot view of the patient's management for an entire hospital stay. Pertinent steps related to care were systematically prioritized into statements, to assist practitioners in appropriate decision making for a specific clinical diagnosis. These chronological steps were called clinical pathways.

Clinical pathways grew in popularity because they emphasized the hallmarks of healthcare in the nineties: treatment based on efficacy and outcomes at reduced cost. By 1993, 57 percent of surveyed hospital administrators claimed to have had a formal process in place for managing patients' hospitalizations (Lumsden and Hagland, 1993). As the trend mushroomed, such plans of care took on many new names: clinical guideline, critical pathway, care path,™ and care map™ to name a few. Key concepts of critical pathways are listed in Table 24.4.

Key to the development of a pathway is standardizing patient care. Recipes unique to the institution are developed to decrease fragmentation of care, embrace practical effectiveness, and eliminate rituals, guesswork, and duplication for patients with comparable medical conditions. Logically developed statements that serve as blueprints for mapping steps of care render consistency in the management of patients because a system-wide patient care plan is utilized.

The general aim of a clinical pathway is to foster collaboration among all members of the patient's care team to design a structured outline or algorithm that:

1. Explicitly determines preferred outcomes. (What are optimal effects of treatment?)
2. Prescribes specific interventions. (What diagnostics, monitors, treatments, medications, nutrition, and

activities are essential to achieve desired outcomes?)

3. Controls resource utilization and reduces cost. (What resources are vital to produce desired effects?)
4. Reduces length of hospital stay. (What is the least amount of time necessary to accomplish goals?)
5. Educates patient and family. (How are patients and family involved in decision making?)
6. Improves patient satisfaction. (Will plan of care reduce patient and family anxiety and promote best outcomes, in a timely fashion, at a reduced cost?)

Clinical pathways generally have four components: collaboration, outcomes, timeline, and comprehensive standardized interventions (Bloyd and Faimon, 1992). Collaboration plays a fundamental role in the development of a clinical pathway. Clinical pathways are a composite of evidence-based research, standing medical orders, protocol, and standards of care. Invigorating dialogue in the team-oriented approach challenges current practices and suggests strategies for constructive change. Variations in practice and process are measured, and a plan is developed that homogenizes care but with enough flexibility to customize individual patient management.

Early decree of the focus of the clinical path facilitates the group process. (Will the path be generalized or specific to a diagnosis or treatment, in an ambulatory or acute care facility?) The team uses specific criteria to determine which diseases or procedures are suitable for a pathway. Diagnoses or procedures that are routinely seen, consume large amounts of resources, and lend to standardization of protocol and resources provide the best medium.

The second component of a clinical pathway is defining target outcomes for the selected diagnosis. Each discipline involved in the care of the patient is responsible for delineating expected results of interventions. Expected outcomes are desired goals following interventions, within a specified time frame defined by physical and behavioral criteria. In addition to clinical outcomes, functional or financial outcomes can be targeted (AORN, 1999). In defining outcomes, performance benchmarks are established for all aspects of care. A benchmark is the level of acceptable performance that is established by comparing practices within the institution or weighing them against external institutions or industries.

The next component of a clinical pathway is a time line. The time line prescribes patient care by sequencing interventions from admission to discharge. All clinically relevant aspects of care are systematically planned along a continuum that ranges from hours to weeks depending on the diagnosis and subsequent care. Interventions are implemented in sequence to provide the most comprehensive care in the shortest time frame. For the surgical patient, the time line would begin with preadmission and end with discharge.

Concomitantly, standardized interventions are prioritized and graphically depicted across the time line (see Figure 24.3). The result is a document that clearly prescribes concise patient care and follows the patient's clinical progress throughout the course of hospitalization. Clinical pathways eliminate the need for specialty providers to document care in separate sections of the patient's record. All activities involved in the management of the patient can be readily found in one document, allowing each discipline to catch sight of how all aspects of care are connected.

Clinical pathways are generally designed in such a way that documenta-

Figure 24.3: Sample Grid for Clinical Pathway

TIMELINE

INTERVENTIONS

	Preadmission	Admission	Preop	Intraop	Postop	Discharge
Consultations						
Laboratory Radiology						
Medications						
Monitors						
Nutrition						
Physical Therapy						
Assessment						
Outcomes						
Patient/Family Education						
Discharge Plan						

(Adapted from clinical pathways with permission from St. Rita's Medical Center, Lima, Ohio.)

tion supports easy identification of variances. Daily tracking of deviations from the prescribed plan holds all disciplines accountable for efficient, comprehensive care of the patient. A variance is any deviation in the prescribed course of the pathway. Variances are categorized as patient/family, practitioner, system, or community (Zander, 1991). For example, a patient variance may be a complication, a practitioner variance may be due to failure to complete a task, there may be operational inefficiencies within the system (equipment failure), or follow-up support (rehabilitation) may not be readily available after discharge (Villaire & Ley,1995). Variances should be addressed as they occur to enhance progression along the pathway. Codes may be developed for system-wide consistency in identifying variances. Codes also provide easy access to information to include in a database for statistical analysis.

Variances should also be analyzed on a regular basis. Aggregate variance analysis is critical to evaluating measures to assess healthcare decisions, services, and outcomes. This creates a quality improvement system whereby care is continuously defined and restructured based on outcomes. Outcomes should be evaluated based on the following: meeting predetermined discharge date, readmission rates, morbidity and mortality, and patient satisfaction (Ebener, Baugh, and Formella, 1996). Villaire and Ley (1995) recommend that 60 percent to 70 percent of patients in the population meet the prescribed outcomes in the pathway; otherwise the plan should be reexamined.

In addition to advancing quality care, clinical pathways can be used to identify activities that reduce costs and shorten hospital stay. For example, at one institution researchers benchmarked the perioperative process in an ambulatory orthopedic surgery setting. The investigators analyzed the effects of regional anesthesia clinical pathway techniques on process efficiency and recovery and determined that clinical pathways that prescribed combined general and femoral nerve block techniques were more effective in reducing costs, resources, labor intensity, and admission rates for patients undergoing anterior cruciate ligament repair at their institution (Williams, DeRiso, Figallo, Anders, Engel, and Sproul, 1998).

Clinical pathways can also be used as patient/family educational tools. Some facilities provide patient clinical pathways that are in tandem with their medical pathways to familiarize them with expected interventions and outcomes. This informed-consent document establishes consistency in educating patients about routine care during their hospitalization.

While the concept of clinical pathways is still emerging in many healthcare facilities, current users of standardized plans of care identify many advantages. Clinical pathways:

- Distill the best evidence to optimize the entire process of patient care.
- Benchmark best therapies.
- Promote practice advancement.

The following are also results of using clinical pathways:

- The team-oriented approach provides a prospective consensus on identifying and implementing interventions for specific patient populations.
- Repetition in all aspects of care is minimized.
- Patient outcomes are improved, ultimately leading to greater patient satisfaction.

As clinical pathways grow in acceptance, anesthesia providers will become integral contributors to developing integrated plans for interventions for surgical patients. These plans will improve patient outcomes by fostering patient safety and reducing error.

PATIENT SAFETY AND REDUCING ERROR

Interest in patient safety and reducing error is not new. Practice safety has long been the goal of the AANA and CRNAs. In fact, one important factor leading to the development of nurse anesthesia as a specialty practice in the United States likely was a concern for patient safety. Many of the early deaths related to anesthesia were the result of carelessness and lack of skill on the part of the person who administered the anesthetic. In the late 1800s, the fact that there were fewer anesthesia-related deaths was attributed in part to the nurses who began to assume the role of anesthetist (Bankert, 1989).

Physician colleagues are concerned with patient safety as well. In 1983, the first formal symposium on morbidity and mortality in anesthesia was held, and in 1984 the American Society of Anesthesiologists Anesthesia Patient Safety Foundation was formed (Sommer, 1999). In 1997, the AMA National Patient Safety Foundation (NPSF), whose mission is to improve patient safety by studying errors in the healthcare system and implementing safeguards to prevent patient injury, was formed. The structure of the NPSF includes a number of working committees whose responsibility is to develop and implement an agenda to improve patient safety. CRNAs are members of these committees, which also include experts in such areas as healthcare, medicine, nursing, law, organizational theory, and engineering.

In response to a number of highly publicized poor patient outcomes, the NPSF joined a multidisciplinary group, which convened at the Annenberg Center for Health Sciences at Eisenhower in Rancho Mirage, California. Dubbed the Annenberg Conference, it was the first error conference in healthcare (Leape et al., 1998). Among the various reports presented at the Annenberg Conference was one generated as a result of forums held by the NPSF, which brought together nurses, physicians, public health officers, dentists, pharmacists, attorneys, consumers, and the media to discuss patient safety. The group identified the following perceptions of existing barriers to patient safety, and themes on what could be done to be more constructive about patient safety (Levy, 1999).

Barriers to Patient Safety

- The culture that exists in the healthcare system was identified as a primary concern. When an event occurs, an individual is targeted for blame. This culture is present at both the societal and institutional level. It is especially so in healthcare given the nature of possible outcomes to patients.
- The systems utilized to report events are often poorly designed. They lack a central location, are not used altogether, or used erroneously, and errors caught and reported through their use are not seen as opportunities to learn, but as punitive in nature. The lack of appropriate structure in this approach promotes a culprit mentality, which feeds the culture of blame. For example, in a study of adverse drug events it was found that only about 7 percent were detected by the conventional method of incident reporting. Fear that disciplinary action would take place against the responsible individual was cited as a reason why the incident report was not filled out (Cullen et al, 1995).
- Unfortunately, the prime focus on error reporting is not as a way to prevent sentinel events. Because of the culture of blame, people fear job loss, litigation, and negative publicity, rather than regard the error as an opportunity to learn.
- The lack of teamwork in the hierarchical system in place at many healthcare institutions does not allow for effective sharing of ideas about how to improve patient safety. Although it is important to have a commitment to patient safety from leadership in the organization, important ideas can be generated from those who work hands-on each day with the actual problems.
- Perhaps important, the healthcare system expects perfection from all individuals all of the time. Both nurses and physicians have stated that this characteristic of their work environment affects their performance. This is a critical barrier, as admitting fallibility is often the first step toward improving system performance and reducing the risk of harm to patients. (Levy, 1999)

Constructive Patient Safety Themes

- The top priority for those in the healthcare community should be the prevention of patient injuries. Learning from past incidents and near misses can make healthcare safer for all. In order to achieve prevention, an open system of communication is needed to actively share solutions and focus proactively on safety.

- Patient/provider relationships play a key role in safety. Patients need to be seen as partners in achieving a safer healthcare system. Patients should be actively involved in the therapeutic decision-making process and apprised of the pros and cons of each suggested approach. This in turn will help reduce the perception of perfection that exists in healthcare.
- The current systems for reporting error need to be changed. Reporting systems should function as safe havens where errors are viewed as opportunities to learn and to work toward the prevention of error.
- Education about patient safety should reach the broadest possible community in order to raise awareness of the issue's importance.
- A strong teamwork culture is critical to the enhancement of patient safety. (Levy, 1999)

Error Management in Other Cultures (Organizations)

There are general lessons to be learned about safety from organizations that have been researching this area for a number of years. In fact, the study of human performance and understanding the human characteristics that define the performance, have long been utilized by the aviation, transportation, and nuclear power industries to prevent errors and mishaps. Understanding the characteristics of human performance—what is required to actually do the job—helps identify strategies to improve performance.

In 1984, a group of social scientists and engineers began investigating industries in which the occurrence of errors or mishaps could result in catastrophic consequences. The design, technological, and management characteristics of the organizations were critiqued. Specifically, banking, U.S. Navy carrier aviation, the commercial marine industry, commercial airlines, hospital intensive care units, hostage and terrorist units, and community emergency services were participants. The investigators found across the organizations that 80 percent of the error rate could be attributed to people and 20 percent to design, technology, and maintenance. Interestingly, the researchers also found that managers continued to direct the majority of their efforts toward correcting errors to the organizational aspects and gave scant attention to the people aspects (Roberts, 1999).

The researchers also determined that organizations that were most successful had certain prevalent characteristics and that a group of management behaviors needed to be part of the organization's culture in order to mitigate the risk of error (Roberts, 1999). Components of the management behaviors were:

- Process auditing, or some system of ongoing checks to identify expected and unexpected errors. The auditing must include testing and safety drills and follow-ups on the errors found during the audits.
- A reward system in which an individual, or organization, receives recognition for specific behavior. The following is an illustration of the reward system described. During review by one of the researchers of a U.S. aircraft carrier that was at sea, a tool was lost on deck. The loss of a tool is critical, especially if it is ingested in a jet aircraft and results in the loss of the aircraft or injury or death of crew. A young seaman informed his chief that the tool was lost, and air operations on the carrier came to an immediate halt until the tool was

found. When the tool was finally found, the officer in charge of air operations called the young seaman and his chief to report immediately to the flight operations deck. When they arrived on the flight operations deck, in front of the crew assembled, the officer praised them for a job well done. This is an example of the type of a reward system that must be in place to ensure error is acknowledged and corrected before a critical incident has the opportunity to occur.

- The quality of the operations of the organization should be reviewed on an ongoing basis against what are acknowledged to be the standards of the system or the industry.
- If there is inherent risk in the work an organization does, the organization must not only acknowledge that risk, but also put in place plans to avoid consequences of the risk involved. For example, it is no longer acceptable for a healthcare organization simply to acknowledge the infection rate for a certain surgical procedure is X percent without putting into place protocols aimed at reducing the infection rate.
- The last component is command and control of management processes. This includes belief in the following: that the person with the most experience should have the greatest influence on decision making, not the person who holds the highest rank; redundancy in both people and hardware so that backups are in place; senior management personnel who have a focus on the big picture and leave the component operations to those best able to complete those tasks; formal rules and procedures to operationalize the job being done; and ongoing training for all involved at all levels of the organization and industry. (Roberts, 1999)

The use of realistic, hands-on simulation to assess not only individual performance, but also the performance of teams, has been a useful model as a safety training tool. Initially used for standard flight training before World War II, simulators have evolved for use in the evaluation of technical performance and intervention management in anesthesiology (Gaba, 1994). Observing people making decisions in real time can enhance our ability to learn about conditions in the environment that affect decision making. While experts may not always be able to articulate their actions that enhance or divert safety, it is possible to unearth the subtle cues that drive and influence behavior. In addition to people retelling an event, orally or in written reports, and making real-time observations, simulation that challenges a person's expertise is useful in the process of error management (Small & Cooper, 1999).

Most recently, simulation has been applied as a learning tool in anesthesia. In this context, the simulation is a model of the environment an anesthesia provider might encounter in the operating room, postanesthesia care unit, intensive care unit, or other area where the delivery of anesthesia services is required. Anesthesia simulators may be realistic or hands-on, and screen-only (computer screen). The use of virtual reality simulation, where the participant wears a head-mounted graphics display that produces three-dimensional images, has not yet been applied to the field of anesthesia (Gaba, 1999). Although the value of simulation in reducing error and enhancing patient safety has yet to be explicitly quantified in research, it is likely that simulation technology will advance and be more widely applied in the future as a learning and measurement tool. In fact, a study by Fallacaro (1998) found that experiential learning is critical to prepare nurse anesthetists to manage untoward events and that full-body patient simulation is a preferred method to address these learning needs.

SUMMARY

In an editorial addressing patient safety, Leape et al (1998) stated eloquently:

> "...patients and physicians in the United States live and interact in a culture characterized by anger, blame, guilt, fear, and distrust.... Clinicians and some health care organizations generally have responded by suppression, stonewalling, and cover-up.... Medical harm ... is not the result of ignorance, malice, laziness, or greed.... The risk of harm is ever present. Systems can be created that will reduce the probability that these mistakes will occur ... thus preventing harm to patients. Error prevention and error detection and correction before harm are the goals. System changes can do that. We now hope to create a predominant culture of error recognition, accountability, honesty, and rapid and fair settlement for injuries, addressing the risk of harm as a systems problem and preventing the problems from occurring again in that or similar settings."

As we evolve through the 21st century, continued emphasis will be placed on our ability as organizations, and as individual practitioners, to provide safe, quality care to our patients. It is hoped that this discussion of the systems and strategies used to improve quality in healthcare will be a helpful guide to practice.

REFERENCES

Association of Operating Room Nurses. (1999). *Standards and Recommended Practices for Operating Room Nurses.* Denver, CO: Author.

Baird, A. (1997). Clinical pathways: A road map to improve care. *Point of View.* August: 10-12.

Baird, A. (1997). Clinical pathways: A road map to improving care Part II. *Point of View.* November: 6-8.

Bankert, M. (1989). *Watchful Care: A History of America's Nurse Anesthetists.* New York, NY: The Continuum Publishing Co.

Bernstein, S.J., et al. (1993). The appropriateness of hysterectomy: A comparison of care in seven health plans. *JAMA.* 269, 2398-2402.

Bidwell-Ceronne, S., Krainovich-Miller, B., Haber, B.A., Penney, N.C. & Carter, E. (1995). Nursing research and patient outcomes: Tools for managing the transformation of the health care delivery system. *The Journal of the New York State Nurses Association.* 26(3), 12-17.

Blumenreich, G.E. (1999). Legal foundations of nurse anesthesia practice. In W. Waugaman, S. Foster & B. Rigor (Eds.), *Principles and Practice of Nurse Anesthesia* (3rd ed., pp. 27-39). Stamford, CT: Appleton & Lange.

Brennan, T., et al. (1991). Incidence of adverse events and negligence in hospitalized patients. *JAMA.* 324, 3170-376.

Chassin, M.R. (1997). Assessing strategies for quality improvement. *Health Affairs.* (3) 151-161. May/June.

Cullen, D.J., et al. (1995). The incident reporting system does not detect adverse drug events: A problem for quality improvement. *Joint Commission Journal on Quality Improvement.* 21 (10), 541-548.

Davies, A.R., Doyle, A.T., Lansky, D., Rutt, W., Stevic, M.O. & Doyle, J.B. (1994). Outcome assessment in clinical settings: A consensus statement on principles and best practices in project management. *Joint Commission Journal on Quality Improvement.* 20 (1), 6-16.

Dettmann, F.G. (1995). The origins and evolution of peer review organizations. *Joint Commission Journal on Quality Improvement.* 21 (7), 322-324.

Ebener, M., Baugh, K. & Formella, N.M. (1996). Proving that less is more: Linking resources to outcomes. *Journal of Nurse Care Quality.* 10 (2), 1-9.

Fallacaro, M.D. (1998). The utilization of full body patient simulation: A preferred method to prepare anesthesia providers in the management of untoward pathophysiologic events. *AANA Journal.* 66 (5), 492-493.

Kennedy, H.L. (1999). The importance of randomized trials and evidence-based medicine: A clinician's view. *Clinical Cardiology.* 22 (1), 6-12.

Lang, N.M. & Marek, K.D. (1995, March). Quality assurance: The foundation of professional care. *The Journal of the New York State Nurses Association.* 26 (1), 48-50.

Leape, L.L., Woods, D.D., Hatlie, J.D., Kizer, K.W., Schroeder, S.A. & Lundberg, G.D. (1998). Promoting patient safety by preventing medical error. *JAMA.* 280 (16), 1444-1447.

Levy, C.A. (1999). The National Patient Safety Foundation regional forums. Enhancing patient safety and reducing errors in health care. National Patient Safety Foundation. Chicago, IL.

Lunsden, K. & Hagland, M. (1993). Mapping care. *Hospitals and Health Networks.* (67) 34-40.

M.J. Field & K.N. Lohrs (Eds.). (1990). *Clinical Practice Guidelines: Directions for a New Program.* Institute of Medicine. Washington, DC: National Academy Press.

Phillips, D.P., Christenfeld, N. & Glynn, L.M. (1998). Increase in U.S. medication-error deaths between 1983 and 1993. *Lancet.* February 28.

Rosenstein, A.H. (1994). Financial risk, accountability, and outcome management: Using data to manage and measure clinical performance. *American Journal of Medical Quality.* 9 (3), 116-121.

The President's Advisory Commission on Consumer Protection and Quality in the Health Care Industry, Final Report. (1998). U.S. Department of Health and Human Services. Washington, D.C.

Small, S.D. & Cooper, J.B. (1999). Confidential interview protocol applied to the study of adverse events in perioperative care and to assess the impact of realistic simulation training. National Patient Safety Foundation (pp. 288-291). Chicago, IL: Author.

Sommer, B. (1999). Patient health and safety. In W. R. Waugaman, S.D. Foster, & B.M. Rigor (Eds.), *Principles and Practice of Nurse Anesthesia* (3rd ed., pp. 81-92). Stamford, CT: Appleton & Lange.

Soumerai, S., et al. (1997). Adverse outcomes because of underuse of beta blockers in elderly survivors of acute myocardial infarction. *JAMA.* 277, 115-121.

The Cardiac Arrhythmia Suppression Trial Investigators. (1989). Preliminary report: Effect of encainide and flecanide on mortality in a randomized trial of arrhythmia suppression after myocardial infarction. *N Engl J Med.* 321, 406-412.

Wennberg, J.E. & Cooper M.M. (1998) *The Dartmouth Atlas of Health Care in the United States.* Chicago, IL: American Hospital Publishing, Inc.

Zander, K. (1991). What's new in managed care and case management. *The New Definition.* 6 (2), 1-2.

Zander, K. (1988). Nursing care management: Strategic management of cost and quality outcomes. *Journal of Nursing Administration.* 18, 23-30.

Zonius, K.M. & Murphy, M. (1995). Use of total quality management sparks staff nurse participation in continuous quality improvement. *The Nursing Clinics of North America.* 30 (1), 1-12.

KEY REFERENCES

Acute Pain Management Panel. (1992). *Acute pain management: Operative or medical procedures and trauma.* Clinical practice guidelines. AHCPR Pub. 92-0032. Rockville, MD: Agency for Health Care Policy and Research, Public Health Service, U.S. Department of Health and Human Services. February 1992.

Batalden, P.B., Nelson, E.C. & Roberts, J.S. (1994). Linking outcomes measurement to continual improvement: The serial "V" way of thinking about improving clinical care. *Joint Commission Journal on Quality Improvement.* 20 (4), 167-177.

Bloyd, B. & Faimon, C. (1997). Finding direction. Clinical pathways guide case managers, healthcare professionals to positive outcomes. *Continuing Care.* June: 24-34.

Centers for Disease Control and Prevention. (1995). Guidelines for isolation precautions in hospitals. *Infection Control and Hospital Epidemiology.* 17, 1.

Evidence-based Medical Working Group. (1992). Evidence-based medicine: A new approach to teaching the practice of medicine. *JAMA.* (268), 2420-2425.

Gaba, D.M. (1994). Human work environment and simulators. In Miller, R.D. (Ed.), *Anesthesia* (4th ed., pp. 2,635-2,679). New York, NY: Churchill Livingston, Inc.

Joint Commission on Accreditation of Healthcare Organizations. (1999). *Accreditation Manual for Hospitals.* Oakbrook Terrace, IL: Author.

Martin-Sheridan, D.M. (1999). Anesthesia outcomes and evaluation. In Waugaman, W.R., Foster, S.D. & Rigor, B.M. (Eds.), *Principles and Practice of Nurse Anesthesia* (3rd ed., pp. 805-816). Stamford, CT: Appleton & Lange.

Roberts, K.H. (1999). Organizational change and a culture of safety. In *Enhancing Patient Safety and Reducing Errors in Health Care* National Patient Safety Foundation. (pp. 25-27). Chicago, IL: Author.

Simpson, K.R. (1999). Strategies for developing an evidence-based approach to perinatal care. *AJMaternal and Child Nursing.* 24 (3), 122-131.

Villaire, M. & Ley, J. (1995). Putting critical pathways on the map. *Critical Care Nurse.* 15 (3), 106-113.

Williams, B.A., et al. (1998). Benchmarking the perioperative process: III, Effects of regional anesthesia clinical pathways techniques on process efficiency and recovery profiles in ambulatory orthopedic sugary. *Journal of Clinical Anesthesia.* (10) 570-578.

STUDY QUESTIONS

1. Discuss two barriers to patient safety and develop realistic strategies to overcome them.

2. Define five components of a CQI process and develop a plan to implement them in your department of anesthesiology.

3. Since accreditation is a voluntary process, why do hospitals choose to comply with JCAHO accreditation standards?

4. Why is it essential for a quality assessment plan to be linked to outcome assessment?

5. Describe how simulation can be applied as a training tool to improve patient safety and outcome.

6. Discuss necessary components to developing evidence-based practice patterns.

7. List references that may be useful to anesthesia providers when developing evidence-based clinical pathways.

8. List the advantages/disadvantages of implementing clinical pathways.

9. Discuss the role of anesthesia providers in clinical pathway development.

INDEX

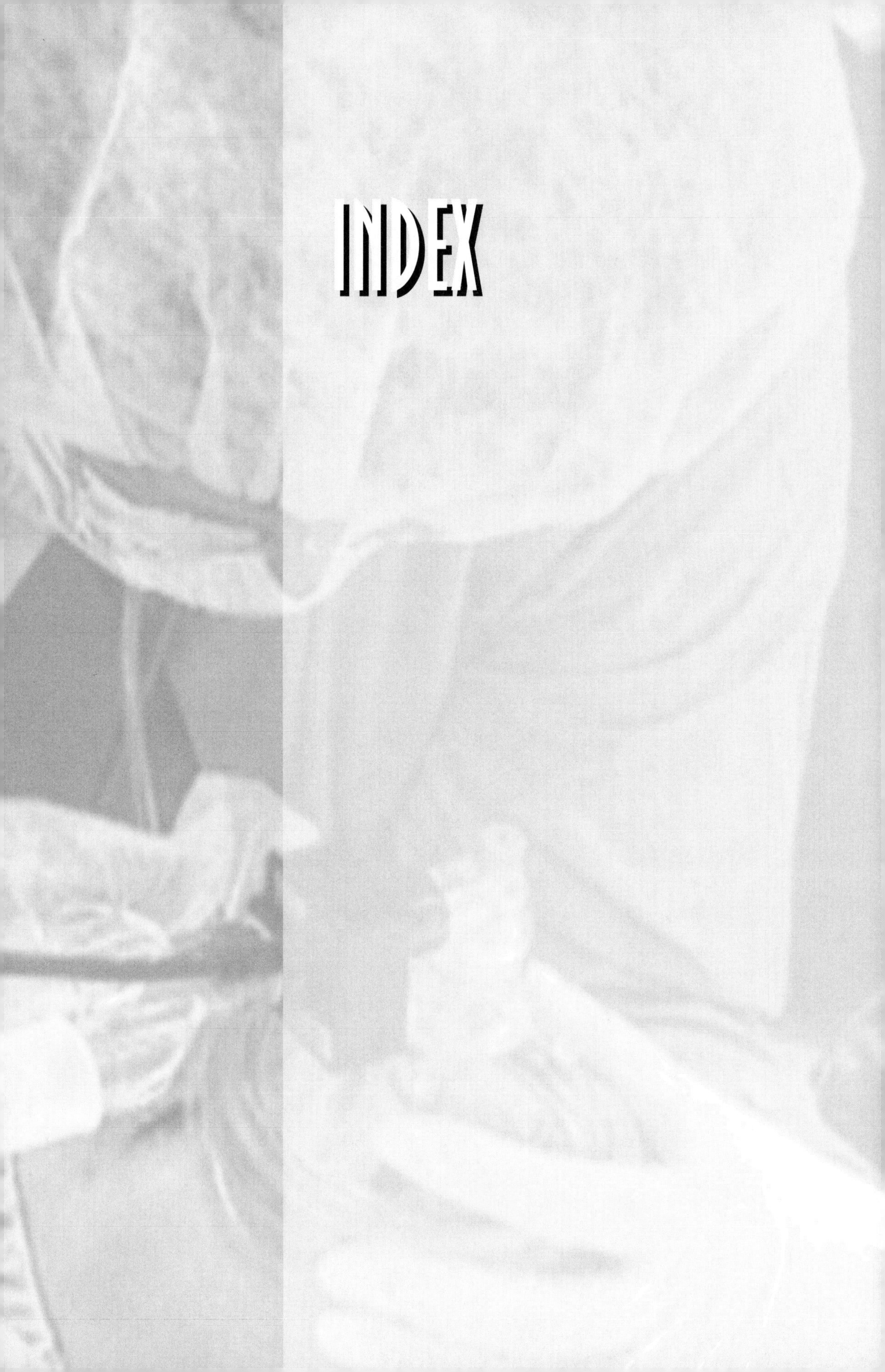

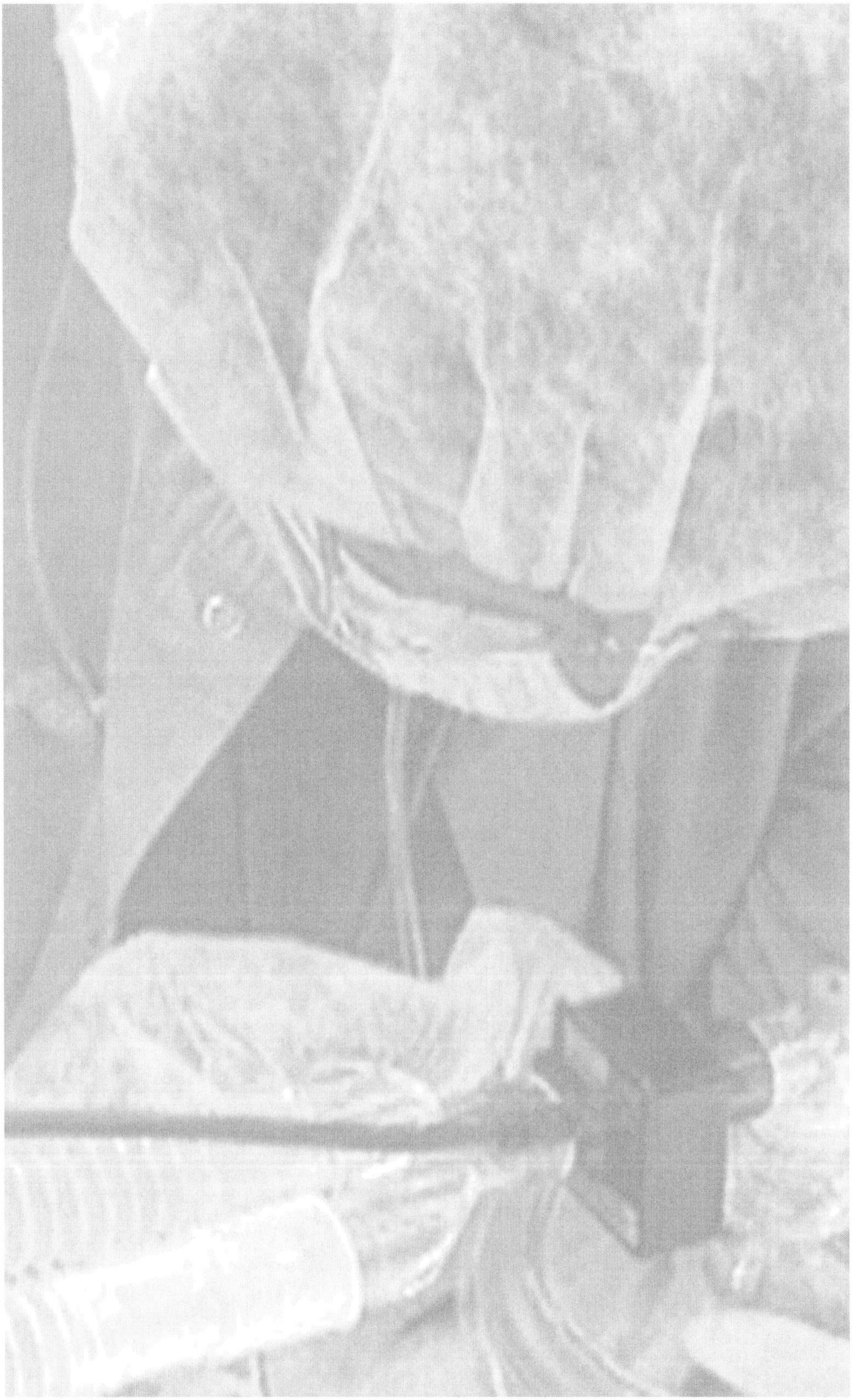

A

B

C

D

E

F

G

H

I

J

K

L

M

Q

R

W

Y